Full View of Yangtze River Pharmaceuticals Group (Taizhou, Jiangsu, China)
扬子江药业集团全景（中国·江苏·泰州）

A Newly Compiled
Practical English-Chinese Library
of Traditional Chinese Medicine
（英汉对照）新编实用中医文库

General Compiler-in-Chief Zuo Yanfu
总主编　左言富

Translators-in-Chief
Zhu Zhongbao Huang Yuezhong Tao Jinwen Li Zhaoguo
总编译　朱忠宝　黄月中　陶锦文　李照国（执行）

Compiled by Nanjing University of
Traditional Chinese Medicine
Translated by Shanghai University
of Traditional Chinese Medicine
南 京 中 医 药 大 学　主编
上 海 中 医 药 大 学　主译

INTERNAL MEDICINE OF TRADITIONAL CHINESE MEDICINE

中 医 内 科 学

Examiner-in-Chief	Zhou Zhongying
Compiler- in-Chief	Wang Yue
Vice-Compiler-in-Chief	Wang Xu
Translators-in-Chief	Huang Yuezhong Xie Jinhua
	Hu Kewu Qin Baichang
Translators	Zhu Jinjiang Huang Xixuan
	He Yingchun Zeng Haiping
	Dai Wenjun Wei Min

主　审　　　周仲瑛
主　编　　　汪　悦
副主编　　　王　旭
主　译　　　黄月中
　　　　　　谢金华
译　者　　　胡克武
　　　覃百长　朱金江
　　　黄熙璇　何迎春
　　　曾海苹　戴文军
　　　　　　魏　敏

PUBLISHING HOUSE OF SHANGHAI UNIVERSITY
OF TRADITIONAL CHINESE MEDICINE
上海中医药大学出版社

Publishing House of Shanghai University of Traditional Chinese Medicine
530 Lingling Road，Shanghai，200032，China

Internal Medicine of Traditional Chinese Medicine
Compiler-in-Chief　Wang Yue　Translators-in-Chief　Huang Yuezhong　Xie Jinhua
(A Newly Compiled Practical English-Chinese Library of TCM General Compiler-in-Chief
Zuo Yanfu)

ISBN 7 - 81010 - 660 - 0/R · 626　paperback
ISBN 7 - 81010 - 682 - 1/R · 647　hardback
Printed in Shanghai Xinhua printing works

图书在版编目(CIP)数据

中医内科学/汪悦主编；黄月中，谢金华主译．—上
海：上海中医药大学出版社，2002
(英汉对照新编实用中医文库/左言富总主编)
ISBN 7 - 81010 - 660 - 0

Ⅰ.中...　Ⅱ.①汪...②黄...③谢...　Ⅲ.中医
内科学—英、汉　Ⅳ.R25

中国版本图书馆 CIP 数据核字(2002)第 058679 号

中医内科学　　主编 汪悦　主译 黄月中 谢金华

上海中医药大学出版社出版发行　　　　　　(零陵路 530 号　邮政编码 200032)
新华书店上海发行所经销　　　　　　　　　　　　　上海新华印刷厂印刷
开本　787mm×1092mm　1/18　印张 29.666　字数 709 千字　印数 1—3 600 册
版次 2002 年 11 月第 1 版　　　　　　　　印次 2002 年 11 月第 1 次印刷

ISBN 7 - 81010 - 660 - 0/R · 626　　　　　　　定价 75.50 元

Compilation Board of the Library

《(英汉对照)新编实用中医文库》编纂委员会

名誉主任　张文康

总 顾 问　陈可冀　徐镜人

顾　　问　（按姓氏笔画为序）

干祖望　尤松鑫　刘再朋　许芝银　孙 桐　宋立人　张民庆　金 实

金妙文　单兆伟　周福贻　施 震　徐景藩　唐蜀华　曹世宏　符为民

外籍顾问

萨利姆（爱尔兰）　亚历山大·古丽（意大利）　卡塞拉·塞肯多（意大利）

雷蒙特·凯·卡罗（澳大利亚）　汤淑兰（英国）　马万里（英国）

大卫·莫罗尼（美国）　施祖谷（美国）　石上博（日本）　赫尔木特（德国）

主　　任　项 平

执 行 主 任　左言富

执行副主任　马 健　杜文东　李照国

副 主 任　黄成惠　吴坤平　刘沈林　吴勉华　陈涤平　蔡宝昌

编　　委　（按姓氏笔画为序）

丁安伟	丁淑华	于 勇	万力生	王 旭
王旭东	王玲玲	王鲁芬	卢子杰	申俊龙
刘 玉	刘跃光	严道南	杨公服	闵仲生
吴昌国	吴拥军	吴建龙	何文彬	何树勋（特邀）
何贵翔	汪 悦	汪受传	沈大庆	张 庆
陈永辉	陈廷汉（特邀）	邵健民	林显增（特邀）	
林端美（特邀）	岳沛平	金宏柱	周礼杲（特邀）	
赵 霞	赵京生	胡 烈	胡 葵	查 炜
姚映芷	袁 颖	夏有兵	夏登杰	倪 云
徐恒泽	郭海英	唐传俭	唐德才	凌桂珍（特邀）
谈 勇	黄桂成	梅晓芸	曹贵珠	蒋中秋
曾庆琪	翟亚春	樊巧玲		

《(英汉对照)新编实用中医文库》编译委员会

顾　　问　邵循道　欧　明

总 编 译　朱忠宝　黄月中　陶锦文

执行总编译　李照国

副 总 编 译　（按姓氏笔画为序）

寻建英　李永安　张庆荣　张登峰　杨洪英　黄国琪　谢金华

编 译 者　（按姓氏笔画为序）

于　新　王瑞辉　田开宇　申　光　兰凤利　成培莉　朱文晓
朱玉琴　朱金江　朱桂香　乐毅敏　刘升鹏　李经蕴　杨　莹
杨明山　何迎春　张　杰　张海峡　张　维　陈仁英　周永明
周素贞　屈榆生　赵俊卿　荆　蓁　胡克武　徐启龙　徐　瑶
郭小民　黄熙璇　曹丽娟　康　勤　董　晶　覃百长　曾海苹
楼建华　赖月珍　鲍　白　裴慧华　薛俊梅　戴文军　魏　敏

编译委员会办公室

主　任　杨明山

秘　书　徐林娣　陈　力

Approval Committee of the Library

Foreword Ⅰ

As we are walking into the 21st century, "health for all" is still an important task for the World Health Organization (WHO) to accomplish in the new century. The realization of "health for all" requires mutual cooperation and concerted efforts of various medical sciences, including traditional medicine. WHO has increasingly emphasized the development of traditional medicine and has made fruitful efforts to promote its development. Currently the spectrum of diseases is changing and an increasing number of diseases are difficult to cure. The side effects of chemical drugs have become more and more evident. Furthermore, both the governments and peoples in all countries are faced with the problem of high cost of medical treatment. Traditional Chinese medicine (TCM), the complete system of traditional medicine in the world with unique theory and excellent clinical curative effects, basically meets the need to solve such problems. Therefore, bringing TCM into full play in medical treatment and healthcare will certainly become one of the hot points in the world medical business in the 21st century.

Various aspects of work need to be done to promote the course of the internationalization of TCM, especially the compilation of works and textbooks suitable for international readers. The impending new century has witnessed the compilation of such a

序　一

人类即将迈入 21 世纪,"人人享有卫生保健"仍然是新世纪世界卫生工作面临的重要任务。实现"人人享有卫生保健"的宏伟目标,需要包括传统医药学在内的多种医学学科的相互协作与共同努力。世界卫生组织越来越重视传统医药学的发展,并为推动其发展做出了卓有成效的工作。目前,疾病谱正在发生变化,难治疾病不断增多,化学药品的毒副作用日益显现,日趋沉重的医疗费用困扰着各国政府和民众。中医药学是世界传统医学体系中最完整的传统医学,其独到的学科理论和突出的临床疗效,较符合当代社会和人们解决上述难题的需要。因此,科学有效地发挥中医药学的医疗保健作用,必将成为 21 世纪世界卫生工作的特点之一。

加快中医药走向世界的步伐,还有很多的工作要做,特别是适合国外读者学习的中医药著作、教材的编写是极其重要的方面。在新千年来临之际,由南京中医药大学

series of books known as *A Newly Compiled Practical English-Chinese Library of Traditional Chinese Medicine* published by the Publishing House of Shanghai University of TCM, compiled by Nanjing University of TCM and translated by Shanghai University of TCM. Professor Zuo Yanfu, the general compiler-in-chief of this Library, is a person who sets his mind on the international dissemination of TCM. He has compiled *General Survey on TCM Abroad*, a monograph on the development and state of TCM abroad. This Library is another important works written by the experts organized by him with the support of Nanjing University of TCM and Shanghai University of TCM. The compilation of this Library is done with consummate ingenuity and according to the development of TCM abroad. The compilers, based on the premise of preserving the genuineness and gist of TCM, have tried to make the contents concise, practical and easy to understand, making great efforts to introduce the abstruse ideas of TCM in a scientific and simple way as well as expounding the prevention and treatment of diseases which are commonly encountered abroad and can be effectively treated by TCM.

This Library encompasses a systematic summarization of the teaching experience accumulated in Nanjing University of TCM and Shanghai University of TCM that run the collaborating centers of traditional medicine and the international training centers on acupuncture and moxibustion set by WHO. I am sure that the publication of this Library will further promote the development of traditional Chinese med-

主编、上海中医药大学主译、上海中医药大学出版社出版的《(英汉对照)新编实用中医文库》的即将问世,正是新世纪中医药国际传播更快发展的预示。本套文库总主编左言富教授是中医药学国际传播事业的有心人,曾主编研究国外中医药发展状况的专著《国外中医药概览》。本套文库的编撰,是他在南京中医药大学和上海中医药大学支持下,组织许多著名专家共同完成的又一重要专著。本套文库的作者们深谙国外的中医药发展现状,编写颇具匠心,在注重真实,不失精华的前提下,突出内容的简明、实用,易于掌握,力求科学而又通俗地介绍中医药学的深奥内容,重点阐述国外常见而中医药颇具疗效的疾病的防治。

本套文库蕴含了南京中医药大学和上海中医药大学作为 WHO 传统医学合作中心、国际针灸培训中心多年留学生教学的实践经验和系统总结,更为全面、系统、准确地向世界传播中医药学。相信本书的出版将对中医更好地走向世界,让世界更好地了解中医产生更

icine abroad and enable the whole world to have a
better understanding of traditional Chinese medicine.

Professor Zhu Qingsheng
Vice-Minister of Health Ministry of the
People's Republic of China

Director of the State Administrative Bureau of
TCM

December 14, 2000 Beijing

为积极的影响。

朱庆生教授
中华人民共和国卫生部副部长

国家中医药管理局局长

2000 年 12 月 14 日于北京

Foreword II

Before the existence of the modern medicine, human beings depended solely on herbal medicines and other therapeutic methods to treat diseases and preserve health. Such a practice gave rise to the establishment of various kinds of traditional medicine with unique theory and practice, such as traditional Chinese medicine, Indian medicine and Arabian medicine, etc. Among these traditional systems of medicine, traditional Chinese medicine is a most extraordinary one based on which traditional Korean medicine and Japanese medicine have evolved.

Even in the 21st century, traditional medicine is still of great vitality. In spite of the fast development of modern medicine, traditional medicine is still disseminated far and wide. In many developing countries, most of the people in the rural areas still depend on traditional medicine and traditional medical practitioners to meet the need for primary health-care. Even in the countries with advanced modern medicine, more and more people have begun to accept traditional medicine and other therapeutic methods, such as homeopathy, osteopathy and naturopathy, etc.

With the change of the economy, culture and living style in various regions as well as the aging in the world population, the disease spectrum has changed. And such a change has paved the way for the new application of traditional medicine. Besides,

序 二

在现代医学形成之前，人类一直依赖草药和其他一些疗法治病强身，从而发展出许多有理论、有实践的传统医学，例如中医学、印度医学、阿拉伯医学等。中医学是世界林林总总的传统医学中的一支奇葩，在它的基础上还衍生出朝鲜传统医学和日本汉方医学。在跨入 21 世纪的今天，古老的传统医学依然焕发着活力，非但没有因现代医学的发展而式微，其影响还有增无减，人们对传统医学的价值也有了更深刻的体会和认识。在许多贫穷国家，大多数农村人口仍然依赖传统医学疗法和传统医务工作者来满足他们对初级卫生保健的需求。在现代医学占主导地位的许多国家，传统医学及其他一些"另类疗法"，诸如顺势疗法、整骨疗法、自然疗法等，也越来越被人们所接受。

伴随着世界各地经济、文化和生活的变革以及世界人口的老龄化，世界疾病谱也发生了变化。传统医学有了新的应用，而新疾病所引起的新需求以及现代医学的成

the new requirements initiated by the new diseases and the achievements and limitations of modern medicine have also created challenges for traditional medicine.

WHO sensed the importance of traditional medicine to human health early in the 1970s and have made great efforts to develop traditional medicine. At the 29th world health congress held in 1976, the item of traditional medicine was adopted in the working plan of WHO. In the following world health congresses, a series of resolutions were passed to demand the member countries to develop, utilize and study traditional medicine according to their specific conditions so as to reduce medical expenses for the realization of "health for all".

WHO has laid great stress on the scientific content, safe and effective application of traditional medicine. It has published and distributed a series of booklets on the scientific, safe and effective use of herbs and acupuncture and moxibustion. It has also made great contributions to the international standardization of traditional medical terms. The safe and effective application of traditional medicine has much to do with the skills of traditional medical practitioners. That is why WHO has made great efforts to train them. WHO has run 27 collaborating centers in the world which have made great contributions to the training of acupuncturists and traditional medical practitioners. Nanjing University of TCM and Shanghai University of TCM run the collaborating centers with WHO. In recent years it has, with the cooperation of WHO and other countries, trained about ten thousand international students from over

就与局限又向传统医学提出了挑战,推动它进一步发展。世界卫生组织早在20世纪70年代就意识到传统医学对人类健康的重要性,并为推动传统医学的发展做了努力。1976年举行的第二十九届世界卫生大会将传统医学项目纳入世界卫生组织的工作计划。其后的各届世界卫生大会又通过了一系列决议,要求各成员国根据本国的条件发展、使用和研究传统医学,以降低医疗费用,促进"人人享有初级卫生保健"这一目标的实现。

世界卫生组织历来重视传统医学的科学、安全和有效使用。它出版和发行了一系列有关科学、安全、有效使用草药和针灸的技术指南,并在专用术语的标准化方面做了许多工作。传统医学的使用是否做到安全和有效,是与使用传统疗法的医务工作者的水平密不可分的。因此,世界卫生组织也十分重视传统医学培训工作。它在全世界有27个传统医学合作中心,这些中心对培训合格的针灸师及使用传统疗法的其他医务工作者做出了积极的贡献。南京中医药大学、上海中医药大学是世界卫生组织传统医学合作中心之一,近年来与世界卫生组织和其他国家合作,培训了近万名来自90多个国

90 countries.

In order to further promote the dissemination of traditional Chinese medicine in the world, *A Newly Compiled Practical English-Chinese Library of Traditional Chinese Medicine*, compiled by Nanjing University of TCM with Professor Zuo Yanfu as the general compiler-in-chief and published by the Publishing House of Shanghai University of TCM, aims at systematic, accurate and concise expounding of traditional Chinese medical theory and introducing clinical therapeutic methods of traditional medicine according to modern medical nomenclature of diseases. Undoubtedly, this series of books will be the practical textbooks for the beginners with certain English level and the international enthusiasts with certain level of Chinese to study traditional Chinese medicine. Besides, this series of books can also serve as reference books for WHO to internationally standardize the nomenclature of acupuncture and moxibustion.

The scientific, safe and effective use of traditional medicine will certainly further promote the development of traditional medicine and traditional medicine will undoubtedly make more and more contributions to human health in the 21st century.

Zhang Xiaorui

WHO Coordination Officer

December, 2000

家和地区的留学生。

在南京中医药大学左言富教授主持下编纂的、由上海中医药大学出版社出版的《(英汉对照)新编实用中医文库》,旨在全面、系统、准确、简要地阐述中医基础理论,并结合西医病名介绍中医临床治疗方法。因此,这套文库可望成为具有一定英语水平的初学中医者和具有一定中文水平的外国中医爱好者学习基础中医学的系列教材。这套文库也可供世界卫生组织在编写国际针灸标准术语时参考。

传统医学的科学、安全、有效使用必将进一步推动传统医学的发展。传统医学一定会在 21 世纪为人类健康做出更大的贡献。

张小瑞

世界卫生组织传统医学协调官员

2000 年 12 月

Preface

The Publishing House of Shanghai University of TCM published *A Practical English-Chinese Library of Traditional Chinese Medicine* in 1990. The Library has been well-known in the world ever since and has made great contributions to the dissemination of traditional Chinese medicine in the world. In view of the fact that 10 years has passed since its publication and that there are certain errors in the explanation of traditional Chinese medicine in the Library, the Publishing House has invited Nanjing University of TCM and Shanghai University of TCM to organize experts to recompile and translate the Library.

Nanjing University of TCM and Shanghai University of TCM are well-known for their advantages in higher education of traditional Chinese medicine and compilation of traditional Chinese medical textbooks. The compilation of *A Newly Compiled Practical English-Chinese Library of Traditional Chinese Medicine* has absorbed the rich experience accumulated by Nanjing University of Traditional Chinese Medicine in training international students of traditional Chinese medicine. Compared with the previous Library, the Newly Compiled Library has made great improvements in many aspects, fully demonstrating the academic system of traditional Chinese medicine. The whole series of books has systematically introduced the basic theory and thera-

前 言

上海中医药大学出版社于 1990 年出版了一套《（英汉对照）实用中医文库》，发行 10 年来，在海内外产生了较大影响，对推动中医学走向世界起了积极作用。考虑到该套丛书发行已久，对中医学术体系的介绍还有一些欠妥之处，因此，上海中医药大学出版社特邀南京中医药大学主编、上海中医药大学主译，组织全国有关专家编译出版《（英汉对照）新编实用中医文库》。

《（英汉对照）新编实用中医文库》的编纂，充分发挥了南京中医药大学和上海中医药大学在高等中医药教育教学和教材编写方面的优势，吸收了作为 WHO 传统医学合作中心之一的两校，多年来从事中医药学国际培训和留学生学历教育的经验，对原《（英汉对照）实用中医文库》整体结构作了大幅度调整，以突出中医学术主体内容。全套丛书系统介绍了中医基础理论和中医辨证论治方法，讲解了中药学和方剂学的基本理论，详细介绍了 236 味中药、152 首常用方剂和 100 种常用中成药；详述

peutic methods based on syndrome differentiation, expounding traditional Chinese pharmacy and prescriptions; explaining 236 herbs, 152 prescriptions and 100 commonly-used patent drugs; elucidating 264 methods for differentiating syndromes and treating commonly-encountered and frequently-encountered diseases in internal medicine, surgery, gynecology, pediatrics, traumatology and orthopedics, ophthalmology and otorhinolaryngology; introducing the basic methods and theory of acupuncture and moxibustion, massage (tuina), life cultivation and rehabilitation, including 70 kinds of diseases suitable for acupuncture and moxibustion, 38 kinds of diseases for massage, examples of life cultivation and over 20 kinds of commonly encountered diseases treated by rehabilitation therapies in traditional Chinese medicine. For better understanding of traditional Chinese medicine, the books are neatly illustrated. There are 296 line graphs and 30 colored pictures in the Library with necessary indexes, making it more comprehensive, accurate and systematic in disseminating traditional Chinese medicine in the countries and regions where English is the official language.

This Library is characterized by following features:

1. Scientific   Based on the development of TCM in education and research in the past 10 years, efforts have been made in the compilation to highlight the gist of TCM through accurate theoretical exposition and clinical practice, aiming at introducing authentic theory and practice to the world.

2. Systematic   This Library contains 14 sepa-

264 种临床内、外、妇、儿、骨伤、眼、耳鼻喉各科常见病与多发病的中医辨证论治方法;系统论述针灸、推拿、中医养生康复的基本理论和基本技能,介绍针灸治疗病种 70 种、推拿治疗病种 38 种、各类养生实例及 20 余种常见病证的中医康复实例。为了更加直观地介绍中医药学术,全书选用线图 296 幅、彩图 30 幅,并附有必要的索引,从而更加全面、系统、准确地向使用英语的国家和地区传播中医学术,推进中医学走向世界,造福全人类。

本丛书主要具有以下特色:(1) 科学性:在充分吸收近 10 余年来中医教学和科学研究最新进展的基础上,坚持突出中医学术精华,理论阐述准确,临床切合实用,向世界各国介绍"原汁原味"的中医药学术;(2) 系统性:本套丛书包括《中医基础理论》、《中医诊断学》、《中药学》、《方剂学》、《中医内

rate fascicles, i. e. *Basic Theory of Traditional Chinese Medicine*, *Diagnostics of Traditional Chinese Medicine*, *Science of Chinese Materia Medica*, *Science of Prescriptions*, *Internal Medicine of Traditional Chinese Medicine*, *Surgery of Traditional Chinese Medicine*, *Gynecology of Traditional Chinese Medicine*, *Pediatrics of Traditional Chinese Medicine*, *Traumatology and Orthopedics of Traditional Chinese Medicine*, *Ophthalmology of Traditional Chinese Medicine*, *Otorhinolaryngology of Traditional Chinese Medicine*, *Chinese Acupuncture and Moxibustion*, *Chinese Tuina (Massage)*, *and Life Cultivation and Rehabilitation of Traditional Chinese Medicine*.

3. Practical   Compared with the previous Library, the Newly Compiled Library has made great improvements and supplements, systematically introducing therapeutic methods for treating over 200 kinds of commonly and frequently encountered diseases, focusing on training basic clinical skills in acupuncture and moxibustion, tuina therapy, life cultivation and rehabilitation with clinical case reports.

4. Standard   This Library is reasonable in structure, distinct in categorization, standard in terminology and accurate in translation with full consideration of habitual expressions used in countries and regions with English language as the mother tongue.

This series of books is not only practical for the beginners with certain competence of English to study TCM, but also can serve as authentic textbooks for international students in universities and colleges of TCM in China to study and practice TCM. For those from TCM field who are going to go

科学》、《中医外科学》、《中医妇科学》、《中医儿科学》、《中医骨伤科学》、《中医眼科学》、《中医耳鼻喉科学》、《中国针灸》、《中国推拿》、《中医养生康复学》14 个分册,系统反映了中医各学科建设与发展的最新成果;(3) 实用性:临床各科由原来的上下两册,根据学科的发展进行大幅度的调整和增补,比较详细地介绍了 200 多种各科常见病、多发病的中医治疗方法,重点突出了针灸、推拿、养生康复等临床基本技能训练,并附有部分临证实例;(4) 规范性:全书结构合理,层次清晰,对中医各学科名词术语表述规范,对中医英语翻译执行了更为严格的标准化方案,同时又充分考虑到使用英语国家和地区人们的语言习惯和表达方式。

本丛书不仅能满足具有一定英语水平的初学中医者系统学习中医之用,而且也为中医院校外国留学生教育及国内外开展中医双语教学提供了目前最具权威的系列教材,同时也是中医出国人员进

abroad to do academic exchange，this series of books will provide them with unexpected convenience.

Professor Xiang Ping, President of Nanjing University of TCM，is the director of the Compilation Board. Professor Zuo Yanfu from Nanjing University of TCM，General Compiler-in-Chief，is in charge of the compilation. Zhang Wenkang, Minister of Health Ministry，is invited to be the honorary director of the Editorial Board. Li Zhenji, Vice-Director of the State Administrative Bureau of TCM，is invited to be the director of the Approval Committee. Chen Keji, academician of China Academy，is invited to be the General Advisor. International advisors invited are Mr. M. S. Khan,Chairman of Ireland Acupuncture and Moxibustion Fund；Miss Alessandra Gulí, Chairman of "Nanjing Association" in Rome, Italy；Doctor Secondo Scarsella, Chief Editor of YI DAO ZA ZHI；President Raymond K. Carroll from Australian Oriental Touching Therapy College；Ms. Shulan Tang, Academic Executive of ATCM in Britain；Mr. Glovanni Maciocia from Britain；Mr. David, Chairman of American Association of TCM；Mr. Tzu Kuo Shih, director of Chinese Medical Technique Center in Connecticut，America；Mr. Helmut Ziegler, director of TCM Center in Germany；and Mr. Isigami Hiroshi from Japan. Chen Ken, official of WHO responsible for the Western Pacific Region，has greatly encouraged the compilers in compiling this series of books. After the accomplishment of the compilation, Professor Zhu Qingsheng, Vice-Minister of Health Ministry and Director of the State Administrative Bureau of TCM, has set a high value on the books in his fore-

行中医药国际交流的重要工具书。

全书由南京中医药大学校长项平教授担任编委会主任、左言富教授任总主编，主持全书的编写。中华人民共和国卫生部张文康部长担任本丛书编委会名誉主任，国家中医药管理局李振吉副局长担任审定委员会主任，陈可冀院士欣然担任本丛书总顾问指导全书的编纂。爱尔兰针灸基金会主席萨利姆先生、意大利罗马"南京协会"主席亚历山大·古丽女士、意大利《医道》杂志主编卡塞拉·塞肯多博士、澳大利亚东方触觉疗法学院雷蒙特·凯·卡罗院长、英国中医药学会学术部长汤淑兰女士、英国马万里先生、美国中医师公会主席大卫先生、美国康州中华医疗技术中心主任施祖谷先生、德国中医中心主任赫尔木特先生、日本石上博先生担任本丛书特邀外籍顾问。世界卫生组织西太平洋地区官员陈恳先生对本丛书的编写给予了热情鼓励。全书完成后，卫生部副部长兼国家中医药管理局局长朱庆生教授给予了高度评价，并欣然为本书作序；WHO传统医学协调官员张小瑞对于本丛书的编写给予高度关注，百忙中也专为本书作序。我国驻外教育机构，特别是中国驻英国曼彻斯特领事张益群先生、中国驻美国休斯敦领事严美华

word for the Library. Zhang Xiaorui, an official
from WHO's Traditional Medicine Program, has
paid great attention to the compilation and written a
foreword for the Library. The officials from the educational organizations of China in other countries
have provided us with some useful materials in our
compilation. They are Mr. Zhang Yiqun, China
Consul to Manchester in Britain; Miss Yan Meihua,
Consul to Houston in America; Mr. Wang Jiping,
First Secretary in the Educational Department in the
Embassy of China to France; and Mr. Gu Shengy-
ing, the Second Secretary in the Educational Department in the Embassy of China to Germany. We are
grateful to them all.

The Compilers
December, 2000

女士、中国驻法国使馆教育处一秘
王季平先生、中国驻德国使馆教育
处二秘郭胜英先生在与我们工作
联系中,间接提供了不少有益资
料。在此一并致以衷心感谢!

编　者
2000 年 12 月

Note for compilation　编写说明

Internal Medicine of Traditional Chinese Medicine (TCM) is a clinical subject dealing especially with traditional Chinese diagnosis and treatment of the diseases and disorders of the viscera of the human body under the guidance of TCM theory. With its systematical theories of syndrome differentiation and treatment, internal medicine of TCM is the basis of various clinical sciences.

This book introduces the basic theories of Chinese internal medicine, the basic knowledge of common internal diseases and the law of syndrome differentiation and treatment. It includes two parts: Introduction and Treatment of Diseases. The former deals with the Classification and Characteristics of Internal Diseases, the Procedure and Principles of Syndrome Differentiation and Treatment, and the Therapeutic Principles and Commonly-used Methods for Internal Diseases of TCM; and the latter, according to TCM theory, are divided into 8 chapters: Syndrome Patterns of the Lung, Syndrome Patterns of the Heart, Syndrome Patterns of the Spleen and Stomach, Syndrome Patterns of the Liver and Gallbladder, Syndrome Patterns of the Kidney, Syndrome Patterns of Qi, Blood, and Body Fluid, General Disease and Acropathy, and Other Diseases. Introduced in the latter part are 47 kinds of syndrome patterns, including the General Description, Essentials for Diagnosis, and Syndrome Differentiation and Treatment. Other Treatments such as Chinese Patent Drugs, Single-

中医内科学是以中医学理论为指导,研究人体内脏疾病,并采用传统中医药治疗方法为主的一门临床学科。它有较系统的辨证论治理论体系,是临床各学科的基础。

本书主要介绍了中医内科学的基础理论、常见内科病证的基本知识及其辨证论治规律。全书分总论和各论两部分。总论主要叙述了内科疾病的分类和病证特点,辨证论治的步骤与基本要求,以及中医内科疾病的治疗原则和常用治法等内容。各论按中医理论,分为肺系病证、心系病证、脾胃病证、肝胆病证、肾系病证、气血津液病证、全身与肢体病证及其他病证八章,分别介绍了临床常见 47 种病证的基本概念、主要病因病机、诊断要点和辨证分型治疗及其他治疗方法。其他治疗方法主要介绍常用中成药、单方验方和各种外治疗法。有关针灸、推拿和养生康复方面的知识由于另有专册介绍,在此不再赘述。

drug or Experiential Prescriptions and External Therapy are also introduced. As for the knowledge of Acupuncture and Moxibustion, Chinese Tuina Therapy, and Life Cultivation and Rehabilitation of Traditional Chinese Medicine, there are specific books to cover these aspects.

Contents

目　录

1 Introduction

TCM internal medicine is a clinical subject dealing with the law of syndrome differentiation and treatment of internal diseases under the guidance of TCM theory. The internal diseases of TCM include two categories: exogenous and endogenous diseases. The exogenous diseases refer to febrile diseases that are mainly caused by the invasion of exogenous cold, wind-heat, summer-heat, damp-heat, etc., and can be differentiated and treated according to the theory of six meridians, theory of wei, qi, ying and blood, and theory of triple energizer. The endogenous diseases include diseases of internal organs and meridian system that are mainly caused by endogenous pathogenic factors. They can be differentiated and treated according to the theory of zang-fu organs, theory of qi, blood and body fluid, and meridian theory.

中医内科学是运用中医学理论研究内科疾病辨证论治规律的一门临床学科。

中医内科疾病主要可以分为外感病和内伤病两大类。一般说来，外感病主要指伤寒、风温、暑温、湿温等急性病，主要根据六经、卫气营血和三焦辨证方法遣治；内伤病包括脏腑经络诸病，主要以脏腑、气血津液、经络等辨证方法论治。

1.1 Classification and Characteristics of Internal Diseases in Traditional Chinese Medicine (TCM)

第一章 中医内科疾病的分类与特点

1.1.1 Classification of Internal Diseases in TCM

第一节 中医内科疾病的分类

For the convenience of clinical application, internal

中医内科疾病的分类从便

diseases are usually classified in the light of their etiology and pathogenesis.

In terms of etiology, internal diseases are divided into two categories: exogenous diseases that are caused by six exogenous pathogenic factors, and endogenous diseases that are caused by seven abnormal emotional factors, improper diet, overstrain, disturbance of distribution of qi, blood and body fluids, and the pathological product secondary to the disturbance.

In terms of pathogenesis, internal diseases can usually also be divided into two categories: exogenous diseases and miscellaneous diseases. This book mainly discusses the miscellaneous diseases, which are chiefly caused by internal damage. Some diseases caused by exogenous pathogenic factors, such as cough, diarrhea, and stranguria, are conventionally discussed under the category of endogenous diseases. This is because most of their manifestations are similar to those of endogenous diseases.

Although the endogenous diseases are varied in types and complicated in pathological changes, their pathogenesis is always limited to the dysfunction of zang-fu organs, disturbance in the production and distribution of qi, blood and body fluid, and the dysfunction of meridian system. To descend to particulars, the lung controls qi and respiration; disorders such as cough and asthma caused by the impaired dispersion of lung qi and dysfunction of respiration belong to diseases of the lung. The heart dominates blood and vessels, and rules the spirit; diseases such as arrhythmia, coronary heart disease and epilepsy are the result of disturbance of blood circulation and abnormality of emotional and mental activities and belong to diseases of the heart. The spleen rules transportation and transformation, and the stomach functions in receiving and digesting food; the dysfunction of the spleen and stomach may

于指导临床应用为出发点,一般多以病因、病机为纲进行分类。

以病因作为分类根据,可分为外感疾病和内伤疾病两大类。外感疾病是由外感六淫之邪等所致;内伤疾病常由七情、饮食劳倦,气血津液敷布失常及其病理代谢产物所致。

就病机分类而言,大体上亦可分为外感与杂病两大类。本书主要介绍杂病。杂病通常由内伤所致,有些由外邪引起的咳嗽、泄泻、淋证等,因其主要临床表现与某些内伤病证相似,习惯上也将它们归入内伤病证范畴。

内伤杂病病种虽多,病理变化亦异常复杂多样,但其病变机制,始终离不开脏腑、经络功能的失调和气血津液的生成、输布的失常。因此,内伤杂病大多根据不同脏腑及气血津液、经络的生理功能和病理变化进行归类。例如,肺主气,司呼吸,故凡肺失宣肃,呼吸功能异常的疾病,如咳嗽、哮喘等都归属于肺系病证。心主血脉,又主神明,所以心的病变主要是血脉运行障碍和情志思维活动的异常,如心律失常、冠状动脉粥样硬化性心脏病、癫痫等。脾主运

lead to gastritis, enteritis and constipation. The liver is a resolute organ, attributed to wood element and responsible for maintaining smooth circulation of qi; the dysfunction of the liver and gallbladder in maintaining smooth circulation of qi may lead to diseases such as hepatitis, hepatocirrhosis and cholecystitis. And endogenous wind due to hyperactivity of liver yang may disturb the head and eyes and lead to dizziness and headache. The kidneys store essence, dominate the development and reproduction, and control water metabolism; therefore diseases affecting the urinary and reproductive systems such as impotence, spermatorrhoea, nephritis and urinary infections can be ascribed to diseases of the kidneys. Diseases such as rheumatoid arthritis and gout are caused by the invasion of pathogenic factors into the meridian system, and should be classified into diseases of the meridian system. By taking the five-zang-organ system as the key link, associating it with the systems of six-fu-organs, meridian, and qi, blood and body fluids, endogenous diseases may be categorized into different patterns. Some diseases such as "xu lao" (consumptive disease) and systemic lupus erythematosus (SLE) may affect two or more organs and should be ascribed to the category of systemic disease.

化,胃主受纳腐熟,若脾胃功能障碍,则可引起胃炎、肠炎、便秘等病证。肝主疏泄,其性刚强,肝为风木之脏,胆附于肝,肝胆疏泄失常,可致肝炎、肝硬化、胆囊炎等病证,或肝阳化风,上扰头目,而致眩晕、头痛等。肾藏精,主生殖,肾主五液,故凡泌尿、生殖方面的病变,如阳痿、遗精、肾炎、泌尿系感染等,皆属肾病证。再如类风湿关节炎、痛风等病证,系肢体经络受邪,属于肢体经络病证。这样,以五脏为主,以脏统腑,辅以经络、气血津液理论进行辨证,就可使大部分内伤杂病的归类各得其所。此外,有些疾病涉及脏腑较多,难以用一脏归类者,则属于全身性病证,如虚劳、系统性红斑狼疮等。

1.1.2 Characteristics of Internal Diseases in TCM

1.1.2.1 Endogenous pathogenic factors — the major causes of internal diseases

Most internal diseases are caused by endogenous pathogenic factors. Emotional damages may cause depressive syndrome, mania-depressive syndrome, wind stroke, vertigo and goiter. Overstrain may cause edema, diabe-

第二节 中医内科疾病的特点

一、病因以内伤为主

内科疾病的病因大都以内伤为主。如情志内伤,可引起郁证、癫狂、中风、眩晕、瘿病等;劳倦过度,可引起水肿、

tes, impotence and spermorrhea. Improper diet may cause stomachache, vomiting, belching and hiccup.

Among the causes of internal diseases, there are some endogenous pathogenic factors secondary to the dysfunction of internal organs. These endogenous pathogenic factors may cause disorders with the manifestations similar to those caused by six exogenous pathogenic factors and they are traditionally called five endogenous pathogenic factors, i. e., endogenous wind, endogenous cold, endogenous dampness, endogenous dryness and endogenous fire. For example, endogenous wind may cause syndromes such as vertigo and apoplexy with the manifestations of dizziness, numbness and convulsion of limbs. Endogenous cold may cause syndromes such as stomachache and abdominal pain with manifestations of cold limbs, pale complexion, vomiting of clear fluid, and abdominal cold pain. Endogenous dryness may bring about the syndromes such as cough and constipation with the manifestations of dry mouth and throat, cough without sputum, dry skin and constipation with dry stools. Endogenous fire may lead to hemorrhagic syndrome, depressive syndrome and wind stroke with manifestations of headache, red eyes, restlessness, irritability, dry and bitter mouth, etc. Endogenous dampness may cause such disorders as diarrhea and epigastric flatulence with manifestations of nausea, vomiting, poor appetite, fullness of abdomen, loose stools, etc.

Also, phlegm and blood stasis are two common endogenous pathogenic factors of internal diseases. They are pathological products due to the dysfunction of zang-fu organs and become secondary pathogenic factors to the human body. Many disorders are associated with these two secondary pathogenic factors. For example, the accu-

消渴、阳痿、遗精等；饮食失宜，常致胃痛、呕吐、呃逆、噎膈之病。

在内科疾病的病因中，还有一类因脏腑功能失调而产生的内风、内寒、内湿、内燥、内火等内生之邪，因其临床表现与外感六淫之邪有相似之处，但究其原因，不是外来之邪，而是由内而生，故又称为"内生五邪"。如"内风"的表现主要是头目昏晕、肢体麻木、四肢抽搐等，常见于眩晕、中风等病证；"内寒"的表现是畏寒肢冷、面色苍白、泛吐清水、脘腹冷痛等，常见于胃痛、腹痛等证；"内燥"的主要表现是口咽干燥、干咳无痰、皮肤干涩、大便干结等，常见于咳嗽、便秘等证；"内火"主要表现是头痛目赤、心烦易怒、口干口苦等，常见于血证、郁证、中风等；"内湿"的表现主要是恶心呕吐、纳呆腹胀、大便溏薄等，常见于泄泻、痞满等病证。

在内科疾病的病因中还有痰饮、瘀血等病邪，也都是因为脏腑功能失调而产生的病理产物。这一类病理产物形成之后，也可成为致病的"病邪"，进一步引起多种病理

mulation of phlegm in the lungs may lead to cough and asthma, and blood stasis may give rise to chest bi-syndrome, abdominal mass, palpitation, stomachache and abdominal pain, etc.

1. 1. 2. 2   Concurrence of cold, heat, deficiency and excess — the pathogenesis of internal diseases

In most cases, internal diseases persist for a relatively long period. They are usually caused by accumulation of pathogenic factors such as cold and heat and by deficiency of qi, blood, yin and yang in the zang-fu organs as well. Thus the pathogenesis of internal diseases is complicated with the concurrence of cold, heat, deficiency and excess. Generally the pathogenesis of internal diseases can be classified into two categories: excess and deficiency. Deficiency of qi, of blood, of yin and of yang, or deficiency of both qi and blood, deficiency of both yin and yang are in the category of deficiency, while qi stagnation, blood stasis, fluid retention, damp-heat and phlegm accumulation are ascribed to the category of excess. To identify whether the case is the heat syndrome or the cold syndrome is to identify the nature of a disease. Generally the cold syndrome and heat syndrome due to internal damage are caused by dysfunction of internal organs and imbalance of yin and yang and they are most likely to be complicated by the syndromes of excess or deficiency.

变化,形成多种病证。如痰饮伏肺,可引起咳嗽、哮喘等病证。瘀血内停可致胸痹、癥积、心悸、胃痛、腹痛等多种病证。

二、病机多寒热虚实错杂

内科疾病由于大多病程较长,既有寒热等病邪内盛的一面,又有脏腑气血阴阳亏虚的一面,所以内科疾病的病机大多寒热虚实错杂。

内科疾病虽多,但究其病理性质不外虚实两类:凡气虚、血虚、阴虚、阳虚,以及气血两虚,阴阳俱损等正气不足之候,皆属虚证;气滞、血瘀、水停、湿热、痰饮等病理产物,其病理过程大多属实证。

寒证与热证,是用以辨明病证的属性。一般而言,内伤疾病中的寒证与热证,多属脏腑功能失调、阴阳失于平衡所致,故其寒热常与其他虚实之象并见,较少单独出现。

1.2 The Procedure and Principles of Diagnosis and Treatment of Internal Diseases in TCM

1.2.1 The Procedure of Diagnosis and Treatment

The procedure of the diagnosis and treatment for internal diseases include the following five steps: to recognize the disease based on the information obtained with the four diagnostic methods, to identify the location and nature of a disease, to infer the cause and judge the pathogenesis of a disease, to design the therapeutic principle and method, and to choose drugs and formulate a prescription.

1.2.1.1 To recognize the disease based on the information obtained with the four diagnostic methods

The complete information about a disease can be collected by four diagnostic methods, i. e., inspection, olfaction and auscultation, interrogation and palpation. It includes the history and manifestations of the disease, and the influence of external environment on the onset and development of the disease. From the information collected, evidence will be provided for differentiating the syndromes, designing the therapeutic principle and organizing a prescription. Therefore the four diagnostic methods are an important procedure for collecting essential information

第二章 中医内科疾病的诊治步骤和基本要求

第一节 中医内科疾病的诊治步骤

中医内科疾病的诊治步骤,一般可归纳为四诊识病、辨性定位、求因审机、确立治法和遣方用药等几个方面。

一、四诊识病

诊治疾病,首先是通过望、闻、问、切四诊,对患者作周密的观察和全面的了解。既要了解患者的病史和临床表现,又要了解患者的外在环境对疾病发生、发展的可能影响。将检查所得,进行分析归纳,运用从外测内、见证推病、以常衡变的方法来判断患者的病情,以此作为辨证、立法、

about the disease and a prerequisite in syndrome differentiation.

Whether the information collected by applying the four diagnostic methods is accurate or not greatly influences the accuracy of syndrome differentiation. So the four diagnostic methods should be performed from different angles to avoid one-sided views and with prominence to the major aspects of the disease.

1. 2. 1. 2 To identify the nature and location of a disease

The fundamental pathogenesis of a disease is the conflict between pathogenic factors and anti-pathogenic qi, which will lead to the imbalance of yin and yang. The excess of yang will cause heat syndrome, while the excess of yin will lead to cold syndrome. For this reason, cold and heat indicate the nature of a disease. On the other hand, the conflict between pathogenic factors and anti-pathogenic qi will also be reflected as excess or deficiency. Therefore all syndromes can be classified into four categories, i. e. , deficiency, excess, cold and heat. And the therapeutic principles such as replenishing deficiency, reducing excess, clearing away heat or warming cold should be applied accordingly. Identifying the nature of a disease is an important step in syndrome differentiation and helps draw an outline of a disease and enables a practitioner to design the general therapeutic principle for a disease.

The location of a disease means the depth, i. e. , exterior and interior; or the site that a disease affects,

处方用药的依据。四诊是辨证论治的第一步,也是最重要的一个环节。

四诊搜集的资料是否准确,是否切合病情,与辨证正确与否有着密切的关系。因此,在进行四诊时,不但要做到全面系统,还要做到重点突出,详而有要,简而不漏,使四诊资料更好地为辨证提供必要依据。

二、辨性定位

辨性,就是辨别病证的性质。疾病发生的根本在于邪正斗争引起的阴阳失调,故其病性无非是阴阳的偏盛偏衰。阳盛则热,阴盛则寒,故病性具体表现在寒热属性上。而虚实是邪正双方消长盛衰的反映,也是构成病变性质的一个重要方面。寒热虚实是一切病变中最基本的性质,各种疾病都离不开这四个方面。由于基本病变是虚实寒热,所以治疗的总原则,就是补虚、泻实、清热、温寒。辨清病变性质的目的,在于对病证有一个基本的认识,治疗上有一个总的原则,因此辨识病证性质是辨证中的一项重要内容。

定位,指判定病变部位。一般包括:表里定位,这在外

i.e., zang-fu organs, qi and blood, or meridian. It is important to identify whether the exterior or interior is involved for the differentiation of exogenous diseases, while it is essential to identify whether the zang-fu organs, the meridians or qi and blood are involved for the differentiation of miscellaneous diseases. Miscellaneous diseases are usually classified into qifen disease and xuefen disease if they are located according to the conditions of qi and blood. Of all the methods for identifying the location of a disease, some are simple, and some are comprehensive. Each has a given scope of application, and may be used alone or together with others according to the clinical situations.

1.2.1.3 To infer the cause and judge the pathogenesis of a disease

In order to refine the diagnosis and syndrome differentiation, it is necessary to infer the cause of the disease from the patient's complaints, the results obtained with the four diagnostic methods and the results of the laboratory tests, and from the time, the season, the environmental factors and climate when the disease develops as well, so as to make a synthetical analysis and find out where the crux lies. By so doing, the treatment principle can be decided with much ground.

1.2.1.4 To design the therapeutic principle and method

The therapeutic principle and method are designed according to the result of syndrome differentiation. For example, the therapeutic principle of clearing away liver fire and lowering the adverse rising lung qi is designed for a cough categorized as syndrome of liver fire invading the lung. The therapeutic principle and method designed must

感病辨证时很重要；脏腑、经络定位,多用于杂病;气血定位,通常杂病要区分气分病、血分病。这些定位方法或简或繁,各有其适用范围,有时需结合应用。

三、求因审机

求因就是审证求因。它是辨证的进一步深化,是根据病人一系列具体证候,包括病人自觉症状、四诊和某些化验检查结果,以及发病的时间、季节、病人所处的环境、气候等,加以综合分析,求得疾病的症结所在,为临床治疗提供确切的依据。

四、确立治法

确立治法,简称"立法", 是根据辨证的结果确立相应的治疗原则和方法。如肝火犯肺的咳嗽,采用清肝肃肺法。立法必须与病机相吻合。

be consistent with the pathogenesis of the disease.

1. 2. 1. 5 To choose drugs and formulate a pre-scription

Syndrome differentiation and therapeutic principle designed are the bases for formulating an appropriate prescription. Usually a traditional prescription is organized for a specific syndrome or disease. It is composed of drugs carefully selected in light of their compatibility and indicated for certain cases. To select an adequate prescription for a clinical case requires the knowledge about the ingredients, organizing principle, compatibility of the ingredients, indications and application of the prescription. Traditional prescriptions are the summary of clinical experience over thousands of years. They reflected the treatment strategy and philosophy created by practitioners from generation to generation for certain diseases under the guidance of TCM theory. And we are encouraged to study, apply and develop these prescriptions in clinical practice. In formulating a prescription for a given disease, simply piecing together the drugs according to a designed therapeutic principle should be avoided and it is better to follow a traditional prescription and modify it as required in actual situation. A traditional prescription is usually chosen based on the pathogenesis of a disease and its reasonable therapeutic principle. Sometimes a prescription may be formulated by selecting drugs simply based on individual conditions, rather than by following any traditional prescription. Nevertheless the therapeutic strategy and philosophy must be embodied in the prescription. Through clinical practice this skill can be gradually gained. Selection of the traditional prescription should be guided by the therapeutic principle and the prescription selected must be consistent with the pathogenesis and the

五、选方遣药

选方是根据辨证立法的结果选用适当的治疗方剂。方剂是因法而立、针对证候而设,具有固定的药物组成与配伍,有其一定的适用范围。因此,要选择好恰当的方剂,必须熟悉方剂的组成、方义和药物配伍关系及其适用范围。方剂是前人临床经验的总结,也是历代医家在有关学术理论指导下,在对某些病证长期实践的基础上,所创造的各种治疗方法的具体应用。临证时应该重视它,学习运用它,并在前人的基础上不断发展和创新。在临床上要防止有法无方、杂药凑合的弊病;也有不拘成方,随证检药而法度井然者,在临床实践中,都必须不断总结和提高。选方必须在治疗法则的指导下进行,所选方剂应符合其病机和治疗法则。

therapeutic principle of the disease.

　　To choose drugs means to modify a selected prescription by adding or deleting drugs according to the individual case. As clinical manifestations are complicated and variable, it is hard to get a traditional prescription that completely fits the clinical situation. Modification to a traditional prescription is often required. Usually drugs are added to or deleted from a traditional prescription to make a modified one, suitable for both the major problem and complications of a disease. And for individual cases, modifications should be made flexibly so as to achieve desired results.

　　In summary, the above five-step procedure is followed in the process of syndrome differentiation and treatment for a disease. Actually it includes the four aspects: *Li* (theory), *Fa* (principle), *Fang* (prescription) and *Yao* (drug). *Li* refers to the etiology and pathogenesis of the disease; *Fa*, the therapeutic principle and method; *Fang*, the traditional prescription; and *Yao*, the drugs in a prescription. The consistency in these four aspects for a specific disease is the premise for good therapeutic effect. Meanwhile this five-step procedure can be divided into two stages, i.e., stage of syndrome differentiation and stage of treatment. Of the five steps, the first three are at the stage of syndrome differentiation, while the rest two at the stage of treatment. It is for the convenience of learning that the procedure in making syndrome differentiation and treatment is divided into five steps or two stages, but clinically it is not necessary to follow it rigidly step by step. When working on a specific disease, a practitioner may follow the procedure in a flexible way. For example, identifying the location and nature of a disease and inferring the cause and judge the pathogenesis of a disease are being conducted when the four diagnostic methods are

　　遣药是在选定方剂的基础上,随证加减药物。由于病证的复杂多变,很难有与具体的病情完全吻合、可直接应用的成方。所以,应根据病证的兼挟情况,针对具体病情加减药物。这是对方剂的灵活应用,使之更能贴切病情。

　　总之,上述各个诊治疾病的步骤包含了辨证论治的全过程,即包括了理、法、方、药各个方面,"理"就是病因病机,"法"即治疗法则,"方"即所选方剂,"药"即所用药物。理、法、方、药必须一致,才能达到良好的治疗效果。以上四诊识病、辨性定位、求因审机的内容,都属于辨证的范围,是辨证论治中的"理";确立治法、选方遣药,则是论治的具体体现。这样,便构成了辨证论治的理、法、方、药的统一。只是为了叙述方便和利于学习、掌握,才分为若干具体的步骤加以表述,在临床应用时,并不是绝对按这样的顺序,有时需相互运用。例如,诊察是搜集临床资料的阶段,是辨证论治的前提,但在诊察过程中,实际已涉及到辨性定

performed to collect the information for analyzing the disease.

1.2.2 Basic Requirements for Diagnosis and Treatment

Internal medicine is the most extensive clinical discipline that covers various categories of internal diseases. Other diseases often present manifestations similar to those of internal diseases at the early stage. Therefore it is important to differentiate them and form a sound judgement. By fulfilling the following requirements, a practitioner may avoid making incorrect diagnosis and delaying treatment for patients.

1. 2. 2. 1   Making an overall analysis of the patient's condition

For making correct syndrome differentiation and diagnosis, it is a premise to collect the complete information by using the four diagnostic methods and referring to the results from physical and laboratory examinations. Inaccurate or incomplete information often leads to an incorrect diagnosis and syndrome differentiation. Clinically the symptoms and signs of internal diseases are complicated and volatile. Some of them are consistent with the

位、求因审机,彼此之间又有着紧密不可分割的联系。所以,在临床上不必拘泥于这种程式或先后次序,可以根据具体病情和自己掌握的熟练程度灵活运用。

第二节　中医内科疾病诊治的基本要求

中医内科疾病是临床各科中范围最广泛的学科,其临床病证的分类也较多,不少非内科疾病的早期表现,也往往反映为内科的证候。因此,对内科的应诊病人,早期进行正确的辨证和诊断,非常重要。它为及时而正确地进行预防和治疗提供依据,对避免误诊和失治,具有十分重要的意义。在辨证论治的过程中,必须要做到以下几点。

一、全面分析病情

全面收集符合实际的"四诊"材料,参考当代实验室检查结果,这是全面分析病情,取得正确辨证和诊断的客观依据。片面和不符合实际的"四诊"材料,往往是辨证错误的原因。内科病证是复杂多变的,有时其临床显现的脉

fundamental nature of the disease, but some are not. When the phenomena (symptoms and signs) are not consistent with the nature of the disease, the inconsistency will appear as false phenomena, e. g., false pulses, false tongue pictures or false symptoms. Therefore a careful and comprehensive analysis of a patient's condition is needed to enable practitioners to identify false phenomena and ensure a correct diagnosis.

The holistic view in TCM is important in making an overall analysis of a patient's condition and directs the syndrome differentiation. It infers a state of completeness and unity, that is, harmony among all parts of the human body and harmony between human beings and the universe. This view postulates that all parts of the human body are associated with each other, and that the skin, muscles, tendons and tissues, meridian system and internal organs are closely associated to form an organic whole. Therefore a regional disease may have systemic manifestations, while a systemic disease may have localized symptoms and signs. An interior disorder may present symptoms and signs on the exterior, while an exterior disease may affect internal organs. The dysfunction of internal organs will lead to the disturbance of emotions, while emotional disorders will injure the internal organs directly. For that reason, regional examination and systemic examinations are equally important. Meanwhile the age, sex, occupation and working conditions of a patient should also be taken into account, as they may be related to the development of certain diseases. Finally it should not be neglected that the nature, including seasons, climates and geographical environments, has a great impact on the human body.

证,有真象也有假象。有时假在脉上,有时假在证上,有时假在舌上,临床上应仔细辨识。如果四诊不全,便得不到全面、确切的资料,辨证分析就难以把握,容易发生误诊、漏诊。

中医的整体观,是全面分析病情,指导内科临床辨证的重要思想方法。整体观在内科临床上的具体应用,可从人体本身与自然环境对人体疾病的影响两方面来说明。因为人体的肌表筋骨和经络与脏腑息息相关,内外相通,彼此联系。人体一旦发生疾病,不论局部和全身,都会出现病理反应,即局部的病变可以影响全身,全身的病变也可以反映于某一局部;内部的病变可以表现于外,外部的病变也可传变入里;情志变化可以影响内脏功能,内脏的病变也可以引起情志活动的异常。所以临证时既要诊察局部,也要审察全身,两者不可偏废。此外,患者的年龄、性别、职业、工作条件等与某些疾病的发生也有一定关系,辨证时均应注意。自然界对人体疾病的影响,包括四时气候与地理环境,也是属于中医整体观的内容,在全面分析病情,进行临

1. 2. 2. 2 Differentiating principal and secondary aspects, insidious and acute conditions

To differentiate principal and secondary aspects is an important step in determining the strategy and priority of treatment. *Biao*, the branch or the secondary aspect of a disease, refers to the manifestation of a disease, and *Ben*, the root or the principal aspect, refers to fundamental nature of a disease. The principal and secondary aspects of diseases are not a fixed pattern. In terms of the cause and manifestation of a disease, the former is the principal aspect, and the latter is the secondary aspect. In term of a disease with two focuses, the primary focus is the principal aspect, and the secondary focus is the secondary aspect. In term of the symptoms of a disease, the primary symptom is the principal aspect, and the secondarily developed symptom is the secondary aspect. In term of the clinical course of a disease, the original disorder is the principal aspect, and the newly developed disorder is the secondary aspect. To differentiate the principal and secondary aspects enables practitioners to find out the essential aspect of the disease, so that they make accurate diagnosis and provide proper treatment.

After the principal and secondary aspects are identified, the priority of treatment may be given to either principal or secondary aspect of the disease according to the severity and urgency of the disease. It is rational to treat the principal aspect first if the principal aspect is urgent and serious, and give the priority of treatment to the secondary aspect or treat principal and secondary aspects simultaneously if the secondary aspect of the disease

床辨证时,对这些因素必须给予重视。

二、辨明标本缓急

审察证候的标本,以定治法的先后逆从,这是辨证的重要内容。“标”是疾病临床表现的标志和现象,“本”是疾病发生的根本。疾病的标本不是固定不变的,它往往随某一种疾病和具体患者而有所不同。以病因而论,引起疾病发生的病因为本,所表现于外的各种临床征象是标;以病变部位而论,原发病变部位为本,继发病变部位是标;以症状本身而论,原发症状是本,继发症状是标;以病之新旧而论,旧病是本,新病是标。病证虽多,但总有其标本关系,一切复杂的证候,都可以分析出它的标与本,从而进行正确的辨证和合理的治疗。

在病证的标本审明之后,在治疗处理上,先治其本,或先治其标,并不是一成不变的,应当视具体病情的轻重缓急而定。一般而论,在本病急、本病重的情况下,当先治其本;在标病急、标病重的情况下,须先治其标,或者标本

appears acute and serious. However, the principal aspect and secondary aspect in a disease may affect each other and transform from one into the other. A treatment for the principal aspect of a disease may benefit the secondary aspect, and vice versa. For instance, strengthening the anti-pathogenic qi, a method of treating the principal aspect, will facilitate eliminating pathogenic factors. Meanwhile treatment of eliminating pathogenic factors will promote the recovery of anti-pathogenic qi.

1.2.2.3　Bringing out the dominant aspect of a disease

Clinically when dealing with a given disease a practitioner should identify the dominant aspect of the disease. The dominant aspect of a disease, which may be brought out only through analyzing the etiology and pathogenesis of the disease, does not necessarily appear frequently or obviously. The dominant aspect is the symptoms or signs that reflect the fundamental pathogenesis, and dominates the development of the disease. Concentration on the dominant symptoms and signs is an important part of a therapeutic strategy.

1.2.2.4　Paying special attention to the transformation of syndromes

A syndrome may change through the course of the disease. A cold syndrome may be transformed into a heat one, a heat syndrome into a cold one, a deficiency syndrome into an excess one, and an excess syndrome into a

同治。但是,由于标本是可逆的,是可互相影响的,所以治标也可以达到治本,治本也可以治标。如临床治疗中扶正以祛邪,治本即所以治标;祛邪以扶正,治标即所以治本。由此可知,病证之标本,本可以及标,标也可以及本,因而在治疗上,也可以本病治标,标病治本。

三、抓住主要矛盾

在诊疗内科某一个具体病证时,应从其临床表现的复杂症候群中,首先辨明它的主症,即抓住它的主要矛盾,这是辨证中的技术关键。怎样判断主症呢? 这不能单从症状出现的多少和明显与否来决定,而是要从病因病机来分析比较,看哪个症是反映其病理本质的,对病情发展起着关键作用的,那么它就是主症。因此,辨明主症,即能抓住主要矛盾,就有助于制定正确的治疗原则。

四、把握转化关系

必须注意,一个证候并不是始终不变的。在一定条件下,寒证可以转化为热证,热证可以转化为寒证;虚证可以

deficiency one. However, the transformation of syndromes depends on various factors such as body constitution of the patient, climate, diet, emotions, drugs used, etc. Some factors may facilitate the transformation and should be carefully monitored. As soon as a transformation is observed, intervention should be given promptly and accordingly.

1. 2. 2. 5　Differentiating cold and heat, true and false

When a series of characteristic and consistent symptoms and signs appear, it is relatively easier for a practitioner to make a conclusive diagnosis. However, the manifestations of many diseases are not typical, and there may be inconsistency or paradox in the symptoms or signs that appear in a disease. Clinically often encountered are false phenomena such as false cold manifestations in a heat syndrome, false heat manifestations in a cold syndrome, false deficiency manifestations in an extreme excess syndrome, and false excess manifestations in an extreme deficiency syndrome. In some cases, the nature of a disease is too complicated to be understood thoroughly, then practitioners should analyze the fundamental nature of the disease carefully, differentiate the true from the false, and the fundamental aspect from the non-fundamental aspect. Probably, many manifestations of a disease are false phenomena and only one or two symptoms and signs reflect its fundamental nature. But it is these symptoms and signs that provide evidence for syndrome differentiation. It is vital not to be confused by the false phenomena. Generally speaking, information from tongue inspection and pulse

转化为实证,实证可以转化为虚证。不过证的转化,是以一定因素作为条件的,包括体质、气候、饮食、情志、药物等各种因素,在密切观察症情变化时,尤应注意促成此一转化的条件,作为分析判断的参考。主症一旦转化,一般应及时思考或调整相应的治疗措施。

五、区分寒热真假

在临床诊断过程中,一些典型的证候,较易认识,但有时某些症状还可能互相矛盾,甚至出现假象,最常见的就是寒热的真假,即所谓"真寒假热"、"真热假寒"、"大实有羸状"、"至虚有盛候"。因此,在不容易看清病证本质的情况下,必须克服片面性和表面性,学会从极其复杂的症群中,透过现象看本质,分清哪些是真的,哪些是假的,哪些是反映疾病本质的,哪些是非本质的。要做到这一点,首先应抓住关键性的证候,不要被假象所迷惑,有时假象很多,而反映本质的症状或体征只有一、两个,但这却是主要的依据。一般说来,舌象、脉象是辨别寒热真假很有参考价值的指征。但问诊也不可忽

taking is indicative of the cold or heat nature of a disease. Of course, the information collected from the interrogation is valuable too. As for indicators of a heat or cold syndrome, they can be obtained by using the four diagnostic methods. Furthermore, factors such as constitution, age, history and course of disease, diet, emotions and administration of medicines, will provide important clues for the differentiation between cold and heat syndromes.

视,从四诊合参之中,找出哪些是关键性指标。其次,要全面分析各种因素,包括从体质、年龄、病史、病程、饮食、情志、服药史等去找线索,进行详细的比较,才能辨明其寒热的真假。

1.3 Therapeutic Principles and Methods of Internal Diseases in TCM

第三章 中医内科疾病的治疗原则和常用治法

1.3.1 Therapeutic Principles

第一节 中医内科疾病的治疗原则

The therapeutic principles are formulated according to the basic theory of TCM and syndrome differentiation. These principles should be followed throughout the process of designing therapeutic methods, selecting prescriptions, and administering drugs.

治疗原则又称治则,治疗法则。它是在中医基本理论和辨证论治精神指导下制定的,对疾病治疗的立法、处方、用药等具有指导意义。

1. 3. 1. 1 Routine treatment and treatment contrary to the routine

一、正治反治

Routine treatment refers to a therapeutic principle of treating a disease with the method and drugs contrary to its nature, i. e., treating heat syndrome with drugs of cold nature, treating cold syndrome with drugs of warm or hot nature, treating deficiency syndrome with replenishing method, and treating excess syndrome with reducing method.

正治也称逆治,是最常用的治法。即指疾病的征象与本质相一致时所采取的治疗原则。寒者温之,热者寒之,虚者补之,实者泻之,均为正治法。

Treatment contrary to the routine refers to a therapeutic principle applied for a specific condition, in which there exist false phenomena against the essential nature of disease. In this case a treatment aiming at the false phenomena is given, i. e., treating the false cold phenomena (in a real heat syndrome) with drugs of cold nature, treating the false heat phenomena (in a real cold

反治也称从治,是在特殊情况下所采取的治疗法则。即指疾病的某些征象与病变的本质不相一致时,采取顺从这些假象而治的法则。但实际上还是逆其疾病本质而治疗。如寒因寒用,热因热用,

syndrome) with drugs of warm or hot nature, treating the false phenomena of stagnation (in a real deficiency syndrome) with replenishing method, and treating diarrhea (in a real excessive heat syndrome) with purging method. These treatments seemingly aim at the false phenomena, e. g., cold method for cold manifestations, and warming method for heat manifestations, but they are directly against the essential pathogenesis of a disease. Clinically Baihu Tang (White Tiger Decoction), which is indicated for excessive heat in yangming meridian or excessive heat in qifen in a febrile disease, is used to treat the patient with false cold phenomena in an excessive heat syndrome; and various Purgative Decoctions are used to treat the patient with false phenomena such as diarrhea and delirium with accumulated heat in the large intestine.

1. 3. 1. 2　Strengthening anti-pathogenic qi and eliminating pathogenic factors

Strengthening anti-pathogenic qi is a therapeutic principle of using replenishing methods for deficiency syndromes; eliminating pathogenic factors is a therapeutic principle of using reducing or removing methods for excess syndromes. The development of a disease is the conflict between the anti-pathogenic qi and pathogenic factors. The disease progresses when pathogenic factors overcome the anti-pathogenic qi, and it subsides when anti-pathogenic qi defeats the pathogenic factors. The treatment of strengthening anti-pathogenic qi and eliminating pathogenic factors will restore the anti-pathogenic qi to resist pathogenic factors, which is conducive to the recovery of diseases.

The methods for strengthening anti-pathogenic qi include replenishing qi, nourishing blood, nourishing yin and invigorating yang. The methods for eliminating patho-

塞因塞用,通因通用,均为反治。再如下利谵语,用通下腑实的诸承气汤治疗;真热假寒证,用寒凉的白虎汤治疗,均是反治的具体运用。

二、扶正祛邪

扶正即补法,用于虚证;祛邪即泻法,用于实证。疾病的过程,在某种意义上可以说是正气与邪气相争的过程,邪胜于正则病进,正胜于邪则病退。因此,扶正祛邪就是改变邪正双方力量的对比,使之有利于疾病向痊愈转化。

用于扶正的补法有益气、养血、滋阴、助阳等;用于祛邪的泻法有发表、攻下、渗湿、利

genic factors include dispelling superficial pathogens, purgation, eliminating dampness, promoting diuresis, promoting digestion, and resolving blood stasis. Being mutually supportive, strengthening anti-pathogenic qi will facilitate resisting pathogenic factors, while eliminating pathogenic factors from the body will help protect and restore anti-pathogenic qi.

Generally methods for strengthening anti-pathogenic qi are used for deficiency syndromes with indistinct pathogenic factors, while methods for eliminating pathogenic factors are used for excess syndromes with indistinct deficiency of anti-pathogenic qi. A complicated syndrome with anti-pathogenic qi deficiency and pathogenic factors accumulation will require a method of both strengthening anti-pathogenic qi and eliminating pathogenic factors. In clinical practice it is necessary to differentiate which is dominant, excess or deficiency, in a complicated syndrome. When deficiency is dominant, serious and acute, the complicated syndrome should be treated with replenishing methods supplemented with a mild eliminating method; while a treatment for eliminating pathogenic factors will be adopted together with a mild replenishing method if the acute and serious excess is the major problem in a complicated syndrome. In a deficiency syndrome complicated with excess, when predominant deficiency does not permit an eliminating treatment, or the eliminating treatment may further damage anti-pathogenic qi, then the eliminating method should be applied only after the anti-pathogenic qi is restored. Likewise, in an excess syndrome complicated with mild deficiency or evident deficiency, the replenishing method may foster the pathogenic factors. In that case replenishing method should be used after the pathogenic factors are eliminated. In short, it is important to avoid the retention of pathogenic factors

水、消导、化瘀等。扶正与祛邪,两者又是相辅相成的,扶正有助于抗御病邪,而祛邪则有利于保存正气和恢复正气。

在一般情况下,扶正适用于正虚邪不盛的病证,而祛邪适用于邪实而正虚不显的病证。扶正祛邪并举,适用于正虚邪实的病证。在具体应用时,也应分清以正虚为主,还是以邪实为主。以正虚较急重者,应以扶正为主,兼顾祛邪;以邪实较急重者,则以祛邪为主,兼顾扶正。若正虚邪实以正虚为主,正气过于虚弱不耐攻伐,倘兼以祛邪反而更伤其正,则应先扶正后祛邪;若邪实而正不甚虚,或虽邪实正虚,倘兼以扶正反会助邪,则应先祛邪后扶正。总之,应以扶正不留邪,祛邪不伤正为原则。

when the method of strengthening anti-pathogenic qi is applied, and not to damage the anti-pathogenic qi when the method for eliminating pathogenic factors is used.

1. 3. 1. 3　Replenishing and eliminating methods for zang-fu organs

As previously discussed, TCM holistic view postulates that the human body is an organic whole, and that zang-fu organs are interrelated physiologically and are affected one another pathologically. Disease of a given organ will affect other organs; and, in turn, disorder of an affected organ may affect the original organ. The replenishing and eliminating methods are given according to the principles defined by the five-element theory among zang-fu organs, e. g. , inter-generation, inter-restriction, and exterior-interior relation. The principles include replenishing the mother-organ for deficiency syndrome and reducing the child-organ for excess syndrome; replenishing water to inhibit pathogenic yang and invigorating fire to eliminate pathogenic yin; and treating the exterior fu-organ to relieve the problem in corresponding interior zang-organ or treating the interior zang-organ to relieve the problem in corresponding exterior fu-organ.

1. 3. 1. 3. 1　Replenishing the mother-organ for deficiency syndrome and reducing the child-organ for excess syndrome

This principle is designed according to the inter-generation and inter-restriction relations among zang-fu organs. By replenishing the mother-organ for deficiency syndrome, it is meant that in treating the deficiency syndrome of a zang-organ, replenishing method can be applied to its mother-organ in addition to replenishing the organ itself directly. By reducing the child-organ for excess syndrome, it is meant that in treating the excess

三、脏腑补泻

由于人体是有机的整体，脏腑之间在生理上相互联系，在病理上相互影响，一脏有病往往影响到他脏，而他脏的情况有了改变，也会反过来影响原发病的脏腑。临床上常应用脏腑之间的生克表里关系，作为补泻治法的原则。这些原则可概括为虚则补其母，实则泻其子；壮水制阳，益火消阴；泻表安里，开里通表，清里润表三个方面。

（一）虚则补其母，实则泻其子

这是将脏腑生克关系运用于临床的治疗原则。所谓虚则补其母，就是当某脏虚弱时，除了直接对该脏进行补法治疗外，也可间接补益它的母脏。实则泻其子，就是某脏之病由于子实而起时，可泻子之实以治母病。

syndrome of a mother-organ caused by the excess of its child-organ, the method for eliminating pathogenic factor in child-organ can be used to reduce the excess of the mother-organ.

1.3.1.3.2　Replenishing water to inhibit pathogenic yang and invigorating fire to eliminate pathogenic yin

These are two important principles from the angle of pathogenesis of the zang-fu organs. The principle of replenishing water to inhibit pathogenic yang means to inhibit relatively hyperactive yang through replenishing kidney water (yin), and is applied for the syndrome of yang hyperactivity due to kidney yin deficiency. The principle of invigorating fire to eliminate the pathogenic yin means to eliminate the accumulated yin and cold pathogens by invigorating kidney fire (yang), and is applied for the deficient cold syndrome due to kidney yang deficiency.

1.3.1.3.3　Purging the exterior fu-organ to calm the interior zang-organ, opening the interior zang-organ to relieve the exterior fu-organ, and clearing the interior zang-organ to lubricate the exterior fu-organ

These principles are designed according to the interior-exterior relations between zang and fu organs, and can be used for the syndrome with zang and fu organs both involved. For instance, there exists an interior-exterior relationship between the lung and large intestine; when excessive heat accumulates in yangming fu-organ (large intestine), which leads to constipation and lung qi obstruction, it is hard to relieve the syndrome by treating the lung alone. Then purging the large intestine (exterior fu-organ) at the same time will relieve the lung qi obstruction (interior zang-organ). Likewise, constipation due to the obstruction of lung qi is hard to relieve by only

(二)壮水制阳和益火消阴

这是从脏腑病机上着手的一种重要治法。壮水制阳,适用于肾之真阴不足的证候,以峻补肾之真阴来消除因肾阴不足不能制阳所引起的一系列阳亢之症。益火消阴,适用于肾之真阳不足的证候,以峻补肾之真阳来消除因肾阳不足、无力温化所引起的一系列阴凝之症。

(三)泻表安里、开里通表和清里润表

这是将脏腑的表里关系运用于治疗上的方法。适用于脏与腑之间表里俱病的情况。如肺与大肠相表里,当阳明实热,大便燥结而肺气壅阻时,只从肺治很难见效,而用泻其大肠之表而安肺之里的方法常能取得明显效果。又如因肺气壅阻不宣,致大便燥结者,只从大肠治亦难见效,在治疗上可采用开肺之里的方法而通大肠之表。再如肺

treating the large intestine, then dispersing lung qi (interior zang-organ) simultaneously will relieve the constipation (in exterior fu-organ). One more example is constipation caused by deficiency of lung yin leading to consumption of body fluid. In this case, clearing away lung heat and nourishing lung yin will lubricate the large intestine and relieve constipation.

1. 3. 1. 4   Different principles for different cases

This means that the principles of treatment should vary with individual cases, climatic conditions, environmental factors, etc.

1. 3. 1. 4. 1   Individuality-concerned treatment

This means that the principles of treatment should be decided according to the individual factors, such as sex, age, constitution, etc. When a female patient is treated, her conditions of menstruation, pregnancy and postpartum period must be taken into account. In general, dosage for young children should be less than that for adults; replenishing methods should be recommended for the elderly; invigorating method with warm drugs should be avoided for the patient with a yang-heat constitution; and cold drugs should be used with caution for the patient with a yin-cold constitution.

1.3.1.4.2 Climate-concerned treatment

Seasonal and climatic conditions exert certain influence on the physiological function and pathological changes of the human body. So the principles of treatment should be decided in accordance with the climate in the season involved. In summer and spring, yang qi dominates in

阴虚而生燥,津液被耗所致大便秘结,在治疗上可采用清肺之里而润大肠之表的方法。

四、异法方宜

异法方宜治则,是指疾病的治疗不能固守一法,对不同的个体、不同的时间、不同的地域等应采取有针对性的、不同的治疗方法,方为适宜。

(一)因人制宜

根据病人的性别、年龄、体质等不同特点,来考虑治疗用药的原则,称“因人制宜”。如妇女有月经、怀孕、产后等生理特点,治疗用药必须加以考虑。一般而言,小儿用量要轻,老年人宜补,阳热之体慎用温补,阴寒之体慎用寒凉等。

(二)因时制宜

四时气候的变化,对人体的生理功能、病理变化均产生一定的影响,根据不同季节的时令特点,以考虑用药的原则,称“因时制宜”。如春夏季

nature, the surface pores on the body are open or loose. Warm and pungent drugs in large dosage should be used cautiously to avoid the damage of qi and yin, whereas in autumn and winter, yin qi dominates in nature, cold and bitter drugs in large dosage should be used cautiously to avoid the consumption of yang qi.

1. 3. 1. 4. 3　Environment-concerned treatment

　　This means that the principles of treatment should be decided in accordance with the environmental factors involved. In northwestern China, a higher altitude region with a cold and dry climate, people are easily affected by pathogenic cold-dryness, and their conditions should be treated with warming method to moisturize the dryness. In southeastern China, a low-lying region with a rainy, humid and warm climate, people tend to have disorders with damp-heat and their conditions should be treated with methods for clearing away heat and resolving dampness. The examples illustrate that spectrums of disease are different in different regions, and different therapeutic principles should be adopted accordingly. Furthermore even if the people suffer from the same disease, the treatments and drug administration should differ for different people in different regions. For example, in cold northwestern China, a larger dose of warm pungent herbs should be used to treat exterior wind cold syndrome while a smaller dose will do in warm southeastern China.

1.3.2　Commonly Used Treatments for Internal Diseases

1.3.2.1　Diaphoretic therapy

　　This is a treatment for expelling pathogenic factors

节，阳气升发，人体腠理疏松发散，应避免开泄太过，耗伤气阴；反之，应慎用寒凉之品，以防苦寒伤阳。

（三）因地制宜

　　根据不同地区的地理环境特点，来考虑治疗用药的原则，称"因地制宜"。如中国西北地区，地势高而寒冷少雨，故其病多燥寒，治宜温润；东南地区，地势低而温热多雨，其病多湿热，治宜清化。说明地区不同，患病亦异，治法应当有别，即使患有相同病证，治疗用药，亦应考虑不同地区的特点，而有轻重之别。如辛温发表药治外感风寒证，在西北严寒地区，药量可以稍重，而东南温热地区，药量就应稍轻。

第二节　中医内科疾病的常用治法

一、汗法

　　汗法又称发汗法，是通过

from the exterior of the body by opening the pores of the skin to induce perspiration. It has the activities of relieving exterior syndrome, subsiding fever and swelling, expelling wind and dampness, and letting out skin eruptions. So it is widely applied for diseases or syndromes with exogenous pathogenic factors on the superficial part of the body, e. g., exogenous exterior syndromes, some acute infectious disease at the early stage, edema and bi-syndrome with the manifestations of exterior syndrome, and measles at the early stage. In order to avoid improper or excessive diaphoresis the dosage of diaphoretic drugs should be carefully controlled.

1.3.2.2　Emetic therapy

This is a treatment for eliminating harmful substances and pathogenic factors from the body by the application of vomitive drugs, or by physical stimuli that can induce vomiting, including potent emesis, mild emesis, emesis by physical stimuli, and gastrolavage. It is used for disorders with the retention of phlegm fluid, undigested food and poisonous substances in the throat, esophagus and stomach, e. g., manic-depressive syndrome, excess syndrome with coma, food poisoning, and over intake of alcohol, but it is contraindicated in the elderly and debilitated patients, critically ill patients, patients with severe cardiovascular diseases, or with history of pneumorrhagia or hemorrhage of upper digestive tract, and pregnant and postpartum women.

1.3.2.3　Purgative therapy

This is a treatment for relieving constipation, eliminating indigested food, excessive heat and pathogenic fluid by the application of purgatives or lubricants, including purgation with drugs of cold nature, that with drugs

开泄腠理,以发汗的形式逐邪外出的一种治法。本法具有解表、退热、消肿、祛风湿、透斑疹等作用,广泛适用于邪遏肌表,宜从汗泄的病证。如外感表证或某些急性传染病的初期;具有表证的水肿、痹证及麻疹将透未透阶段。运用汗法时不宜过汗、妄汗,注意个体差异,掌握用药的峻缓。

二、吐法

吐法又称涌吐法,是运用具有催吐作用的方药,或以物探导,通过引发呕吐反应,促使有害病邪排出体外的治法。本法主要包括峻吐法、缓吐法、探吐法、洗胃法,适用于痰涎、宿食、毒物滞留在咽喉、胸膈、胃脘等病证。如癫狂、昏迷实证、误食毒物、过食酒食等。对年老体弱、病危、严重心脏病或有肺出血、上消化道出血病史者,以及妊娠和产后者,应禁用本法。

三、下法

下法又称攻下法,是运用有泻下或润下作用的药物,以通导大便,消除积滞,荡涤实热,攻逐水饮的治法。本法有

of warm nature, that with lubricants, and drastic purgation to eliminate retained fluid. It can be applied to various interior-excess syndromes, for instance, obstruction in the stomach and intestines such as constipation, retention of undigested food, malnutrition due to parasitic infestation, blood stasis, retention of phlegm, etc.; or to the disorders like endogenous heat accumulation, dysentery at the early stage, food or drug poisoning, etc. The timing is very important in using purgation. And the intensity of purgation should be carefully controlled to the appropriate extent.

1.3.2.4 Regulating therapy

This is a treatment for eliminating pathogenic factors from Shaoyang meridian, strengthening anti-pathogenic qi to conduct pathogenic factors out of the body, and coordinating the functions of the viscera. It can be used to coordinate the interior and the exterior, and the yingfen and weifen for exogenous febrile disease, but mainly used to coordinate the functions of the liver and spleen, of the gallbladder and stomach, and of the stomach and intestine for endogenous diseases. Though the drugs used in regulating therapy are mild in nature, this therapy should by no means be abused.

1.3.2.5 Warming therapy

Warming therapy is a treatment to invigorate yangqi and dispel pathogenic cold by the application of drugs of warm or hot nature. It can revive yang for resuscitation, warm the middle energizer to dispel cold and warm the meridians to activate yang. Therefore, it is widely used for interior cold syndromes such as vomiting, diarrhea, cold limbs and intolerance to cold, and spasmodic pain. The therapy should be used with cautions for patients with

寒下、温下、润下及逐水之别，具有通便、下积、泻火、逐水等作用，广泛适用于有各种里实证的患者，如燥屎秘结、食积、虫积、蓄血、痰饮等阻于肠胃者；内热壅盛、痢疾初期、食物或药物中毒等病证者。使用下法应把握时机，权衡攻下之峻缓，以邪去为度，不宜过量。

四、和法

和法是和解少阳、扶正达邪、协调内脏功能的一种治法。和法的内容丰富，应用广泛，如外感疾病宜采用和解表里、和解营卫，内伤杂病则主要采用调和肝脾、调和胆胃以及调和胃肠诸法。运用和法时应掌握适应证，不可认为和法药性平稳而滥用。

五、温法

温法又称温里法，是使用温性或热性的药物，以祛除寒邪，补益阳气的一种治法。本法具有回阳救逆、温中散寒、温经通阳等作用，广泛应用于因寒邪所致的呕逆泄泻、肢冷畏寒、拘挛疼痛的里寒病证。素体阴虚、咽喉干燥者，或有

yin deficiency constitution, and dry throat and mouth, or patients with a history of hemorrhage such as haematemesis and epistaxis.

1.3.2.6 Heat-clearing therapy

Heat-clearing therapy is a treatment to clear away pathogenic heat by the application of drugs of cold or cool nature, including clearing away heat from qifen, clearing away heat from yingfen and cooling blood, clearing away heat and toxic material, clearing away heat from the viscera, and clearing away heat to conserve yin and body fluid. It is widely used for disorders due to heat pathogenic factors such as fever, hyperfunction of the viscera, restlessness, bleedings, rashes, and ulceration and pyogenic infection of the skin. Attention should be paid to the differentiation of true or false cold or heat, of deficient fire or excessive fire, and to the differentiation of syndromes and differentiation of individuality of patients as well.

1.3.2.7 Resolving therapy

Resolving therapy is a treatment to resolve the accumulation of tangible pathogenic factors by the application of drugs effective for promoting digestion, promoting the flow of qi and blood circulation, resolving phlegm, and softening hard masses. It is indicated for retention of indigested food, abdominal mass, subcutaneous nodule, scrofula, calculus, ulcer and pyogenic infection of the skin. It should be used with caution for patients with qi and blood deficiency, and patients with cold syndrome due to deficiency of kidney yang and spleen yang.

1.3.2.8 Invigorating therapy

Invigorating therapy is a treatment to replenish qi, blood, yin and yang, or nourish the viscera of the human

吐血、衄血等出血病史者,应慎用本法。

六、清法

清法又称清热法,是采用寒凉泄热的药物和措施,以消除热证的治法。本法具有清气分热、清营凉血、清热解毒、清脏腑热、保津存阴等作用,广泛应用于因温热病邪所致的发热、脏腑功能亢进、烦躁、出血斑疹、疮疡等病证。运用清法时注意辨别寒热真假、虚火、实火,审证而清,因人而清,以防伤正。

七、消法

消法又称消导或消散法,即使用具有消导、消散、软坚、散结等功效的方药,治疗有形积滞的一种治法。本法应用广泛,适用于饮食停滞、癥积肿块、痰核瘰疬、结石疮痈等病证。消法用药多为克伐之剂,对气血虚弱、脾肾虚寒者应慎用。

八、补法

补法又称补益法,是用具有补益作用的药物,补益人体

body by the application of tonics. It is widely used for congenital and postnatal deficiency, and deficiency of qi, blood, yin, yang and body fluid after a prolonged illness or serious illness. It is also applied to protecting the anti-pathogenic qi of the patient undergoing purgative or resolving therapies. When this therapy is applied, consideration should be given simultaneously to qi and blood, yin and yang, and the five zang-organs should be invigorated accordingly. Any unconsidered or excessive use of invigorating treatments should be avoided.

阴阳气血的不足,或补益某一脏腑之虚损的治法。本法有补气、补血、补阴、补阳等作用,广泛适用于先天不足,或后天失调,或久病、重病后证见气、血、阴、阳、津液等不足之虚证,或应用攻伐之剂而须固护正气者。运用补法时应兼顾气血,调补阴阳,五脏分补,不可妄补、滥补。

2 Treatment of Diseases

2.1 Syndrome Patterns of the Lung

2.1.1 Colds

General Description

Colds are virus-infected diseases in the upper respiratory tract and classified as common cold and influenza. They are mainly manifested as nasal stuffiness and nasal discharge, sneezing, cough, aversion to cold, fever, headache and general aching. Common cold, usually mild, results from rhinovirus infection and is characterized mainly by nasal symptoms. With a high morbidity and repeated infection tendency, common cold may occur all the year round but mostly in winter and spring. But influenza, usually widespread, is due to influenza virus infection and has pronounced systemic toxic symptoms.

Colds fall into the categories of "shang feng" (common cold), "shi xing gan mao" (influenza), etc. in TCM according to the clinical manifestations. The chief pathogenic factors are pathogenic wind and pestilential toxicity and the main pathogenesis includes pathogenic factors invading the body surface and disharmony between weifen and the exterior. The syndrome mostly seen is exterior excess of the lung and weifen.

Essentials for Diagnosis

(1) Cold contact history, acute onset.

各 论

第一章 肺系病证

第一节 感冒

【概述】

感冒主要是由病毒引起的上呼吸道感染性疾病,分为普通感冒与流行性感冒两种。临床主要表现为鼻塞,流涕,喷嚏,咳嗽,恶寒发热,头身疼痛等。普通感冒主要由鼻病毒所引起,以鼻咽部证候为主,一般病情较轻微;流行性感冒是由流感病毒引起,全身中毒证候明显,易引起大流行。本病发病率高,具有反复感染的特点,一年四季均可发生,尤以冬春多见。

根据本病的临床表现,属于中医学"伤风"、"时行感冒"等范畴。其病因主要为外感风邪疫毒。主要病机为邪侵肺卫,卫表不和,一般以肺卫表实证居多。

【诊断要点】

(1) 有与感冒病人接触

(2) Nasal discharge and obstruction, sneezing, itching or sore throat, cough, aversion to cold, fever, little or no sweating, headache and general aching or discomfort.

(3) Influenza should be considered when cold has a wide spreading tendency and patients have high fever, severe headache and sore limbs, which may be accompanied by nausea, vomiting, diarrhea, nasal discharge, sore throat and severe cough.

(4) Laboratory examination shows total leukocyte count normal or slightly reduced, neutrophil decreased and lymphocyte increased. Higher leukocyte count may be seen in patients complicated with bacterial infection.

Syndrome Differentiation and Treatment

Syndrome differentiation for this disease mainly focuses on differentiating between the exterior cold and exterior heat. Patients with more chills, less fever and no sweating mostly belong to the exterior cold syndrome, whereas those with less chill, more fever, sweating, red and swelling throat mainly pertain to the exterior heat syndrome. Clinically colds have four types of syndromes that are wind-cold, wind-heat, exterior cold and interior heat, and summer-heat and dampness. The therapeutic principle for cold is to relieve exterior syndrome through elimination of pathogenic factors. Wind-cold syndrome is treated by diaphoresis with pungent and warm herbs; wind-heat by clearing heat with pungent and cool herbs; exterior cold and interior heat by expelling cold and clearing heat; and summer-heat and dampness by clearing summer-heat and removing dampness.

1. Wind-cold Type

Chief Manifestations: Severe chill, mild fever, no

史,起病多急。

(2)鼻塞流涕,喷嚏,咽痒或痛,咳嗽,恶寒发热,无汗或少汗,头痛,身体酸楚。

(3)高热、头痛及四肢酸痛较重,或伴恶心呕吐、腹泻、流涕、咽痛,咳嗽较甚,又有流行趋势者,应考虑患流行性感冒的可能。

(4)实验室检查可见血液白细胞总数正常或偏低,中性粒细胞减少,淋巴细胞相对增多。若由细菌感染引起的,白细胞总数可以增高。

【辨证论治】

本病辨证主要是辨其表寒和表热。恶寒重,发热轻,无汗者,多属表寒;恶寒轻,发热重,有汗,咽喉红肿者,多属表热。临床主要分为风寒证、风热证、表寒里热证和暑湿证。治疗当采取解表达邪的原则,风寒治以辛温发汗,风热治以辛凉清解,表寒里热治以散寒清热,暑湿挟感者又当清暑祛湿解表。

1. 风寒证

主要证候 恶寒重,发热

sweating, headache, sore limbs, stuffy nose, muffled voice, thin nasal discharge, throat itching, cough with clear and thin sputum, white and thin tongue coating, and superficial or superficial and tense pulse.

Therapeutic Method: To relieve exterior syndrome with pungent and warm herbs.

Prescription: Modified Jing Fang Baidu San (Antiphlogistic Powder with Schizonepetae and Saposhnikoviae), composed of Jingjie (*Herba Schizonepetae*) 10 g, Fangfeng (*Radix Saposhnikoviae*) 10 g, Qianhu (*Radix Peucedani*) 10 g, Xingren (*Semen Armeniacae Amarum*) 10 g, Zhike (*Fructus Aurantii*) 10 g, Chuanxiong (*Rhizoma Chuanxiong*) 10 g, Zisuye (*Folium Perillae*) 10 g, Guizhi (*Ramulus Cinnamomi*) 6 g, Gancao (*Radix Glycyrrhizae*) 5 g and Shengjiang (*Rhizoma Zingiberis Recens*) 5 g.

Modifications: For severe chills and no sweating, add Mahuang (*Herba Ephedrae*) 6 g and Jiegeng (*Radix Platycodi*) 6 g; for severe headache and general aching resulting from wind-cold combined with dampness, add Baizhi (*Radix Angelicae Dahuricae*) 10 g and Qianghuo (*Rhizoma et Radix Notoperygii*) 6 g; for stuffy and running nose, add Cang'erzi (*Fructus Xanthii*) 10 g and Xinyi (*Flos Magnoliae*) 6 g; for general discomfort and lassitude, forceless cough, pale tongue coating and superficial and weak pulse, add Dangshen (*Radix Codonopsis*) 10 g, Fuling (*Poria*) 10 g and Gegen (*Radix Puerariae*) 10 g.

2. Wind-heat Type

Chief Manifestations: Severe fever, slight chill, obstructed sweating, distending pain in the head, dry and sore throat, or red and swelling tonsil, thirst with a desire to drink, stuffy nose with sticky discharge, cough with yellow sputum, red tongue tip, thin and yellow

轻,无汗,头痛,肢体酸疼,鼻塞声重,流涕清稀,喉痒咳嗽,痰吐稀薄,舌苔薄白,脉浮或浮紧。

治　法　辛温解表。

方　药　荆防败毒散加减:荆芥10 g,防风10 g,前胡10 g,杏仁10 g,枳壳10 g,川芎10 g,紫苏叶10 g,桂枝6 g,甘草5 g,生姜5 g。

加　减　恶寒重,无汗等表寒症状重者,加麻黄6 g,桔梗6 g;挟湿而头痛身痛较重者,加白芷10 g,羌活6 g;鼻塞流清涕者,加苍耳子10 g,辛夷6 g;伴见身楚倦怠,咳痰无力,舌苔淡白,脉浮无力者,加党参10 g,茯苓10 g,葛根10 g。

2. 风热证

主要证候　发热重,微恶风寒,汗出不畅,头胀痛,咽干咽痛或咽喉乳蛾红肿疼痛,口渴欲饮,鼻塞流浊涕,咳嗽痰黄,舌尖红,苔薄黄,脉浮数。

tongue coating, and superficial and rapid pulse.

Therapeutic Method: To relieve exterior syndrome with pungent and cool herbs.

Prescription: Modified Yin Qiao San (Lonicerae and Forsythiae Powder) and Cong Chi Jiegeng Tang (Decoction of Shallot, Sojae Preparatum and Platycodi), composed of Jinyinhua (*Flos Lonicerae*) 15 g, Lianqiao (*Fructus Forsythiae*) 15 g, Dandouchi (*Semen Sojae Preparatum*) 12 g, Bohe (*Herba Menthae*, to be decocted later) 5 g, Niubangzi (*Fructus Arctii*) 10 g, Xingren (*Semen Armeniacae Amarum*) 10 g, Jiegeng (*Radix Platycodi*) 6 g and Gancao (*Radix Glycyrrhizae*) 5 g.

Modifications: For severe distending pain in the head, add Manjingzi (*Fructus Viticis*) 10 g, Sangye (*Folium Mori*) 10 g and Juhua (*Flos Chrysanthemi*) 10 g; for abundant sputum, add Zhebeimu (*Bulbus Fritillariae Thunbergii*) 10 g and Gualoupi (*Pericarpium Trichosanthis*) 15 g; for sore, swelling and red throat, add Xuanshen (*Radix Scrophulariae*) 10 g, Tuniuxi (*Radix Achyranthis Bidentatae*) 15 g and Yizhi Huanghua (*Herba Solidaginis Decurentis*) 15 g; for severe fever and thirst, add Zhimu (*Rhizoma Anemarrhenae*) 10 g and Tianhuafen (*Radix Trichosanthis*) 15 g; for pronounced manifestations due to toxic heat, add Daqingye (*Folium Isatidis*) 30 g, Banlangen (*Radix Isatidis*) 30 g and Caoheche (*Rhizoma Paridis*) 30 g; for patients attacked by autumnal dryness manifested as cough with little sputum, dry throat, nose and lips, dry and thin tongue coating, add Nanshashen (*Radix Adenophorae*) 12 g, Tianhuafen (*Radix Trichosanthis*) 15 g and Lipi (*Pericarpium Pyri*) 10 g; for patients complicated with dizziness, restlessness, cough with little sputum, red tongue with little coating and thready and rapid

治　法　辛凉解表。

方　药　银翘散合葱豉桔梗汤加减：金银花15 g,连翘15 g,淡豆豉12 g,薄荷(后下)5 g,牛蒡子10 g,杏仁10 g,桔梗6 g,甘草5 g。

加　减　头胀痛甚者,加蔓荆子10 g,桑叶10 g,菊花10 g;咳嗽痰多者,加浙贝母10 g,瓜蒌皮15 g;咽痛红肿者,加玄参10 g,土牛膝15 g,一枝黄花15 g;高热口渴甚者,加知母10 g,天花粉15 g;时行热毒主要证候明显者,加大青叶30 g,板蓝根30 g,草河车30 g;秋季兼燥邪伤人,伴有咳呛痰少,口咽鼻唇干燥,苔薄少津者,加南沙参12 g,天花粉15 g,梨皮10 g;兼见头昏心烦,干咳痰少,舌红少苔,脉细数者,加玉竹10 g,白薇10 g。

pulse, add Yuzhu (*Rhizoma Polygonati Odorati*) 10 g
and Baiwei (*Radix Cynanchi Atrati*) 10 g.

3. Exterior Cold and Interior Heat Type

Chief Manifestations: Fever, aversion to cold, no
sweating, thirst, stuffy nose, muffled voice, cough, rapid
breathing, yellow, sticky and thick sputum, brown urine,
constipation, red tongue tip and margins with yellow and
white coating, and superficial and rapid pulse.

Therapeutic Methods: To disperse wind and release lung qi, expel cold and clear away heat.

Prescription: Modified Ma Xing Shi Gan Tang (Decoction of Ephedrae, Armeniacae Amarum, Gypsum Fibrosum and Glycyrrhizae), composed of Mahuang (*Herba
Ephedrae*) 6 g, Xingren (*Semen Armeniacae Amarum*) 10 g, Fangfeng (*Radix Saposhnikoviae*) 10 g,
Jingjie (*Herba Schizonepetae*) 10 g, Huangqin (*Radix
Scutellariae*) 10 g, Zhizi (*Fructus Gardeniae*) 10 g,
Lianqiao (*Fructus Forsythiae*) 10 g, Shengshigao (*Gypsum Fibrosum*, to be decocted first) 30 g, Jiegeng (*Radix Platycodi*) 5 g, Bohe (*Herba Menthae*, to be decocted later) 5 g and Shenggancao (*Radix Glycyrrhizae*)
5 g.

Modifications: For aversion to cold and pain in the
bones and joints due to severe external pathogenic cold,
add Zisuye (*Folium Perillae*) 10 g and Jiegeng (*Radix
Platycodi*) 8 g; for red, swelling and sore throat due to
severe endogenous heat, add Banlangen (*Radix Isatidis*)
30 g and Tuniuxi (*Radix Achyranthis Bidentatae*) 15 g;
for constipation, add Zhidahuang (*Radix et Rhizoma
Rhei Preparata*) 5 - 10 g; for persistent high fever, restlessness, thirst, or even coma or delirium, crimson
tongue with yellow and dry coating and rapid pulse due to
transformation of wind and cold into the interior, add
Shuiniujiao (*Cornu Bubali*, to be decocted first) 30 g,

3. 表寒里热证

主要证候　发热恶寒,无
汗口渴,鼻塞声重,咽痛,咳嗽
气急,痰黄黏稠,尿黄便秘,舌
边尖红,苔黄白相兼,脉浮数。

治　法　疏风宣肺,散寒
清热。

方　药　麻杏石甘汤加
减:麻黄6 g,杏仁10 g,防风
10 g,荆芥10 g,黄芩10 g,栀子
10 g,连翘10 g,生石膏(先煎)
30 g,桔梗5 g,薄荷(后下)5 g,
生甘草5 g。

加　减　外感较甚,恶寒
骨节疼痛者,加紫苏叶10 g,桔
梗8 g;里热较甚,咽喉红肿疼
痛者,加板蓝根30 g,土牛膝
15 g;大便秘结不通者,加制大
黄5～10 g;如风寒化热入里,
症见高热不退,心烦口渴,甚
则神昏谵语,舌苔黄少津,舌
质红绛,脉数者,宜用水牛角
(先煎)30 g,生地黄15 g,竹叶
10 g,连翘12 g,金银花15 g,玄
参12 g,黄连6 g,黄芩10 g,石

Shengdihuang (*Radix Rehmanniae*) 15 g, Zhuye (*Herba Lophatheri*) 10 g, Lianqiao (*Fructus Forsythiae*) 12 g, Jinyinhua (*Flos Lonicerae*) 15 g, Xuanshen (*Radix Scrophulariae*) 12 g, Huanglian (*Rhizoma Coptidis*) 6 g, Huangqin (*Radix Scutellariae*) 10 g, Shichangpu (*Rhizoma Acori Tatarinowii*) 10 g and Gancao (*Radix Glycyrrhizae*) 3 g.

4. Summer-heat and Dampness Type

Chief Manifestations: Fever, slight aversion to cold, little sweating, or sweating without relieving fever, heavy or sore limbs, dizziness, heavy and distending sensation of the head, cough with sticky sputum, sticky nasal discharge, restlessness, thirst without much desire to drink, feeling of oppression in the chest, acid regurgitation, scanty dark urine, thin, yellow and greasy tongue coating, and soft-superficial and rapid pulse.

Therapeutic Methods: To clear away summer-heat, resolve dampness and relieve exterior syndrome.

Prescription: Modified Xinjia Xiangru Yin (Newly Modified Mosla Decoction), composed of Xiangru (*Herba Moslae*) 6 g, Jinyinhua (*Flos Lonicerae*) 10 g, Biandouhua (*Flos Lablab Album*, fresh) 10 g, Lianqiao (*Fructus Forsythiae*) 10 g, Heye (*Folium Nelumbinis*, fresh) 10 g, Houpo (*Cortex Magnoliae Officinalis*) 8 g, Lugen (*Rhizoma Phragmitis*) 15 g and Shenggancao (*Radix Glycyrrhizae*) 5 g.

Modifications: For predominant summer-heat, add Huanglian (*Rhizoma Coptidis*) 5 g and Qinghao (*Herba Artemisiae Annuae*) 6 g; for dampness attacking weifen and the exterior, add Doujuan (*Semen Glycines Siccus*) 10 g and Peilan (*Herba Eupatorii*) 10 g; for predominant endogenous dampness, add Cangzhu (*Rhizoma Atractylodis*) 10 g, Baikouren (*Semen Amomi Rotundus*, to be decocted later) 5 g; for scanty and dark urine, add Liuyi

菖蒲10 g,甘草3 g。

4. 暑湿证

主要证候 身热,微恶风,汗少或汗出热不解,肢体酸重或疼痛,头昏重胀痛,咳嗽痰黏,鼻流浊涕,心烦口渴,渴不多饮,胸闷泛恶,小便短赤,舌苔薄黄而腻,脉濡数。

治 法 清暑祛湿解表。

方 药 新加香薷饮加减:香薷6 g,金银花10 g,鲜扁豆花10 g,连翘10 g,鲜荷叶10 g,厚朴8 g,芦根15 g,生甘草5 g。

加 减 暑热偏盛,加黄连5 g,青蒿6 g;湿困卫表,加豆卷10 g,佩兰10 g;里湿偏重,加苍术10 g,白蔻仁(后下)5 g;小便短赤,加六一散(包煎)10 g,茯苓15 g。

San (Six to One Powder, wrapped) 10 g and Fuling (*Poria*) 15 g.

Other Treatments

1. Chinese Patent Drugs

(1) Yin Qiao Jiedu Pian (Lonicerae and Forsythiae Tablet for Removing Toxic Substance): 4 - 6 tablets each time, thrice daily; applicable to the cold of wind-heat type.

(2) Sang Ju Ganmao Chongji (Mori and Chrysanthemi Granule for Common Cold): 1 sachet each time, thrice daily; applicable to cold of wind-heat type.

(3) Yin Huang Koufuye (Oral Liquid of Lonicerae and Coptidis): 10 - 20 ml each time, thrice daily; applicable to influenza, upper respiratory tract infection, and acute tonsillitis, etc.

(4) Wushi Cha (Lunch-Time Tea): 10 g each time, thrice daily; applicable to the cold of wind-cold type and internal injury by improper diet.

(5) Jiang Zao Quhan Chongji (Zingiberis and Jujubae Granule for Expelling Cold): 15 - 30 g each time, thrice daily; applicable to the cold of wind-cold type.

(6) Huoxiang Zhengqi Wan (Agastache Pill for Restoring Healthy Qi): 3 - 5 g each time, thrice daily; applicable to the cold of summer-heat and dampness type.

(7) Xiao Chaihu Chongji (Bupleurum Granule for Shaoyang Syndrome): 10 g each time, thrice daily; applicable to influenza and common cold, manifested as alternate chills and fever, feeling of fullness and discomfort in the chest and hypochondrium.

(8) Banlangen Chongji (Isatis Granule): 15 g each time, thrice daily; applicable to the cold of wind-heat type and the prevention of influenza.

2. Single-drug or Experiential Prescriptions

(1) Yejuhua (*Flos Chrysanthemi Indici*) or Banlan-

【其他疗法】

1. 中成药

(1) 银翘解毒片　每服 4～6片,每日 3 次。适用于风热感冒。

(2) 桑菊感冒冲剂　每服 1 包,每日 3 次。适用于风热感冒。

(3) 银黄口服液　每服 10～20 ml,每日 3 次。适用于流感及上呼吸道感染,急性扁桃体炎等。

(4) 午时茶　每服10 g, 每日 3 次。适用于感冒外感风寒,内伤饮食者。

(5) 姜枣祛寒冲剂　每服 15～30 g,每日 3 次。适用于风寒感冒。

(6) 藿香正气丸　每服 3～5 g,每日 3 次。适用于暑湿感冒。

(7) 小柴胡冲剂　每服 10 g,每日 3 次。适用于流行性感冒和普通感冒,症见寒热往来,胸胁苦满者。

(8) 板蓝根冲剂　每服 15 g,每日 3 次。适用于风热感冒及预防时行感冒。

2. 单验方

(1) 野菊花或板蓝根

gen (*Radix Isatidis*) 10 – 30 g. Decoct the drug with water, use the decoction as gargle or spray to wash or moisten the mouth and throat, 3 – 5 times daily. This is applicable to the cold of wind-heat type with pronounced sore throat.

(2) Jiangmo (Ginger powder) 6 g, Conghua (*Shallot*) 6 g and adequate amount of brown sugar. Soak the drugs in boiling water to make tea. This is applicable to cold due to wind-cold attacking the exterior.

(3) Daqingye (*Folium Isatidis*) 30 g, Yuxingcao (*Herba Houttuyniae*) 15 g, Longkui (*Herba Solani Nigri*) 15 g and Shegan (*Rhizoma Belamcandae*) 15 g. Decoct the drugs with 600 ml of water and concentrate the decoction to 200 ml, add adequate amount of white sugar or honey, take the decoction in two divided doses daily. This is applicable to cold due to wind-heat.

(4) Fangfeng (*Radix Saposhnikoviae*) 10 g, Congbai (*Bulbus Allii Fistulosi*) 10 g, Shengjiang (*Rhizoma Zingiberis Recens*) 10 g and 30 g of rice. Decoct Fangfeng (*Radix Saposhnikoviae*), Congbai (*Bulbus Allii Fistulosi*) and Shengjiang (*Rhizoma Zingiberis Recens*) with water and cook the rice into watery porridge and then mix the decoction and porridge. Take the porridge warm, once daily. Mild sweating suggests a good effect. This is applicable to the cold of wind-cold type.

(5) Fresh Heye (*Folium Nelumbinis*) 24 g or dry Heye (*Folium Nelumbinis*) 10 g, Juhua (*Flos Chrysanthemi*) 12 g and Yiyiren (*Semen Coicis*) 30 g. Decoct the drugs with adequate amount of water. Take the decoction in 2 – 3 divided doses daily. This is applicable to cold due to attack of the summer heat and dampness.

3. External Therapy

(1) Bohe (*Herba Menthae*) 6 g, Dasuan (*Bulbus Allii*) 6 g and Shengjiang (*Rhizoma Zingiberis Recens*)

10～30 g,水煎含漱,或喷润咽喉,每日 3～5 次。适用于风热感冒咽痛明显者。

(2) 姜末6 g,葱花6 g,红糖适量,沸水冲泡代茶饮。适用于风寒束表感冒者。

(3) 大青叶30 g,鱼腥草15 g,龙葵15 g,射干15 g。加水600 ml,煎至200 ml,加白糖或蜂蜜适量,分 2 次服,每日 2 剂。适用于风热感冒。

(4) 防风10 g,葱白10 g,生姜10 g,大米30 g。先将防风、葱、姜水煎,取汁备用。再将大米煮为稀粥,待熟时调入药汁,趁热服用,以微微汗出为佳,每日 1 剂,1 次服完。适用于风寒感冒。

(5) 鲜荷叶24 g(或干荷叶10 g),菊花 12 g,薏苡仁30 g。加水适量,煎汤,去渣服用。每日 1 剂,分 2～3 次服。适用于暑湿袭表之感冒。

3. 外治法

(1) 薄荷6 g,大蒜6 g,生姜6 g。将诸药捣烂如膏,贴敷

6 g. Mash the drugs into paste, apply the paste on Dazhui (GV 14) and Taiyang (EX-HE5) acupoints, cover them with gauze and fix the gauze with adhesive plaster. Then apply the paste onto bilateral Laogong (PC 8) acupoints, close both hands and put the hands in between the two thighs for about 30 minutes. This method is suitable for cold at the early stage with symptoms as aversion to cold and headache, and mild sweating suggests a good effect. For patients with pronounced general aching caused by wind-cold, add Xixin (*Herba Asari*) 3 g into herbs above, mash and stir-bake with a few drops of wine, apply the warmed mixture externally; or conduct moxibustion with moxa rolls above Dazhui (GV 14) and Taiyang (EX-HE5) that are covered with the mashed herbs to induce sweating.

(2) Mash garlic bulbs, collect the juice and concoct 10% garlic solution for nasal drip, 1 - 2 drops, twice or thrice daily. It is applicable to the cold of wind-cold type.

(3) Jingjie (*Herba Schizonepetae*) 10 g, Fangfeng (*Radix Saposhnikoviae*) 10 g, Qianhu (*Radix Peucedani*) 10 g, Qianghuo (*Rhizoma et Radix Notoperygii*) 10 g, Chaihu (*Radix Bupleuri*) 12 g, Shengjiang (*Rhizoma Zingiberis Recens*) 10 g and Duhuo (*Radix Angelicae Pubescentis*) 10 g. Decoct the drugs with 3,000 ml of water, boil them for 10 minutes, pour the decoction into an enamel washbasin, steam and wash the face and head for 30 minutes, twice daily, one dose per day. Wipe the face and head dry immediately after the treatment. This is suitable for the cold of wind-cold type.

2.1.2 Cough

General Description
Cough is a main symptom in pulmonary diseases.

于大椎、太阳穴，以纱布覆盖，用胶布固定。两手劳宫穴贴药合掌，夹于两腿之间，约30分钟。本法对感冒初起有恶寒头痛者，若微汗出即效。风寒感冒全身酸痛明显者，上药加细辛3 g同捣，并加酒数滴炒热贴敷；或用艾卷隔药悬灸大椎、太阳穴，促使汗出可愈。

（2）将大蒜捣烂取液汁，配成10%大蒜液，每次1～2滴，每日2～3次，滴鼻。适用于风寒感冒。

（3）荆芥10 g，防风10 g，前胡10 g，羌活10 g，柴胡12 g，生姜10 g，独活10 g。将上药加水3 000 ml，煮沸10分钟，去渣取汁，倒入搪瓷盆中，薰洗头面部，每次30分钟，每日1剂，薰洗2次。洗后用毛巾将水擦干，避风。适用于感冒属风寒者。

第二节　咳嗽

【概述】
咳嗽是肺系疾病的主要

Generally, cough with a sound but without sputum is called "ke", while cough with sputum but without sound is called "sou". Since a cough usually with both sound and sputum, they are simply called "ke sou" clinically. Cough is a common symptom of various diseases as well as an independent disease. From the point of etiology, cough can be divided into two types: exogenous and endogenous. The former is caused by the six exogenous pathogenic factors invading the lung while the latter is due to dysfunction of the zang-fu organs leading to disturbance of the lung by endogenous pathogenic factors. Whether the pathogenic factors are exogenous or endogenous, they would impair the purifying and descending function of the lung and induce abnormal rising of lung qi, thus causing cough. In western medicine, cough is the main symptom in diseases such as upper respiratory tract infection, acute and chronic bronchitis, bronchiectasis, pneumonia and pulmonary tuberculosis.

Essentials for Diagnosis

(1) Cough with a sound, or accompanied by itching throat and expectoration.

(2) Exogenous cough is characterized by an acute onset, often accompanied by aversion to cold, fever and other exterior symptoms. Endogenous cough has a long duration, with repeated attacks and complicated with other syndromes resulting from the dysfunction of zang-fu organs.

(3) Auscultation reveals hoarse breathing sounds and dry and moist rales.

(4) Laboratory examination reveals a high count of total leukocyte and neutrophil at the acute stage.

(5) Chest X-ray shows normal or increased bronchovascular shadows.

证候之一。一般认为,有声无痰为咳,有痰无声为嗽,但临床多为痰声并具,难以截然分开,故一般通称咳嗽。咳嗽既是独立性的病症,又是多种疾病的一个常见症状。究其成因,不外外感、内伤两大类。外感咳嗽为六淫外邪侵袭于肺;内伤咳嗽为脏腑功能失调,内邪干肺。不论邪从外入,或自内而发,均可引起肺失宣肃,肺气上逆作咳。

西医学的上呼吸道感染、急慢性支气管炎、支气管扩张、肺炎、肺结核等疾病均可表现以咳嗽为主症。

【诊断要点】

(1) 咳逆作声,或伴咽痒咳痰。

(2) 外感咳嗽,起病急,可伴有恶寒发热等外感表证。内伤咳嗽,多反复发作,病程较长,伴有其他脏腑功能失调的证候。

(3) 两肺听诊可闻及呼吸音增粗,或伴有干湿性啰音。

(4) 实验室检查急性期血白细胞总数和中性粒细胞增高。

(5) 肺部 X 线摄片检查,肺纹理正常或增多、增粗等。

Syndrome Differentiation and Treatment

Cough is clinically classified into two categories: exogenous and endogenous. The former mainly includes syndromes such as wind-cold attacking the lung, wind-heat attacking the lung, warm-dryness impairing the lung and cool-dryness impairing the lung. The latter principally includes syndromes as retention of phlegm-dampness in the lung, accumulation of phlegm-heat in the lung, liver fire attacking the lung, consumption of lung yin and deficiency of lung qi. In the treatment, the healthy qi and the pathogenic factors, and the deficiency and excess should be distinguished first. Exogenous cough should be treated by eliminating the pathogenic factors to benefit the lung, while endogenous cough should be treated by strengthening the body resistance as well as eliminating pathogenic factors, that is, the treatment for the principal and secondary aspects must be taken into consideration simultaneously.

1. Exogenous Cough

(1) Wind-cold Attacking the Lung

Chief Manifestations: Hoarse cough with thin and white sputum, itching throat, nasal obstruction and discharge, or accompanied by headache, general aching, aversion to cold, fever, no sweating, sore limbs, thin and white tongue coating, and superficial and tense pulse.

Therapeutic Methods: To disperse wind, expel cold, release lung qi and stop cough.

Prescription: Modified Zhisou San (Powder for Relieving Cough) and San'ao Tang (Three Crude-Drug Decoction), composed of Mahuang (*Herba Ephedrae*) 6 g, Xingren (*Semen Armeniacae Amarum*) 10 g, Jingjie (*Herba Schizonepetae*) 10 g, Ziwan (*Radix Asteris*) 10 g, Baibu (*Radix Stemonae*) 10 g, Zisuye (*Folium Perillae*) 10 g, Baiqian (*Rhizoma Cynanchi*

【辨证论治】

本病证临床分为外感咳嗽与内伤咳嗽两大类。前者主要包括风寒袭肺证、风热犯肺证、温燥伤肺证、凉燥伤肺证；后者主要包括痰湿蕴肺证、痰热郁肺证、肝火犯肺证、肺阴亏耗证、肺气亏虚证。治疗应分清邪正虚实。外感咳嗽，治以祛邪利肺；内伤咳嗽治以祛邪扶正，标本兼顾。

1. 外感咳嗽

（1）风寒袭肺证

主要证候　咳嗽声重，咳痰稀薄色白，气急咽痒，鼻塞流涕，或伴头痛身痛，恶寒发热，无汗，肢体酸楚，舌苔薄白，脉浮紧。

治　法　疏风散寒，宣肺止咳。

方　药　止嗽散合三拗汤加减：麻黄6 g，杏仁10 g，荆芥10 g，紫菀10 g，百部10 g，紫苏叶10 g，白前10 g，桔梗6 g，甘草6 g。

Stauntonii) 10 g, Jiegeng (*Radix Platycodi*) 6 g and
Gancao (*Radix Glycyrrhizae*) 6 g.

Modifications: For severe exogenous wind-cold,
add Fangfeng (*Radix Saposhnikoviae*) 6 g and Qianghuo
(*Rhizoma et Radix Notoperygii*) 10 g; for exogenous
cold and endogenous heat, remove Baiqian (*Rhizoma
Cynanchi Stauntonii*) and Ziwan (*Radix Asteris*) and
add Shengshigao (*Gypsum Fibrosum*, to be decocted
first) 20 g, Sangbaipi (*Cortex Mori*) 15 g and Huangqin
(*Radix Scutellariae*) 10 g; for severe cough, add Jinfei-
cao (*Herba Inulae*) 10 g; for severe headache, add Chuanxiong (*Rhizoma Chuanxiong*) 10 g and Baizhi (*Radix
Angelicae Dahuricae*) 10 g.

(2) Wind-heat Attacking the Lung

Chief Manifestations: Hoarse cough with white or
yellow sputum, dry and sore throat, or cough with hoarse
voice, or fever, slight aversion to wind and cold, yellow
nasal discharge, thirst, headache, red tongue tip, thin
and yellow coating, and superficial and rapid pulse.

Therapeutic Methods: To dispel wind, clear away
heat, release lung qi and resolve phlegm.

Prescription: Modified Sang Ju Yin (Mori and Chrysanthemi Decoction), composed of Sangye (*Folium Mor-
i*) 10 g, Juhua (*Flos Chrysanthemi*) 10 g, Xingren (*Semen Armeniacae Amarum*) 10 g, Jiegeng (*Radix
Platycodi*) 10 g, Lugen (*Rhizoma Phragmitis*) 15 g,
Lianqiao (*Fructus Forsythiae*) 12 g, Bohe (*Herba Menthae*, to be decocted later) 6 g and Gancao (*Radix Glycyrrhizae*) 6 g.

Modifications: For severe cough, add Zhebeimu
(*Bulbus Fritillariae Thunbergii*) 10 g, Pipaye (*Folium Eriobotryae*, wrapped) 10 g and Qianhu (*Radix Peucedani*) 10 g; for pronounced fever and thirst, add Huangqin (*Radix Scutellariae*) 10 g, Zhimu (*Rhizoma

加 减 风寒表证重者，
加防风6 g，羌活10 g；外寒内
热者，去白前、紫菀，加生石膏
（先煎）20 g，桑白皮15 g，黄芩
10 g；咳嗽较重者，加金沸草
10 g；头痛甚者，加川芎10 g，
白芷10 g。

（2）风热犯肺证
主要证候 咳嗽气粗，咯
痰色白或黄，喉燥咽痛，或咳
声嘶哑，或有发热，微恶风寒、
鼻流黄涕、口渴，头痛，舌尖
红，苔薄黄，脉浮数。
治 法 疏风清热，肃肺
化痰。
方 药 桑菊饮加减：
桑叶10 g，菊花10 g，杏仁10 g，
桔梗10 g，芦根15 g，连翘12 g，
薄荷（后下）6 g，甘草6 g。

加 减 咳嗽重者，加浙
贝母10 g，枇杷叶（包煎）10 g，
前胡10 g；发热口渴明显者，加
黄芩10 g，知母10 g，瓜蒌皮
10 g；咽痛声嘎者，加射干10 g，

Anemarrhenae) 10 g and Gualoupi (*Pericarpium Trichosanthis*) 10 g; for sore throat with hoarse voice, add Shegan (*Rhizoma Belamcandae*) 10 g, Chishaoyao (*Radix Paeoniae Rubra*) 10 g and Guajindeng (*Herba Physalis Peruvianae*) 5 g; for dry mouth and red tongue, add Nanshashen (*Radix Adenophorae*) 10 g and Tianhuafen (*Radix Trichosanthis*) 10 g; for summer-heat, add Liuyi San (Six to One Powder, wrapped) 10 g and Heye (*Folium Nelumbinis*, fresh) 10 g.

(3) Warm-dryness Attacking the Lung

Chief Manifestations: Cough with little sputum which is difficult to expectorate, dry and sore throat, dry nose and mouth, red tongue tip, thin and yellow tongue coating with little moisture, thready and rapid pulse.

Therapeutic Methods: To dispel wind, clear away lung heat, moisten the lung and stop cough.

Prescription: Modified Sang Xing Tang (Mori and Armaniacae Decoction), composed of Sangye (*Folium Mori*) 10 g, Xingren (*Semen Armeniacae Amarum*) 10 g, Nanshashen (*Radix Adenophorae*) 10 g, Zhebeimu (*Bulbus Fritillariae Thunbergii*) 10 g, Qianhu (*Radix Peucedani*) 10 g, Zhizi (*Fructus Gardeniae*) 6 g, Dandouchi (*Semen Sojae Preparatum*) 6 g and Lipi (*Pericarpium Pyri*) 6 g.

Modifications: For pronounced dryness-heat, add Shigao (*Gypsum Fibrosum*, to be decocted first) 30 g and Zhimu (*Rhizoma Anemarrhenae*) 8 g; for severe sore throat, add Xuanshen (*Radix Scrophulariae*) 10 g and Mabo (*Lasiosphaera seu Calvatia*) 10 g; for epistaxis or blood-stained sputum, add Baimaogen (*Rhizoma Imperatae*) 15 g and Shengdihuang (*Radix Rehmanniae*) 10 g; for severe consumption of body fluid, add Maimendong (*Radix Ophiopogonis*) 10 g and Yuzhu (*Rhizoma Polygonati Odorati*) 10 g.

(4) Cool-dryness Attacking the Lung

Chief Manifestations: Cough with little or no spu-

赤芍药10 g,挂金灯5 g;口干少津,舌质红者,加南沙参10 g,天花粉10 g;夏季挟暑者,加六一散(包煎)10 g,鲜荷叶10 g。

(3) 温燥伤肺证

主要证候　干咳少痰,咯痰不爽,咽喉干痛,鼻燥咽干,口干,舌尖红,苔薄黄少津,脉细数。

治　法　疏风清肺,润燥止咳。

方　药　桑杏汤加减:桑叶10 g,杏仁10 g,南沙参10 g,浙贝母10 g,前胡10 g,栀子6 g,淡豆豉6 g,梨皮6 g。

加　减　燥热明显者,加石膏(先煎)30 g,知母8 g;咽痛明显者,加玄参10 g,马勃10 g;鼻衄或痰中挟血者,加白茅根15 g,生地黄10 g;津伤较甚者,加麦门冬10 g,玉竹10 g。

(4) 凉燥伤肺证

主要证候　咳嗽,痰少或

tum, itching throat, dry nose and lips, headache, aversion to cold, fever, no sweating, thin, white and dry tongue coating, and superficial and tense pulse.

Therapeutic Methods: To dispel wind and cold, moisten the lung and stop cough.

Prescription: Modified Xingsu San (Powder of Armeniacae Amarum and Perillae), composed of Xingren (*Semen Armeniacae Amarum*) 10 g, Zisuye (*Folium Perillae*) 10 g, Jiegeng (*Radix Platycodi*) 10 g, Baiqian (*Rhizoma Cynanchi Stauntonii*) 10 g, Baibu (*Radix Stemonae*) 10 g, Ziwan (*Radix Asteris*) 10 g, Kuandonghua (*Flos Farfarae*) 10 g, Chenpi (*Pericarpium Citri Reticulatae*) 6 g and Gancao (*Radix Glycyrrhizae*) 6 g.

Modification: For severe aversion to cold, add Jingjie (*Herba Schizonepetae*) 10 g and Fangfeng (*Radix Saposhnikoviae*) 10 g.

2. Endogenous Cough

(1) Retention of Phlegm-dampness in the Lung

Chief Manifestations: Cough with muffled sound, profuse white sticky sputum, or thick sputum in lumps, which is aggravated in the morning or after intake of sweet and greasy food, distending sensation in the chest and abdomen, nausea, poor appetite, lassitude, white and greasy tongue coating, and soft, superficial and smooth pulse.

Therapeutic Methods: To invigorate the spleen, dry dampness, resolve phlegm and stop cough.

Prescription: Modified Erchen Tang (Erchen Decoction) and Sanzi Yangqin Tang (*Decoction of Perillae, Sinapis and Coicis*), composed of Chenpi (*Pericarpium Citri Reticulatae*) 10 g, Fabanxia (*Rhizoma Pinelliae Preparata*) 10 g, Cangzhu (*Rhizoma Atrac-*

无痰,喉痒,咽干唇燥,头痛,恶寒发热,无汗,舌苔薄白而干,脉浮紧。

治　法　疏散风寒,润肺止咳。

方　药　杏苏散加减:杏仁10 g,紫苏叶10 g,桔梗10 g,白前10 g,百部10 g,紫菀10 g,款冬花10 g,陈皮6 g,甘草6 g。

加　减　恶寒甚者,加荆芥10 g,防风10 g。

2. 内伤咳嗽

(1) 痰湿蕴肺证

主要证候　咳嗽痰多,咳声重沉,晨起为甚,痰黏腻或稠厚成块,色白量多,食甘甜油腻食物加重,胸闷脘痞,呕恶食少,体倦,舌白腻,脉濡滑。

治　法　健脾燥湿,化痰止咳。

方　药　二陈汤合三子养亲汤加减:陈皮10 g,法半夏10 g,苍术6 g,厚朴6 g,茯苓15 g,紫苏子10 g,白芥子10 g,莱菔子10 g,薏苡仁20 g。

tylodis) 6 g, Houpo (*Cortex Magnoliae Officinalis*) 6 g, Fuling (*Poria*) 15 g, Zisuzi (*Fructus Perillae*) 10 g, Baijiezi (*Semen Sinapis*) 10 g, Laifuzi (*Semen Raphani*) 10 g and Yiyiren (*Semen Coicis*) 20 g.

Modifications: For severe cold-phlegm, white, sticky and foamy sputum and aversion to cold, add Ganjiang (*Rhizoma Zingiberis*) 6 g and Xixin (*Herba Asari*) 3 g; for lassitude due to spleen deficiency in prolonged cases, add Dangshen (*Radix Codonopsis*) 10 g and Baizhu (*Rhizoma Atractylodis Macrocephalae*) 10 g; for yellow sputum due to transformation of phlegm-dampness into heat, add Huangqin (*Radix Scutellariae*) 6 g and Gualoupi (*Pericarpium Trichosanthis*) 10 g.

(2) Accumulation of Phlegm-heat in the Lung

Chief Manifestations: Cough with hoarse breath, profuse sputum which is sticky and yellow or hot and stinking, or blood-stained and difficult expectoration, distending sensation in the chest and hypochondrium, chest pain induced by cough, flushed face, fever, dry mouth with a desire to drink, red tongue with yellow and greasy coating, and smooth and rapid pulse.

Therapeutic Methods: To clear away heat, resolve phlegm, release lung qi and stop cough.

Prescription: Modified Qingjin Huatan Tang (Decoction for Clearing away Lung Heat and Resolving Phlegm), composed of Sangbaipi (*Cortex Mori*) 15 g, Huangqin (*Radix Scutellariae*) 10 g, Zhizi (*Fructus Gardeniae*) 10 g, Zhebeimu (*Bulbus Fritillariae Thunbergii*) 10 g, Zhimu (*Rhizoma Anemarrhenae*) 10 g, Jiegeng (*Radix Platycodi*) 10 g, Quangualou (*Fructus Trichosanthis*) 15 g, Juhong (*Exocarpium Citri Rubrum*) 6 g and Gancao (*Radix Glycyrrhizae*) 6 g.

Modifications: For purulent or yellow sputum, add

加　减　寒痰较重,痰黏白如沫,怕冷者,加干姜6 g,细辛3 g;久病脾虚,神倦者,加党参10 g,白术10 g;痰湿化热,痰转黄者,加黄芩6 g,瓜蒌皮10 g。

（2）痰热郁肺证

主要证候　咳嗽气粗,痰多质稠,色黄难咯,或有热腥味或吐血痰,胸肋胀满,咳时引痛,面赤或有身热,口干欲饮,舌质红,苔黄腻,脉滑数。

治　法　清热化痰,肃肺止咳。

方　药　清金化痰汤加减:桑白皮15 g,黄芩10 g,栀子10 g,浙贝母10 g,知母10 g,桔梗10 g,全瓜蒌15 g,橘红6 g,甘草6 g。

加　减　痰黄如脓或腥

Yuxingcao (*Herba Houttuyniae*) 30 g, Jinqiaomai (*Rhizoma Fagopyri Cymosi*) 30 g and Dongguazi (*Semen Benincasae*) 15 g; for the feeling of oppression in the chest, severe cough, profuse sputum and constipation, add Tinglizi (*Semen Lepidii seu Descurainiae*) 10 g and unprepared Dahuang (*Radix et Rhizoma Rhei*, to be decocted later) 6 g; for severe thirst due to body fluid consumption, add Nanshashen (*Radix Adenophorae*) 10 g, Maimendong (*Radix Ophiopogonis*) 10 g and Tianhuafen (*Radix Trichosanthis*) 10 g.

(3) Liver Fire Attacking the Lung

Chief Manifestations: Paroxysmal irritable cough with pain in hypochondriac region, flushed face, conjunctival congestion, dry throat, restlessness, bitter mouth, feeling of the throat obstructed by phlegm which is scanty and sticky and difficult to expectorate, thin and yellow tongue coating with little moisture, and smooth and rapid pulse.

Therapeutic Methods: To clear away lung heat, soothe the liver, lower qi and purge fire.

Prescription: Modified Xiebai San (Powder for Clearing away Lung Heat) and Dai Ge San (Powder of Indigo Naturalis and Concha Meretricis seu Cyclinae), composed of Sangbaipi (*Cortex Mori*) 15 g, Digupi (*Cortex Lycii*) 15 g, Qingdai (*Indigo Naturalis*, to be infused separately) 6 g, Haigeke (*Concha Meretricis seu Cyclinae*) 10 g, Huangqin (*Radix Scutellariae*) 10 g, Zhimu (*Rhizoma Anemarrhenae*) 10 g, Tianhuafen (*Radix Trichosanthis*) 10 g and Gancao (*Radix Glycyrrhizae*) 6 g.

Modification: For frequent cough due to predominant heat, add Mudanpi (*Cortex Moutan Radicis*) 10 g and Zhizi (*Fructus Gardeniae*) 10 g.

(4) Deficiency of Lung Qi

Chief Manifestations: Long-standing cough with

臭者,加鱼腥草30 g,金荞麦30 g,冬瓜子15 g;胸满,咳逆痰涌,便秘者,加葶苈子10 g,生大黄(后下)6 g;津伤口渴甚者,加南沙参10 g,麦门冬10 g,天花粉10 g。

（3）肝火犯肺证

主要证候　咳呛气逆阵作,咳时胁痛,面红目赤,咽喉干燥,心烦口苦,常感痰滞咽喉,咯之难出,量少质黏,舌苔薄黄少津,脉弦数。

治　法　清肺平肝,顺气降火。

方　药　加减泻白散合黛蛤散加减:桑白皮15 g,地骨皮15 g,青黛(另冲)6 g,海蛤壳10 g,黄芩10 g,知母10 g,天花粉10 g,甘草6 g。

加　减　火热较盛,咳嗽频作者,加牡丹皮10 g,栀子10 g。

（4）肺气亏虚证

主要证候　病久咳声低

low sound and asthmatic breathing, white and thin sputum, poor appetite, shortness of breath, feeling of oppression in the chest, tiredness, spontaneous sweating, aversion to cold, pale and tender tongue with white coating, and thready and weak pulse.

Therapeutic Methods: To replenish lung qi, resolve phlegm and stop cough.

Prescription: Modified Bufei Tang (Decoction for Replenishing Lung Qi), composed of Huangqi (*Radix Astragali*) 15 g, Dangshen (*Radix Codonopsis*) 10 g, Ziwan (*Radix Asteris*) 10 g, Sangbaipi (*Cortex Mori*) 10 g, Wuweizi (*Fructus Schisandrae*) 6 g, Fabanxia (*Rhizoma Pinelliae Preparata*) 10 g, Fuling (*Poria*) 10 g, Baizhu (*Rhizoma Atractylodis Macrocephalae*) 10 g, Chenpi (*Pericarpium Citri Reticulatae*) 6 g and Gancao (*Radix Glycyrrhizae*) 6 g.

Modifications: For white and foamy sputum, add Ganjiang (*Rhizoma Zingiberis*) 6 g, Xixin (*Herba Asari*) 3 g and Wuzhuyu (*Fructus Evodiae*) 6 g; for severe cough and shortness of breath, add Hezi (*Fructus Chebulae*) 6 g and Buguzhi (*Fructus Psoraleae*) 10 g; for aversion to cold and cold limbs, add Rougui (*Cortex Cinnamomi*, to be decocted later) 3 g and Zhifuzi (*Radix Aconiti Lateralis Preparata*) 6 g.

(5) Consumption of Lung Yin

Chief Manifestations: General dryness, cough in short bursts with sticky and scanty white sputum, or blood-stained sputum, dry mouth and throat, feverish sensation in the palms and soles, night sweating, red tongue with little coating, and thready and rapid pulse.

Therapeutic Methods: To nourish yin, moisten the lung, stop cough and resolve phlegm.

Prescription: Modified Shashen Maidong Tang (Glehniae and Ophiopogonis Decoction), composed of Nan-

微,咳而伴喘,咯痰稀薄色白,食少,气短胸闷,神倦乏力,自汗畏寒,舌淡嫩,苔白,脉细弱。

治　法　补益肺气,化痰止咳。

方　药　补肺汤加减:黄芪15 g,党参10 g,紫菀10 g,桑白皮10 g,五味子6 g,法半夏10 g,茯苓10 g,白术10 g,陈皮6 g,甘草6 g。

加　减　痰多呈白沫者,加干姜6 g,细辛3 g,吴茱萸6 g;咳逆气短者加诃子6 g,补骨脂10 g;畏寒,肢冷者,加肉桂(后下)3 g,制附子6 g。

(5) 肺阴亏耗证

主要证候　干燥,咳声短促,痰少黏白,或痰中带血,咽干口燥,手足心热,夜寐盗汗,舌质红、少苔,脉细数。

治　法　滋阴润肺,止咳化痰。

方　药　沙参麦冬汤加减:南沙参15 g,麦门冬12 g,

shashen (*Radix Adenophorae*) 15 g, Maimendong (*Radix Ophiopogonis*) 12 g, Yuzhu (*Rhizoma Polygonati Odorati*) 12 g, Baihe (*Bulbus Lilii*) 12 g, Tianhuafen (*Radix Trichosanthis*) 12 g, Chuanbeimu (*Bulbus Fritillariae Cirrhosae*) 10 g, Xingren (*Semen Armeniacae Amarum*) 10 g, Sangye (*Folium Mori*) 10 g and Gancao (*Radix Glycyrrhizae*) 6 g.

Modifications: For tidal fever, add Biejia (*Carapax Trionycis*, to be decocted first) 15 g, Shidagonglaoye (*Folium Mahoniae*) 10 g, Digupi (*Cortex Lycii*) 10 g and Qinghao (*Herba Artemisiae Annuae*) 6 g; for cough with shortness of breath, add Wuweizi (*Fructus Mume*) 10 g and Hezi (*Fructus Chebula*) 10 g; for profuse night sweating, add Wumei (*Fructus Mume*) 6 g, Bietaogan (*Fructus Pruni Immaturus*) 15 g and Fuxiaomai (*Fructus Tritici Levis*) 15 g; for cough with yellow sputum, add Haigeke (*Concha Meretricis seu Cyclinae*) 15 g, Zhimu (*Rhizoma Anemarrhenae*) 10 g and Huangqin (*Radix Scutellariae*) 10 g; for blood-stained sputum, add Mudanpi (*Cortex Moutan Radicis*) 10 g, Zhizi (*Fructus Gardeniae*) 10 g and Oujie (*Nodus Nelumbinis Rhizomatis*) 10 g.

Other Treatments
1. Chinese Patent Drugs
(1) Sang Ju Ganmao Pian (Mori and Chrysanthemi Tablet for Common Cold): 4 - 8 tablets each time, twice or thrice daily; applicable to cough due to wind-heat or dry heat.

(2) Shedan Chuanbei Ye (Oral Liquid of Snake's Bile and Fritillariae Cirrhosae): 1 vial each time, thrice daily; applicable to cough due to lung heat.

(3) Qingqi Huatan Wan (Pill for Clearing away Lung Heat and Resolving Phlegm): 6 - 9 g each time, thrice daily; applicable to cough due to phlegm-heat and fire.

玉竹12 g,百合12 g,天花粉12 g,川贝母10 g,杏仁10 g,桑叶10 g,甘草6 g。

加 减 潮热者,加鳖甲(先煎)15 g,十大功劳叶10 g,地骨皮10 g,青蒿6 g;咳而气促者,加五味子10 g,诃子10 g;盗汗量多者,加乌梅6 g,瘪桃干15 g,浮小麦15 g;咯吐黄痰者,加海蛤壳15 g,知母10 g,黄芩10 g;痰中带血者,加牡丹皮10 g,栀子10 g,藕节10 g。

【其他疗法】
1. 中成药
(1) 桑菊感冒片 每服4～8 片,每日 2～3 次。适用于风热咳嗽,燥热咳嗽。

(2) 蛇胆川贝液 每服1支,每日 3 次。适用于肺热咳嗽。

(3) 清气化痰丸 每服6～9 g,每日 3 次。适用于痰热咳嗽及气火咳嗽。

(4) Xing Su Erchen Wan (Erchen Pill with Armeniacae Amarum and Perillae): 6 - 9 g each time, twice daily; applicable to cough due to phlegm-dampness.

(5) Mujingyou Jiaowan (Capsule of Oleum Viticis Negundo): 1 - 2 capsule(s) each time, thrice daily; applicable to chronic cough and dyspnea.

(6) Fufang Gancao Pian (Compound Glycyrrhizae Tablet): 2 - 3 tablets each time, thrice daily. Chew and swallow the tablet or dissolve the tablet in the mouth. It is applicable to cough caused by common cold.

2. Single-drug or Experiential Prescriptions

(1) Yuxingcao (*Herba Houttuyniae*) 3 g, Jiegeng (*Radix Platycodi*) 9 g and Gancao (*Radix Glycyrrhizae*) 6 g. Decoct all the drugs with water and take the decocton. It is applicable to cough due to lung heat.

(2) Nanshashen (*Radix Adenophorae*) 15 g, Chuanbeimu (*Bulbus Fritillariae Cirrhosae*) 9 g and Baihe (*Bulbus Lilii*) 15 g. Decoct all the drugs with water and take the decoction. It is applicable to cough due to deficiency of lung yin.

(3) Dangshen (*Radix Codonopsis*) 60 g, Dongchongxiacao (*Cordyceps*) 30 g, Wuweizi (*Fructus Schisandrae*) 15 g and Gejie (*Gecko*) 1 pair. Pulverize all the drugs and take the fine powder with warm boiled water, 3 g each time, thrice daily. It is applicable to chronic cough and dyspnea due to qi deficiency.

(4) Pipaye (*Folium Eriobotryae*) 10 g. Brush away its hairs, decoct the drug with water and take the decoction three times daily. It is applicable to cough due to phlegm-heat.

(5) Hongdoukou (*Fructus Galangae*) 3 g, Laifuzi (*Semen Raphani*) 6 g and Zisuzi (*Fructus Perillae*) 6 g. Decoct the drugs with water and take the decoction in two divided doses. It is applicable to cough and asthma

（4）杏苏二陈丸　每服6～9g,每日 2 次。适用于痰湿咳嗽。

（5）牡荆油胶丸　每服1～2 丸 ,每日 3 次。适用于慢性咳嗽、气喘。

（6）复方甘草片　每服2～3 片,每日 3 次,嚼碎服或含服。适用于感冒引起的咳嗽。

2. 单验方

（1）鱼腥草3 g,桔梗9 g,甘草6 g,水煎服。适用于肺热咳嗽。

（2）南沙参15 g,川贝母9 g,百合15 g,水煎服。适用于肺阴虚咳嗽。

（3）党参60 g,冬虫夏草30 g,五味子15 g,蛤蚧 1 对,共为细末,每服3 g,每日 3 次,温水送服。适用于慢性气虚咳嗽伴气喘者。

（4）枇杷叶10 g,刷去毛洗净,放小锅中煎汁,其色如茶,每日服 3 次。适用于痰热之咳嗽。

（5）红豆蔻3 g,莱菔子6 g,紫苏子6 g,水煎,每日 2 次分服。适用于咯痰不爽的咳喘。

with difficult expectoration.

(6) Shishuang (*Mannosum Kaki*) 12 – 18 g. Dissolve it in warm water and take the solution in divided doses every day. It is applicable to dry cough and sore throat.

3. External Therapy

(1) Mahuang (*Herba Ephedrae*) 12 g, Guizhi (*Ramulus Cinnamomi*) 10 g, Shigao (*Gypsum Fibrosum*) 20 g, Zhishi (*Fructus Aurantii Immaturus*) 6 g, Ziwan (*Radix Asteris*) 8 g and Zisuye (*Folium Perillae*) 20 g. Pulverize the drugs, mix the powder with sesame oil or with vaseline and make it into an ointment. Apply cupping or point pricking therapy on the selected acupoints first and then cover the ointment on these points and fix the ointment with gauze and adhesive plaster. Points used are Feishu (BL 13), Tanzhong (CV 17), Dazhui (GV 14) and Quchi (LI 11). For wind-cold cough, add Jianjing (GB 21) and Chengshan (GB 57); for wind-heat cough, add Zhongfu (LU 1) and Zhongwan (CV 12).

(2) Baijiezi (*Semen Sinapis*). Stir-bake it until it turns crisp, then pulverize it, mix the fine powder with warm water or ginger juice, stir the mixture into paste. Apply the paste on Tanzhong (CV 17), Dazhui (GV 14), Feishu (BL 13) and Yongquan (KI 1), etc., cover the paste with foil paper, and fix with gauze and adhesive plaster. Remove the paste as soon as a burning sensation and blisters occur. Do not break the blisters. This treatment may be used once daily, 7 days as a treatment course, applicable to wind-cold and chronic cough.

(3) Dilong (*Pheretima*) Extract (1 : 1) and Congbai (*Bulbus Allii Fistulosi*) Extract (1 : 1). Take 8 ml of each extract and mix them in a dropping bottle. This may be used for nasal drip, 1 – 3 drops each time, 10 – 30

(6) 柿霜12～18 g,温水化服,每日分次服。适用于干咳喉痛者。

3. 外治法

(1) 麻黄12 g,桂枝10 g,石膏20 g,枳实6 g,紫菀8 g,紫苏叶20 g。将药物共研细末,以麻油或凡士林调拌成膏。先在所选穴位处拔罐或刺血,再敷上药膏,用纱布、胶布固定。选穴肺俞、膻中、大椎、曲池。风寒咳嗽,加肩井、承山;风热咳嗽加中府、中脘。

(2) 白芥子单味炒黄,炒香,研极细末,过筛,备用。将药末用温水或姜汁调成糊膏,选敷于膻中、大椎、肺俞、涌泉等穴之上,盖以铂纸,纱布、胶布固定。局部有烧灼样痛感和起水泡时去掉。水泡不要弄破。每日1次,7日为1个疗程。适用于风寒咳嗽、慢性咳嗽。

(3) 地龙提取液(1 : 1)、葱白提取液(1 : 1)各8 ml。药液混合装眼药瓶内,每服1～3滴,滴鼻腔内,每日 10 ～ 30

times daily with 10 days as a treatment course and 2 - 3 consecutive courses are recommended. It is applicable to persistent cough.

次。10 日为 1 个疗程,连续 2～3个疗程。适用于久咳。

2.1.3 Asthma

General Description

Asthma, also called bronchial asthma, is defined as a chronic inflammatory disorder of the airways, involving various cells particularly mastocyte, eosinophilic granulocyte and T-lymphocyte. It is manifested as paroxysmal wheeze, chest distress and /or cough, which usually occur at night and /or at early morning and may remit spontaneously or by treatment. According to pathogenesis, it may be classified as exogenous asthma and endogenous asthma. The incidence of bronchial asthma is very high, which is a great threat to public health. There are about 100 million patients of asthma in the world, and in China it affects 1% of the population.

This disease belongs to the category of "xiao zheng" (wheezing syndrome) in TCM. Its pathogenic factors include endopathic and exopathic aspects. The former refers to congenital defect, kidney qi deficiency and weak constitution, or allergic constitution, or the lung obstructed by long-retained phlegm. The latter is related to invasion by exogenous pathogenic factors, improper diet, emotional disturbance, over strain, etc. Phlegm, as the principal pathogenic factor, accumulates in the lung and becomes an "obstinate root" of this disease. Because of this, an acute attack of disease may be induced by sudden change of climate, aspiraton of allergen, improper diet, emotional disdorder or over strain. Repeated attacks of

第三节   哮喘

【概述】

哮喘是支气管哮喘的简称,是由多种细胞特别是肥大细胞、嗜酸性白细胞和 T 淋巴细胞参与的慢性气道炎症。主要表现为反复发作的喘息、气促、胸闷和(或)咳嗽等症状,多在夜间和(或)凌晨发生,症状可自行或经治疗缓解。根据病因的不同,可分为外源性哮喘和内源性哮喘两型。本病发病率甚高,全世界约有 1 亿哮喘患者,我国哮喘的患病率约为 1%,是一种严重威胁公众健康的慢性疾病。

本病属于中医学"哮证"的范畴。其病因有内外两个方面的因素。内因是先天不足,肾气虚弱,素体不强,或具有过敏体质,或宿痰伏肺;外因有外感、饮食、情志、劳倦等。病理因素以痰为主,痰伏于肺,成为本病的"夙根"。在此基础上,适逢气候突变、吸入致敏物质、饮食不当、情志失调、劳累等诱因,即可促使本病急性发作。若长期反复发作,可致肺脾肾三脏受损。肺

asthma for long periods can weaken the lung, spleen and kidney. Lung qi deficiency may results in failure of weiqi to protect the body against diseases and the disease is more likely to recur due to exogenous pathogenic factors. Spleen deficiency may bring about failure in transporting function and produce phlegm in the lung. Kidney deficiency may cause failure of receiving qi by the kidney; and kidney yang deficiency causes accumulation of pathogenic fluid that may transform into phlegm, while kidney yin deficiency induces hyperactive fire to scorch the body fluid into phlegm, which moves upwards and stays in the lung, thus worsening the condition.

气虚弱,卫外失固,则更易感受外邪而诱发;脾失健运,又可生痰渍肺;肾虚不能纳气,而且阳虚则水泛为痰,阴虚则火旺灼津成痰,上干于肺,从而加重病情。

Essentials for Diagnosis

（1）Inquiry for predisposing causes including inhaling of allergic or non-allergic substances, infection, climatic change, certain medicines and food, and emotional irritation should be made.

（2）Paroxysmal expiratory dyspnea accompanied by wheezing is the typical symptom. At the early stage, patients often experience itching nose and throat, sneezing, nasal discharge and cough. Then expiratory dyspnea occurs abruptly with difficult and prolonged expiration accompanied by wheezing. Abundant white sticky sputum may appear at the resolving stage, while purulent sputum may occur after bacterial infection.

（3）Physical signs include orthopnea, nares flaring, shoulders heave, chest undulation, distention of jugular vein, over-inflated chest, hyperresonant thoracic percussion note, reduced border of cardiac dullness, diminution of breathing sounds, prolonged expiration, wheezing sound in the whole chest (appearing mainly at the expiratory stage, also at the inspiratory period in deteriorated cases). When the condition gets worse, dyspnea becomes more severe but wheezing sounds are reduced.

【诊断要点】

（1）追询发病前有无抗原或非抗原性物质吸入及感染、气候改变、服用某些药物和饮食、精神刺激等诱发因素。

（2）典型症状为发作性呼气性呼吸困难,伴哮鸣音。发作前有鼻咽发痒、喷嚏、流涕、咳嗽等,随后突然发作以呼气为主的呼吸困难,呼气延长费力伴哮鸣。发作好转时咳大量白色黏稠痰,细菌感染时咳脓性痰。

（3）体征为端坐呼吸,鼻翼煽动,两肩耸动,胸部起伏,颈静脉怒张,胸廓胀满呈吸气状。叩诊胸部呈过清音,心浊音界缩小。呼吸音减弱,呼气延长,双肺满布哮鸣音,呼气期为主,加重时吸气期亦存在;严重时呼吸困难加剧,哮鸣音反而减少。

(4) High total leukocyte and neutrophil count in the peripheral blood when complicated by infection, high eosinophil count, Charcot-Leyden crystals formed by the membrane protein of eosinophilic granulocyte appearing in sputum, and high count of serum IgE and IgG in exogenous asthma.

(5) Senstinogen skin test and inspiratory provocative test can be applied to detect the senstinogen.

Syndrome Differentiation and Treatment

Since the pathogenic factors are prevailing in the stage of attack, the therapeutic principle at this stage is to eliminate the pathogenic factors as a symptomatic treatment. The treatment should be focused on eliminating these factors and resolving phlegm. Cold-phlegm should be warmed and resolved so as to release lung qi, whereas warm-phlegm should be cleared and resolved in order to lower lung qi. Since the body resistance is weakened at the remission stage, the treatment should be based on the principle of strengthening the body resistance as a causative treatment. Cases with yang deficiency should be treated by invigorating therapy, while those with yin insufficiency by nourishing treatment. According to the involvement of the zang organs, methods of nourishing the lung, invigorating the spleen or strengthening the kidney are applied accordingly.

1. Stage of Attack

(1) Retention of Cold-phlegm in the Lung

Chief Manifestations: Dyspnea with wheezing induced usually by cold, white, thin and clear sputum, suffocative feeling in the chest, dark and bluish complexion, no thirst, or thirst with preference to warm drink, cold limbs, aversion to cold, tendency of occurrence in cold weather or after cold attack, pale tongue with white

（4）外周血白细胞总数及中性粒细胞在感染时升高,嗜酸性粒细胞升高,痰液中有嗜酸性白细胞膜蛋白所组成的夏科-雷登结晶。外源型哮喘血清 IgE 和 IgG 增高。

（5）可采用过敏原皮试及吸入激发试验,以确定过敏原。

【辨证论治】

本病发作期一般以邪实为主。根据发时祛邪治标的原则,重在祛邪化痰,寒痰宜温化宣肺,热痰宜清化肃肺。哮喘缓解期一般以正虚为主,治疗以扶正治本为原则,阳气虚弱者应温补,阴液不足者宜滋养,并根据病变脏器的不同,分别给予补肺、健脾、益肾之治法。

1. 发作期

（1）寒痰蕴肺证

主要证候　喘促气急,喉中哮鸣有声,痰多清稀色白,胸膈满闷如塞,面色晦滞带青,口不渴,或渴喜热饮,形寒怕冷,每遇天冷或受寒易发,舌质淡,苔白滑,脉弦紧。

and smooth coating, and wiry and tense pulse.

Therapeutic Methods: To warm the lung, dispel cold, resolve phlegm and relieve asthma.

Prescription: Modified Shegan Mahuang Tang (Belamcandae and Ephedrae Decoction), composed of Shegan (*Rhizoma Belamcandae*) 10 g, Mahuang (*Herba Ephedrae*) 6 g, Ganjiang (*Rhizoma Zingiberis*) 3 g, Xixin (*Herba Asari*) 3 g, Zhibanxia (*Rhizoma Pinelliae Preparata*) 10 g, Houpo (*Cortex Magnoliae Officinalis*) 10 g, Baiqian (*Rhizoma Cynanchi Stauntonii*) 10 g, Xingren (*Semen Armeniacae Amarum*) 10 g, Ziwan (*Radix Asteris*) 10 g and Kuandonghua (*Flos Farfarae*) 10 g.

Modifications: For severe dyspnea with abundant sputum and inability to lie flat, add Tinglizi (*Semen Lepidii seu Descurainiae*) 10 g and Baijiezi (*Semen Sinapis*) 10 g; for aversion to cold, fever and headache, add Jingjie (*Herba Schizonepetae*) 6 g, Fangfeng (*Radix Saposhnikoviae*) 6 g, Dandouchi (*Semen Sojae Preparatum*) 6 g, Guizhi (*Ramulus Cinnamomi*) 5 g, Baizhi (*Radix Angelicae Dahuricae*) 6 g and Zisuye (*Folium Perillae*) 10 g; for itching nose, nasal obstruction, clear and thin nasal discharge and frequent sneezing, add Xinyihua (*Flos Magnoliae*) 6 g and Chantui (*Periostracum Cicadae*) 5 g.

(2) Retention of Phlegm-heat in the Lung

Chief Manifestations: Dyspnea with hoarse voice, wheezing sound in the throat, over inflated chest, frequent irritable cough, abundant yellow and thick sputum, irritability, flushed face, thirst with a desire to drink, red tongue with yellow and greasy coating, and smooth and rapid pulse.

Therapeutic Methods: To clear away heat, resolve phlegm, release lung qi and relieve asthma.

治　法　温肺散寒,化痰平喘。

方　药　射干麻黄汤加减:射干10 g,麻黄6 g,干姜3 g,细辛3 g,制半夏10 g,厚朴10 g,白前10 g,杏仁10 g,紫菀10 g,款冬花10 g。

加　减　痰涌喘逆不得卧者,加葶苈子10 g,白芥子10 g;恶寒、发热、头痛者,加荆芥6 g,防风6 g,淡豆豉6 g,桂枝5 g,白芷6 g,紫苏叶10 g;鼻痒鼻塞,清涕较多,喷嚏频作者,加辛夷花6 g,蝉蜕5 g。

(2)痰热壅肺证

主要证候　呼吸气粗息涌,喉中痰鸣如吼,胸高胁胀,咳呛阵作,咳痰量多色黄稠厚,烦躁不安,面赤,口渴欲饮,舌红,苔黄腻,脉滑数。

治　法　清热化痰,肃肺定喘。

Prescription: Modified Dingchuan Tang (Decoction for Relieving Asthma), composed of Sangbaipi (*Cortex Mori*) 12 g, Huangqin (*Radix Scutellariae*) 10 g, Zhimahuang (*Herba Ephedrae*, roasted) 10 g, Xingren (*Semen Armeniacae Amarum*) 10 g, Zisuzi (*Fructus Perillae*) 10 g, Baiguo (*Semen Ginkgo*) 6 g, Beimu (*Bulbus Fritillariae*) 10 g, Gualou (*Fructus Trichosanthis*) 10 g and Kuandonghua (*Flos Farfarae*) 10 g.

Modifications: For severe dyspnea with inability to lie flat due to obstruction of lung qi, add Tinglizi (*Semen Lepidii seu Descurainiae*) 10 g; for dry and hard stool due to qi obstruction in the fu-organs, add Shengdahuang (*Radix et Rhizoma Rhei*, to be decocted later) 6 g and Mangxiao (*Natrii Sulfas*, to be infused separately) 10 g; for abundant yellow and fishy sputum, add Yuxingcao (*Herba Houttuyniae*) 15 g, Jinqiaomai (*Rhizoma Fagopyri Cymosi*) 15 g, Dongguazi (*Semen Benincasae*) 12 g, Yiyiren (*Semen Coicis*) 12 g and Lugen (*Rhizoma Phragmitis*) 20 g; for predominant heat in the lung, add Shigao (*Gypsum Fibrosum*, to be decocted first) 30 g.

(3) Blockage of Phlegm in the Lung

Chief Manifestations: Dyspnea, feeling of oppression in the chest, wheezing sound in the throat, cough with abundant thick and white sputum aggravated in the early morning, nausea, sticky and greasy sensation in the mouth, thick and greasy tongue coating, and smooth pulse.

Therapeutic Methods: To remove phlegm, dredge aperture, lower adverse lung qi and stop asthma.

Prescription: Modified Erchen Tang (Erchen Decoction) and Sanzi Yangqin Tang (Decoction of Perillae, Sinapis and Coicis), composed of Zhibanxia (*Rhizoma Pinelliae Preparata*) 10 g, Chenpi (*Pericarpium Citri Reticulatae*) 6 g, Fuling (*Poria*) 12 g, Zisuzi

方　药　定喘汤加减:桑白皮12 g,黄芩10 g,炙麻黄5 g,杏仁10 g,紫苏子10 g,白果6 g,贝母10 g,瓜蒌10 g,款冬花10 g。

加　减　肺气壅实,痰鸣息涌不得卧者,加葶苈子10 g;大便干结,腑气不通者,加生大黄(后下)6 g,芒硝(另冲)10 g;痰多稠黄有腥味者,加鱼腥草15 g,金荞麦15 g,冬瓜子12 g,薏苡仁12 g,芦根20 g;肺热内盛者,加石膏(先煎)30 g。

(3) 痰浊阻肺证

主要证候　喘促,胸闷,喉中痰鸣如曳锯,咳嗽痰多,稠厚色白,晨起尤甚,兼有恶心,口中黏腻,舌苔厚腻,脉滑。

治　法　涤痰利窍,降气平喘。

方　药　二陈汤合三子养亲汤加减:制半夏10 g,陈皮6 g,茯苓12 g,紫苏子10 g,莱菔子10 g,苍术10 g,厚朴10 g,杏仁10 g。

(*Fructus Perillae*) 10 g, Laifuzi (*Semen Raphani*) 10 g, Cangzhu (*Rhizoma Atractylodis*) 10 g, Houpo (*Cortex Magnoliae Officinalis*) 10 g and Xingren (*Semen Armeniacae Amarum*) 10 g.

Modifications: For poor appetite, add Jiaoshanzha (*Fructus Crataegi*, charred) 10 g, Chaoshenqu (*Massa Medicata Fermentata*, stir-baked) 10 g, Guya (*Fructus Setariae Germinatus*) 12 g and Maiya (*Fructus Hordei Germinatus*) 2 g; for predominant dampness, add Sharen (*Fructus Amomi*, to be decocted later) 3 g.

(4) Attack on the Lung by Stagnated Liver Qi

Chief Manifestations: Dyspnea with wheezing sound in the throat, suffocative sensation in the chest, abdominal distension, which are induced by emotional irritation and relieved by belching or by passing flatus, thin and white tongue coating, and wiry pulse.

Therapeutic Methods: To soothe the liver, regulate qi circulation, lower the adverse lung qi and stop asthma.

Prescription: Modified Chaihu Shugan San (Bupleuri Powder for Soothing Liver Qi), composed of Chaihu (*Radix Bupleuri*) 6 g, Zhike (*Fructus Aurantii*) 10 g, Baishaoyao (*Radix Paeoniae Alba*) 12 g, Xiangfu (*Rhizoma Cyperi*) 10 g, Chenxiang (*Lignum Aquilariae Resinatum*) 6 g, Muxiang (*Radix Aucklandiae*) 10 g, Yujin (*Radix Curcumae*) 10 g and Qingpi (*Pericarpium Citri Reticulatae Viride*) 6 g.

Modifications: For palpitation and insomnia, add Hehuanhua (*Flos Albiziae*) 10 g, Suanzaoren (*Semen Ziziphi Spinosae*) 10 g, Yuanzhi (*Radix Polygalae*) 6 g and Yejiaoteng (*Caulis et Folium Polygoni Multiflori*) 12 g; for irritability, add Mudanpi (*Cortex Moutan Radicis*) 10 g and Zhizi (*Fructus Gardeniae*) 10 g.

加　减　食欲不振者,加焦山楂10 g,炒神曲12 g,谷芽12 g,麦芽12 g;湿重者,加砂仁(后下)3 g。

（4）肝气犯肺证

主要证候　每遇情志刺激遂发,呼吸急促,喉中痰鸣,胸闷如窒,脘腹胀满,嗳气或矢气后则诸症稍宽,舌苔薄白,脉弦。

治　法　疏肝开郁,降气平喘。

方　药　柴胡疏肝散加减:柴胡6 g,枳壳10 g,白芍药12 g,香附10 g,沉香6 g,木香10 g,郁金10 g,青皮6 g。

加　减　心悸、失眠者,加合欢花10 g,酸枣仁10 g,远志6 g,夜交藤12 g;性情急躁易怒者,加牡丹皮10 g,栀子10 g。

2. Stage of Remission

(1) Lung Deficiency Syndrome

Chief Manifestations: Frequent spontaneous sweating, aversion to wind, liability to catching cold which is frequently induced by climate changes, dyspnea, low voice, mild rale in the throat, cough with thin and white sputum, pale and lusterless complexion, pale tongue with thin and white coating, and thready and weak pulse.

Therapeutic Methods: To tonify the lung and strengthen weifen.

Prescription: Modified Yupingfeng San (Jade Screen Powder), composed of Huangqi (*Radix Astragali*) 12 g, Baizhu (*Rhizoma Atractylodis Macrocephalae*) 10 g, Fangfeng (*Radix Saposhnikoviae*) 6 g, Dangshen (*Radix Codonopsis*) 10 g, Wuweizi (*Fructus Schisandrae*) 6 g, Hutaorou (*Semen Ouglandis*) 10 g and Shanyao (*Rhizoma Dioscoreae*) 12 g.

Modifications: For pronounced aversion to cold, add Guizhi (*Ramulus Cinnamomi*) 6 g, Baishaoyao (*Radix Paeoniae Alba*) 12 g, Shengjiang (*Rhizoma Zingiberis Recens*) 3 g and Dazao (*Fructus Jujubae*) 10 pcs; for irritable cough with little sticky sputum due to the deficiency of both qi and yin, add Nanshashen (*Radix Adenophorae*) 10 g, Maimendong (*Radix Ophiopogonis*) 10 g, Yuzhu (*Rhizoma Polygonati Odorati*) 10 g, Baihe (*Bulbus Lilii*) 12 g, Chuanbeimu (*Bulbus Fritillariae Cirrhosae*) 6 g and Xingren (*Semen Armeniacae Amarum*) 10 g.

(2) Spleen Deficiency Syndrome

Chief Manifestations: Poor appetite and abdominal distension, formless stools, diarrhea induced by intake of greasy food, shortness of breath, spiritlessness, lassitude, cough with white thick, clotted sputum in the morning, pale and swollen tongue with teeth marks on the

2. 缓解期

(1) 肺虚证

主要证候 经常自汗,恶风,易感冒,每因气候变化而诱发,气喘声低,喉中有轻度哮鸣,咳痰清稀色白,面色淡白无华,舌质淡,苔薄白,脉细弱。

治 法 补肺固卫。

方 药 玉屏风散加减:黄芪12 g,白术10 g,防风6 g,党参10 g,五味子6 g,胡桃肉10 g,山药12 g。

加 减 畏寒明显者,加桂枝6 g,白芍药12 g,生姜3 g,大枣 10 枚;气阴两虚,呛咳痰少质黏者,加南沙参10 g,麦门冬10 g,玉竹10 g,百合12 g,川贝母6 g,杏仁10 g。

(2) 脾虚证

主要证候 食少腹胀,大便不成形,食油腻则易腹泻,气短不足以息,神疲倦怠,晨起咯痰稠白成块,常因饮食不当而引发本病,舌质淡胖,苔

margins, and thready and soft-superficial pulse. This syndrome is often induced by improper diet.

Therapeutic Methods: To strengthen the spleen and resolve phlegm.

Prescription: Modified Liujunzi Tang (Six Mild-Drug Decoction), composed of Dangshen (*Radix Codonopsis*) 10 g, Baizhu (*Rhizoma Atractylodis Macrocephalae*) 10 g, Fuling (*Poria*) 12 g, Zhigancao (*Radix Glycyrrhizae, roasted*) 3 g, Zhibanxia (*Rhizoma Pinelliae Preparata*) 10 g, Chenpi (*Pericarpium Citri Reticulatae*) 6 g, Cangzhu (*Rhizoma Atractylodis*) 10 g and Houpo (*Cortex Magnoliae Officinalis*) 10 g.

Modifications: For diarrhea due to spleen deficiency, add Yiyiren (*Semen Coicis*) 12 g, Shanyao (*Rhizoma Dioscoreae*) 10 g and Biandou (*Semen Dolichoris*) 10 g; for abdominal distension due to food stagnation, add Laifuzi (*Semen Raphani*) 10 g, Jiaoshanzha (*Fructus Crataegi*, charred) 10 g, Shenqu (*Massa Medicata Fermentata*) 12 g, Chaomaiya (*Fructus Hordei Germinatus*, stir-baked) 12 g; for spleen yang deficiency, add Ganjiang (*Rhizoma Zingiberis*) 3 g and Shufuzi (*Radix Aconiti Lateralis Preparata*) 6 g.

(3) Kidney Deficiency Syndrome

Chief Manifestations: Shortness of breath induced and worsened by exertion, tinnitus, soreness in the lower back; or aversion to cold, cold limbs, pale complexion, pale and tender tongue with thin and white coating, and deep and thready pulse; or flushed cheeks, dysphoria with feverish sensation in the five centers (chest, palms and soles), night sweating, red tongue with little coating, and thready and rapid pulse. This syndrome is often induced by overstrain.

Therapeutic Method: To invigorate the kidney to receive lung qi.

薄白,舌边有齿痕,脉细濡。

治　法　健脾化痰。

方　药　六君子汤加减:党参10 g,白术10 g,茯苓12 g,炙甘草3 g,制半夏10 g,陈皮6 g,苍术10 g,厚朴10 g。

加　减　脾虚腹泻者,加薏苡仁12 g,山药10 g,扁豆10 g;食滞腹胀者,加莱菔子10 g,焦山楂10 g,神曲12 g,炒麦芽12 g;脾阳虚弱者,加干姜3 g,熟附子6 g。

(3)肾虚证
主要证候　短气息促,动则尤甚,耳鸣,腰酸,每因劳累而引发本病。或畏寒肢冷,面色苍白,舌质淡胖嫩,苔薄白,脉沉细;或颧红,五心烦热,盗汗,舌红少苔,脉细数。

治　法　补肾纳气。

Prescription: Modified Jingui Shenqi Wan (Pill for Invigorating Kidney Qi from *Golden Cabinet*), composed of Shufuzi (*Radix Aconiti Lateralis Preparata*) 6 g, Rougui (*Cortex Cinnamomi*) 3 g, Shudihuang (*Radix Rehmanniae Preparata*) 12 g, Shanyao (*Rhizoma Dioscoreae*) 12 g, Shanzhuyu (*Fructus Corni*) 10 g, Mudanpi (*Cortex Moutan Radicis*) 10 g, Zexie (*Rhizoma Alismatis*) 12 g and Fuling (*Poria*) 12 g.

Modifications: For predominant yang deficiency, add Buguzhi (*Fructus Psoraleae*) 10 g, Lujiao Pian (*Cornu Cervi*, sliced) 10 g, Roucongrong (*Semen Myristicae*) 10 g and Yinyanghuo (*Herba Epimedii*) 10 g; for yin deficiency, add Maimendong (*Radix Ophiopogonis*) 10 g, Baihe (*Bulbus Lilii*) 10 g, Beishashen (*Radix Glehniae*) 12 g, Zishiying (*Fluoritum*) 15 g, Guibanjiao (*Colla Plastri Testudinis*, to be melted and infused separately) 15 g and Danggui (*Radix Angelicae Sinensis*) 10 g.

Other Treatments

1. Chinese Patent Drugs

(1) Zhike Pingchuan Pian (Tablet for Relieving Cough and Asthma): 2 - 4 tablets each time, thrice daily; applicable to bronchial asthma with an acute onset.

(2) Jiming Dingchuan Wan (Rooster-Crowing Bolus for Relieving Asthma): 1 bolus each time, twice daily; applicable to asthma with headache, general aching, fever, aversion to cold and other exterior symptoms due to wind-cold.

(3) Wuwei Zhike Pian (Five-Drug Tablet for Relieving Cough): 6 - 8 tablets each time, twice daily; applicable to asthma with cough, blood-stained sputum, dyspneal fullness and wheezing sound in the throat due to prolonged stagnation of lung heat.

(4) Mahuang Zhichuan Wan (Ephedra Bolus for

方　药　《金匮》肾气丸加减：熟附子6 g,肉桂3 g,熟地黄12 g,山药12 g,山茱萸10 g,牡丹皮10 g,泽泻12 g,茯苓12 g。

加　减　阳虚明显者,加补骨脂10 g,鹿角片10 g,肉苁蓉10 g,淫羊藿10 g;阴虚者,加麦门冬10 g,百合10 g,北沙参12 g,紫石英15 g,龟版胶(烊化冲服)15 g,当归10 g。

【其他疗法】

1. 中成药

(1) 止咳平喘片　每服2~4片,每日3次。适用于支气管哮喘急性发作。

(2) 鸡鸣定喘丸　每服1丸,每日2次。适用于哮喘伴头痛体痛、发热恶寒等风寒表证。

(3) 五味止咳片　每次6~8片,每日2次。适用于肺热久瘀,咳嗽喘满,痰中带血,气逆痰鸣。

(4) 麻黄止喘丸　每服1

Relieving Asthma): 1 bolus each time, twice daily; applicable to bronchial asthma with abundant sputum and short breath.

2. Single-drug or Experiential Prescriptions

(1) Yuyan Dan (Scolopendra Pill): composed of Youyan (*Scolopendra*) 20 pcs, Zhebeimu (*Bulbus Fritillariae Thunbergii*) 15 g and Mahuang (*Herba Ephedrae*) 10 g. Dry and pulverize Youyan (*Scolopendra*) and Zhebeimu (*Bulbus Fritillariae Thunbergii*) first, mix the powder with Mahuang decoction and prepare it into pills, 3 g each time, thrice daily. It is applicable to bronchial asthma due to abundant phlegm-heat.

(2) Jiangqi Pingchuan Tang (Decoction for Lowering Lung Qi and Relieving Asthma): composed of Shegan (*Rhizoma Belamcandae*) 12 g, Mahuang (*Herba Ephedrae*) 6 g, Dilong (*Pheretima*) 12 g, Zisuzi (*Fructus Perillae*) 12 g, Tinglizi (*Semen Lepidii seu Descurainiae*) 15 g, Xixin (*Herba Asari*) 3 g, Sangbaipi (*Cortex Mori*) 20 g, Xuchangqing (*Radix Cynanchi Paniculati*) 20 g and Gancao (*Radix Glycyrrhizae*) 6 g. Decoct the drugs with water, 1 dose daily. It is applicable to asthma of excess type.

(3) Huotan Quyu Jiangqi Tang (Decoction for Eliminating Phlegm, Removing Blood Stasis and Lowering Lung Qi): composed of Zisuzi (*Fructus Perillae*) 15 g, Laifuzi (*Semen Raphani*) 15 g, Shuizhi (*Hirudo*) 9 g, Baijiezi (*Semen Sinapis*) 9 g, Danshen (*Radix Salviae Miltiorrhizae*) 20 g, Dilong (*Pheretima*) 20 g, Danggui (*Radix Angelicae Sinensis*) 12 g, Tinglizi (*Semen Lepidii seu Descurainiae*) 10 g, Taoren (*Semen Persicae*) 10 g, Kushen (*Radix Sophorae Flavescentis*) 10 g and Xingren (*Semen Armeniacae Amarum*) 10 g. Decoct the drugs with water, 1 dose daily. It is applicable to protracted asthma with stagnation of phlegm and blood in the lung.

丸,每日 2 次。适用于支气管哮喘痰多气促者。

2. 单验方

(1) 玉蜓丹　蚰蜓 20 条,浙贝母 15 g,麻黄 10 g。先将蚰蜓、浙贝母捣烂晒干为末,再以麻黄 10 g 煎汤,拌和为丸。每次口服 3 g,每日 3 次。适用于支气管哮喘痰热偏盛者。

(2) 降气平喘汤　射干 12 g,麻黄 6 g,地龙 12 g,紫苏子 12 g,葶苈子 15 g,细辛 3 g,桑白皮 20 g,徐长卿 20 g,甘草 6 g。水煎服,每日 1 剂。适用于哮喘实证。

(3) 豁痰祛瘀降气汤　紫苏子 15 g,莱菔子 15 g,水蛭 9 g,白芥子 9 g,丹参 20 g,地龙 20 g,当归 12 g,葶苈子 10 g,桃仁 10 g,苦参 10 g,杏仁 10 g。水煎服,每日 1 剂。适用于哮喘久发,痰瘀阻肺。

（4）Lengxiao Yin（Decoction for Asthma of Cold Type）: composed of Zhimahuang（*Herba Ephedrae*, roasted）12 g, Jingjie（*Herba Schizonepetae*）9 g, Fangfeng（*Radix Saposhnikoviae*）9 g, Baiguo（*Semen Ginkgo*）10 g, Guizhi（*Ramulus Cinnamomi*）9 g, Shegan（*Rhizoma Belamcandae*）10 g, Jiangbanxia（*Rhizoma Pinelliae*, ginger prepared）10 g, Fuling（*Poria*）10 g, Chenpi（*Pericarpium Citri Reticulatae*）10 g, Yinyanghuo（*Herba Epimedii*）15 g, Xixin（*Herba Asari*）3 g, Gancao（*Radix Glycyrrhizae*）5 g and Shengjiang（*Rhizoma Zingiberis Recens*）6 g. Decoct the drugs with water, 1 dose daily. It is applicable to cold asthma with symptoms of sneezing, nasal obstruction and discharge, cough, feeling of oppression in the chest, wheezing sound in the throat, etc.

（5）Rexiao Yin（Decoction for Asthma of Heat Type）: composed of Jinyinhua（*Flos Lonicerae*）30 g, Lianqiao（*Fructus Forsythiae*）15 g, Huangqin（*Radix Scutellariae*）15 g, Yuxingcao（*Herba Houttuyniae*）30 g, Zhimahuang（*Herba Ephedrae*, roasted）10 g, Baiguo（*Semen Ginkgo*）12 g, Dilong（*Pheretima*）10 g, Gualou（*Fructus Trichosanthis*）18 g, Jiangbanxia（*Rhizoma Pinelliae*, ginger prepared）10 g, Chenpi（*Pericarpium Citri Reticulatae*）10 g, Shengshigao（*Gypsum Fibrosum*, to be decocted first）24 g and Gancao（*Radix Glycyrrhizae*）6 g. Decoct the drugs with water, 1 dose daily. It is applicable to heat-asthma with symptoms as wheezing sound in the throat, sticky nasal discharge, red tongue with thin and yellow coating, and smooth and rapid pulse.

（6）Qutan Huayu Tongfu Tang（Decoction for Resolving Phlegm, Removing Blood Stasis and Regulating Intestines）: composed of Tinglizi（*Semen Lepidii seu Descurainiae*）15 g, Kuandonghua（*Flos Farfarae*）

（4）冷哮饮　炙麻黄12 g, 荆芥9 g, 防风9 g, 白果10 g, 桂枝9 g, 射干10 g, 姜半夏10 g, 茯苓10 g, 陈皮10 g, 淫羊藿15 g, 细辛3 g, 甘草5 g, 生姜6 g。水煎服, 每日1剂。适用于寒哮, 症见喷嚏、鼻塞流涕、咳嗽、胸闷、喉中哮鸣等。

（5）热哮饮　金银花30 g, 连翘15 g, 黄芩15 g, 鱼腥草30 g, 炙麻黄10 g, 白果12 g, 地龙10 g, 瓜蒌18 g, 姜半夏10 g, 陈皮10 g, 生石膏（先煎）24 g, 甘草6 g。水煎服, 每日1剂。适用于热哮, 症见喉中痰鸣、鼻流浊涕、舌红、苔薄黄、脉滑数等。

（6）祛痰化瘀通腑汤　葶苈子15 g, 款冬花12 g, 大黄10 g, 桃仁10 g, 蚤休10 g, 百部10 g, 枳实10 g, 麻黄10 g, 杏仁

12 g, Dahuang (*Radix et Rhizoma Rhei*) 10 g, Taoren (*Semen Persicae*) 10 g, Zaoxiu (*Rhizoma Paridis*) 10 g, Baibu (*Radix Stemonae*) 10 g, Zhishi (*Fructus Aurantii Immaturus*) 10 g, Mahuang (*Herba Ephedrae*) 10 g, Xingren (*Semen Armeniacae Amarum*) 10 g and Dilong (*Pheretima*) 10 g. Decoct the drugs with water, 1 dose daily. It is applicable to the attack stage of asthma with blockage of phlegm and blood stasis in the lung and obstruction in fu organs.

(7) Jiejing Pingchuan Tang (Decoction for Relieving Spasm and Asthma): composed of Quanxie (*Scorpio*, to be pulverized and swallowed) 3 g, Mayi (*Formica*, to be pulverized and swallowed) 3 g, Zhibanxia (*Rhizoma Pinelliae Preparata*) 10 g, Mahuang (*Herba Ephedrae*) 6 g, Xing ren (*Semen Armeniacae Amarum*) 10 g, Zisuzi (*Fructus Perillae*) 10 g, Maimendong (*Radix Ophiopogonis*) 10 g and Gancao (*Radix Glycyrrhizae*) 4 g. Decoct the drugs with water, 1 dose daily. It is applicable to severe asthmatic cough.

(8) Ma Xing Su Cha Tang (Decoction of Ephedrae, Armeniacae Amarum, Perillae and Camelliae Sinensis): composed of Mahuang (*Herba Ephedrae*) 9 g, Xing-ren (*Semen Armeniacae Amarum*) 10 g, Zisuzi (*Fructus Perillae*) 10 g, Chaye (*Camelliae Sinensis*) 6 g, Jiegeng (*Radix Platycodi*) 6 g, Ganjiang (*Rhizoma Zingiberis*) 3 g, Hezi (*Fructus Chebulae*) 6 g and Zhigancao (*Radix Glycyrrhizae*, roasted) 3 g. Decoct the drugs with water, 1 dose daily. It is applicable to prolonged bronchial asthma.

3. External Therapy

(1) Baijiezi (*Semen Sinapis Albae*) 15 g, Fabanxia (*Rhizoma Pinelliae Preparata*) 15 g, Guixin (*Cortex Cinnamomi*) 15 g, Yanhusuo (*Rhizoma Corydalis*) 12 g, Chenxiang (*Lignum Aquilariae Resinatum*) 3 g

10 g,地龙10 g。水煎服,每日 1剂。适用于哮喘发作期痰瘀阻肺,腑气不通者。

(7)解痉平喘汤　全蝎(研末吞服)3 g,蚂蚁(研末吞服)3 g,制半夏10 g,麻黄6 g,杏仁10 g,紫苏子10 g,麦门冬10 g,甘草4g。水煎服,每日1剂。适用于咳喘明显者。

(8)麻杏苏茶汤　麻黄9 g,杏仁10 g,紫苏子10 g,茶叶6 g,桔梗6 g,干姜3 g,诃子6 g,炙甘草3 g。水煎服,每日1剂。适用于支气管哮喘病程日久者。

3. 外治法

(1)取双肺俞、双风门、双厥阴俞六穴,将白芥子、法半夏、桂心各15 g,延胡索12 g,沉香、甘遂各3 g,共研细末,用

and Gansui (*Radix Kansui*) 3 g. Pulverize the drugs and mix the powder with ginger juice, prepare it into paste, and divide it into six portions. Apply the paste onto bilateral Feishu (BL 13), Fengmen (BL 12) and Jueyinshu (BL 14) respectively, cover the paste with oilpaper and fix with adhesive plaster for 12 hours, once daily, with 3 times as a treatment course. It is applicable to patients without pronounced cold and heat manifestations.

(2) Baijiezi (*Semen Sinapis Albae*) 200 g, Gansui (*Radix Kansui*) 100 g, Yuanhua (*Flos Genkwa*) 50 g, Xixin (*Herba Asari*) 30 g and Shegan (*Rhizoma Belamcandae*) 50 g. Pulverize the drugs, and mix the medicated powder with 200 g of fresh loess and honey into a paste. Apply the paste onto the chest and back for 24 hours, and change the dressing every other day. It is applicable to asthma.

(3) Baijiezi (*Semen Sinapis*) 30 g, Yanhusuo (*Rhizoma Corydalis*) 30 g, Xixin (*Herba Asari*) 15 g, Gansui (*Radix Kansui*) 15 g, Mahuang (*Herba Ephedrae*) 15 g, Cang'erzi (*Fructus Xanthii*) 10 g, Rougui (*Cortex Cinnamomi*) 10 g, Dingxiang (*Gemma Caryophylli*) 6 g and Ganjiang (*Rhizoma zingiberis*) 30 g. Grind the drugs into dust and mix it with ginger juice to form a paste and put it evenly on a 4 cm × 5 cm oilpaper. During the three ten-day periods of hot season, apply the paste on bilateral Bailao (EX), Feishu (BL 13) and Gaohuang (BL 43), and fix them with adhesive plaster, once every 10 days and 4 - 8 hours each time. After the hot season, conduct moxibustion with moxa stick for 10 minutes over bilateral Kongzui (LU 6), Lieque (LU 7), Tiantu (CV 22) and Zusanli (ST 36), and then apply the paste on these points, once every month, 4 - 8 hours each time, until the Beginning of Winter (19th solar term,

老姜汁调成糊状。将药糊分成 6 份贴敷于穴位上,用油纸覆盖,胶布固定。贴 12 小时后去药洗净,然后隔 12 小时再贴,共贴 3 次。适用于无明显寒热表现的哮喘。

(2) 白芥子 200 g,甘遂 100 g,芫花 50 g,细辛 30 g,射干 50 g,共研细面,加新鲜黄土 200 g,用蜂蜜调成糊状,敷于胸背部,每次敷 24 小时,隔日换药 1 次。适用于哮喘。

(3) 白芥子 30 g,延胡索 30 g,细辛 15 g,甘遂 15 g,麻黄 15 g,苍耳子 10 g,肉桂 10 g,丁香 6 g,干姜 30 g,共研细末。临用时以生姜汁适量调膏,摊于 4 cm × 5 cm 油纸上,伏天贴于双侧百劳、肺俞、膏肓穴,胶布固定。伏天过后改贴双孔最、列缺、天突、足三里,贴前用艾条悬灸俞穴 10 分钟。贴药时间为伏天内每隔 10 日贴 1 次,3 次后,每月 1 次,至立冬,共贴 6 次,每次 4~8 小时,连贴 3 年为 1 个疗程。适用于支气管哮喘。

Nov. 7 or 8). Continuous application of three years makes up a treatment course. It is applicable to bronchial asthma.

(4) Mahuang (*Herba Ephedrae*) 5 g, Xingren (*Semen Armeniacae Amarum*) 10 g, Shengshigao (*Gypsum Fibrosum*, to be decocted first) 30 g, Huangqin (*Radix Scutellariae*) 10 g, Sangbaipi (*Cortex Mori*) 15 g and Jinyinhua (*Flos Lonicerae*) 20 g. Decoct the drugs with water twice, filter and concentrate the decoction into 50 ml, bottle the solution and seal the bottle. Inhale the vapour of the solution through an ultrasonic aerosol inhalator for 40 minutes. It is applicable to asthma of the heat type.

(5) Mahuang (*Herba Ephedrae*) 10 g, Guizhi (*Ramulus Cinnamomi*) 10 g, Xingren (*Semen Armeniacae Amarum*) 10 g, Zisuzi (*Fructus Perillae*) 10 g, Juhong (*Exocarpium Citri Rubrum*) 5 g and Gancao (*Radix Glycyrrhizae*) 10 g. Decoct the drugs with water twice, filter and concentrate the decoction into 50 ml, bottle the solution and seal the bottle, inhale the vapour of the solution through ultrasonic aerosol inhalator for 40 minutes. It is applicable to asthma due to cold-phlegm.

(6) Badouren (*Fructus Crotonis*) 2 pcs, Chenpi (*Pericarpium Citri Reticulatae*) 5 g and adequate amount of Shengjiang (*Rhizoma Zingiberis Recens*) Juice. Crush and deoil Badouren (*Fructus Crotonis*) with alcohol to make fine powder. Mix the powder with fresh ginger juice and mold it as a stick and wrap the stick with gauze. Soak the stick together with Chenpi (*Pericarpium Citri Reticulatae*) in water for 10 minutes, and insert it into one nostril for 15 minutes and the other nostril a few minutes later. It is applicable to asthma of excess type.

(4) 麻黄5 g,杏仁10 g,生石膏(先煎)30 g,黄芩10 g,桑白皮15 g,金银花20 g。上药加水煎 2 次,再浓煎反复过滤,沉淀取液 50 ml,装瓶封口备用。临用时用超声雾化器口腔雾化吸入,每次雾化时间为 40 分钟左右。适用于哮喘属于热证者。

(5) 麻黄10 g,桂枝10 g,杏仁10 g,紫苏子10 g,橘红5 g,甘草10 g。上药加水煎 2 次,再浓煎反复过滤,沉淀取液50 ml,装瓶封口备用。临用时用超声雾化器进行口腔雾化吸入,每次雾化时间为 40 分钟。适用于寒痰型哮喘。

(6) 巴豆仁 2 粒,陈皮5 g,生姜汁适量。先将巴豆仁压碎,用酒精去油法制成巴豆霜。用鲜生姜汁调成膏,捏成圆柱状,纱布包裹,再加陈皮用水浸泡 10 分钟,塞入一侧鼻孔,15 分钟后取出,休息数分钟,再塞另一侧鼻孔。适用于哮喘属于实证者。

2.1.4 Lung Cancer

General Description

Lung cancer, also called primary bronchogenic carcinoma, is a malignant pulmonary tumor primarily originating from bronchial mucosa and glands, manifested mainly by irritable cough, blood-stained sputum or hemoptysis, chest pain and oppression, shortness of breath, fever, etc. Its incidence is the highest of all tumors in males and takes the second place in females. With an ominous prognosis, it has a very high mortality. Its average survival rate of five years is about 10% after various treatments.

The etiology and mechanism of lung cancer is not completely clear. It is believed that the disease is related to some inherent factors of the body and some environmental factors; and in particular, the lung is the organ exposed to the environment, so environmental factors should not be ignored. It is already known that all the carcinogenic factors can cause lung cancer, for instance, cigarette smoking, air pollution, occupational carcinogenic factors, ionizing radiation, etc. Other factors related to it, to some degree, are immunologic hypofunction, metabolic disorder, endocrine dysfunction and heredity.

In TCM, according to its clinical manifestations, lung cancer belongs to the categories of "ka xue" (hemoptysis), "fei ji" (lung mass), "xi ben" (hypochondrium lumps), "xu lao" (consumptive disease), etc. The exopathic factors are the six exogenous pathogenic factors that invade the lung. The endopathic ones include weak constitution, smoking and drinking, dust, emotional upset

第四节 肺癌

【概述】

原发性支气管肺癌(简称肺癌)是起源于支气管黏膜和腺体的肺部原发性恶性肿瘤。临床主要表现为刺激性咳嗽,痰中带血或咯血,胸痛,胸闷,气急,发热等。肺癌发病率在男性肿瘤中占首位,在女性肿瘤中占第二位。本病死亡率高,预后不良,经各种治疗平均5年生存率为10%左右。

肺癌的病因和发病机理至今尚不十分明确,多数学者认为可能与机体内在因素和周围环境因素有关,特别由于肺是一个开放性器官,因此外界环境因素更是一个不可忽视的问题。已知所有的致癌因素大多可致肺癌。其发病的高危因素主要有吸烟、空气污染、职业致癌因子、电离辐射等,此外与机体免疫功能低下、代谢失常、内分泌功能紊乱、遗传因素也有一定的关系。

根据本病的临床表现,属于中医学"咯血"、"肺积"、"息贲"、"虚劳"等范畴。其外因为六淫邪毒,侵袭于肺,内因与平素体虚、嗜食烟酒、环境多尘、情志所伤、劳倦太过等有关。主要病机为正气内虚,

and overstrain. The main pathogenesis involves deficiency of anti-pathogenic factors with accumulation of phlegm and blood stasis in the lung. Generally, this disease is characterized by principal deficiency and secondary excess. The excess refers to qi accumulation, blood stasis, phlegm, dampness and toxic fire in the lung locally, and the deficiency denotes disorder of the whole body involving qi, blood, yin and yang.

Essentials for Diagnosis

(1) Irritable cough, blood stained sputum or hemoptysis, chest pain and oppression, shortness of breath and fever are the chief manifestations.

(2) Exfoliated cell examination in sputum may find cancer cells. If hydrothorax exists, cancer cells may be found in the smear of centrifuged and precipitated pleural effusion.

(3) Space-occupying lesions found in X-ray, CT, and bronchography are helpful to diagnosis; bronchoscopy, isotope scanning, and biopsy examination are also helpful.

(4) Males above 30 years with a long smoking history should be taken into consideration.

Syndrome Differentiation and Treatment

Syndromes of this disease are clinically classified as yin deficiency and toxic heat, deficiency of lung qi and spleen qi, accumulation of phlegm-dampness in the lung, qi stagnation and blood stasis, deficiency of qi and yin, and deficiency of yin and yang. The therapeutic principle is strengthening the body resistance and eliminating the pathogenic factors. According to the state of the deficiency of body resistance or the excess of pathogenic factors, treatment methods such as clearing away heat and resolving phlegm, activating collaterals and dissipating blood

痰浊瘀毒胶结于肺所致。总属本虚标实,实为局部,虚为整体。其实者,多由气滞血瘀及痰、湿、火毒凝聚于肺;其虚者,每见全身气血阴阳的虚衰。

【诊断要点】

(1) 以刺激性咳嗽,痰中带血或咯血,胸痛、胸闷、气急、发热等为主要证候。

(2) 痰液脱落细胞检查可发现癌细胞;如有胸水者,抽胸水离心沉淀,涂片可找到癌细胞。

(3) 胸部平片、CT、支气管造影等,如发现占位性病变,可协助诊断;支气管镜、同位素扫描及活体组织检查有助确诊。

(4) 30 岁以上有长期吸烟史的男性更应注意。

【辨证论治】

本病临床主要分为阴虚毒热证、肺脾气虚证、痰湿壅肺证、气滞血瘀证、气阴两虚证和阴阳两虚证。治疗以扶正祛邪为原则,根据邪正虚实的主次,分别采用清化痰热、和络化瘀、解毒软坚、养阴润肺、益气温阳法治疗。

stasis, removing toxic substance and softening hard masses, nourishing yin and moistening the lung, and invigorating qi and warming yang are used respectively.

1. Yin Deficiency and Toxic Heat

Chief Manifestations: Dry cough with little or no
sputum, or blood-stained sputum, or frequent hemoptysis, low fever, night sweating, dry mouth, yellow urine,
constipation, red tongue with little or no coating, and
thready and rapid pulse.

Therapeutic Methods: To nourish yin, clear away
heat, remove toxic substance and diminish stagnation.

Prescription: Modified Shashen Maidong Tang (Glehniae and Ophiopogonis Decoction) and Baihe Gujin Tang
(Lilii Decoction for Strengthening Lung), composed of
Beishashen (*Radix Glehniae*) 15 g, Maimendong (*Radix Ophiopogonis*) 15 g, Tianmendong (*Radix Asparagi*) 15 g, Shengdihuang (*Radix Rehmanniae*) 15 g,
Baihe (*Bulbus Lilii*) 15 g, Xuanshen (*Radix Scrophulariae*) 15 g, Zhebeimu (*Bulbus Fritillariae Thunbergii*) 15 g, Huangqin (*Radix Scutellariae*) 10 g, Digupi
(*Cortex Lycii*) 10 g, Zhibiejia (*Carapax Trionycis*,
roasted, to be decocted first) 15 g, Madouling (*Fructus
Aristolochiae*) 10 g, Longkui (*Herba Solani Nigri*)
30 g, Shancigu (*Pseudobulbus Cremastrae seu Pleiones*)
10 g, Yuxingcao (*Herba Houttuyniae*) 30 g, Banzhilian
(*Herba Scutellariae Barbatae*) 30 g and Baihuasheshecao (*Herba Hedyotis Diffusae*) 30 g.

Modifications: For prolonged high fever, add Jinyinhua (*Flos Lonicerae*) 30 g, Daqingye (*Folium Isatidis*) 30 g and Shengshigao (*Gypsum Fibrosum*) 30 g;
for persistent blood expectoration, add Baimaogen (*Rhizoma Imperatae*) 30 g, Xianhecao (*Herba Agrimoniae*)
30 g, Ejiao (*Colla Corii Asini*, to be melted and infused
separately) 10 g and Sanqifen (*Radix Notoginseng*,

1. 阴虚毒热证

主要证候 干咳无痰或
少痰,或痰中带血,或咯血时
作,低热盗汗,口干舌燥,尿黄
便结,舌质红,少苔或光红无
苔,脉细数。

治 法 滋阴清热,解毒
散结。

方 药 沙参麦冬汤合
百合固金汤加减:北沙参
15 g,麦门冬15 g,天门冬15 g,
生地黄15 g,百合15 g,玄参
15 g,浙贝母15 g,黄芩10 g,地
骨皮10 g,炙鳖甲(先煎)15 g,
马兜铃10 g,龙葵30 g,山慈姑
10 g,鱼腥草30 g,半枝莲30 g,
白花蛇舌草30 g。

加 减 高热不退者,加
金银花30 g,大青叶30 g,生石
膏30 g;咯血不止者,加白茅根
30 g,仙鹤草30 g,阿胶(烊化
冲服)10 g,三七粉(另冲)3 g;
痰多难出者,加海浮石30 g,鹅
管石30 g,葶苈子10 g,杏仁

powdered and to be infused separately) 3 g; for abundant sputum with difficult expectoration, add Haifushi (*Os Costaziae*) 30 g, Eguanshi (*Stalactitum*) 30 g, Tinglizi (*Semen Lepidii seu Descurainiae*) 10 g and Xingren (*Semen Armeniacae Amarum*) 10 g; for spontaneous sweating and shortness of breath, add Renshen (*Radix Ginseng*, to be decocted separately) 10 g, Dongchongxia-cao (*Cordyceps*, to be decocted separately) 5 g, Huangqi (*Radix Astragali*) 12 g, Maimendong (*Radix Ophiopog-onis*) 12 g and Wuweizi (*Fructus Schisandrae*) 12 g; for constipation, add Zhidahuang (*Radix et Rhizoma Rhei Preparata*) 10 g, Shengdihuang (*Radix Reh-manniae*) 10 g, Huomaren (*Semen Cannabis*) 10 g and Yuliren (*Semen Pruni*) 10 g.

2. Deficiency of Lung Qi and Spleen Qi Syndrome

Chief Manifestations: Shortness of breath, cough with abundant white sputum, lassitude, feeling of oppression in the chest, poor appetite, abdominal distension, loose stools, sweating on exertion, pale tongue with teeth marks on lateral sides, white and greasy tongue coating, and thready or soft-superficial and smooth pulse.

Therapeutic Methods: To replenish qi, invigorate the spleen, regulate qi and resolve phlegm.

Prescription: Modified Xiang Sha Liujunzi Tang (Six Mild-Drug Decoction with Cyperi and Amomi), composed of Taizishen (*Radix Pseudostellariae*) 15 g, Ziheche (*Placenta Hominis*) 15 g, Fuling (*Poria*) 15 g, Huangjing (*Rhizoma Polygonati*) 15 g, Huangqi (*Radix Astragali*) 15 g, Baizhu (*Rhizoma Atractylodis Macro-cephalae*) 10 g, Wuweizi (*Fructus Schisandrae*) 10 g, Fabanxia (*Rhizoma Pinelliae Preparata*) 10 g, Jiegeng (*Radix Platycodi*) 10 g, Jupi (*Pericarpium Citri Reticulatae*) 6 g, Zhixiangfu (*Rhizoma Cyperi Preparata*)

10 g；自汗短气者,加人参(另煎)10 g,冬虫夏草(另煎)5 g,黄芪12 g,麦门冬12 g,五味子12 g;大便秘结者,加制大黄10 g,生地黄10 g,火麻仁10 g,郁李仁10 g。

2. 肺脾气虚证

主要证候 咳嗽气短,痰多色白,神疲乏力,胸闷纳少,腹胀便溏,动则汗出,舌质淡边有齿痕,苔白腻,脉细或濡滑。

治 法 益气健脾,理气化痰。

方 药 香砂六君子汤加减:太子参15 g,紫河车15 g,茯苓15 g,黄精15 g,黄芪15 g,白术10 g,五味子10 g,法半夏10 g,桔梗10 g,橘皮6 g,制香附10 g,砂仁(后下)3 g,炙甘草6 g。

10 g, Sharen (*Fructus Amomi*, to be decocted later) 3 g
and Zhigancao (*Radix Glycyrrhizae*, roasted) 6 g.

Modifications: For severe dyspnea and cough due to
qi deficiency, add Xiyangshen (*Radix Panacis Quinquefolii*, to be decocted separately) 10 g, Dongchongxiacao
(*Cordyceps*, to be decocted separately) 10 g and Shanhai-
luo (*Concha Rapanae Thomasianae*) 30 g; for mingled
phlegm and blood stasis, add Lufengfang (*Nidus Vespae*)
10 g, Baijiangcan (*Bombyx Batryticatus*) 10 g and
Taoren (*Semen Persicae*) 10 g; for retention of toxic
heat in the lung, add Banzhilian (*Herba Scutellariae
Barbatae*) 30 g, Maozhuacao (*Radix Ranunculi Terna-
ti*) 30 g and Baihuasheshecao (*Herba Hedyotis Diffusae*)
30 g.

3. Accumulation of Phlegm-Dampness in the Lung

Chief Manifestations: Shortness of breath, wheezing sound in the throat, cough with difficult expectoration
of sticky sputum, distending pain in the chest and hypochondriac region, pale tongue with white and greasy or
yellow and greasy coating, wiry and smooth or smooth and
rapid pulse.

Therapeutic Methods: To resolve phlegm, eliminate turbidity, remove toxic substance and clear the lung.

Prescription: Modified Daotan Tang (Decoction for
Expelling Phlegm) and Tingli Dazao Xiefei Tang (Lepidii
seu Descurainiae and Jujubae Decoction for Clearing away
Lung Heat), composed of Fabanxia (*Rhizoma Pinelliae
Preparata*) 10 g, Chenpi (*Pericarpium Citri Reticula-
tae*) 10 g, Baizhu (*Rhizoma Atractylodis Macrocepha-
lae*) 10 g, Zhishi (*Fructus Aurantii Immaturus*) 10 g,
Zhinanxing (*Rhizoma Arisaema cum Bile*) 10 g,
Xingren (*Semen Armeniacae Amarum*) 10 g, Taoren
(*Semen Persicae*) 10 g, Tinglizi (*Semen Lepidii seu

加　减　气虚喘咳甚者,
加西洋参(另煎)10 g,冬虫夏
草(另煎)10 g,山海螺30 g;痰
毒瘀结者,加露蜂房10 g,白僵
蚕10 g,桃仁10 g;热毒恋肺
者,加半枝莲30 g,猫爪草
30 g,白花蛇舌草30 g。

3. 痰湿壅肺证

主要证候　咳嗽气喘,喉
中痰鸣,痰黏难咯,胸胁支满
疼痛,舌质淡,苔白腻或黄腻,
脉弦滑或滑数。

治　法　化痰祛浊,解毒
清肺。

方　药　导痰汤合葶苈
大枣泻肺汤加减:法半夏
10 g,陈皮10 g,白术10 g,枳实
10 g,制南星10 g,杏仁10 g,桃
仁10 g,葶苈子10 g,茯苓30 g,
薏苡仁30 g,半枝莲30 g,白花
蛇舌草30 g,大枣10 g。

Descurainiae) 10 g, Fuling (*Poria*) 30 g, Yiyiren (*Semen Coicis*) 30 g, Banzhilian (*Herba Scutellariae Barbatae*) 30 g, Baihuasheshecao (*Herba Hedyotis Diffusae*) 30 g and Dazao (*Fructus Jujubae*) 10 g.

Modifications: For blood-stained sputum, add Baimaogen (*Rhizoma Imperatae*) 30 g, Dai Ge San (*Powder of Indigo Naturalis and Concha Meretricis seu Cyclinae*, wrapped) 30 g, Xianhecao (*Herba Agrimoniae*) 30 g, Xueyutan (*Crinis Carbonisatus*) 10 g, Oujie (*Nodus Nelumbinis Rhizomatis*) 10 g; for distending pain in the chest and hypochondriac region, add Quangualou (*Fructus Trichosanthis*) 15 g, Yanhusuo (*Rhizoma Corydalis*) 15 g, Zhiruxiang (*Olibanum Preparata*) 10 g and Zhimoyao (*Myrrha Preparata*) 10 g.

4. Stagnation of Qi and Blood Stasis

Chief Manifestations: Stabbing pain and oppression in the chest, shortness of breath, rough cough with darkish blood in sputum, purplish lips, crimson tongue with ecchymotic spots on its surface, thin yellow tongue coating, and thready and unsmooth or wiry and thready pulse.

Therapeutic Methods: To promote the circulation of qi and blood, resolve phlegm and soften hard masses.

Prescription: Modified Tao Hong Siwu Tang (Four-Ingredient Decoction with Persicae and Carthami) and Wuling San (Faeces Trogopterori Powder), composed of Taoren (*Semen Persicae*) 10 g, Honghua (*Flos Carthama*) 10 g, Shudihuang (*Radix Rehmanniae Preparata*) 10 g, Danggui (*Radix Angelicae Sinensis*) 10 g, Puhuang (*Pollen Typhae*, wrapped) 10 g, Wulingzhi (*Faces Trogopterori*) 10 g, Sanqifen (*Radix Notoginseng*, powdered and to be swallowed separately) 3 g, Chuanbeimu (*Bulbus Fritillariae Cirrhosae*) 10 g, Chenpi (*Pericarpium Citri Reticulatae*) 10 g, Zhishi (*Fructus Aurantii Immaturus*) 10 g, Xiakucao (*Spica*

加　减　痰中带血者,加白茅根30 g,黛蛤散(包煎)30 g,仙鹤草30 g,血余炭10 g,藕节10 g;胸胁胀痛者,加全瓜蒌15 g,延胡索15 g,制乳香10 g,制没药10 g。

4. 气滞血瘀证

主要证候　胸部疼痛,痛如针刺,或胸闷气急,咳嗽不畅,便秘口干,痰血暗红,唇暗舌绛,舌瘀斑点,舌苔薄黄,脉细涩或弦细。

治　法　行气活血,化痰软坚。

方　药　桃红四物汤合五灵散加减:桃仁10 g,红花10 g,熟地黄10 g,当归10 g,蒲黄(包煎)10 g,五灵脂10 g,三七粉(另包吞服)3 g,川贝母10 g,陈皮10 g,枳实10 g,夏枯草15 g,赤芍药15 g,全瓜蒌15 g。

Prunellae) 15 g, Chishaoyao (*Radix Paeoniae Rubra*) 15 g and Quangualou (*Fructus Trichosanthis*) 15 g.

Modifications: For severe chest pain, add Sanleng (*Rhizoma Sparganii*) 10 g, Ezhu (*Rhizoma Curcumae*) 10 g, Lufengfang (*Nidus Vespae*) 10 g, Zhiruxiang (*Olibanum* Preparata) 6 g and Zhimoyao (*Myrrha Preparata*) 6 g; for fever due to blood stasis, add Lianqiao (*Fructus Forsythiae*) 10 g, Huangqin (*Radix Scutellariae*) 10 g, Qiyeyizhihua (*Rhizoma Paridis*) 30 g and Baihuasheshecao (*Herba Hedyotis Diffusae*) 30 g; for dyspneic cough, add Weibaiguo (*Semen Ginkgo*, roasted in hot cinders) 10 g, Kuandonghua (*Flos Farfarae*) 10 g, Xingren (*Semen Armeniacae Amarum*) 10 g and Chenxiang Fen (*Lignum Aquilariae Resinatum*, powdered) 6 g; for hydrothorax, add Tinglizi (*Semen Lepidii seu Descurainiae*) 10 g, Chixiaodou (*Semen Phaseoli*) 10 g, Sangbaipi (*Cortex Mori*) 10 g, Dongguapi (*Exocarpium Benicasae*) 10 g and Dongguazi (*Semen Benicasae*) 20 g; for shortness of breath and lassitude, remove Puhuang (*Pollen Typhae*), Wulingzhi (*Faces Trogopterori*) and add Dangshen (*Radix Codonopsis*) 20 g, Maimendong (*Radix Ophiopogonis*) 12 g, Wuweizi (*Fructus Schisandrae*) 10 g, Dongchongxiacao (*Cordyceps*, to be decocted separately) 10 g and Shenghuangqi (*Radix Astragali*) 20 g.

5. Deficiency of Qi and Yin

Chief Manifestations: Dull pain in the chest and back, cough with low sound, lassitude, dysphoria with feverish sensation in the chest, palms and soles, spontaneous sweating, night sweating, red tongue with little coatings, and deep, thready and rapid pulse.

Therapeutic Methods: To replenish qi, nourish yin, clear away lung heat and remove toxic substance.

Prescription: Modified Sijunzi Tang (Four Mild-

加　减　胸痛甚者,加三棱10 g,莪术10 g,露蜂房10 g,制乳香6 g,制没药6 g;血瘀发热者,加连翘10 g,黄芩10 g,七叶一枝花30 g,白花蛇舌草30 g;喘咳气急者,加煨白果10 g,款冬花10 g,杏仁10 g,沉香粉6 g;胸腔积水者,加葶苈子10 g,赤小豆10 g,桑白皮10 g,冬瓜皮10 g,冬瓜子20 g;短气乏力者,去蒲黄、五灵脂,加党参20 g,麦门冬12 g,五味子10 g,冬虫夏草(另煎)10 g,生黄芪20 g。

5. 气阴两虚证

主要证候　胸背隐隐作痛,咳声低微,神疲乏力,五心烦热,自汗盗汗,舌质红苔少,脉沉细数。

治　法　益气养阴,清肺解毒。

方　药　四君子汤合清

Drug Decoction) and Qingzao Jiufei Tang (Decoction for
Expelling Dryness of the Lung), composed of Taizishen
(*Radix Pseudostellariae*) 15 g, Baizhu (*Rhizoma At-
ractylodis Macrocephalae*) 15 g, Fuling (*Poria*) 15 g,
Nanshashen (*Radix Adenophorae*) 15 g, Maimendong
(*Radix Ophiopogonis*) 15 g, Shengdihuang (*Radix Reh-
manniae*) 15 g, Yuzhu (*Rhizoma Polygonati Odorati*)
15 g, Shihu (*Herba Dendrobii*) 30 g, Lugen (*Rhizoma
Phragmitis*) 30 g, Tianhuafen (*Radix Trichosanthis*)
30 g, Yuxingcao (*Herba Houttuyniae*) 30 g, Xiakucao
(*Spica Prunellae*) 30 g, Banzhilian (*Herba Scutellariae
Barbatae*) 30 g, Sharen (*Fructus Amomi*, to be decocted later) 6 g and Zhigancao (*Radix Glycyrrhizae*, roasted) 6 g.

Modifications: For dry cough with little sputum,
fever, night sweating and hoarse voice, add Baihe (*Bulbus Lilii*) 10 g, Xuanshen (*Radix Scrophulariae*) 10 g,
Chuanbeimu (*Bulbus Fritillariae Cirrhosae*) 10 g,
Jiegeng (*Radix Platycodi*) 10 g, Huangqin (*Radix
Scutellariae*) 10 g and Wuweizi (*Fructus Schisandrae*)
10 g; for persistent chest pain, add Gualoupi (*Pericarpium Trichosanthis*) 10 g, Juluo (*Vascular Aurantii
Citri Tangerinea*) 10 g, Zhiruxiang (*Olibanum
Preparata*) 10 g and Zhimoyao (*Myrrha Preparata*)
10 g.

6. Deficiency of Yin and Yang

Chief Manifestations: Pale complexion, cough
with little sputum, feeling of oppression in the chest,
shortness of breath, dyspnea on exertion, sweating, tinnitus, lumbago and weak legs, aversion to cold, cold
limbs, pale tongue with thin and white coating, and deep
and thready pulse.

Therapeutic Methods: To invigorate the lung and
kidney, and regulate both yin and yang.

燥救肺汤加减：太子参15 g，
白术15 g，茯苓15 g，南沙参
15 g，麦门冬15 g，生地黄15 g，
玉竹15 g，石斛30 g，芦根30 g，
天花粉30 g，鱼腥草30 g，夏枯
草30 g，半枝莲30 g，砂仁（后
下）6 g，炙甘草6 g。

加 减　干咳少痰，发热
盗汗，声音嘶哑者，加百合
10 g，玄参10 g，川贝母10 g，桔
梗10 g，黄芩10 g，五味子10 g；
胸痛不止者，加瓜蒌皮10 g，橘
络10 g，制乳香10 g，制没药
10 g。

6. 阴阳两虚证

主要证候　面色㿠白，咳
嗽痰少，胸闷气急，动则喘促，
汗出气短，耳鸣如蝉，腰膝酸
软，畏寒肢冷，舌淡，苔薄白，
脉沉细。

治 法　补肺益肾，阴阳
两调。

Prescription: Modified Shengmai Yin (Decoction for Reinforcing Qi and Nourishing Yin) and Erxian Tang (Epimedii and Curculiginis Decoction), composed of Taizishen (*Radix Pseudostellariae*) 15 g, Tianmendong (*Radix Asparagi*) 10 g, Maimendong (*Radix Ophiopogonis*) 10 g, Wuweizi (*Fructus Schisandrae*) 10 g, Yinyanghuo (*Herba Epimedii*) 10 g, Xianmao (*Rhizoma Curculiginis*) 10 g, Bajirou (*Radix Morindae Officinalis*) 10 g, Shanzhuyu (*Fructus Corni*) 10 g, Buguzhi (*Fructus Psoraleae*) 10 g, Chanpi (*Periostracum Bufonis*) 6 g and Banzhilian (*Herba Scutellariae Barbatae*) 30 g.

Modifications: For dyspnea with inability to lie flat, add Zhongrushi (*Stalactitum*) 10 g and Zishiying (*Fluoritum*) 15 g; for cough with abundant sputum, add Ziwan (*Radix Asteris*) 12 g, Kuandonghua (*Flos Farfarae*) 12 g and Zhibaijiangcan (*Bombyx Batryticatus*, roasted) 10 g; for weak voice and spontaneous sweating, add Huangqi (*Radix Astragali*) 12 g, Gancao (*Radix Glycyrrhizae*) 3 g and Baizhu (*Rhizoma Atractylodis Macrocephalae*) 10 g; for dysphoria with feverish sensation in the chest, palms and soles and pronounced dry mouth, add Guiban (*Plastrum Testudinis*, to be decocted first) 15 g, Huangjing (*Rhizoma Polygonati*) 10 g and Nüzhenzi (*Fructus Ligustri Lucidi*) 10 g.

Other Treatments
1. Chinese Patent Drugs

(1) Xi Huang Wan (Pill of Cornu Rhinocerotis Asiatici and Rehmanniae): 3 g each time, once or twice daily; applicable to lung cancer with pronounced pain.

(2) Meihua Dianshe Dan (Antiphlogistic Pill): 30 pills each time, thrice daily; applicable to intermediate and late lung cancer with pronounced pain.

(3) Shen Lian Jiaonang (Ginseng and Nelumbinis Capsule): 6 capsules each time, thrice daily; applicable to

方 药 生脉饮合二仙汤加减：太子参15 g，天门冬10 g，麦门冬10 g，五味子10 g，淫羊藿10 g，仙茅10 g，巴戟肉10 g，山茱萸10 g，补骨脂10 g，蟾皮6 g，半枝莲30 g。

加 减 气喘不能平卧加钟乳石10 g，紫石英15 g；咯痰量多者，加紫菀12 g，款冬花12 g，炙白僵蚕10 g；言语无力、自汗者，加黄芪12 g，甘草3 g，白术10 g；五心烦热，口干明显者，加龟版（先煎）15 g，黄精10 g，女贞子10 g。

【其他疗法】
1. 中成药

（1）犀黄丸 每服3 g，每日1～2 次。适用于肺癌疼痛明显者。

（2）梅花点舌丹 每日30 粒，每日 3 次。适用于肺癌中晚期疼痛者。

（3）参莲胶囊 每服 6粒，每日 3 次。适用于中晚期

intermediate and late lung cancer.

(4) Yulu Baofei Wan (Jade-like Dew Bolus for Protecting Lung): 1 bolus each time, thrice daily; applicable
to lung cancer with lung heat caused by yin deficiency.

(5) Fufang Yuxingcao Koufuye (Compound Houttuyniae
Oral Liquid): 1 vial each time, thrice daily; applicable to
lung cancer, particularly for patients with radiotherapy
and chemotherapy.

2. Single-drug or Experiential Prescriptions

(1) Xiaojin San (Powder for Removing Lung Mass):
composed of Chilianshefen (*Dinodon Rufozonatum*,
powdered) 30 g, Tiannanxing (*Rhizoma Arisaematis*)
30 g, Baiji (*Rhizoma Bletillae*) 30 g, Fenghuangyi
(*Membrana Follicularis Ovi*) 30 g, Guangchenpi (*Pericarpium Citri Reticulatae*) 30 g, Quangualou (*Fructus
Trichosanthis*) 30 g, Beishashen (*Radix Glehniae*)
60 g, Xiyangshen (*Radix Panacis Quinquefolii*) 15 g,
Zhibiejia (*Carapax Trionycis*, roasted) 45 g, Zhiruxiang
(*Olibanum Preparata*) 10 g, Zhimoyao (*Myrrha
Preparata*) 10 g and Zhusha (*Cinnabaris*) 12 g. Pulverize the drugs and take 1 g with boiled water, thrice daily.
This is applicable to patients with yin deficiency, blood
stasis and phlegm accumulation.

(2) Longkui (*Herba Solani Nigri*, fresh) 30 g. Decoct it with water for oral use, once daily. This is applicable to various kinds of lung cancer with hydrothorax.

(3) Leigongtenggen (Rhizoma Tripterygii Wilfordii,
coarse cortex and inner membrane removed, xylem for
use) 15 - 21 g. Decoct it with water for 2 hours and take
the decoction in two divided doses daily, 10 days making
up a course of treatment. It is applicable to lung cancer
with pain.

(4) Xiaoji San (Powder for Removing Mass): composed of Daimao (*Carapax Eretmochelydis*) 15 g, Gui-

肺癌。

(4) 玉露保肺丸　每服1
丸,每日3次。适用于肺癌阴
虚肺热者。

(5) 复方鱼腥草口服液
每服1支,每日3次。适用于
肺癌,尤其配合放疗、化疗
更佳。

2. 单验方

(1) 消金散　赤练蛇粉
30 g,天南星30 g,白及30 g,凤
凰衣30 g,广陈皮30 g,全瓜蒌
30 g,北沙参60 g,西洋参15 g,
炙鳖甲45 g,炙乳香10 g,炙没
药10 g,朱砂12 g。共研细末,
每服1 g,每日3次,冲服。适
用于肺癌阴虚血瘀痰聚者。

(2) 鲜龙葵30 g,每日1
次,水煎温服。适用于各型肺
癌有胸水者。

(3) 雷公藤根(去粗皮及
内衣,用木质部入药),每日
15～21 g,煎煮2小时,分2次
服,10日为1个疗程。适用于
肺癌疼痛者。

(4) 消积散　玳瑁15 g,
龟版(先煎)15 g,海藻15 g,露

ban (*Plastrum Testudinis*, to be decocted first) 15 g, Haizao (*Sargassum*) 15 g, Lufengfang (*Nidus Vespae*) 10 g, Yadanzi (*Fructus Bruceae*) 10 g and Chansu (*Venenum Bufonis*) 1 piece. Pulverize the drugs and take the powder with boiled water, 1 g each time, twice daily. It is applicable to patients with lung mass.

(5) Fei'ai Fangliaoqi Fang (Decoction for Lung Cancer Patient with Radiotherapy Treatment): composed of Zhuling (*Polyporus*) 15 g, Taizishen (*Radix Pseudostellariae*) 15 g, Danshen (*Radix Salviae Miltiorrhizae*) 15 g, Fuling (*Poria*) 15 g, Yiyiren (*Semen Coicis*) 15 g, Maimendong (*Radix Ophiopogonis*) 10 g, Nanshashen (*Radix Adenophorae*) 10 g, Huangjing (*Rhizoma Polygonati*) 10 g, Gouqizi (*Fructus Lycii*) 10 g, Jinyinhua (*Flos Lonicerae*) 10 g, Pipaye (*Folium Eriobotryae*, wrapped) 10 g, Chuanbeimu (*Bulbus Fritillariae Cirrhosae*) 10 g, Fangfeng (*Radix Saposhnikoviae*) 6 g and Gancao (*Radix Glycyrrhizae*) 6 g. Modify the formula according to individual cases. Decoct the drugs with water for oral use, 1 dose daily. It is applicable to patients with general deficiency during the stage of radiotherapy and chemotherapy.

(6) Fei'ai Shuhou Fang (Decoction for Postoperative Patient of Lung Cancer): composed of Zhuling (*Polyporus*) 15 g, Taizishen (*Radix Pseudostellariae*) 15 g, Fuling (*Poria*) 15 g, Shenghuangqi (*Radix Astragali*) 12 g, Maimendong (*Radix Ophiopogonis*) 12 g, Jiaogulan (*Rhizoma seu Herba Gynostemmatis Pentaphylli*) 12 g, Nanshashen (*Radix Adenophorae*) 10 g, Gouqizi (*Fructus Lycii*) 10 g, Shihu (*Herba Dendrobii*) 10 g, Pipaye (*Folium Eriobotryae*, wrapped) 10 g, Chuanbeimu (*Bulbus Fritillariae Cirrhosae*) 10 g, Xing-ren (*Semen Armeniacae Amarum*) 10 g, Baihe (*Bulbus Lilii*) 10 g, Baihuasheshecao (*Herba Hedyotis Diffusae*) 30 g

蜂房10 g, 鸦胆子10 g, 蟾酥 1 个。研成粉剂, 每服1 g, 每日 2 次, 白开水送下。适用于肺癌而有积块者。

(5) 肺癌放疗期方　猪苓 15 g, 太子参15 g, 丹参15 g, 茯苓15 g, 薏苡仁15 g, 麦门冬 10 g, 南沙参10 g, 黄精10 g, 枸杞子10 g, 金银花10 g, 枇杷叶 (包煎)10 g, 川贝母10 g, 防风 6 g, 甘草6 g。随证加减。水煎分服, 每日 1 剂。适用于肺癌放疗或化疗期间体质虚弱者。

(6) 肺癌术后方　猪苓 15 g, 太子参15 g, 茯苓15 g, 生黄芪12 g, 麦门冬12 g, 绞股蓝 12 g, 南沙参10 g, 枸杞子10 g, 石斛10 g, 枇杷叶 (包煎)10 g, 川贝母10 g, 杏仁10 g, 百合 10 g, 白花蛇舌草30 g, 西洋参 6 g。水煎分服, 每日 1 剂。适用于肺癌术后正虚阴伤者。

and Xiyangshen (*Radix Panacis Quinquefolii*) 6 g. Decoct the drugs with water for oral use, 1 dose daily. It is applicable to postoperative patients with deficient healthy qi and impaired yin.

3. External Therapy

(1) Shannai (*Rhizoma Kacmpferiae*) 20 g, Ruxiang (*Olibanum*) 20 g, Moyao (*Myrrha*) 20 g, Jianghuang (*Rhizoma Curcumae Longae*) 20 g, Zhizi (*Fructus Gardeniae*) 20 g, Baizhi (*Radix Angelicae Dahuricae*) 20 g, Huangqin (*Radix Scutellariae*) 20 g, Xiaohuixiang (*Fructus Foeniculi*) 15 g, Gongdingxiang (*Gemma Caryophylli*) 15 g, Chishaoyao (*Radix Paeoniae Rubra*) 15 g, Muxiang (*Radix Aucklandiae*) 15 g, Huangbo (*Cortex Phellodendri*) 15 g and Bimaren (*Semen Ricini*) 20 pcs. Pulverize the drugs and mix the powder with egg white thoroughly, then apply the mixture on acupoint Rugen (ST 18), change the dressing every 6 hours. It is applicable to patients with severe pain.

(2) Sangye (*Folium Mori*) 10 g, Juhua (*Flos Chrysanthemi*) 10 g, Jiegeng (*Radix Platycodi*) 6 g, Xingren (*Semen Armeniacae Amarum*) 10 g, Yuxingcao (*Herba Houttuyniae*) 15 g, Huangqin (*Radix Scutellariae*) 10 g, Banzhilian (*Herba Scutellariae Barbatae*) 15 g and Bingpian (*Borneolum Syntheticum*) 3 g. Decoct the drugs with water, inhale the vapor of the decoction intermittently for 15 - 20 minutes, 3 - 4 times daily. It is applicable to patients with dry mouth and nose, hoarse voice, syspneic cough with difficulty to expectorate sticky sputum.

3. 外治法

（1）山奈20 g,乳香20 g,没药20 g,姜黄20 g,栀子20 g,白芷20 g,黄芩20 g,小茴香15 g,公丁香15 g,赤芍药15 g,木香15 g,黄柏15 g,蓖麻仁20粒。上药共研细末,用鸡蛋清调匀外敷乳根穴,6小时换药1次。适用于肺癌疼痛者。

（2）桑叶10 g,菊花10 g,桔梗6 g,杏仁10 g,鱼腥草15 g,黄芩10 g,半枝莲15 g,冰片3 g,加水煮沸,频频吸入蒸气,每日3~4次,每次15~20分钟。适用于肺癌患者见咽干鼻燥,声音嘶哑,咳嗽气喘,痰黏难咯等症。

2.2 Syndrome Patterns of the Heart

2.2.1 Insomnia

General Description

Insomnia is characterized by inability to acquire normal sleep, which results from the heart being deprived of nourishment or from mental disturbance. It is manifested as insufficient sleep, shallow sleep and failure to relieve fatigue and restore the physical and mental strength by sleep. Mild insomnia refers to difficulty to fall asleep, or broken sleep, or inability to resume sleep once waking up, while severe insomnia refers to inability to fall asleep the whole night.

The causes of insomnia include emotional disorder, improper diet, weak constitution after illness, infirmity of age, congenital insufficiency and timidness. It involves the heart and closely related to stagnation of liver qi, deficiency of the gallbladder, spleen and kidney and dysfunction of stomach qi. Its main pathogenesis associates with imbalance between yin and yang and disorder of qi and blood in the heart, gallbladder, spleen and kidney, resulting in the inadequate nourishment of the heart or mental disturbance.

The following description on the syndrome differentiation and treatment for insomnia can serve as reference for the diseases with insomnia as the chief symptom in Western medicine, such as neurosis, menopausal syndrome, sequela of brain concussion, hypertension,

第二章 心系病证

第一节 失眠

【概述】

失眠是由于心神失养或不安而引起经常不能获得正常睡眠为特征的一类病证。主要表现为睡眠时间、深度的不足,以及醒后不能消除疲劳、恢复体力与精力,轻者入睡困难,或寐而不酣,时寐时醒,或醒后不能再寐,重则彻夜不寐。

引起失眠的原因有情志所伤、饮食不节、病后体虚、年迈体弱、禀赋不足与心虚胆怯。病位在心,与肝郁、胆怯、脾肾亏虚、胃失和降密切相关。主要病机不外心、胆、脾、肾的阴阳失调,气血失和,以致心神失养或心神不安。

西医学中诸如神经官能症、更年期综合征、脑震荡后遗症,以及高血压病、肝病、甲状腺功能亢进症、贫血、脑动脉硬化、慢性中毒、精神分裂

hepatopathy, hyperthyroidism, anemia, cerebral arterio-sclerosis, chronic intoxication and schizophrenia in the early stage.

Essentials for Diagnosis

(1) Mild cases have difficulty to fall asleep, or liability to wake up, or inability to fall asleep again after waking up, for over 3 weeks. Severe cases cannot get to sleep all night.

(2) It is usually accompanied by headache, dizziness, palpitation, amnesia, lassitude, restlessness and dream-fulness.

(3) Some organic diseases with dyssomnia should be excluded by laboratory examinations.

Syndrome Differentiation and Treatment

It is important to differentiate between the deficiency type and excess type of insomnia. Syndromes such as hyperactivity of heart fire, liver qi stagnation turning into fire, and internal disturbance of phlegm-heat belong to the excess, while those such as hyperactivity of fire due to yin deficiency, deficiency of the heart and spleen, and deficiency of heart qi and gallbladder qi pertain to the deficiency. Treatments should be based on the principles of replenishing deficiency and purging excess, regulating yin and yang, and calming the heart and tranquilizing the mind. Patients of deficiency type should be treated with methods of reinforcing qi and nourishing blood, and tonifying the liver and kidney, while those of the excess type should be treated with methods of eliminating food retention and regulating the spleen and stomach, and clearing away fire and resolving phlegm. For patients complicated by both the deficiency and excess, the method of reinforcing and purging should be used in combination.

1. Hyperactivity of Heart Fire

Chief Manifestations: Restlessness, insomnia, anxiety, dry mouth and tongue, scanty dark urine, aph-

症早期患者等,以失眠为主要临床表现者,均可参考本节内容辨证论治。

【诊断要点】

(1) 轻者入寐困难或睡而易醒,醒后不寐连续 3 周以上,重者彻夜难眠。

(2) 常伴有头痛头昏、心悸健忘、神疲乏力、心神不宁、多梦等。

(3) 实验室检查排除妨碍睡眠的其他器质性病变。

【辨证论治】

本病临床主要辨其虚实。心火炽盛、肝郁化火和痰热内扰证属实,阴虚火旺、心脾两虚和心胆气虚证属虚。治疗当以补虚泻实,调整阴阳,宁心安神为原则。虚者宜补其不足,益气养血,滋补肝肾;实者宜泻其有余,消导和中,清火化痰。虚实夹杂者,应补泻兼顾。

1. 心火炽盛证

主要证候 心烦不寐,躁扰不宁,口干舌燥,小便短赤,

thous stomatitis, red tongue tip, yellow thin tongue coating, and forceful and rapid or thready and rapid pulse.

Therapeutic Methods: To clear away heart fire, tranquilize the mind and soothe the heart.

Prescription: Modified Zhusha Anshen Wan (Cinnabaris Pill for Tranquilizing Mind), composed of Huanglian (*Rhizoma Coptidis*) 5 g, Shengdihuang (*Radix Rehmanniae*) 12 g, Zhizi (*Fructus Gardeniae*) 10 g, Huangqin (*Radix Scutellariae*) 10 g, Lianqiao (*Fructus Forsythiae*) 10 g, Danggui (*Radix Angelicae Sinensis*) 10 g and Zhufushen (*Sclerotium Poriae Circum Radicem Pini*, *prepared with Cinnabaris*) 12 g.

Modifications: For anxiety, feeling of oppression in the chest and nausea, add Dandouchi (*Semen Sojae Preparatum*) 10 g and Zhuru (*Caulis Bambuswae in taeniam*) 6 g; for constipation and dark colored urine, add Zhidahuang (*Radix et Rhizoma Rhei Preparata*) 6 g, Danzhuye (*Herba Lophatheri*) 10 g and Hupo (*Succinum*, to be infused in the decoction) 1 g.

2. Liver Qi Stagnation Turning into Fire

Chief Manifestations: Anxiety, irritability, dreamful sleep or even inability to fall asleep all night, accompanied by dizziness, distending sensation in the head, conjunctival congestion, tinnitus, dry and bitter mouth, poor appetite, constipation, dark urine, red tongue with yellow coating, and wiry and rapid pulse.

Therapeutic Methods: To clear the liver, reduce fire, and tranquilize the mind.

Prescription: Modified Longdan Xiegan Tang (Gentiana Decoction for Purging Liver Fire), composed of Longdancao (*Radix Gentianae*) 6 g, Chaihu (*Radix Bupleuri*) 6 g, Huangqin (*Radix Scutellariae*) 10 g, Mutong (*Caulis Akebiae*) 6 g, Zhizi (*Fructus Gardeniae*) 10 g, Zexie (*Rhizoma Alismatis*) 10 g, Cheqianzi (*Se-

口舌生疮,舌尖红,苔薄黄,脉数有力或细数。

治　法　清心泻火,安神宁心。

方　药　朱砂安神丸加减:黄连5 g,生地黄12 g,栀子10 g,黄芩10 g,连翘10 g,当归10 g,朱茯神12 g。

加　减　胸中懊恼,胸闷泛恶者,加淡豆豉10 g,竹茹6 g;便秘溲赤,加制大黄6 g,淡竹叶10 g,琥珀(冲服)1 g。

2. 肝郁化火证

主要证候　急躁易怒,不寐多梦,甚至彻夜不眠,伴有头晕头胀,目赤耳鸣,口干而苦,不思饮食,便秘溲赤,舌红苔黄,脉弦而数。

治　法　清肝泻火,镇心安神。

方　药　龙胆泻肝汤加减:龙胆草6 g,柴胡6 g,黄芩10 g,木通6 g,栀子10 g,泽泻10 g,车前子(包煎)10 g,当归10 g,生地黄10 g,龙骨(先煎)15 g,牡蛎(先煎)15 g。

men Plataginis, wrapped) 10 g, Danggui (*Radix Angelicae Sinensis*) 10 g, Shengdihuang (*Radix Rehmanniae*) 10 g, Longgu (*Os Draconis*, to be decocted first) 15 g and Muli (*Concha Ostreae*, to be decocted first) 15 g.

Modifications: For distending pain in the chest and hypochondriac region and frequent sighing, add Xiangfu (*Rhizoma Cyperi*) 10 g and Yujin (*Radix Curcumae*) 10 g; for dizziness, splitting headache, insomnia, hysteria and constipation, add Mudanpi (*Cortex Moutan Radicis*) 10 g and Shengdahuang (*Radix et Rhizoma Rhei*, to be decocted later) 5 - 10 g.

3. Internal Disturbance of Phlegm-heat

Chief Manifestations: Feeling of oppression in the chest, restlessness, insomnia, nausea, belching, accompanied by heavy sensation in the head, dizziness, bitter mouth, red tongue with yellow greasy coating, and wiry and rapid pulse.

Therapeutic Methods: To clear away heat, resolve phlegm, regulate the stomach and tranquilize the mind.

Prescription: Modified Wendan Tang (Decoction for Clearing away Gallbladder Heat), composed of Huanglian (*Rhizoma Coptidis*) 5 g, Zhizi (*Fructus Gardeniae*) 10 g, Chenpi (*Pericarpium Citri Reticulatae*) 6 g, Zhibanxia (*Rhizoma Pinelliae Preparata*) 10 g, Fuling (*Poria*) 15 g, Zhuru (*Caulis Bambuswae in taeniam*) 10 g, Zhike (*Fructus Aurantii*) 10 g, Danshen (*Radix Salviae Miltiorrhizae*) 10 g, Yuanzhi (*Radix Polygalae*) 6 g, Shenqu (*Massa Medicata Fermentata*) 10 g, Dazao (*Fructus Jujubae*) 5 pcs and Gancao (*Radix Glycyrrhizae*) 5 g.

Modifications: For palpitation and fright, add Zhenzhumu (*Concha Margaritifera Usta*, to be decocted

加　减　胸闷胁胀,善太息者,加香附10 g,郁金10 g;头晕目眩,头痛欲裂,不寐欲狂,大便秘结者,加牡丹皮10 g,生大黄(后下)5~10 g。

3. 痰热内扰证

主要证候　胸闷,心烦不寐,泛恶,嗳气,伴有头重目眩,口苦,舌红,苔黄腻,脉滑数。

治　法　清化痰热,和中安神。

方　药　温胆汤加减:黄连5 g,栀子10 g,陈皮6 g,制半夏10 g,茯苓15 g,竹茹10 g,枳壳10 g,丹参10 g,远志6 g,神曲10 g,大枣 5 枚,甘草5 g。

加　减　心悸动甚,惊惕不安者,加珍珠母(先煎)30 g,

first) 30 g and Cishi (*Magnetitum*, to be decocted first) 30 g; for difficulty to fall asleep or inability to sleep all night, and constipation, add Zhidahuang (*Radix et Rhizoma Rhei Preparata*) 10 g; for severe retention of food, add Jineijin (*Endothelium Corneum Gigeriae Galli*) 10 g and Jiaoshanzha (*Fructus Crataegi*, charred) 10 g.

4. Hyperactivity of Fire due to Yin Deficiency

Chief Manifestations: Palpitation, restlessness, insomnia, lumbago, weak legs, dizziness, tinnitus, poor memory, seminal emission, dry mouth, dysphoria with feverish sensation in the chest, palms and soles, red tongue with little coating, and thready rapid pulse.

Therapeutic Methods: To nourish yin, reduce fire, clear heart fire and tranquilize the mind.

Prescription: Modified Liuwei Dihuang Wan (Bolus of Six Drugs Containing Rehmanniae) and Huanglian Ejiao Tang (Coptidis and Colla Corii Asini Decoction), composed of Shengdihuang (*Radix Rehmanniae*) 10 g, Huanglian (*Rhizoma Coptidis*) 5 g, Ejiao (*Colla Corii Asini*, to be melted and infused separately) 10 g, Baishaoyao (*Radix Paeoniae Alba*) 10 g, Tianmendong (*Radix Asparagi*) 10 g, Maimendong (*Radix Ophiopogonis*) 10 g, Xuanshen (*Radix Scrophulariae*) 10 g, Danshen (*Radix Salviae Miltiorrhizae*) 10 g, Danggui (*Radix Angelicae Sinensis*) 10 g, Fushen (*Sclerotium Poriae Circum Radicem Pini*) 15 g, Wuweizi (*Fructus Schisandrae*) 10 g and Suanzaoren (*Semen Ziziphi Spinosae*) 15 g.

Modifications: For restlessness, palpitation and nocturnal emission, add Rougui (*Cortex Cinnamomi*, to be decocted later) 2 g and Huanglian (*Rhizoma Coptidis*) 4 g; for constipation and dry mouth due to severe yin consumption, add Zhimu (*Rhizoma Anemarrhenae*) 10 g,

磁石(先煎)30 g;经久不寐,或彻夜不寐,大便秘结者,加制大黄10 g;宿食积滞较甚者,加鸡内金10 g,焦山楂10 g。

4. 阴虚火旺证

主要证候　心悸不安,心烦不寐,腰酸足软,伴头晕,耳鸣,健忘,遗精,口干津少,五心烦热,舌红少苔,脉细而数。

治　法　滋阴降火,清心安神。

方　药　六味地黄丸合黄连阿胶汤加减:生地黄10 g,黄连5 g,阿胶(烊化冲服)10 g,白芍药10 g,天门冬10 g,麦门冬10 g,玄参10 g,丹参10 g,当归10 g,茯神15 g,五味子10 g,酸枣仁15 g。

加　减　心烦心悸,梦遗失精者,加肉桂(后下)2 g,黄连4 g;便秘,口干,阴伤甚者,加知母10 g,何首乌10 g,夜交藤15 g;心烦不寐,彻夜不眠

Heshouwu (*Radix Polygoni Multiflori*) 10 g and Yejiao-
teng (*Caulis et Folium Polygoni Multiflori*) 15 g; for
restlessness and sleeplessness for the whole night, add
Longgu (*Os Draconis*, to be decocted first) 25 g, Muli
(*Concha Ostreae*, to be decocted first) 25 g and Cishi
(*Magnetitum*, to be decocted first) 20 g .

5. Deficiency of the Heart and Spleen

Chief manifestation: Dreamful and restless sleep,
palpitation, amnesia, poor appetite, dizziness, tired
limbs, pale complexion, pale tongue with thin coating,
and weak pulse.

Therapeutic Methods: To nourish the heart, invigorate the spleen and tranquilize the mind.

Prescription: Modified Guipi Tang (Decoction for
Invigorating Spleen and Nourishing Heart), composed of
Huangqi (*Radix Astragali*) 15 g, Dangshen (*Radix
Codonopsis*) 10 g, Baizhu (*Rhizoma Atractylodis Mac-
rocephalae*) 10 g, Danggui (*Radix Angelicae Sinensis*)
10 g, Fushen (*Sclerotium Poriae Circum Radicem Pi-
ni*) 10 g, Yuanzhi (*Radix Polygalae*) 6 g, Suanzaoren
(*Semen Ziziphi Spinosae*) 10 g, Guiyuanrou (*Arillus
Longan*) 10 g and Zhigancao (*Radix Glycyrrhizae*,
roasted) 5 g.

Modifications: For severe blood deficiency, add
Shudihuang (*Radix Rehmanniae Preparata*) 10 g,
Baishaoyao (*Radix Paeoniae Alba*) 10 g and Ejiao (*Colla
Corii Asini*, to be melted and infused separately) 10 g;
for severe insomnia, add Wuweizi (*Fructus Schisandrae*) 10 g, Yejiaoteng (*Caulis et Folium Polygoni Multiflori*) 15 g, Hehuanpi (*Cortex Albiziae*) 10 g and Baiziren (*Semen Platycladi*) 10 g; for abdominal distention, poor appetite and greasy tongue coating, add Zhibanxia (*Rhizoma Pinelliae Preparata*) 10 g, Chenpi
(*Pericarpium Citri Reticulatae*) 6 g, Fuling (*Poria*)

者,加龙骨(先煎)25 g,牡蛎
(先煎)25 g,磁石(先煎)20 g。

5. 心脾两虚证

主要证候 多梦易醒,心
悸健忘,神疲食少,头晕目眩,
四肢倦怠,面色少华,舌质淡,
苔薄,脉细无力。

治 法 补益心脾,养心
安神。

方 药 归脾汤加减:
黄芪15 g,党参10 g,白术10 g,
当归10 g,茯神10 g,远志6 g,
酸枣仁10 g,桂圆肉10 g,炙甘
草5 g。

加 减 血虚较甚者,加
熟地黄10 g,白芍药10 g,阿胶
(烊化冲服)10 g;失眠较重者,
加五味子10 g,夜交藤15 g,合
欢皮10 g,柏子仁10 g;脘闷纳
呆,苔腻者,加制半夏10 g,陈
皮6 g,茯苓10 g,厚朴6 g。

10 g and Houpo (*Cortex Magnoliae Officinalis*) 6 g.

6. Deficiency of Heart Qi and Gallbladder Qi

Chief Manifestations: Restlessness, insomnia, dreamful and restless sleep, frightened palpitation, shortness of breath, spontaneous sweating, lassitude, pale tongue and wiry and thready pulse.

Therapeutic Methods: To replenish qi, relieve frightened palpitation and tranquilize the mind.

Prescription: Modified Anshen Dingzhi Wan (Pill for Tranquilizing Mind) and Suanzaoren Tang (Ziziphi Spinosae Decoction), composed of Dangshen (*Radix Codonopsis*) 10 g, Fushen (*Sclerotium Poriae Circum Radicem Pini*) 10 g, Yuanzhi (*Radix Polygalae*) 6 g, Shichangpu (*Rhizoma Acori Tatarinowii*) 6 g, Suanzao-ren (*Semen Ziziphi Spinosae*) 15 g, Wuweizi (*Fructus Schisandrae*) 10 g, Shenglongchi (*Dens Draconis*, to be decocted first) 25 g and Shengmuli (*Concha Ostreae*, to be decocted first) 25 g.

Modification: For severe frightened palpitation, and restlessness, add Cishi (*Magnetitum*, to be decocted first) 20 g.

Other Treatments
1. Chinese Patent Drugs

(1) Tianwang Buxin Dan (Tianwang Bolus for Tonifying Heart): 1 bolus each time, twice daily; applicable to insomnia due to deficiency of heart yin.

(2) Zhusha Anshen Wan (Cinnabaris Bolus for Tranquilizing Mind): 1 bolus each time, twice daily; applicable to insomnia due to deficiency of heart blood. This bolus should not be taken for a long time.

(3) Baizi Yangxin Wan (Platycladi Pill for Nourishing Heart): 6 g each time, thrice daily; applicable to insomnia due to deficiency of the heart and spleen.

(4) Naolejing Tangjiang (Syrup for Tranquillizing

6. 心胆气虚证

主要证候 心烦不寐,多梦易醒,胆怯心悸,触事易惊,伴有气短自汗,倦怠乏力,舌质淡,脉弦细。

治 法 益气镇惊,安神定志。

方 药 安神定志丸合酸枣仁汤加减:党参10 g,茯神10 g,远志6 g,石菖蒲6 g,酸枣仁15 g,五味子10 g,生龙齿(先煎)25 g,生牡蛎(先煎)25 g。

加 减 心悸甚,惊惕不安者,加磁石(先煎)20 g。

【其他疗法】
1. 中成药

(1) 天王补心丹 每服1丸,每日2次。适用于失眠证属心阴不足者。

(2) 朱砂安神丸 每服1丸,每日2次。适用于失眠证属心血不足,心火亢盛者。本品不宜久服。

(3) 柏子养心丸 每服6 g,每日3次。适用于失眠证属心脾两虚者。

(4) 脑乐静糖浆 每服

Mind): 30 ml each time, thrice daily; applicable to insomnia with mental disarrangement due to deficiency of heart qi.

(5) Ciwujia Pian (Acanthopanacis Senticosi Tablet): 4 tablets each time, thrice daily; applicable to insomnia due to deficiency of heart blood.

2. Single-drug or Experiential Prescriptions

(1) Chaosuanzaoren (*Semen Ziziphi Spinosae*, *stir-baked*) 4.5 g and Wuweizi (*Fructus Schisandrae*) 1.2 g. Mash the drugs and take the mixture with water 1 hour before going to bed. It is applicable to insomnia due to yin and blood deficiency of the liver and kidney.

(2) Danggui (*Radix Angelicae Sinensis*) 20 g, Suanzaoren (*Semen Ziziphi Spinosae*) 20 g, Yanhusuo (*Rhizoma Corydalis*) 20 g, Heshouwu (*Radix Polygoni Multiflori*) 15 g and Kushen (*Radix Sophorae Flavescentis*) 12 g. Decoct the drugs with water, take the decoction half an hour before going to bed. It is applicable to insomnia due to blood deficiency.

(3) Danshen (*Radix Salviae Miltiorrhizae*) 20 - 45 g, Sanleng (*Rhizoma Sparganii*) 20 - 45 g, Muxiang (*Radix Aucklandiae*) 10 - 25 g, Xiangfu (*Rhizoma Cyperi*) 10 - 25 g, Danggui (*Radix Angelicae Sinensis*) 10 - 25 g and Zhizi (*Fructus Gardeniae*) 10 - 25 g. Decoct the drugs with water and take the decoction, 1 dose daily, 20 days as a treatment course. It is applicable to various kinds of insomnia.

(4) Suanzaoshugen (*Radix Ziziphi Spinosae*, with cortex) 30 g and Danshen (*Radix Salviae Miltiorrhizae*) 12 g. Decoct the drugs with water for 1 - 2 hours, take the decoction before taking a nap at noon and before going to bed in the evening, 1 dose daily. It is applicable to various kinds of insomnia.

3. External Therapy

(1) Wuzhuyu (*Fructus Evodiae*) 9 g and adequate

---

30 ml,每日 3 次。适用于失眠证属心气不足,神不守舍者。

(5)刺五加片 每服 4 片,每日 3 次。适用于失眠证属心气虚弱者。

2. 单验方

(1)炒酸枣仁4.5 g,五味子1.2 g,共捣碎,每晚睡前 1 小时冲服。适用于失眠证属肝肾阴血不足者。

(2)当归20 g,酸枣仁20 g,延胡索20 g,何首乌15 g,苦参12 g。水煎浓缩,睡前半小时服。适用于失眠证属血虚者。

(3)丹参20~45 g,三棱20~45 g,木香10~25 g,香附10~25 g,当归10~25 g,栀子10~25 g。水煎服,每服 1 剂,20 日为 1 个疗程。适用于失眠各种证型。

(4)酸枣树根(连皮)30 g,丹参12 g,水煎 1~2 小时,在午休及晚上临睡前各服 1 次,每日 1 剂。适用于失眠各种证型。

3. 外治法

(1)吴茱萸9 g,米醋适

amount of vinegar. Pulverize Wuzhuyu, mix it with vinegar into paste, apply the paste on both Yongquan (KI 1) acupoints, cover it with gauze and fix it with adhesive plaster, once daily. This is applicable to insomnia due to incoordination between the heart and kidney.

(2) Cishi (*Magnetitum*) 20 g, Fushen (*Sclerotium Poriae Circum Radicem Pini*) 15 g, Wuweizi (*Fructus Schisandrae*) 10 g and Ciwujia (*Radix Acanthopanacis Senticosi*) 20 g. Boil Cishi (*Magnetitum*) first for 30 minutes, add in the others and boil for another 30 minutes; remove the dregs, soak the clean gauze in the decoction, apply the warm gauze on the forehead and Taiyang (EX-HE5) acupoint for 20 minutes every evening. This is applicable to various kinds of insomnia.

(3) Qingpi (*Pericarpium Citri Reticulatae Viride*, fresh) 1 piece. Warm it on wood-fire and rub the eyelids with it for 20 minutes when it is still warm, once daily. This is applicable to various kinds of insomnia.

(4) Juhua (*Flos Chrysanthemi*) 1,000 g, Chuanxiong (*Rhizoma Chuanxiong*) 400 g, Mudanpi (*Cortex Moutan Radicis*) 200 g and Baizhi (*Radix Angelicae Dahuricae*) 200 g. Put the drugs in a cotton bag and make it a medicated pillow. This is applicable to insomnia with headache due to transformation of fire from liver qi stagnation.

(5) Immerse the feet in warm water in a basin for 10 minutes before sleep, once daily. This is applicable to various kinds of insomnia.

2.2.2 Arrhythmia

General Description

Arrhythmia refers to any disturbance in the rhythm

量。吴茱萸研成细末,米醋调成糊状,敷于两足涌泉穴,盖以纱布,胶布固定,每日 1 次。适用于失眠证属心肾不交者。

(2) 磁石20 g,茯神15 g,五味子10 g,刺五加20 g。先煎煮磁石 30 分钟,然后再入其余药物再煎煮 30 分钟,去渣取汁,将洁净纱布浸泡于药汁中,趁热敷患者前额及太阳穴,每晚 1 次,每次 20 分钟。适用于失眠各证型。

(3) 新青皮 1 块。青皮置于柴火上烘热,趁热熨擦两眼之上下两睑。每次进行 20 分钟左右,每日 1 次。适用于失眠各证型。

(4) 菊花1 000 g,川芎400 g,牡 丹 皮 200 g,白 芷200 g。用布缝制一枕头,装入上药,睡眠时以此为枕头。适用于失眠证属肝郁化火伴头痛者。

(5) 热水一盆,患者睡前热水洗足 10 分钟。每日 1 次。适用于失眠各证型。

第二节 心律失常

【概述】

心律失常是指患者出现

of the heartbeat, manifested clinically as pale complexion, lassitude, chest pain or oppression, palpitation, insomnia and excessive sweating. There may appear rapid, slow, rapid-irregular, slow-irregular and intermittent pulses in arrhythmia cases. In some mild cases, there may not be clinical symptoms; but in severe cases, symptoms such as dizziness, chest pain, shortness of breath, profuse sweating, cold limbs, even collapse may also be seen.

Some causes of arrhythmia are still not very clear, but it is known that many heart diseases, including sick sinus syndrome, pre-excitation syndrome, heart failure and cardioneurosis, may give rise to various forms of arrhythmia such as achycardia, bradycardia, premature systole, auricular fibrillation or flutter, and atrioventricular block.

According to its clinical manifestations, arrhythmia is categorized as "xin ji" (palpitation), "zheng chong" (severe palpitation), "xuan yun" (dizziness), "yun jue" (syncope) and "mai jie dai" (slow-irregular and intermittent pulse) in TCM. Its pathogenic factors include delicate constitution, improper diet, overstrain, emotional upset, exogenous factors and drug intoxication. Its pathologic changes involve deficiency and excess. The former refers to deficiency of qi, blood, yin and yang; the latter includes phlegm-fire disturbing the heart, excessive fluid attacking the heart, blood stasis obstructing collaterals and stagnation of qi and blood.

Essentials for Diagnosis

(1) The manifestations include palpitation, uncontrollable nervousness, and paroxysmal or persistent change of heart beat in velocity rhythm and strength, or various pulse conditions such as rapid, swift, rapid-irreg-

心率和节律的异常改变。其临床表现轻者可无自觉症状，通常可伴见面色少华、体倦乏力、胸闷或痛、心悸怔忡、失眠、多汗等症，心律则失常可有数脉、迟脉、促脉、结脉、代脉等之分；重症心律失常除心律失常外，可见头晕目眩、胸痛气促、汗泄肢冷，甚至虚脱而危及生命。

本病见于各种原因引起的心律失常，如心动过速、心动过缓、期前收缩、房颤或房扑、房室传导阻滞、病态窦房结综合征、预激综合征、心功能不全、神经官能症等，但仍有部分原因尚未明确。

根据本病的临床表现，属于中医学"心悸"、"怔忡"、"眩晕"、"晕厥"、"脉结代"范畴。病因主要与体质虚弱、饮食劳倦、七情所伤、感受外邪和药物中毒有关。病理变化有虚实两方面，虚者为气血阴阳亏损，心神失养所致；实者多由痰火扰心、水饮凌心，以及瘀血阻脉，气血运行不畅而引起。

【诊断要点】

（1）自觉心慌、心跳，神情紧张，不能自主，心搏或快或慢，或心跳过重，或忽跳忽止，呈阵发性或持续不止。或见

ular, slow-irregular, intermittent, deep or slow pulse.

(2) Determination of the presence of infection, oxygen deficit, acid-base dysequilibrium, electrolyte disorder, drug reaction, and vegetative nerve functional disturbance, etc. is helpful to the differentiation of the functional and organic arrhythmia.

(3) Examinations of electrocardiogram, sphygmometer, chest X-ray and blood pressure determination are helpful to the diagnosis.

Syndrome Differentiation and Treatment

This disease has the deficiency and excess syndromes. Syndromes such as excessive fluid attacking the heart, blood stasis blocking the heart and phlegm-fire disturbing the heart belong to the excess, while syndromes such as deficiency of the heart and gallbladder, deficiency of the heart and spleen, fire hyperactivity due to yin deficiency, and inactivity of heart yang pertain to the deficiency. The therapeutic principles include replenishing qi and nourishing blood, replenishing yin and warming yang, activating qi and removing blood stasis, clearing fire and resolving phlegm, eliminating excessive fluid and inducing diuresis, and nourishing the heart and tranquilizing the mind.

1. Deficiency of the Heart and Gallbladder

Chief Manifestations: Palpitation, restlessness, timidity, shallow and dreamful sleep, poor appetite, aversion to noise, white thin tongue coating, and thready and rapid or thready and wiry pulse.

Therapeutic Methods: To calm emotions, nourish the heart and tranquilize the mind.

Prescription: Modified Anshen Dingzhi Wan (Pill for Tranquilizing Mind), composed of Dangshen (*Radix Codonopsis*) 10 g, Fuling (*Poria*) 10 g, Yuanzhi (*Radix*

脉象数、疾、促、结、代、沉、迟等变化。

（2）了解发病因素，排除各种诱因，如有无感染、缺氧、电解质或酸碱平衡失调、药物反应和植物神经功能失调等，区别功能和器质性病变。

（3）心电图检查、脉象图、血压检测、X线胸部摄片有助于诊断。

【辨证论治】

本病有虚有实，水饮凌心、心血瘀阻证和痰火扰心证属实；心虚胆怯、心脾两虚、阴虚火旺和心阳不振证属虚。治疗以益气养血、滋阴温阳、行气化瘀、清火化痰、涤饮利水以及养心安神、重镇安神为大法。

1. 心虚胆怯证

主要证候　心悸不宁，善惊易恐，坐卧不安，少寐多梦而易惊醒，食少纳呆，恶闻声响，苔薄白，脉细略数或细弦。

治　法　镇惊定志，养心安神。

方　药　安神定志丸加减：党参10 g，茯苓10 g，远志6 g，石菖蒲10 g，酸枣仁15 g，

Polygalae) 6 g, Shichangpu (*Rhizoma Acori Tatari-nowii*) 10 g, Suanzaoren (*Semen Ziziphi Spinosae*) 15 g, Wuweizi (*Fructus Schisandrae*) 10 g, Baiziren (*Semen Platycladi*) 10 g and Zhigancao (*Radix Glycyr-rhizae*, roasted) 6 g.

Modifications: For spontaneous sweating, add Mahuanggen (*Radix Ephedrae*) 10 g, Fuxiaomai (*Fructus Tritici Levis*) 10 g, Shanzhuyu (*Fructus Corni*) 10 g and Wumei (*Fructus Mume*) 10 g; for qi deficiency with blood stasis, add Danshen (*Radix Salviae Miltior-rhizae*) 10 g, Taoren (*Semen Persicae*) 10 g and Hong-hua (*Flos Carthama*) 10 g; for insufficiency of heart blood, add Shudihuang (*Radix Rehmanniae Preparata*) 12 g and Ejiao (*Colla Corii Asini*, to be melted and in-fused separately) 10 g; for palpitation, restlessness, mental depression, pain in the chest and hypochondriac region, add Chaihu (*Radix Bupleuri*) 6 g, Yujin (*Radix Curcumae*) 10 g, Hehuanpi (*Cortex Albiziae*) 10 g and Lü'emei (*Flos Mume*) 6 g.

2. Deficiency of the Heart and Spleen

Chief Manifestations: Palpitation, shortness of breath, dizziness, blurred vision, pale complexion, lassi-tude, poor appetite, abdomenal distention, loose stool, dreamful sleep, insomnia, pale tongue, and thready and weak pulse.

Therapeutic Methods: To replenish blood, nourish the heart, supplement qi and tranquilize the mind.

Prescription: Modified Guipi Tang (Decoction for Invigorating Spleen and Nourishing Heart), composed of Huangqi (*Radix Astragali*) 30 g, Dangshen (*Radix Codonopsis*) 10 g, Baizhu (*Rhizoma Atractylodis Mac-rocephalae*) 10 g, Danggui (*Radix Angelicae Sinensis*) 10 g, Fushen (*Sclerotium Poriae Circum Radicem Pi-ni*) 10 g, Yuanzhi (*Radix Polygalae*) 6 g, Suanzaoren

五味子10 g,柏子仁10 g,炙甘草6 g。

加　减　自汗加麻黄根10 g,浮小麦10 g,山茱萸10 g,乌梅10 g;气虚挟瘀,加丹参10 g,桃仁10 g,红花10 g;兼心血不足,加熟地黄12 g,阿胶(烊化冲服)10 g;若心气郁结,心悸烦闷,精神抑郁,胸胁时痛者,加柴胡6 g,郁金10 g,合欢皮10 g,绿萼梅6 g。

2. 心脾两虚证

主要证候　心悸气短,头晕目眩,面色无华,神疲乏力,纳呆食少,腹胀便溏,少寐多梦,健忘,舌淡红,脉细弱。

治　法　补血养心,益气安神。

方　药　归脾汤加减:黄芪30 g,党参10 g,白术10 g,当归10 g,茯神10 g,远志6 g,酸枣仁10 g,桂圆肉10 g,炙甘草5 g,木香10 g,熟地黄10 g。

(*Semen Ziziphi Spinosae*) 10 g, Guiyuanrou (*Arillus Longan*) 10 g, Zhigancao (*Radix Glycyrrhizae*, roasted) 5 g, Muxiang (*Radix Aucklandiae*) 10 g and Shudihuang (*Radix Rehmanniae Preparata*) 10 g.

Modifications: For palpitation with irregular pulse, add Guizhi (*Ramulus Cinnamomi*) 10 g and increase the amount of Zhigancao (*Radix Glycyrrhizae*, roasted) to 10 g; for spontaneous sweating and night sweating, add Mahuanggen (*Radix Ephedrae*) 10 g, Shanzhuyu (*Fructus Corni*) 10 g, Duanlonggu (*Os Draconis Usta*, to be decocted first) 30 g, Duanmuli (*Concha Ostreae Usta*, to be decocted first) 30 g and Nuodaogen (*Rhizxoma et Radix Oryzae Glutinosae*) 20 g; for poor appetite and abdomenal distention, add Chenpi (*Pericarpium Citri Reticulatae*) 10 g, Guya (*Fructus Setariae Germinatus*) 12 g, Maiya (*Fructus Hordei Germinatus*) 12 g and Jineijin (*Endothelium Corneum Gigeriae Galli*) 10 g; for insomnia and dreamful sleep, add Hehuanpi (*Cortex Albiziae*) 10 g, Yejiaoteng (*Caulis et Folium Polygoni Multiflori*) 15 g, Wuweizi (*Fructus Schisandrae*) 10 g and Baiziren (*Semen Platycladi*) 10 g; for restlessness, dry mouth and red tongue, add Maimendong (*Radix Ophiopogonis*) 10 g and Yuzhu (*Rhizoma Polygonati Odorati*) 10 g.

3. Fire Hyperactivity due to Yin Deficiency
Chief Manifestations: Palpitation worsened by strain, timidity, restlessness, insomnia, feverish sensation in the chest, palms and soles, dry mouth, night sweating, tinnitus, lumbago, dizziness, blurred vision, red tongue with little fluid, little tongue coating, and thready and rapid pulse.

Therapeutic Methods: To replenish yin, clear fire, nourish the heart and tranquilize the mind.

Prescription: Modified Tianwang Buxin Dan (Tian-

加 减 心动悸而脉结代者,加桂枝10 g,重用炙甘草10 g;自汗、盗汗者,加麻黄根10 g,山茱萸10 g,煅龙骨(先煎)30 g,煅牡蛎(先煎)30 g,糯稻根20 g;纳呆,腹胀者,加陈皮10 g,谷芽12 g,麦芽12 g,鸡内金10 g;失眠多梦者,加合欢皮10 g,夜交藤15 g,五味子10 g,柏子仁10 g;心烦,口干,舌红者,加麦门冬10 g,玉竹10 g。

3. 阴虚火旺证
主要证候 心悸易惊,心烦失眠,五心烦热,口干,盗汗,思虑劳心则加重,耳鸣腰酸,头晕目眩,舌红少津,苔少或无,脉象细数。

治 法 滋阴清火,养心安神。

方 药 天王补心丹加

wang Bolus for Tonifying Heart), composed of Maimendong (*Radix Ophiopogonis*) 10 g, Shengdihuang (*Radix Rehmanniae*) 10 g, Yuzhu (*Rhizoma Polygonati Odorati*) 10 g, Danshen (*Radix Salviae Miltiorrhizae*) 15 g, Huanglian (*Rhizoma Coptidis*) 5 g, Zhizi (*Fructus Gardeniae*) 10 g, Suanzaoren (*Semen Ziziphi Spinosae*) 10 g, Baiziren (*Semen Platycladi*) 10 g, Cishi (*Magnetitum*, to be decocted first) 25 g, Zhenzhumu (*Cincha Margaritifera Usta*, to be decocted first) 30 g.

Modifications: For seminal emission and lumbago due to deficiency of kidney yin and disturbance of deficient fire, add Guiban (*Plastrum Testudinis*, to be decocted first) 15 g, Shudihuang (*Radix Rehmanniae Preparata*) 12 g, Zhimu (*Rhizoma Anemarrhenae*) 10 g and Huangbai (*Cortex Phellodendri*) 10 g; for restlessness and dizziness, add Baishaoyao (*Radix Paeoniae Alba*) 10 g, Heshouwu (*Radix Polygoni Multiflori*) 10 g and Gouqizi (*Fructus Lycii*) 10 g.

4. Deficiency of Heart Yang

Chief Manifestations: Palpitation worsened by exertion, restlessness, feeling of oppression in the chest, shortness of breath, pale complexion, cold limbs, pale tongue with white coating, and weak or forceless deep and thready pulse.

Therapeutic Methods: To warm and replenish heart yang and tranquilize the mind.

Prescription: Modified Guizhi Gancao Longgu Muli Tang (Decoction of Cinnamomi, Glycyrrhizae, Os Draconis and Concha Ostreae), composed of Guizhi (*Ramulus Cinnamomi*) 10 g, Zhigancao (*Radix Glycyrrhizae*, roasted) 10 g, Dangshen (*Radix Codonopsis*) 30 g, Yinyanghuo (*Herba Epimedii*) 10 g, Xianmao (*Rhizoma Curculiginis*) 10 g, Shudihuang (*Radix Rehmanniae*

减：麦门冬 10 g，生地黄 10 g，玉竹 10 g，丹参 15 g，黄连 5 g，栀子 10 g，酸枣仁 10 g，柏子仁 10 g，磁石（先煎）25 g，珍珠母（先煎）30 g。

　　加　减　肾阴亏虚，虚火妄动，遗精腰酸者，加龟版（先煎）15 g，熟地黄 12 g，知母 10 g，黄柏 10 g；虚烦头晕者，加白芍药 10 g，何首乌 10 g，枸杞子 10 g。

4. 心阳不振证

　　主要证候　心悸不安，胸闷气短，动则尤甚，面色苍白，形寒肢冷，舌质淡，苔白，脉虚弱，或沉细无力。

　　治　法　温补心阳，安神定悸。

　　方　药　桂枝甘草龙骨牡蛎汤加减：桂枝 10 g，炙甘草 10 g，党参 30 g，淫羊藿 10 g，仙茅 10 g，熟地黄 15 g，当归 10 g，山茱萸 12 g，五味子 6 g。

Preparata) 15 g, Danggui (*Radix Angelicae Sinensis*) 10 g, Shanzhuyu (*Fructus Corni*) 12 g and Wuweizi (*Fructus Schisandrae*) 6 g.

Modifications: For cold limbs due to insufficiency of heart yang, add Huangqi (*Radix Astragali*) 30 g, Dangshen (*Radix Codonopsis*) 15 g and Zhifuzi (*Radix Aconiti Lateralis Preparata*) 10 g; for excessive sweating, add Hongshen (*Radix Ginseng Rubra*, to be decocted separately) 10 g, Duanlonggu (*Os Draconis Usta*, to be decocted first) 30 g and Duanmuli (*Concha Ostreae Usta*, to be decocted first) 30 g; for dizziness, nausea and vomiting due to upward attack of excessive fluid, add Zhibanxia (*Rhizoma Pinelliae Preparata*) 10 g, Fuling (*Poria*) 15 g and Chenpi (*Pericarpium Citri Reticulatae*) 10 g; for edema and scanty urine, add Fuling (*Poria*) 15 g, Zhuling (*Polyporus*) 10 g, Zexie (*Rhizoma Alismatis*) 15 g, Wannianqinggen (*Radix et Rhizoma Rohdeae Japonicae*) 10 g and Cheqianzi (*Semen Plataginis*, wrapped) 10 g; for purple lips, tongue and nails, and a mass in the right hypochondriac region with distending pain, add Danshen (*Radix Salviae Miltiorrhizae*) 10 g, Chishaoyao (*Radix Paeoniae Rubra*) 10 g, Taoren (*Semen Persicae*) 10 g, Honghua (*Flos Carthama*) 10 g and Zelan (*Herba Lycopi*) 10 g; for red tongue and thready rapid pulse due to pronounced yin consumption, add Maimendong (*Radix Ophiopogonis*) 10 g, Yuzhu (*Rhizoma Polygonati Odorati*) 10 g and Wuweizi (*Fructus Schisandrae*) 6 g; for bradycardia due to yang deficiency, add Zhimahuang (*Herba Ephedrae*, roasted) 10 g, Buguzhi (*Fructus Psoraleae*) 10 g and Zhifuzi (*Radix Aconiti Lateralis Preparata*) 10 g.

5. Excessive Fluid Attacking the Heart

Chief Manifestations: Palpitation, feeling of oppression in the chest, thirst without a desire to drink,

加　减　心阳不足,形寒肢冷者,加黄芪30 g,党参15 g,制附子10 g;大汗出者,加红参(另煎)10 g,煅龙骨(先煎)30 g,煅牡蛎(先煎)30 g;饮邪上逆,头晕目眩,恶心呕吐者,加制半夏10 g,茯苓15 g,陈皮10 g;肢体浮肿,尿少者,加茯苓15 g,猪苓10 g,泽泻15 g,万年青根10 g,车前子(包煎)10 g;唇舌爪甲青紫,右胁痞块胀痛者,加丹参10 g,赤芍药10 g,桃仁10 g,红花10 g,泽兰10 g;阴伤明显,舌红,脉细数者,加麦门冬10 g,玉竹10 g,五味子6 g;若心阳不振,以心动过缓为著者,酌加炙麻黄10 g,补骨脂10 g,制附子10 g。

5. 水饮凌心证

主要证候　心悸怔忡,胸闷痞满,渴不欲饮,小便短少,

scanty urine, edema of lower limbs, cold limbs, dizziness, nausea, vomiting, productive expectoration, pale tongue with smooth coating, and wiry and smooth or deep, thready and wiry pulse.

Therapeutic Methods: To activate heart yang, promote qi circulation and induce diuresis.

Prescription: Modified Ling Gui Zhu Gan Tang (Decoction of Poria, Cinnamomi, Atractylodis Macrocephalae and Glycyrrhizae), composed of Fuling (*Poria*) 15 g, Guizhi (*Ramulus Cinnamomi*) 10 g, Zhigancao (*Radix Glycyrrhizae*, roasted) 6 g, Baizhu (*Rhizoma Atractylodis Macrocephalae*) 15 g, Zexie (*Rhizoma Alismatis*) 15 g, Zhibanxia (*Rhizoma Pinelliae Preparata*) 10 g, Chenpi (*Pericarpium Citri Reticulatae*) 10 g, Sangbaipi (*Cortex Mori*) 10 g and Yuanzhi (*Radix Polygalae*) 10 g.

Modifications: For scanty urine and edema of limbs, add Zhuling (*Polyporus*) 10 g, Fangji (*Radix Stephaniae Tetrandra*) 10 g, Tinglizi (*Semen Lepidii seu Descurainiae*) 10 g, Dafupi (*Pericarpium Arecae*) 10 g and Cheqianzi (*Semen Plataginis, wrapped*) 10 g; for dyspneic cough, add Xingren (*Semen Armeniacae Amarum*) 10 g, Qianhu (*Radix Peucedani*) 10 g, Jiegeng (*Radix Platycodi*) 6 g and Fangji (*Radix Stephaniae Tetrandra*) 10 g; for vomiting, add Sharen (*Fructus Amomi*, to be decocted later) 3 g and Shengjiang (*Rhizoma Zingiberis Recens*) 5 g.

6. Blood Stasis Blocking the Heart

Chief Manifestations: Palpitation, chest distress, intermittent stinging pain in the chest, purple lips and nails, purple tongue with ecchymosis, unsmooth or slow-irregular or intermittent pulse.

Therapeutic Methods: To promote blood circulation, remove blood stasis, regulate qi and activate the col-

下肢浮肿,形寒肢冷,头目眩晕,恶心呕吐,咳吐痰涎,舌质淡,苔滑,脉弦滑或沉细而滑。

治 法 振奋心阳,化气利水。

方 药 苓桂术甘汤加减:茯苓15 g,桂枝10 g,炙甘草6 g,白术15 g,泽泻15 g,制半夏10 g,陈皮10 g,桑白皮10 g,远志10 g。

加 减 尿少,肢肿,加猪苓10 g,防己10 g,葶苈子10 g,大腹皮10 g,车前子(包煎)10 g;咳喘者,加杏仁10 g,前胡10 g,桔梗6 g,防己10 g;呕恶者,加砂仁(后下)3 g,生姜5 g。

6. 心血瘀阻证

主要证候 心悸怔忡,胸闷不适,心痛时作,痛如针刺,唇甲青紫,舌质紫暗或有瘀斑,脉涩或结或代。

治 法 活血化瘀,理气通络。

laterals.

Prescription: Modified Taoren Honghua Jian (Persicae and Carthami Decoction for Removing Blood Stasis), composed of Taoren (*Semen Persicae*) 10 g, Honghua (*Flos Carthama*) 10 g, Danshen (*Radix Salviae Miltiorrhizae*) 10 g, Chishaoyao (*Radix Paeoniae Rubra*) 10 g, Chuanxiong (*Rhizoma Chuanxiong*) 10 g, Yanhusuo (*Rhizoma Corydalis*) 10 g, Xiangfu (*Rhizoma Cyperi*) 10 g, Qingpi (*Pericarpium Citri Reticulatae Viride*) 10 g, Shengdihuang (*Radix Rehmanniae*) 10 g and Danggui (*Radix Angelicae Sinensis*) 10 g.

Modifications: For stagnation of qi and blood, add Chaihu (*Radix Bupleuri*) 6 g and Zhike (*Fructus Aurantii*) 10 g; for shortness of breath and lassitude due to qi deficiency and blood stasis, add Huangqi (*Radix Astragali*) 15 g, Dangshen (*Radix Codonopsis*) 10 g and Huangjing (*Rhizoma Polygonati*) 10 g; for dizziness and pale complexion, add Heshouwu (*Radix Polygoni Multiflori*) 10 g, Gouqizi (*Fructus Lycii*) 10 g and Shudihuang (*Radix Rehmanniae Preparata*) 10 g; for dry mouth, red tongue with little coating, add Maimendong (*Radix Ophiopogonis*) 10 g, Yuzhu (*Rhizoma Polygonati Odorati*) 10 g and Nüzhenzi (*Fructus Ligustri Lucidi*) 10 g; for lumbago, cold limbs and intolerance to cold, add Zhifuzi (*Radix Aconiti Lateralis Preparata*) 10 g, Rougui (*Cortex Cinnamomi*, to be decocted later) 3 g and Yinyanghuo (*Herba Epimedii*) 10 g; for suffocative sensation in the chest due to blockage of collaterals, remove Shengdihuang (*Radix Rehmanniae*) and add Chenxiang (*Lignum Aquilariae Resinatum*) 3 g, Tanxiang (*Lignum Santali Albi*) 10 g and Jiangxiang (*Lignum Dalbergiae Odoriferae*) 10 g; for distending pain in the chest and greasy tongue coating resulting from turbid phlegm, add Gualou (*Fructus Trichosanthis*) 10 g, Xie-

方　药　桃仁红花煎加减：桃仁10 g,红花10 g,丹参10 g,赤芍药10 g,川芎10 g,延胡索10 g,香附10 g,青皮10 g,生地黄10 g,当归10 g。

加　减　气滞血瘀者,加柴胡6 g,枳壳10 g;因虚致瘀,气短乏力者,加黄芪15 g,党参10 g,黄精10 g;头昏目眩,面色无华者,加何首乌10 g,枸杞子10 g,熟地黄10 g;口干,舌红,少苔者,加麦门冬10 g,玉竹10 g,女贞子10 g;腰酸膝冷,畏寒怕冷者,加制附子10 g,肉桂(后下)3 g,淫羊藿10 g;络脉痹阻,胸部窒闷者,去生地黄,加沉香3 g,檀香10 g,降香10 g;挟有痰浊,胸满闷痛,苔浊腻者,加瓜蒌10 g,薤白6 g,制半夏10 g;胸痛甚者,加乳香10 g,没药10 g,五灵脂10 g,蒲黄(包煎)10 g,三七粉(另冲)3 g。

bai (*Bulbus Allii Macrostemi*) 6 g and Zhibanxia (*Rhizoma Pinelliae Preparata*) 10 g; for severe chest pain, add Ruxiang (*Olibanum*) 10 g, Moyao (*Myrrha*) 10 g, Wulingzhi (*Faces Trogopterori*) 10 g, Puhuang (*Pollen Typhae*, wrapped) 10 g and Sanqifen (*Radix Notoginseng*, powdered and to be infused separately) 3 g.

7. Phlegm-fire Disturbing the Heart

Chief Manifestations: Paroxysmal palpitation easily induced by scare, feeling of oppression in the chest, restlessness, insomnia, dreamfulness, constipation, dry and bitter mouth, dark scanty urine, red tongue with yellow greasy coating, and wiry and smooth pulse.

Therapeutic Methods: To clear away heat, resolve phlegm and tranquilize the mind.

Prescription: Modified Huanglian Wendan Tang (Coptidis Decoction for Clearing away Gallbladder Heat), composed of Huanglian (*Rhizoma Coptidis*) 5 g, Chenpi (*Pericarpium Citri Reticulatae*) 10 g, Zhibanxia (*Rhizoma Pinelliae Preparata*) 10 g, Fuling (*Poria*) 15 g, Zhuru (*Caulis Bambuswae in Taeniam*) 10 g, Zhishi (*Fructus Aurantii Immaturus*) 10 g, Danshen (*Radix Salviae Miltiorrhizae*) 10 g, Yuanzhi (*Radix Polygalae*) 6 g, Zhizi (*Fructus Gardeniae*) 10 g, Huangqin (*Radix Scutellariae*) 10 g, Chendanxing (*Arisaema cum Bile*) 10 g, Shenqu (*Massa Medicata Fermentata*) 10 g, Dazao (*Fructus Jujubae*) 5 pcs and Gancao (*Radix Glycyrrhizae*) 5 g.

Modifications: For constipation due to combination of phlegm and fire, add Shengdahuang (*Radix et Rhizoma Rhei*, to be decocted later) 5 -10 g; for severe palpitation, add Yuanzhi (*Radix Polygalae*) 6 g, Shichangpu (*Rhizoma Acori Tatarinowii*) 6 g, Suanzaoren (*Semen Ziziphi Spinosae*) 10 g, Shenglonggu (*Os Draconis*, to be decocted first) 30 g and Shengmuli (*Concha Ostreae*,

7. 痰火扰心证

主要证候　心悸时发时止,受惊易作,胸闷烦躁,失眠多梦,口干口苦,大便秘结,小便短赤,舌质红,苔黄腻,脉弦滑。

治　法　清热化痰,宁心安神。

方　药　黄连温胆汤加减:黄连5 g,陈皮10 g,制半夏10 g,茯苓15 g,竹茹10 g,枳实10 g,丹参10 g,远志6 g,栀子10 g,黄芩10 g,陈胆星10 g,神曲10 g,大枣 5 枚,甘草5 g。

加　减　痰火互结,大便秘结者,加生大黄(后下)5～10 g;心悸重症,加远志6 g,石菖蒲 6 g,酸枣仁10 g,生龙骨(先煎)30 g,生牡蛎(先煎)30 g;火郁伤阴,舌红少苔者,加沙参10 g,麦门冬10 g,玉竹

to be decocted first) 30 g; for red tongue with little coating due to stagnated fire impairing yin, add Shashen (*Radix Glehniae*) 10 g, Maimendong (*Radix Ophiopogonis*) 10 g, Yuzhu (*Rhizoma Polygonati Odorati*) 10 g, Tianmendong (*Radix Asparagi*) 10 g and Shengdihuang (*Radix Rehmanniae*) 10 g.

Other Treatments

1. Chinese Patent Drugs

(1) Suanzaoren Heji (Ziziphi Spinosa Mixture): 10 ml each time, thrice daily; applicable to arrhythmia due to yin and blood deficiency of the heart and liver.

(2) Dingxin Wan (Pill for Tranquillizing Mind): 6 g each time, twice daily; applicable to arrhythmia due to predominant deficiency of qi and yin. This drug should not be taken for a long time in order to avoid mercurial intoxication.

(3) Zhusha Anshen Wan (Cinnabaris Bolus for Tranquiling Mind): 1 bolus each time, twice daily; applicable to arrhythmia due to insufficiency of heart blood and hyperactivity of heart fire. This drug should not be taken for long otherwise mercurial intoxication may occur.

(4) Baizi Yangxin Wan (Platycladi Pill for Nourishing Heart): 6 g each time, thrice daily; applicable to arrhythmia due to qi deficiency of the heart and spleen.

(5) Shen Rong Anshen Wan (Ginseng and Cervi Pantotrichum Pill for Tranquilizing Mind): 10 g each time, twice daily; applicable to arrhythmia due to qi deficiency of the spleen and kidney.

(6) Zixinyin Koufuye (Oral Liquid for Nourishing Heart Yin): 10 ml each time, thrice daily; applicable to arrhythmia due to deficiency of heart yin.

(7) Buxinqi Koufuye (Oral Liquid for Replenishing Heart Qi): 10 ml each time, thrice daily; applicable to arrhythmia due to deficiency of heart qi.

10 g,天门冬10 g,生地黄10 g。

【其他疗法】

1. 中成药

(1) 酸枣仁合剂　每服10 ml,每日3次。适用于心律失常心肝阴血不足者。

(2) 定心丸　每服6 g,每日2次。适用于心律失常偏气阴两虚者。本品不可过量长期服用,以防汞中毒。

(3) 朱砂安神丸　每服1丸,每日2次。适用于心律失常证属心血不足,心火亢盛者。本品不宜久服。

(4) 柏子养心丸　每服6 g,每日3次。适用于心律失常证属心脾两虚者。

(5) 参茸安神丸　每服10 g,每日2次。适用于心律失常脾肾两虚者。

(6) 滋心阴口服液　每服10 ml,每日3次。适用于心律失常心阴不足者。

(7) 补心气口服液　每服10 ml,每日3次。适用于心律失常心气不足者。

2. Single-drug or Experiential Prescriptions

（1）Kushen (*Radix Sophorae Flavescentis*) 20 g. Decoct it with water, and take the decoction orally, 1 dose daily. It is applicable to arrhythmia with rapid or rapid-irregular pulse.

（2）Hongshen (*Radix Ginseng Rubra*) 10 g, Danggui (*Radix Angelicae Sinensis*) 10 g, Chishaoyao (*Radix Paeoniae Rubra*) 15 g, Fuling (*Poria*) 15 g, Zhigancao (*Radix Glycyrrhizae*, roasted) 20 g and Guizhi (*Ramulus Cinnamomi*) 10 g. Decoct the drugs with water and take the decoction in 2 divided doses daily. It is applicable to arrhythmia resulting from yang deficiency.

（3）Dangshen (*Radix Codonopsis*) 30 g, Danshen (*Radix Salviae Miltiorrhizae*) 30 g, Kushen (*Radix Sophorae Flavescentis*) 20 g, Zhigancao (*Radix Glycyrrhizae*, roasted) 15 g, Baiziren (*Semen Platycladi*) 10 g and Changshan (*Radix Dichroae*) 10 g. Decoct the drugs with water and take the decoction in 2 divided doses daily. It is applicable to arrhythmia with restlessness.

（4）Chaihu (*Radix Bupleuri*) 10 g, Zhike (*Fructus Aurantii*) 10 g, Dangshen (*Radix Codonopsis*) 10 g, Danshen (*Radix Salviae Miltiorrhizae*) 20 g, Cheqianzi (*Semen Plataginis*, wrapped) 10 g, Gualoupi (*Pericarpium Trichosanthis*) 10 g and Beiwujiapi (*Cortex Acanthopanacis*) 3 - 10 g. Decoct the drugs with water and take the decoction in 2 divided doses daily. It is applicable to palpitation due to the excessive fluid attacking the heart.

（5）Dangshen (*Radix Codonopsis*) 30 g, Danshen (*Radix Salviae Miltiorrhizae*) 30 g, Huangqi (*Radix Astragali*) 30 g, Maimendong (*Radix Ophiopogonis*) 15 g, Gouqizi (*Fructus Lycii*) 15 g, Yuzhu (*Rhizoma Polygonati Odorati*) 15 g, Wuweizi (*Fructus Schisandrae*) 10 g and Taizishen (*Radix Pseudostellariae*) 30 g.

2. 单验方

（1）苦参20 g,水煎服,每日1剂。适用于心悸而脉数或促的患者。

（2）红参10 g,当归10 g,赤芍药15 g,茯苓15 g,炙甘草20 g,桂枝10 g。水煎服,每日1剂,分2次服。适用于心律失常阳虚者。

（3）党参30 g,丹参30 g,苦参20 g,炙甘草15 g,柏子仁10 g,常山10 g。水煎服,每日1剂,分2次服。适用于心律失常,心烦不安者。

（4）柴胡10 g,枳壳10 g,党参10 g,丹参20 g,车前子(包煎)10 g,瓜蒌皮10 g,北五加皮3～10 g。水煎服,每日1剂,分2次服。适用于惊悸水气凌心者。

（5）党参30 g,丹参30 g,黄芪30 g,麦门冬15 g,枸杞子15 g,玉竹15 g,五味子10 g,太子参30 g。水煎服,每日1剂,分2次服。适用于心悸属气血两虚者。

Decoct the drugs with water and take the decoction in 2 divided doses daily. It is applicable to palpitation due to deficiency of qi and blood.

3. External Therapy

(1) Nanxing (*Rhizoma Arisaematis*) 10 g and Chuanwu (*Radix Aconiti*) 10 g. Pulverize the drugs and mix them with melted yellow wax, apply the mixture onto centers of the palms and soles upon sleeping, once daily, 10 days as a treatment course. It is applicable to palpitation due to deficiency of heart yang and blood stasis blocking in collaterals.

(2) Shengdihuang (*Radix Rehmanniae*) 45 g, Wuweizi (*Fructus Schisandrae*) 30 g, Maimendong (*Radix Ophiopogonis*) 20 g, Zhuye (*Herba Lophatheri*) 10 g and Dangshen (*Radix Codonopsis*) 20 g. Decoct the drugs with 3,000 ml of water for 30 minutes, remove the dregs, immerse the feet in the warm decoction for 30 minutes, once every 2 days, 7 days as a treatment course. It is applicable to palpitation, feeling of oppression in the chest, precordial dull pain, shortness of breath and dislike of speaking.

2.2.3 Coronary Arteriosclerotic Cardiopathy

General Description

Coronary arteriosclerotic cardiopathy, called coronary heart disease (CHD) for short, is characterized by paroxysmal oppressed sensation or pain in the chest, pale complexion, anxiety or irritability, palpitation, shortness of breath, and severe pain with sweating. Clinically it is manifested as latent CHD, angina pectoris, myocardial infarction, myocardial sclerosis and sudden death. Among

3. 外治法

(1) 南星10 g,川乌10 g,共为细末,用黄蜡融化摊于手、足心。每日 1 次,晚敷晨取,10 日为 1 个疗程。适用于心悸心阳衰弱、瘀血阻络者。

(2) 生地黄45 g,五味子30 g,麦门冬20 g,竹叶10 g,党参20 g。上药加水3 000 ml,煮沸 30 分钟,去渣取药液,待药温后浸浴双足,每次 30 分钟,每日 1 次,7 日为 1 个疗程,每剂可用 2 日。适用于心悸胸闷,心前区隐痛,气短懒言者。

第三节 冠状动脉粥样硬化性心脏病

【概述】

冠状动脉粥样硬化性心脏病,简称"冠心病"。临床主要表现为突然阵发性的胸骨后压榨感或疼痛,面色苍白,表情焦虑或烦躁,心悸不宁,心慌气短,疼痛剧烈时可伴出汗。临床分为隐性冠心病、心

them angina pectoris and myocardial infarction are most commonly encountered. CHD often occurs among the people aged above forty. More males suffer from this disease than females and most patients are mental workers. Nowadays, it is one of the most common heart diseases in Europe and America, and about 5.7 millions in U. S. A. (2.5% of the population) suffer from this disease. In China its incidence is increasing in recent years and it has become one of the most dangerous diseases threatening people's lives.

The disease is associated with hypertension, hyperlipidemia, diabetes, obesity, cigarette smoking, and social and psychological factors. As atheromatous plaque formed in the inner wall of coronary artery causes stenosis or obstruction of the blood vessel and block of blood flow, and results in myocardial ischemia, hypoxia and even necrosis, the disease is also called ischaemic heart disease. About 90% of CHDs result from coronary atheroclerosis and about 5%-10% from coronary vasospasm.

According to the clinical manifestations, it belongs the categories of "xiong bi" (thoracic obstruction of qi), "xin tong" (cardialgia), "xin ji" (palpitation), "jue xin tong" (precordial pain with cold limbs) and "zhen xin tong" (angina pectoris) in TCM. Its pathogenic factors include inward attack of exogenous pathogenic cold, improper diet, emotional disharmony, and aging and debility. Its pathogenesis is involved with the deficiency and excess. The former refers to deficiency of the heart, spleen and kidney and nutritional deficiency of blood vessel; the latter to stagnation of cold, qi and blood, and phlegm obstructing pectoral yang and heart vessels. If the

绞痛、心肌梗死、心肌硬化、猝死五大类型,其中以心绞痛、心肌梗死较为常见。本病多发生在 40 岁以上的人,男性多于女性,且以脑力劳动者为多。在欧美国家是最常见的心脏病,在美国约有 570 万人患本病,占人口的 2.5%。我国近年发病率有增多趋势,已成为危害人民健康的主要疾病之一。

本病的发生一般认为与高血压、高脂血症、糖尿病、肥胖、吸烟、社会心理因素等有关。由于粥样硬化斑块形成于冠状动脉内壁,血管腔的狭窄或梗阻使血流受阻,导致心肌缺血、缺氧,甚至坏死,故又称缺血性心脏病。其中 90% 以上为粥样硬化所致,5%~10% 为冠状动脉痉挛所引起。

根据本病的临床表现,属于中医学"胸痹"、"心痛"、"心悸"、"厥心痛"、"真心痛"的范畴。本病的发生多与寒邪内侵、饮食不当、情志失调、年老体虚等因素有关。其病机有虚实两方面:实为寒凝、气滞、血瘀、痰阻,痹遏胸阳,阻滞心脉;虚为心脾肝肾亏虚,心脉失养。如果病情进一步发展,瘀血闭阻心脉,可致心肌梗死。

blockage of heart vessels by blood stasis occurs, it may give rise to myocardial infarction and the prognosis may be unfavourable.

Essentials for Diagnosis

(1) Typical symptoms of angina pectoris or myocardial infarction.

(2) Pronounced myocardial ischemic signs revealed by ECGs during rest time; or positive result of ECG exercise test without other explanation in male aged above 40, or female above 45, asymptomatic CHD can be made if clinical symptoms are absent.

(3) In males aged above 40 and females above 45 with primary cardiac arrest that can be excluded from other diseases, CHD can be diagnosed. If the primary cardiac arrest cannot be excluded completely from other diseases, the diagnosis of asymptomatic CHD can be made.

(4) In males aged above 40 and females above 45, if heart failure with cardiac dilatation, dysfunction of papillary muscles and severe arrhythmia can not be explained by other reasons, the diagnosis of CHD can be made with reference to other risk factors such as hypertension, hyperlipidemia and diabetes.

(5) ECG is normal at rest, but the apperance of transient acute ischemic change of ST-T segment, or T wave turning erection from inversion, or transient abnormal q wave and ST-T segment elevation, and various kinds of intraventricular conductional disturbances during or after the attack may support the diagnosis. Furthermore, myocardial ischemia and arrhythmia revealed by ECG after exercise and food intake are helpful to the diagnosis.

(6) Acute myocardial infarction is often complicated

【诊断要点】

(1) 有典型心绞痛或心肌梗死症状。

(2) 休息时心电图有明显心肌缺血型表现,或男性 40 岁以上,女性 45 岁以上,心电图运动试验阳性,无其他原因可查者。如无有关临床症状,可确诊为无症状性冠心病。

(3) 男性 40 岁以上,女性 45 岁以上,发生原发性心脏骤停,并能排除其他原因者,可确诊为冠心病,如不可能完全排除者,则为可疑冠心病。

(4) 男性 40 岁以上,女性 45 岁以上,心脏扩大伴心力衰竭,乳头肌功能失调,严重心律失常,不能用其他原因解释者,结合易患因素(高血压、高血脂、糖尿病),可确诊为冠心病。

(5) 平时心电图大多为正常。发作时或发作后短暂出现的急性缺血型 ST－T 改变,或见 T 波由倒置转为直立,或短暂出现异常 q 波、ST 段抬高、各种室内传导异常等,有助于本病的诊断。此外,运动、饱餐等负荷实验后出现缺血性心电图及心律失常,亦有助于诊断。

(6) 急性心肌梗死常合并

with arrhythmia, cardiac insufficiency and shock, so dynamic ECG, peripheral WBC count, blood sedimentation rate and serum zymologic tests are helpful to further comfirmation of diagnosis.

Syndrome Differentiation and Treatment

Whether the secondary or the principal aspects and the deficiency or the excess is predominant or not should be determined first. The secondary excess predominates in syndromes such as stagnation of heart blood, obstruction of turbid phlegm and accumulation of yin cold, and the principal deficiency in those such as yin deficiency of the heart and kidney, deficiency of qi and yin and deficiency of yang qi. The idea of "Treating the secondary first and the principal later" should be followed as the therapeutic principle. Treatment methods for the secondary excess include expelling cold, eliminating phlegm, promoting blood circulation and removing blood stasis, and those for the principal deficiency include invigorating qi, warming yang and nourishing yin which are applied to relevant organs. In the case of intermingled deficiency and excess, treatment should be mainly on the pincipal aspect.

1. Stagnation of Heart Blood

Chief Manifestations: Localized stabbing chest pain aggravated at night, palpitation, restlessness, dark purple tongue, and deep and unsmooth pulse.

Therapeutic Methods: To promote blood circulation to remove blood stasis and dredge collaterals to relieve pain.

Prescription: Modified Xuefu Zhuyu Tang (Decoction for Removing Blood Stasis in Chest), composed of Danggui (*Radix Angelicae Sinensis*) 10 g, Chuanxiong (*Rhizoma Chuanxiong*) 12 g, Zhike (*Fructus Aurantii*) 12 g, Taoren (*Semen Persicae*) 12 g, Honghua

心律失常、心功能不全及休克,应配合心电图动态观察及白细胞总数、血沉、血清酶学检查,以进一步明确诊断。

【辨证论治】

本病临床首先要辨其标本虚实的主次。心脉瘀阻、痰浊壅塞、阴寒凝结证以标实为主;心肾阴虚、气阴两虚和阳气虚衰证以本虚为主。治疗以"先顾其标,后顾其本"为原则。标实者,当予祛寒、豁痰、活血化瘀;本虚者,分别脏器予以益气、温阳、滋阴。若虚实夹杂者,可分清主次,适当兼顾。

1. 心脉瘀阻证

主要证候 胸部刺痛,固定不移,入夜更甚,心悸不宁,舌质紫暗,脉象沉涩。

治 法 活血化瘀,通络止痛。

方 药 血府逐瘀汤加减:当归10 g,川芎12 g,枳壳12 g,桃仁12 g,红花12 g,柴胡10 g,丹参30 g,桔梗10 g,赤芍药15 g,生地黄15 g,牛膝10 g,

(*Flos Carthama*) 12 g, Chaihu (*Radix Bupleuri*) 10 g, Danshen (*Radix Salviae Miltiorrhizae*) 30 g, Jiegeng (*Radix Platycodi*) 10 g, Chishaoyao (*Radix Paeoniae Rubra*) 15 g, Shengdihuang (*Radix Rehmanniae*) 15 g, Niuxi (*Radix Achyranthis Bidentatae*) 10 g and Gancao (*Radix Glycyrrhizae*) 6 g.

Modifications: For severe chest pain, add Jiangxiang (*Lignum Dalbergiae Odoriferae*) 6 g, Yujin (*Radix Curcumae*) 10 g and Yanhusuo (*Rhizoma Corydalis*) 10 g; for severe pain, aversion to cold and cold limbs, add Xixin (*Herba Asari*) 3 g, Guizhi (*Ramulus Cinnamomi*) 10 g and Gaoliangjiang (*Rhizoma Alpiniae Officinarum*) 6 g; for mild cases with blood stagnation, use Danshen Yin (Salviae Miltiorrhiza Decoction).

2. Obstruction of Turbid Phlegm

Chief Manifestations: Suffocative sensation in the chest, chest pain radiating toward the shoulder and back, shortness of breath, general heavy sensation, obesity, profuse sputum, turbid and greasy tongue coating, and smooth pulse.

Therapeutic Methods: To activate yang, purge turbidity, eliminate phlegm and relieve stagnation.

Prescription: Modified Gualou Xiebai Banxia Tang (Decoction of Trichosanthis, Allii Macrostemi and Pinelliae), composed of Gualou (*Fructus Trichosanthis*) 10 g, Xiebai (*Bulbus Allii Macrostemi*) 10 g, Zhibanxia (*Rhizoma Pinelliae Preparata*) 10 g, Ganjiang (*Rhizoma Zingiberis*) 5 g, Chenpi (*Pericarpium Citri Reticulatae*) 10 g, Baikouren (*Semen Amomi Rotundus*, to be decocted later) 5 g, Shichangpu (*Rhizoma Acori Tatarinowii*) 10 g, Yujin (*Radix Curcumae*) 10 g and Gancao (*Radix Glycyrrhizae*) 6 g.

Modifications: For feeling of oppression in the chest and abdominal distention due to pronounced turbid

甘草6 g。

加 减 胸痛较甚者,酌加降香6 g,郁金10 g,延胡索10 g;痛剧并伴恶寒肢冷者,加细辛3 g,桂枝10 g,高良姜6 g;血瘀轻证可用丹参饮。

2. 痰浊壅塞证

主要证候 胸闷如塞而痛,或痛引肩背,气短喘促,肢体沉重,形体肥胖,痰多,苔浊腻,脉滑。

治 法 通阳泄浊,豁痰开结。

方 药 瓜蒌薤白半夏汤加减:瓜蒌10 g,薤白10 g,制半夏10 g,干姜5 g,陈皮10 g,白蔻仁(后下)5 g,石菖蒲10 g,郁金10 g,甘草6 g。

加 减 痰浊较甚,胸闷脘胀者,加枳实10 g,厚朴

phlegm, add Zhishi (*Fructus Aurantii Immaturus*) 10 g and Houpo (*Cortex Magnoliae Officinalis*) 10 g; for cough with profuse sputum, add Xingren (*Semen Armeniacae Amarum*) 10 g and Fuling (*Poria*) 10 g; for yellow sputum, yellow greasy tongue coating and smooth, rapid pulse, remove Xiebai (*Bulbus Allii macrostemi*) and add Zhuru (*Caulis Bambuswae in Taeniam*) 10 g, Huangqin (*Radix Scutellariae*) 10 g, Huanglian (*Rhizoma Coptidis*) 5 g, Tianzhuhuang (*Concretio Silicea Bambusae*) 10 g and Danxing (*Arisaema cum Bile*) 10 g.

3. Accumulation of Yin Cold

Chief Manifestations: Chest pain radiating to the back aggravated by cold, feeling of oppression in the chest, palpitation, shortness of breath with inability to lie flat in severe cases, pale complexion, extremely cold limbs, white tongue coating, and deep and thready pulse.

Therapeutic Methods: To activate yang with pungent-warm drugs, remove obstruction and expel cold.

Prescription: Modified Gualou Xiebai Guizhi Tang (Decoction of Trichosanthis, Allii Macrostemi and Cinnamomi), composed of Quangualou (*Fructus Trichosanthis*) 10 g, Xiebai (*Bulbus Allii Macrostemi*) 10 g, Zhishi (*Fructus Aurantii Immaturus*) 10 g, Guizhi (*Ramulus Cinnamomi*) 10 g, Zhifuzi (*Radix Aconiti Lateralis Preparata*, to be decocted first) 10 g, Danshen (*Radix Salviae Miltiorrhizae*) 15 g and Gancao (*Radix Glycyrrhizae*) 10 g.

Modifications: For severe yin cold, add Zhichuanwu (*Radix Aconiti Preparata*) 6 g and Xixin (*Herba Asari*) 3 g or add Suhexiang Wan (Bolus of Styrax) 1 bolus; for chest pain and cough with sputum due to accumulation of turbid phlegm, add Shengjiang (*Rhizoma Zingiberis Recens*) 5 g, Chenpi (*Pericarpium Citri*

10 g；咳嗽痰多者,加杏仁 10 g,茯苓10 g；痰黄,舌苔黄 腻,脉滑数者,去薤白,加竹茹 10 g,黄芩10 g,黄连5 g,天竺 黄10 g,胆星10 g。

3. 阴寒凝结证

主要证候 胸痛彻背,感 寒痛甚,胸闷气短,心悸,重则 喘息不能平卧,面色苍白,四 肢厥冷,舌苔白,脉沉细。

治 法 辛温通阳,开痹 散寒。

方 药 瓜蒌薤白桂枝 汤加减：全瓜蒌10 g,薤白 10 g,枳实10 g,桂枝10 g,制附 子(先煎)10 g,丹参15 g,甘草 10 g。

加 减 阴寒严重者,加 制川乌6 g,细辛3 g；或加苏合 香丸 1 粒口服。痰浊内盛,胸 痛伴咳唾痰涎者,加生姜5 g, 陈皮10 g,茯苓10 g,杏仁10 g。

Reticulatae) 10 g, Fuling (*Poria*) 10 g and Xingren
(*Semen Armeniacae Amarum*) 10 g.

4. Yin Deficiency of the Heart and Kidney

Chief Manifestations: Chest pain and oppression,
restlessness, insomnia, palpitation, night sweating, lumbago, weak waist and knees, dizziness, tinnitus, red
tongue with ecchymosis, and thready and rapid or thready
and unsmooth pulse.

Therapeutic Methods: To replenish yin, tonifiy the
kidney, nourish the heart and tranquilize the mind.

Prescription: Modified Zuogui Yin (Decoction for
Replenishing Kidney Yin), composed of Shudihuang (*Ra-
dix Rehmanniae Preparata*) 15 g, Shanzhuyu (*Fructus
Corni*) 10 g, Gouqizi (*Fructus Lycii*) 10 g, Shanyao
(*Rhizoma Dioscoreae*) 15 g, Fuling (*Poria*) 10 g, Wu-
weizi (*Fructus Schisandrae*) 10 g, Baiziren (*Semen
Platycladi*) 10 g, Yuanzhi (*Radix Polygalae*) 6 g and
Gancao (*Radix Glycyrrhizae*) 10 g.

Modifications: For palpitation, night sweating,
restlessness and insomnia due to deficiency of heart yin,
add Maimendong (*Radix Ophiopogonis*) 10 g, Wuweizi
(*Fructus Schisandrae*) 10 g, Baiziren (*Semen Platycladi*) 10 g and Suanzaoren (*Semen Ziziphi Spinosae*)
10 g; for chest pain and oppression, add Danggui (*Radix
Angelicae Sinensis*) 10 g, Danshen (*Radix Salviae
Miltiorrhizae*) 15 g, Chuanxiong (*Rhizoma Chuanxiong*) 10 g and Yujin (*Radix Curcumae*) 15 g; for dizziness, numbness of tongue and limbs and hot sensation of
face due to deficient yin causing hyperactive yang, add
Zhiheshouwu (*Radix Polygoni Multiflori Preparata*)
10 g, Nüzhenzi (*Fructus Ligustri Lucidi*) 10 g, Gouteng (*Ramulus Uncariae cum Uncis*, to be decocted
later) 10 g, Shengshijueming (*Concha Haliotidis*, to be
decocted first) 25 g, Muli (*Concha Ostreae*, to be decoc-

4. 心肾阴虚证

主要证候 胸闷且痛,心
烦不寐,心悸盗汗,腰膝酸软,
头晕耳鸣,舌质红或有紫斑,
脉细带数或见细涩。

治 法 滋阴益肾,养心
安神。

方 药 左归饮加减:
熟地黄15 g,山茱萸10 g,枸杞
子10 g,山药15 g,茯苓10 g,五
味子10 g,柏子仁10 g,远志
6 g,甘草10 g。

加 减 心阴亏虚而见
心悸、盗汗、心烦不寐者,加麦
门冬10 g,五味子10 g,柏子仁
10 g,酸枣仁10 g;胸闷且痛
者,加当归10 g,丹参15 g,川
芎10 g,郁金15 g;阴虚阳亢而
见头晕目眩,舌麻肢麻,面部
烘热者,加制何首乌10 g,女贞
子10 g,钩藤(后下)10 g,生石
决明(先煎)25 g,牡蛎(先煎)
25 g,鳖甲(先煎)15 g。

ted first) 25 g and Biejia (*Carapax Trionycis*, to be decocted first) 15 g.

5. Deficiency of Qi and Yin

Chief Manifestations: Feeling of oppression in the chest, shortness of breath, paroxysmal dull pain in the chest which is aggravated by exertion, palpitation, lassitude, dizziness, reddish tongue with teeth marks, and thready and weak, slow-irregular or intermittent pulse.

Therapeutic Methods: To replenish qi, nourish yin, promote blood circulation and activate collaterals.

Prescription: Modified Shengmai San (Powder for Reinforcing Qi and Nourishing Yin) and Renshen Yang-ying Tang (Ginseng Decoction for Nourishing Blood), composed of Taizishen (*Radix Pseudostellariae*) 10 g, Huangqi (*Radix Astragali*) 30 g, Baizhu (*Rhizoma Atractylodis Macrocephalae*) 10 g, Fuling (*Poria*) 10 g, Maimendong (*Radix Ophiopogonis*) 10 g, Danggui (*Radix Angelicae Sinensis*) 10 g, Baishaoyao (*Radix Paeoniae Alba*) 15 g, Yuanzhi (*Radix Polygalae*) 6 g, Wuweizi (*Fructus Schisandrae*) 6 g, Shengdihuang (*Radix Rehmanniae*) 15 g, Chenpi (*Pericarpium Citri Reticulatae*) 10 g, Rougui (*Cortex Cinnamomi*, to be decocted later) 3 g and Gancao (*Radix Glycyrrhizae*) 5 g.

Modification: For chest pain and oppression, add Danshen (*Radix Salviae Miltiorrhizae*) 15 g, Sanqifen (*Radix Notoginseng*, powdered and to be infused separately) 3 g, Yimucao (*Herba Leonuri*) 10 g, Yujin (*Radix Curcumae*) 10 g and Wulingzhi (*Faeces Trogopterori*) 10 g.

6. Deficiency of Yang Qi

Chief Manifestations: Feeling of oppression in the chest, shortness of breath, chest pain radiating toward the back, palpitation, sweating, aversion to cold, cold

5. 气阴两虚证

主要证候 胸闷气短,间有隐痛,遇劳更甚,心悸气短,倦怠懒言,面色少华,头晕目眩,舌偏红或有齿印,脉细弱无力,或结代。

治 法 益气养阴,活血通络。

方 药 生脉散合人参养营汤加减:太子参10 g,黄芪30 g,白术10 g,茯苓10 g,麦门冬10 g,当归10 g,白芍药15 g,远志6 g,五味子6 g,生地黄15 g,陈皮10 g,肉桂(后下)3 g,甘草5 g。

加 减 胸闷、胸痛者,加丹参15 g,三七粉(另冲)3 g,益母草10 g,郁金10 g,五灵脂10 g。

6. 阳气虚衰证

主要证候 胸闷气短,甚则胸痛彻背,心悸汗出,畏寒肢冷,腰酸乏力,面色苍白,唇

limbs, pale complexion, pale or purple lips, nails and tongue, deep and thready or deep and indistinct pulse.

Therapeutic Methods: To warm yang, supplement qi, promote blood circulation and activate collaterals.

Prescription: Modified Shen Fu Tang (Decoction of Ginseng Rubra and Aconiti Lateralis) and Yougui Yin (Decoction for Replenishing Kidney Yang), composed of Hongshen (*Radix Ginseng Rubra*, to be decocted separately) 10 g, Zhifupian (*Radix Aconiti Lateralis Preparata*, sliced) 10 g, Rougui (*Cortex Cinnamomi*, to be decocted later) 3 g, Shudihuang (*Radix Rehmanniae Preparata*) 15 g, Shanzhuyu (*Fructus Corni*) 10 g, Gouqizi (*Fructus Lycii*) 10 g, Duzhong (*Cortex Eucommiae*) 10 g, Shanyao (*Rhizoma Dioscoreae*) 15 g and Gancao (*Radix Glycyrrhizae*) 6 g.

Modification: For purple complexion, lips and nails, excessive sweating, extremely cold limbs and indistinct pulse, use Hongshen (*Radix Ginseng Rubra*) 15 g and Zhifuzi (*Radix Aconiti Lateralis Preparata*) 15 g, add Longgu (*Os Draconis*, to be decocted first) 20 g and Muli (*Concha Ostreae*, to be decocted first) 20 g.

Other Treatments

1. Chinese Patent Drugs

(1) Huoxin Wan (Pill for Activating Heart): 20–40 mg each time, 1 to 3 times daily; applicable to CHD with stagnation of heart blood and used with caution for women in pregnancy and menstrual periods.

(2) Jiuxin Dan (Pill for Saving Heart): 25–50 mg each time, twice daily, taken sublingually or orally, or taken immediately when pain attacks; applicable to angina pectoris but contraindicated to pregnant women. Discontinue the treatment to avoid consuming qi and impairing yin when the condition gets stable.

甲淡白或青紫,舌淡白或紫暗,脉沉细或沉微欲绝。

治　法　温阳益气,活血通络。

方　药　参附汤合右归饮加减:红参(另煎)5 g,制附片10 g,肉桂(后下)3 g,熟地黄15 g,山茱萸10 g,枸杞子10 g,杜仲10 g,山药15 g,甘草6 g。

加　减　面色唇甲青紫,大汗出,四肢厥冷,脉微细欲绝者,可重用红参15 g,制附子10 g,并加龙骨(先煎)20 g,牡蛎(先煎)20 g。

【其他疗法】

1. 中成药

(1) 活心丸　每服20～40 mg,每日1～3次。适用于冠心病心血瘀阻者。孕妇、妇女经期慎用。

(2) 救心丹　每服25～50 mg,每日2次,舌下含服或口服,或疼痛发作时立即含服。适用于冠心病心绞痛者。疼痛消失后停药,不宜长服久服,以免耗气伤阴。孕妇忌用。

(3) Shanhai Dan (Shanhai Pill): 2.5 g each time, thrice daily; applicable to angina pectoris.

(4) Suxiao Jiuxin Wan (Quick-Action Pill for Saving Heart): 10 pills, taken sublingually during the attack; applicable to angina pectoris with severe pain.

(5) Fufang Danshen Pian (Compound Salviae Miltiorrhizae Tablet): 3 tablets each time, thrice daily; applicable to CHD with stagnation of qi and blood.

(6) Jingzhi Guanxin Pian (Refined Tablet for Angina Pectoris): 6 - 8 tablets each time, thrice daily; applicable to angina pectoris.

(7) Di'ao Xinxuekang (Di'ao Capsule for Treating Heart and Blood-vessel Diseases): 100 - 200 mg each time, thrice daily; applicable to CHD with deficiency of heart blood and interior blockage of blood stasis.

(8) Buxinqi Koufuye (Oral Liquid for Replenishing Heart Qi): 10 ml each time, twice daily; applicable to CHD with deficiency of heart qi.

(9) Buxinyin Koufuye (Oral Liquid for Replenishing Heart Yin): 10 ml each time, twice daily; applicable to CHD with deficiency of heart qin.

2. Single-drug or Experiential Prescriptions

(1) Maodongqing (*Radix Ilicis Pubescentis*) 100 g. Soak it in water for 24 hours, then decoct it for 4 hours and concentrate the decoction to 20 ml, take 10 ml twice daily. It is applicable to various types of CHD.

(2) Shanzha (*Fructus Crataegi*) 20 g and Caojueming (*Semen Cassiae*) 30 g. Decoct the drugs with water, take the decoction in 2 divided doses daily. It is applicable to various types of CHD.

(3) Wulingzhi (*Faces Trogopterori*, vinegar prepared) 10 g and Shengjiang (*Rhizoma Zingiberis Re-*

（3）山海丹　每服2.5 g，每日 3 次。适用于冠心病心痛者。

（4）速效救心丸　胸痛发作时含服 10 丸。适用于冠心病心痛明显者。

（5）复方丹参片　每服 3 片，每日 3 次。适用于冠心病属气滞血瘀者。

（6）精制冠心片　每服 6～8 片，每日 3 次。适用于冠心病心绞痛者。

（7）地奥心血康　每服 100～200 mg，每日 3 次。适用于冠心病心血不足，瘀血内阻者。

（8）补心气口服液　每服 10 ml，每日 2 次。适用于冠心病心气不足者。

（9）补心阴口服液　每服 10 ml，每日 2 次。适用于冠心病心阴不足者。

2. 单验方

（1）毛冬青100 g。用水浸泡 24 小时，煎 4 小时后，浓缩成20 ml，每日 1 剂，分 2 次服。适用于冠心病各证型。

（2）山楂 20 g，草决明 30 g。水煎服，每日 1 剂，分 2 次服。适用于冠心病各证型。

（3）五灵脂（醋制）10 g，生姜3 g。共捣碎，每服3 g，冲

cens) 3 g. Mash and mix the drugs, take 3 g of the mixture after it is infused in water, once or twice daily. It is applicable to CHD with blockage of blood stasis.

(4) Dangshen (*Radix Codonopsis*) 15 g, Huangqi (*Radix Astragali*) 15 g, Danggui (*Radix Angelicae Sinensis*) 15 g, Shudihuang (*Radix Rehmanniae Preparata*) 15 g, Danshen (*Radix Salviae Miltiorrhizae*) 15 g, Maimendong (*Radix Ophiopogonis*) 10 g, Chuanlianzi (*Fructus Meliae Toosendan*) 10 g, Guiyuanrou (*Arillus Longan*) 10 g, Shenglonggu (*Os Draconis*) 30 g, Shengmuli (*Concha Ostreae*) 30 g, Jiaoshanzha (*Fructus Crataegi*, charrred) 15 g and Yuanzhi (*Radix Polygalae*) 10 g. Decoct the drugs with water, concentrate the decoction to 300 ml, sterilize it with high pressure and have it bottled. Take 100 ml each time, thrice daily. It is applicable to various types of CHD.

(5) Chaozhizi (*Fructus Gardeniae*, stir-baked) 10 g, Baishaoyao (*Radix Paeoniae Alba*) 30 g, Muxiang (*Radix Aucklandiae*) 6 g, Shichangpu (*Rhizoma Acori Tatarinowii*) 6 g, Gegen (*Radix Puerariae*) 10 g, Shengshanzha (*Fructus Crataegi*) 10 g, and Zhiheshouwu (*Radix Polygoni Multiflori Preparata*) 15 g. Decoct the drugs with water, take half the decoction orally in the morning and the rest in the evening daily, 15 days as a treatment course. It is applicable to angina pectoris.

(6) Shuizhi (*Hirudo*) 3 g, Jiuxiangchong (*Aspongopus*) 3 g, Zhechong (*Eupolyphaga seu Steleophaga*) 3 g, Yujin (*Radix Curcumae*) 9 g and Yinchen (*Herba Artemisiae Scopariae*) 30 g. Decoct the drugs with water, concentrate the decoction into paste and add appropiate amount of excipient to prepare tablets, 0.5 g each (equivalent to 2 g of crude herbs). Take 4-8 tablets each time, thrice daily. It is applicable to CHD due to blockage

服,每日 1～2 次。适用于冠心病瘀血阻滞者。

(4) 党参15 g,黄芪15 g,当归15 g,熟地黄15 g,丹参15 g,麦门冬10 g,川楝子10 g,桂圆肉10 g,生龙骨30 g,生牡蛎30 g,焦山楂15 g,远志10 g。浓煎 300 ml,装瓶高压,消毒备用,每服 100 ml,每日 3 次。适用于冠心病各证型。

(5) 炒栀子10 g,白芍药30 g,木香6 g,石菖蒲6 g,葛根10 g,生山楂10 g,制何首乌15 g。上药水煎服,每日 1 剂,分早晚 2 次服,15 日为 1 个疗程。适用于冠心病心绞痛者。

(6) 水蛭3 g,九香虫3 g,蟅虫3 g,郁金9 g,茵陈30 g。将上药经水煎去渣浓缩成膏,加入适量赋形药制成片剂,每片 0.5 g,相当于生药 2 g,每次服4～8 片,每日 3 次。适用于冠心病瘀血阻滞者。

in the collaterals by blood stasis.

(7) Zhibanxia (*Rhizoma Pinelliae Preparata*) 9 g, Maimendong (*Fructus Hordei Germinatus*) 9 g, Wuweizi (*Fructus Schisandrae*) 9 g, Chaozhishi (*Fructus Aurantii Immaturus, stir-baked*) 15 g, Danshen (*Radix Salviae Miltiorrhizae*) 15 g, Beishashen (*Radix Glehniae*) 15 g, Fuling (*Poria*) 30 g, Chuanxiong (*Rhizoma Chuanxiong*) 12 g and Chishaoyao (*Radix Paeoniae Rubra*) 12 g. Decoct the drugs with water and take the decoction in two divided doses daily. It is applicable to CHD with predominate deficiency of yin.

（7）制半夏9 g,麦门冬9 g,五味子9 g,炒枳实15 g,丹参15 g,北沙参15 g,茯苓30 g,川芎12 g,赤芍药12 g。水煎服,每日1剂,分2次服。适用于冠心病偏阴虚者。

(8) Danshen (*Radix Salviae Miltiorrhizae*) 40 g, Chuanxiong (*Rhizoma Chuanxiong*) 25 g, Chishaoyao (*Radix Paeoniae Rubra*) 20 g, Honghua (*Flos Carthama*) 10 g and Maodongqing (*Radix Ilicis Pubescentis, pounded and to be decocted first*) 40 g. Decoct the drugs with water and take the decoction in two divided doses daily. It is applicable to CHD with stagnation of heart blood.

（8）丹参40 g,川芎25 g,赤芍药20 g,红花10 g,毛冬青(砸碎,先下)40 g,水煎服,每日1剂,分2次服。适用于冠心病心血瘀阻者。

3. External Therapy

(1) Jianghuang (*Rhizoma Curcumae Longae*) 10 g, Wutou (*Radix Aconiti Kusnezoffii or Radix Aconiti*) 5 g, Xuejie (*Resina Draconis*) 5 g, Hujiao (*Fructus Piperis*) 1 g, Shensanqi (*Radix Notoginseng*) 3 g, Guizhi (*Ramulus Cinnamomi*) 5 g, Shexiang (*Moschus*) 0.1 g, Chuanxiong (*Rhizoma Chuanxiong*) 5 g and Xiebai (*Bulbus Allii Macrostemi*) 10 g. Pulverize the drugs and mix the powder with excipient to prepare small plasters (1.5 g drugs each), apply the plasters onto Tanzhong (CV 17) and Xinshu (BL 15). This is applicable to angina pectoris.

3. 外治法

（1）姜黄10 g,乌头5 g,血竭5 g,胡椒1 g,参三七3 g,桂枝5 g,麝香0.1 g,川芎5 g,薤白10 g。研末,加入赋形剂,制成每张重1.5 g小膏药待用,贴敷膻中、心俞穴。适用于冠心病心绞痛者。

(2) Zhizi (*Fructus Gardeniae*) 12 g, Taoren (*Semen Persicae*) 12 g and honey 30 g. Pulverize the drugs and mix the powder with honey to make paste. Ap-

（2）栀子12 g,桃仁12 g,炼蜜30 g。上两药研末,加炼蜜调成糊状,摊敷在心前区,

ply the paste of about 7 cm × 15 cm in size onto the pre-
cardial region, cover it with gauze. In the beginning,
change the dressing once every 3 days for two times, then
change it once every 7 days afterwards, 6 times as a
treatment course. This is applicable to various types of
CHD.

(3) Chuanxiong (*Rhizoma Chuanxiong*) 4.8 g, Wu-
tou (*Radix Aconiti*) 15 g, Xixin (*Herba Asari*) 15 g,
Zhifuzi (*Radix Aconiti Lateralis Preparata*) 15 g,
Qianghuo (*Rhizoma et Radix Notopterygii*) 15 g, Guixin
(*Cortex Cinnamomi*) 15 g and Shujiao (*Pericarpium
Zanthoxyli*) 15 g. Pulverize the drugs, sift the powder
and wrap it with a piece of silk cloth, warm it over mild
fire and press the back with it till the chest pain stops.
This is applicable to suffocative pain in the chest and
back.

2.2.4　Viral Myocarditis

General Description

Viral myocarditis is characterized by myocardial inflammatory changes resulting from viral infection. In mild
cases, only localized lesions exist and no clinical symptoms can be found. In serious cases, however, edema and
necrosis appear extensively in cardiac muscle cells, which
may cause arrhythmia, heart failure and sudden death or
may develop into a chronic problem. This disease usually
occurs in summer and autumn and affects the people aged
20 to 30, more common in males than in females.

It is caused mostly by the infection of Coxsackie virus, ECHO virus, poliovirus and enterovirus. Generally,
the pathologic changes are simply caused by viruses at the
early stage, but associated with immune response at the

摊敷的面积约7 cm×15 cm,然
后纱布敷盖,初用时,每 3 日
换药 1 次;2 次后,7 日换药 1
次,6 次为 1 个疗程。适用于
冠心病各证型。

(3) 川芎4.8 g,乌头15 g,
细辛 15 g,制附子15 g,羌活
15 g,桂心15 g,蜀椒15 g。上
药研末,过筛,帛裹微火烤,热
熨背上,胸痛止则停止。适用
于胸背闷痛者。

第四节　病毒性心肌炎

【概述】

病毒性心肌炎系病毒感
染引起的以心肌炎性病变为
主要表现的疾病。轻者成灶
性病变,可无症状;重者大片
心肌细胞水肿、坏死,可致心
律失常、心力衰竭、猝死或转
为慢性。本病多见 20～30
岁,男性多于女性,发病以夏
秋季节为高。

本病的病因以柯萨奇病
毒、埃可病毒、脊髓灰质病毒、
肠道病毒为常见。一般认为
本病早期以病毒直接作用为

later stage or in the chronic period.

According to the clinical manifestations, viral myocarditis belongs to the categories of "shi re du" (epidemic dampness heat), "shi xing du" (seasonal contagious toxin), "wen du" (epidemic heat syndrome), "xin ji" (palpitation) and "zheng chong" (severe palpitation), etc. in TCM. Its pathogenic factors are exogenous pathogenic toxic heat, improper diet, overstrain, and congenital insufficiency. Its main pathogenesis is healthy qi deficiency causing invasion of pathogenic factors to the lung, intestines and heart, followed by qi and yin deficiency of the heart, blockage of blood stasis in blood vessels, interior retention of fluid, and collapse of heart yang ultimately.

Essentials for Diagnosis

(1) History of viral infection, such as upper respiratory tract infection or diarrhea 1 - 3 weeks prior to the attack.

(2) Newly developed symptoms of palpitation, shortness of breath and chest distress, and signs of arrhythmia, gallop rhythm, low heart sounds and enlarged cardiac dullness area. No history of heart disease.

(3) Laboratory examinations show detachment of virus from the pharynx or feces, 4-time increased ratio of antibody neutral titer of serum Coxsackie virus when compared with the first division of serum (or the ratio of the first antibody titer ≥1 : 640), positive serum anti-cardiac-muscle antibody (1 : 10), and possible increase of serum GOT, LDH, CPK and its isoenzymes.

(4) ECG shows nonspecific changes of ST segment, flattened, biphasic, or inverted T wave, various arrhythmias, ventricular hypertrophy, prolonged QT segment and low voltage. X-ray may reveal normal heart shadow in

主,后期及慢性期与免疫反应有关。

根据本病的临床表现,属中医学"湿热毒"、"时行毒"、"温毒"、"心悸"、"怔忡"等范畴。其病因为外感温热邪毒,内伤饮食,劳倦太过,先天禀赋不足;主要病机为正气不足,邪毒入内,犯肺、侵肠、损心,继之心之气阴亏虚,血脉瘀阻,痰饮内停,终见心阳气衰脱之证。

【诊断要点】

(1) 病前 1~3 个星期有上呼吸道感染或腹泻等病毒感染史。

(2) 既往无心脏病而近期出现心悸、气短、胸闷不适等症状和心律失常、奔马律、心音低钝、心界扩大等体征。

(3) 实验室检查咽部或粪便中可分离出病毒;血清柯萨奇病毒中和抗体滴定效价较第一份血清升高 4 倍,或首次抗体效价≥1 : 640;血抗心肌抗体阳性(1 : 10);部分病人血清 GOT、LDH、CPK 及其同工酶增高。

(4) 心电图检查,最常见非特异性的 ST 段移位、T 波平坦、双相或倒置。可出现各种心律失常。也可有心室肥

localized myocarditis, or enlarged shadow and decreased pulsation in extensive myocarditis or cases complicated by pericarditis, and pulmonary congestion or edema in severe cases. Besides, ultrasound cardiogram and nuclein test are helpful to diagnosis.

大、QT 间期延长、低电压等。X 线检查,局灶性心肌炎者心影可无改变,病变广泛者或合并心包炎可见心影增大、搏动减弱,严重者可见肺瘀血或肺水肿。此外,超声心动图、核素检查均有助于诊断。

Syndrome Differentiation and Treatment

Syndrome differentiation should be focused on the determination of deficiency and excess. The former includes collapse of yang and depletion of qi, deficiency of both qi and yin, and deficiency of both yin and yang; the latter involves toxic heat disturbing the heart, interior stagnation of phlegm and damp, and blockage of heart vessel by blood stasis. So the treatment method is to clear away toxic heat in the heart and yingfen and to reinforce qi and nourish yin. But for different cases, the methods should vary: to promote blood circulation and remove blood stasis for prolonged blockage of blood stasis; to recuperate depleted yang and stop collapse for severe cases with heart yang tending to collapse; to tonify healthy qi and strengthen the body resistance for cases with absence of pathogenic factors and presence of healthy qi deficiency after illness.

【辨证论治】

本病辨证以辨虚实为主,热毒侵心、痰湿内阻和心脉瘀阻证属实;阳虚气脱、气阴两虚和阴阳两虚证属虚。治疗以清解心营热毒为主,兼以益气养阴为其大法。若病久瘀阻者,应活血化瘀;病情危重,心阳欲脱者,急宜回阳固脱;病后邪去正虚者,应扶正固本。

1. Toxic-heat Disturbing the Heart

Chief Manifestations: Fever, general aching, nasal obstruction and discharge, itching and sore throat, cough with sputum, abdominal pain, diarrhea, discomfort of muscles and limbs, palpitation, feeling of oppression in the chest, shortness of breath, red tongue with thin yellow or greasy coating, thready and rapid or slow-irregular and intermittent pulse.

Therapeutic Methods: To clear away heat, remove toxic substances and nourish heart yin.

1. 热毒侵心证

主要证候 发热身痛,鼻塞流涕,咽痒喉痛,咳嗽咯痰,腹痛泄泻,肌痛肢楚,继之心悸惕动,胸闷气短,舌质红、苔薄黄或腻,脉细数或结代。

治 法 清热解毒,滋养心阴。

Prescription: Modified Yin Qiao San (Lonicerae and Forsythiae Powder), composed of Jinyinhua (*Flos Lonicerae*) 10 g, Lianqiao (*Fructus Forsythiae*) 12 g, Jingjie (*Herba Schizonepetae*) 10 g, Dandouchi (*Semen Sojae Preparatum*) 10 g, Jiegeng (*Radix Platycodi*) 6 g, Gancao (*Radix Glycyrrhizae*) 6 g, Zhuye (*Herba Lophatheri*) 12 g and Lugen (*Rhizoma Phragmitis*) 30 g.

Modifications: For pronounced swelling and sore throat, add Shandougen (*Radix Sophorae Tonkinensis*) 10 g and Qingdai (*Indigo Naturalis*, to be infused separately) 6 g; for high fever and irritability, add Shengshigao (*Gypsum Fibrosum*, to be decocted first) 30 g, Zhimu (*Rhizoma Anemarrhenae*) 10 g and Huangqin (*Radix Scutellariae*) 6 g; for feeling of oppression in the chest, vomiting, yellow and greasy tongue coating, add Ganlu Xiaodu Dan (Sweet Dew Detoxification Pill, wrapped) 15 g, Huang lian (*Rhizoma Coptidis*) 6 g, Baishaoyao (*Radix Paeoniae Alba*) 10 g, Fuling (*Poria*) 10 g and Muxiang (*Radix Aucklandiae*) 10 g; for feeling of oppression in the chest, add Danshen (*Radix Salviae Miltiorrhizae*) 15 g, Taoren (*Semen Persicae*) 12 g and Jiangxiang (*Lignum Dalbergiae Odoriferae*) 6 g; for palpitation, add Chaosuanzaoren (*Semen Jujubae*, stirbaked) 15 g and Baiziren (*Semen Platycladi*) 15 g.

2. Collapse of Yang and Depletion of qi

Chief Manifestations: Acute onset, shortness of breath and palpitation with difficulty in lying on the back, purple lips, irritability, spontaneous sweating, extremely cold limbs, pale or grayish tongue with thin coating, indistinct, thready and intermittent or thready and extremely faint pulse.

Therapeutic Methods: To recuperate yang, replenish qi and relieve collapse.

方 药 银翘散加减: 金银花10g,连翘12g,荆芥 10g,淡豆豉10g,桔梗6g,甘 草6g,竹叶12g,芦根30g。

加 减 咽喉肿痛明显 者,加山豆根10g,青黛(冲服) 6g;壮热心烦者,加生石膏(先 煎)30g,知母10g,黄芩6g;胸 闷呕吐,舌苔黄腻者,加甘露 消毒丹(包煎)15g,黄连6g, 白芍药10g,茯苓10g,木香 10g;胸闷痛者,加丹参15g, 桃仁12g,降香6g;心悸怔忡 者,加炒酸枣仁15g,柏子仁 15g。

2. 阳虚气脱证

主要证候 起病急骤,气 喘心悸,倚息不得卧,口唇青 紫,烦躁不安,自汗不止,四肢 厥冷,舌质淡白或舌暗,苔薄, 脉微细代,或脉细欲绝。

治 法 回阳益气固脱。

Prescription: Modified Shen Fu Long Mu Tang (Decoction of Ginseng Rubra, Aconiti Lateralis, Os Draconis and Concha Ostreae), composed of Hongshen (*Radix Ginseng Rubra*, to be decocted separately) 10 g, Zhifuzi (*Radix Aconiti Lateralis Preparata*, to be decocted first) 10 g, Zhigancao (*Radix Glycyrrhizae, roasted*) 6 g, Shenglonggu (*Os Draconis*, to be decocted first) 25 g and Shengmuli (*Concha Ostreae*, to be decocted first) 25 g.

Modifications: For cases at critical stage with sudden faint and cold limbs due to pathogenic factors invading pericardium resulting in internal obstruction and external exhaustion, use Zhibao Dan (Bolus of Precious Drugs) 1 bolus and Zixue Dan (Purple Snow Bolus) 1 bolus or Suhexiang Wan (Styrax Bolus) 1 bolus.

3. Deficiency of Both Qi and Yin

Chief Manifestations: Palpitation, shortness of breath, felling of oppression in the chest and spontaneous sweating which are aggravated by exertion, lassitude, insomnia, dreamfulness, dry mouth and tongue, discomfort of throat, red tongue with little fluid, and thready and rapid or slow-irregular or intermittent pulse.

Therapeutic Methods: To replenish qi, nourish yin, and tranquilize the mind.

Prescription: Modified Zhigancao Tang (Glycyrrhizae Preparata Decoction) and Shengmai San (Powder for Reinforcing Qi and Nourishing Yin), composed of Zhigancao (*Radix Glycyrrhizae*, roasted) 12 g, Shengjiang (*Rhizoma Zingiberis Recens*) 10 g, Taizishen (*Radix Pseudostellariae*) 12 g, Guizhi (*Ramulus Cinnamomi*) 10 g, Shendihuang (*Radix Rehmanniae*) 30 g, Ejiao (*Colla Corii Asini*, to be melted and infused separately) 6 g, Maimendong (*Fructus Hordei Germinatus*) 10 g and Dazao (*Fructus Jujubae*) 5 pcs.

方　药　参附龙牡汤加减：红参(另煎)10 g,制附子(先煎)10 g,炙甘草6 g,生龙骨(先煎)25 g,生牡蛎(先煎)25 g。

加　减　急性期突见晕厥肢冷,乃属邪陷心包,内闭外脱者,可合用至宝丹、紫雪丹或苏合香丸各1粒。

3. 气阴两虚证

主要证候　心悸气短,胸闷自汗,动则尤甚,神疲乏力,失眠多梦,口舌干燥,咽部不适,舌红少津,脉细数或结代。

治　法　益气养阴,养心安神。

方　药　炙甘草汤合生脉散加减：炙甘草12 g,生姜10 g,太子参12 g,桂枝10 g,生地黄30 g,阿胶(烊化冲服)6 g,麦门冬10 g,大枣5枚。

Modifications: For lassitude and pronounced spontaneous sweating, add Huangqi (*Radix Astragali*) 15 g and Baizhu (*Rhizoma Atractylodis Macrocephalae*) 12 g; for feverish sensation in the chest, palms and soles, tidal fever, night sweating, flushed cheeks and dry mouth, add Xuanshen (*Radix Scrophulariae*) 15 g, Shashen (*Radix Glehniae*) 12 g and Wuweizi (*Fructus Schisandrae*) 10 g; for palpitation and restlessness, add Suanzaoren (*Semen Ziziphi Spinosae*) 15 g, Baiziren (*Semen Platycladi*) 15 g, Shenglonggu (*Os Draconis*, to be decocted first) 25 g, Shengmuli (*Concha Ostreae*, to be decocted first) 25 g and Zhenzhumu (*Concha Margaritifera Usta*, to be decocted first) 20 g.

4. Interior Stagnation of Phlegm and Dampness

Chief Manifestations: Chest pain and oppression, shortness of breath, palpitation, dizziness, abdominal fullness, poor appetite, pale and swollen tongue with pale and greasy coating, and soft-superficial and smooth or slow-irregular and intermittent pulse.

Therapeutic Methods: To resolve phlegm, eliminate dampness, warm and activate heart yang.

Prescription: Modified Gualou Xiebai Banxia Tang (Decoction of Trichosanthis, Allii Macrostemi and Pinelliae), composed of Gualou (*Fructus Trichosanthis*) 20 g, Banxia (*Rhizoma Pinelliae*) 6 g, Xiebai (*Bulbus Allii Macrostemi*) 10 g, Ganjiang (*Rhizoma Zingiberis*) 6 g, Chenpi (*Pericarpium Citri Reticulatae*) 10 g and Baikouren (*Semen Amomi Rotundus*, to be decocted later) 3 g.

Modifications: For pronounced palpitation, add Fuling (*Poria*) 12 g, Xingren (*Semen Armeniacae Amarum*) 10 g, and Gancao (*Radix Glycyrrhizae*) 6 g; for suffocative sensation in the chest, dyspnea with inability to lie flat, add Zhike (*Fructus Aurantii*) 10 g, Tinglizi

加　减　肢体倦怠,乏力,自汗明显者,加黄芪15 g,白术12 g;五心烦热,潮热,盗汗,颧红,口干者,加玄参15 g,沙参12 g,五味子10 g;心悸不宁者,加酸枣仁15 g,柏子仁15 g,生龙骨(先煎)25 g,生牡蛎(先煎)25 g,珍珠母(先煎)20 g。

4. 痰湿内阻证

主要证候　胸闷憋气,胸痛心悸,头晕目眩,脘痞纳呆,舌体淡胖,舌苔白腻,脉濡滑或结代。

治　法　化痰逐湿,温通心阳。

方　药　瓜蒌薤白半夏汤加减:瓜蒌20 g,半夏10 g,薤白6 g,干姜6 g,陈皮10 g,白蔻仁(后下)3 g。

加　减　胸闷,心悸明显者,加茯苓12 g,杏仁10 g,甘草6 g;气憋,喘促不能平卧者,加枳壳10 g,葶苈子15 g,大枣5枚。

(*Semen Lepidii seu Descurainiae*) 15 g and Dazao
(*Fructus Jujubae*) 5 pcs.

5. Blockage of Heart Vessel by Blood Stasis

Chief Manifestations: Localized chest pain sometimes with stabbing sensation, palpitation, purple lips,
shortness of breath, dark tongue with occasional ecchymosis and petechiae, thready, unsmooth and slow-irregular or intermittent pulse.

Therapeutic Methods: To promote blood circulation to remove blood stasis, dredge collaterals and tranquilize the mind.

Prescription: Modified Xuefu Zhuyu Tang (Decoc-
tion for Removing Blood Stasis in Chest), composed of
Taoren (*Semen Persicae*) 12 g, Honghua (*Flos Cartha-
ma*) 10 g, Danggui (*Radix Angelicae Sinensis*) 15 g,
Shendihuang (*Radix Rehmanniae*) 15 g, Chishaoyao
(*Radix Paeoniae Rubra*) 12 g, Chuanxiong (*Rhizoma
Chuanxiong*) 12 g, Jiegeng (*Radix Platycodi*) 6 g,
Zhike (*Fructus Aurantii*) 6 g, Niuxi (*Radix Achyran-
this Bidentatae*) 12 g and Gancao (*Radix Glycyrrhizae*)
6 g.

Modifications: For pronounced shortness of breath
and lassitude, add Dangshen (*Radix Codonopsis*) 15 g
and Huangqi (*Radix Astragali*) 12 g; for precordial stabbing pain radiating to the shoulder and back, add Zhichuanwu (*Radix Aconiti, Preparata*) 6 g, Guizhi (*Ramulus
Cinnamomi*) 6 g and Yiyiren (*Semen Coicis*) 30 g.

6. Deficiency of Both Yin and Yang

Chief Manifestations: Palpitation, shortness of
breath, lassitude, pale complexion, cold limbs, loose
stool, soreness of lower back, pale tongue with thin and
white coating, and deep and thready or slow-irregular and
intermittent pulse.

Therapeutic Methods: To warm yang, replenish

5. 心脉瘀阻证

主要证候 心悸,胸痛,
痛有定处,可有刺痛,唇甲青
紫,气短微喘,舌质偏暗,或有
瘀点、瘀斑,脉细涩结代。

治 法 活血化瘀,通络
宁心。

方 药 血府逐瘀汤加
减:桃仁12 g,红花10 g,当归
15 g,生地黄15 g,赤芍药12 g,
川芎12 g,桔梗6 g,枳壳6 g,牛
膝12 g,甘草6 g。

加 减 气短,乏力明显
者,加党参15 g,黄芪12 g;心
前区刺痛,胸痛彻背者,加制
川乌6 g,桂枝6 g,薏苡仁30 g。

6. 阴阳两虚证

主要证候 心悸怔忡,气
短乏力,面色㿠白,四肢清冷,
大便溏泄,腰酸乏力,舌质淡,
苔薄白,脉沉细或结代。

治 法 温阳益气,滋阴

qi, nourish yin and recuperate pulse.

Prescription: Modified Shen Fu Yangying Tang (Decoction of Ginseng Rubra and Aconiti Lateralis for Nourishing Blood), composed of Hongshen (*Radix Ginseng Rubra*, to be decocted separately) 10 g, Guizhi (*Ramulus Cinnamomi*) 10 g, Zhifuzi (*Radix Aconiti Lateralis Preparata*) 10 g, Ganjiang (*Rhizoma Zingiberis*) 5 g, Shendihuang (*Radix Rehmanniae*) 20 g, Dang-gui (*Radix Angelicae Sinensis*) 15 g, Baishaoyao (*Radix Paeoniae Alba*) 12 g, Maimendong (*Fructus Hordei Germinatus*) 10 g, Beishashen (*Radix Glehniae*) 15 g and Huangqi (*Radix Astragali*) 15 g.

Modification: For pronounced chest pain, add Yujin (*Radix Curcumae*) 15 g, Yanhusuo (*Rhizoma Corydalis*) 10 g and Chuanlianzi (*Fructus Meliae Toosendan*) 10 g.

Other Treatments

1. Chinese Patent Drugs

(1) Jinyinhua Lu (Lonicerae Syrup): 10 - 15 ml each time, thrice daily; applicable to acute myocarditis and to prevent for exogenous diseases.

(2) Banlangen ChongJi (Isatidis Granule): 15 g each time, thrice daily; applicable to acute myocarditis.

(3) Fufang Yin Huang Koufuye (Compound Lonicerae and Coptidis Oral Liquid): 10 ml each time, thrice daily; applicable to acute or chronic myocarditis complicated by affection of exogenous pathogenic factors.

(4) Danshen Zhusheye (Salviae Miltiorrhiza Injection): 20 ml in 5% glucose solution for intravenous drop, once daily, 10 - 15 days as a treatment course; applicable to myocarditis with pronounced symptoms of blood stagnation such as palpitation and feeling of oppression in the chest.

复脉。

方药 参附养营汤加减：红参（另煎）10 g，桂枝10 g，制附子10 g，干姜5 g，生地黄20 g，当归15 g，白芍药12 g，麦门冬10 g，北沙参15 g，黄芪15 g。

加减 胸痛明显者，加郁金15 g，延胡索10 g，川楝子10 g。

【其他疗法】

1. 中成药

（1）金银花露 每服10～15 ml，每日3次。适用于预防外感、心肌炎急性期。

（2）板蓝根冲剂 每服15 g，每日3次。适用于心肌炎急性期。

（3）复方银黄口服液 每服10 ml，每日3次。适用于本病急性期或慢性期复感外邪。

（4）丹参注射液 20 ml加入5%葡萄糖溶液中静脉滴注。每日1次，10～15日为1个疗程。适用于心肌炎心悸、胸闷等瘀血证候明显者。

(5) Yupingfeng Koufuye (Jade Screen Oral Liquid):
10 ml each time, twice daily; applicable to chronic myocarditis cases who are debilitated and subject to colds.

(6) Shuanghuanglian Koufuye (Oral Liquid of Coptidis and Phellodendri): 10 ml each time, thrice daily; applicable to myocarditis at acute stage or with repeated attacks of exogenous pathogenic factors.

(7) Shengmai Yin (Decoction for Reinforcing Qi and
Nourishing Yin): 10 - 20 ml each time, twice daily; applicable to myocarditis at chronic stage or at convalescent
stage with deficient healthy qi.

2. Single-drug or Experiential Prescriptions

(1) Jingjie (*Herba Schizonepetae*) 15 g, Fangfeng
(*Radix Saposhnikoviae*) 15 g, Huangqi (*Radix Astra-
gali*) 15 g, Jinyinhua (*Flos Lonicerae*) 15 g, Lianqiao
(*Fructus Forsythiae*) 15 g, Dangshen (*Radix Codonopsis*) 10 g, Zhigancao (*Radix Glycyrrhizae*, roasted)
10 g, Maimendong (*Fructus Ophiopogonis*) 10 g,
Shendihuang (*Radix Rehmanniae*) 10 g, Ejiao (*Colla
Corii Asini*, to be melted) 10 g, Huomaren (*Semen
Cannabis*) 10 g and Baiziren (*Semen Platycladi*) 10 g.
Decoct the drugs with water for 15 minutes, filter and
collect the decoction and then decoct the dregs with water
for 20 minutes. Mix both decoctions thoroughly and take
in several times, 1 - 2 doses daily. This is applicable to
acute or chronic myocarditis complicated with affection of
exogenous pathogenic factors.

(2) Xuanshen (*Radix Scrophulariae*) 20 g and
Shengdihuang (*Radix Rehmanniae*) 20 g. Decoct the
drugs with water and take the decoction, 1 dose daily.
This is applicable to chronic myocarditis cases subject to
exogenous diseases.

(3) Jinyinhua (*Flos Lonicerae*) 30 g, Banlangen
(*Radix Isatidis*) 30 g, Lianqiao (*Fructus Forsythiae*)

（5）玉屏风口服液　每服
10 ml,每日 2 次。适用于心肌
炎慢性期体弱易于外感者。

（6）双黄连口服液　每服
10 ml,每日 3 次。适用于心肌
炎反复外感或急性期。

（7）生脉饮　每服 10～
20 ml,每日 2 次。适用于心肌
炎慢性期或恢复期正气较
虚者。

2. 单验方

（1）荆芥15 g,防风15 g,
黄芪15 g,金银花15 g,连翘
15 g,党参10 g,炙甘草10 g,麦
门冬 10 g,生地黄 10 g,阿胶
(烊化)10 g,火麻仁10 g,柏子
仁10 g。加水煎 15 分钟,滤出
药液,再加水煎 20 分钟,去
渣,两煎所得药液兑匀,分服,
每日 1～2 剂。适用于本病急
性期或慢性期复感外邪。

（2）玄参20 g,生地黄
20 g。水煎服,每日 1 剂。适
用于心肌炎慢性期体弱易于
外感者。

（3）金银花30 g,板蓝根
30 g,连翘18 g,大青叶18 g,芦

18 g, Daqingye (*Folium Isatidis*) 18 g, Lugen (*Rhizoma Phragmitis*) 18 g, Shengdihuang (*Radix Rehmanniae*) 18 g, Maimendong (*Fructus Ophiopogonis*) 18 g, Mudanpi (*Cortex Moutan Radicis*) 12 g and Xuanshen (*Radix Scrophulariae*) 12 g. Decoct the drugs with water and take the decoction, 1 dose daily. This is applicable to acute or chronic myocarditis complicated with affection of exogenous pathogenic factors.

(4) Fuling (*Poria*) 15 g, Rougui (*Cortex Cinnamomi*, to be decocted later) 15 g, Baizhu (*Rhizoma Atractylodis Macrocephalae*) 15 g, Zhigancao (*Radix Glycyrrhizae*, roasted) 15 g, Dangshen (*Radix Codonopsis*) 15 g, Shendihuang (*Radix Rehmanniae*) 15 g, Guizhi (*Ramulus Cinnamomi*) 9 g, Maren (*Semen Cannabis*) 9 g, Ejiao (*Colla Corii Asini*, to be melted) 9 g and Dazao (*Fructus Jujubae*) 5 pcs. Decoct the drugs with water and take the decoction, 1 dose daily. This is applicable to myocarditis.

3. External Therapy

(1) Wannianqing (*Radix et Rhizoma Rohdeae Japonicae*) 10 g, Kushen (*Radix Sophorae Flavescentis*) 10 g, Shashen (*Radix Adenophorae*) 10 g, Danshen (*Radix Salviae Miltiorrhizae*) 10 g and Dangshen (*Radix Codonopsis*) 10 g. Decoct the drugs with 3,000 ml of water for 20 minutes, remove the dregs and pour the decoction into a basin, add in 3,500 ml of water, and bathe the whole body for 30 minutes, 7 days as a treatment course. This is applicable to myocarditis with constant chest pain and oppression, palpitation and shortness of breath.

(2) Nanxing (*Rhizoma Arisaematis*) 10 g and Chuanwu (*Radix Aconiti*) 10 g. Pulverize the drugs and mix the powder with melted yellow wax, apply it onto the centers of palms and soles in the evening and remove it

根18 g,生地黄18 g,麦门冬18 g,牡丹皮12 g,玄参12 g。水煎服,每日1剂。适用于本病急性期或慢性期复感外邪。

(4) 茯苓15 g,肉桂(后下)15 g,白术15 g,炙甘草15 g,党参15 g,生地黄15 g,桂枝9 g,麻仁9 g,阿胶(烊化)9 g,大枣5枚。水煎服,每日1剂。适用于心肌炎患者。

3. 外治法

(1) 万年青10 g,苦参10 g,沙参10 g,丹参10 g,党参10 g。上药加水3 000 ml,煮沸20分钟,去渣取汁,倒入盆中,兑水3 500 ml浸洗全身,每次30分钟,7 日为1个疗程。适用于病毒性心肌炎胸闷时痛,心悸气短者。

(2) 南星10 g,川乌10 g,共为细末,用黄蜡融化摊于手、足心。每日1次,晚敷晨取,10 日为1个疗程。适用于

the next morning, once daily, 10 days as a treatment course. This is applicable to myocarditis with palpitation due to deficiency of heart yang and obstruction of collaterals by blood stasis.

心悸心阳衰弱、瘀血阻络者。

2.2.5　Epilepsy

General Description

Epilepsy, a common chronic paroxysmal disease in nervous system, is a clinical syndrome characterized by sudden transient cerebral dysfunction resulting from repeated abnormal electric discharge of neuron, manifested mainly as motorial, sensory, mental and behavioral disorders and vegetative nerve functional disturbance. The disease occurs in people of all ages from the new-born to the aged, most likely in those around 5 years old and teenages, and more common in males than in female, its incidence being 0.3%–0.7%.

This disease is usually associated with genetic and acquired factors. The former refers to congenital defect, and the latter includes craniocerebral injury, various kinds of cerebritis, meningitis, cerebroma, cerebrovascular disease, parasitosis, metabolic disturbance and intoxication.

In view of the clinical manifestations, it belongs to the categories of "dian xian" (epilepsy), "xian zheng" (epileptic syndrome) and "yang xian feng" (informal term of epilepsy) in TCM. Its causative factors are emotional disorder, congenital defect and drastic fright, and its pathogeneses are phlegm accumulation, adverse flow of qi and wind-phlegm obstruction. The diseased zang-organs are the heart and liver, with the spleen and kidney also

第五节　癫痫

【概述】

癫痫为常见的神经系统慢性发作性疾病,是以在病程中有反复发作的神经元异常放电引致的、暂时性突发性大脑功能失常为特征的一组临床综合征。临床主要表现为运动、感觉、意识、行为及植物神经障碍的现象。自新生儿至老年均可发病,尤以5岁前后和青春期为发病高峰,男性多于女性,其发病率为0.3%~0.7%。

本病的发生多与遗传因素和获得性因素有关。获得性因素包括先天性发育异常、颅脑损伤、各种脑炎、脑膜炎、脑瘤、脑血管病、寄生虫病、代谢障碍和中毒等。

根据本病的临床表现,属中医学"癫痫"、"痫证"、"羊痫风"范畴。其病因与情志失调、先天不足、大惊大恐等因素有关。发病机理为痰聚气逆,风痰闭阻;病变脏器主要在于心、肝,涉及脾、肾;久发不愈,邪伤精气,可致心肾

involved. If the disease lasts long, healthy qi may be impaired by pathogenic factors, resulting in deficiency of the heart and kidney.

Essentials for Diagnosis

(1) Acute onset with dizziness, chest distress and sighing are the premonitory symptoms. In typical cases, the patient may fall on the ground suddenly, lose consciousness, stare upwards, spit foamy saliva, scream with strange sound and convulse. The patient may regain consciousness shortly after the attack and behaves like ordinary people, feeling very tired. In other cases, the patient may only stop activities suddenly, drop things unexpectedly, or lower the head suddenly then raise it soon afterwards, or stare up for a few seconds to several minutes. The patient knows nothing of what has happened after the attack.

(2) Many patients, especially those whose first attack began in childhood, may have congenital defect or family history of epilepsy. The attack is often induced by fright, strain, emotional upsets, improper or contaminated diet, head trauma, or indulgence in sexual relations.

(3) Electroencephalograph may show epileptic waves (spike, sharp, or spike-slow wave). Craniocerebral CT and MRI are helpful to the diagnosis.

Syndrome Differentiation and Treatment

There are syndromes of deficiency and excess in this disease. Syndromes such as obstruction of wind-phlegm, excessive internal phlegm-fire and internal blockage of blood stasis belong to the excess, while deficiency of the heart and kidney, and deficiency of the liver yin and kidney yin pertain to the deficiency. The secondary and the principal aspects and the deficiency and excess syndromes

亏虚。

【诊断要点】

（1）起病多骤急，发作前常有眩晕、胸闷、叹息等先兆。典型病例发则突然仆倒，不省人事，两目上视，口吐涎沫，四肢抽搐，或口中怪叫。移时苏醒，除疲乏无力外，一如常人。也有动作中断，手中物件落地，或头突然向前倾下而后迅速抬起，或两目上吊，多在数秒至数分钟即可恢复，对上述主要证候在发作后全然无知。

（2）多有先天因素或家族史，尤其与病发于幼年者的关系密切。每因惊恐、劳累、情志过极、饮食不节或不洁，或头部外伤，或劳欲过度等诱发。

（3）实验室检查脑电图可发现癫痫样波（棘波、尖波、棘慢复合波），必要时颅脑 CT、MRI 检查有助于明确诊断。

【辨证论治】

本病有虚有实，风痰闭阻、痰火内盛和瘀血内阻证属实；心肾亏虚和肝肾阴虚证属虚。治疗时需分清标本虚实。发作时以治标为主，着重豁痰顺气，熄风开窍；平时则以治本为重，宜补益肝肾，养心健

should be differentiated before the treatment is given. During the attack, the secondary aspect must be treated first, with the treatment focusing on eliminating phlegm and regulating qi, and suppressing wind and opening the orifices. During the remission, the principal aspect should be treated, with the treatment focusing on tonifying the liver and kidney, nourishing the heart and invigorating the spleen, together with resolving phlegm and dredging collaterals.

1. Obstruction of Wind-phlegm

Chief Manifestations: Falling down suddenly, unconsciousness, convulsions, upward staring, clenched jaws, spitting foamy saliva, and screaming during the attack, dizziness, chest distress and lassitude before the attack, white greasy tongue coating, and wiry and smooth pulse.

Therapeutic Methods: To eliminate phlegm, suppress wind, cause resuscitation and arrest convulsion.

Prescription: Modified Dingxian Wan (Pill for Relieving Epilepsy), composed of Zhuli (*Succus Bambusae*) 10 g, Shichangpu (*Rhizoma Acori Tatarinowii*) 10 g, Danxing (*Arisaema cum Bile*) 10 g, Qingbanxia (*Rhizoma Pinelliae*) 10 g, Tianma (*Rhizoma Gastrodiae*) 10 g, Quanxie (*Scorpio*) 5 g, Baijiangcan (*Bombyx Batryticatus*) 10 g, Hupofen (*Succinum*, to be powdered and infused separately) 1 g, Fushen (*Sclerotium Poriae Circum Radicem Pini*) 10 g, Yuanzhi (*Radix Polygalae*) 10 g and Zhigancao (*Radix Glycyrrhizae*, roasted) 5 g.

Modifications: For conjunctivitis, constipation and forceful rapid pulse due to stagnated phlegm transforming into fire, add Huanglian (*Rhizoma Coptidis*) 4 g and Longdancao (*Radix Gentianae*) 6 g; for the persistent attack of epilepsy and convulsion, add Shijueming (*Concha Haliotidis*, to be decocted first) 30 g, Gouteng

脾,佐以化痰通络。

1. 风痰闭阻证

主要证候 发时突然跌倒,神志不清,抽搐,两目上视,口噤,口吐涎沫,并有吼叫声,发作前有眩晕、胸闷、乏力,舌苔白腻,脉象弦滑。

治　法 涤痰熄风,开窍定痫。

方　药 定痫丸加减:竹沥10 g,石菖蒲10 g,胆星10 g,清半夏10 g,天麻10 g,全蝎5 g,白僵蚕10 g,琥珀粉(另冲)1 g,茯神10 g,远志10 g,炙甘草5 g。

加　减 若痰郁化火,目赤,便秘,脉数有力者,可酌加黄连4 g,龙胆草6 g;若痫证持续发作,抽搐不止,可加石决明(先煎)30 g,钩藤10 g,羚羊角粉(另冲)1 g。

(*Ramulus Uncariae cum Uncis*) 10 g and Ling-yangjiaofen (*Cornu Saigae Tataricae*, powdered and to be infused separately) 1 g.

2. Excessive Internal Phlegm-fire

Chief Manifestations: Falling down suddenly, unconsciousness, convulsions, splitting foamy saliva and screaming during the attack, impatience, restlessness, insomnia, bitter and dry mouth, difficult expectoration of sputum, constipation, red tongue with yellow greasy coating, and wiry, smooth and rapid pulse during the remission.

Therapeutic Methods: To purge liver fire, resolve phlegm and cause resuscitation.

Prescription: Modified Longdan Xiegan Tang (Gentianae Decoction for Purging Liver Fire) and Ditan Tang (Decoction for Eliminating Phlegm), composed of Longdancao (*Radix Gentianae*) 6 g, Shichangpu (*Rhizoma Acori Tatarinowii*) 10 g, Huangqin (*Radix Scutellariae*) 10 g, Zhizi (*Fructus Gardeniae*) 10 g, Mutong (*Caulis Akebiae*) 5 g, Juhong (*Exocarpium Citri Rubrum*) 10 g, Qingbanxia (*Rhizoma Pinelliae*) 10 g, Fuling (*Poria*) 10 g, Danxing (*Arisaema cum Bile*) 10 g and Zhigancao (*Radix Glycyrrhizae*, roasted) 5 g.

Modifications: For constipation due to excessive phlegm-fire, add Zhishi (*Fructus Aurantii Immaturus*) 10 g, Mengshi (*Lapis Chloriti*, to be decocted first) 15 g and Shengdahuang (*Radix et Rhizoma Rhei*, to be decocted later) 5 - 10 g; for dry mouth with desire to drink and red tongue with little coating due to excessive fire impairing body fluid, add Maimendong (*Radix Ophiopogonis*) 12 g and Nanshashen (*Radix Adenophorae*) 12 g.

3. Internal Blockage by Blood Stasis

Chief Manifestations: Suddenly falling down, unconsciousness, convulsions, or possible muscle contrac-

2. 痰火内盛证

主要证候 发作时昏仆、抽搐、吐涎、吼叫,平时性情急躁,心烦失眠,口苦而干,咯痰不爽,便秘,舌红,苔黄腻,脉弦滑数。

治 法 清肝泻火,化痰开窍。

方 药 龙胆泻肝汤合涤痰汤加减:龙胆草6 g,石菖蒲10 g,黄芩10 g,栀子10 g,木通5 g,橘红10 g,清半夏10 g,茯苓10 g,胆星10 g,炙甘草5 g。

加 减 痰火内盛,大便秘结,加枳实10 g,礞石(先煎)15 g,生大黄(后下)5～10 g;火盛伤津,出现口干欲饮,舌红少苔者,加麦门冬12 g,南沙参12 g。

3. 瘀血内阻证

主要证候 发则卒然昏仆,抽搐,或仅有口角、眼角、

tions of mouth, eyes and limbs, and purple complexion and lips during the attack; dizziness, localized headache, dark red tongue with occasional ecchymosis, thin and white tongue coating, and unsmooth pulse during the remission. These manifestations are usually secondary to craniocerebral injury, birth trauma and intracranial infection.

Therapeutic Methods: To promote blood circulation to remove blood stasis, suppress wind and activate collaterals.

Prescription: Modified Xuefu Zhuyu Tang (Decoction for Removing Blood Stasis in Chest), composed of Taoren (*Semen Persicae*) 10 g, Honghua (*Flos Carthama*) 10 g, Danggui (*Radix Angelicae Sinensis*) 10 g, Chuanxiong (*Rhizoma Chuanxiong*) 10 g, Chishaoyao (*Radix Paeoniae Rubra*) 10 g, Chuanniuxi (*Radix Cyathulae*) 10 g, Jiegeng (*Radix Platycodi*) 6 g, Chaihu (*Radix Bupleuri*) 6 g, Zhike (*Fructus Aurantii*) 10 g, Shendihuang (*Radix Rehmanniae*) 10 g and Gancao (*Radix Glycyrrhizae*) 6 g.

Modifications: For cases complicated with phlegm, add Zhibanxia (*Rhizoma Pinelliae Preparata*) 10 g, Danxing (*Arisaema cum Bile*) 10 g and Zhuru (*Caulis Bambuswae in Taeniam*) 10 g; for pronounced convulsions, add Gouteng (*Ramulus Uncariae cum Uncis*, to be decocted later) 10 g, Dilong (*Pheretima*) 10 g and Quanxie (*Scorpio*) 5 g; for severe blood stagnation, add Shuizhi (*Hirudo*) 3 g and Mengchong (*Tabanus*) 6 g.

4. Deficiency of the Heart and Kidney

Chief Manifestations: Frequent recurrence, palpitation, amnesia, dizziness, soreness and weakness in the lumbar region and knees, lassitude, thin tongue coating, and thready and weak pulse.

Therapeutic Methods: To nourish the heart and

肢体抽搐,颜面口唇青紫,平素多有头昏头痛,痛有定处,舌质暗红或有瘀斑,苔薄白,脉涩。多继发于颅脑外伤、产伤、颅内感染性疾患等。

治 法 活血化瘀,熄风通络。

方 药 血府逐瘀汤加减:桃仁10 g,红花10 g,当归10 g,川芎10 g,赤芍药10 g,川牛膝10 g,桔梗6 g,柴胡6 g,枳壳10 g,生地黄10 g,甘草6 g。

加 减 挟痰者,加制半夏10 g,胆星10 g,竹茹10 g;抽搐明显者,加钩藤(后下)10 g,地龙10 g,全蝎5 g;瘀血重者,加水蛭3 g,虻虫6 g。

4. 心肾亏虚证

主要证候 癫痫反复发作,心悸健忘,头晕目眩,腰膝酸软,神疲乏力,苔薄腻,脉细弱。

治 法 补益心肾,健脾

kidney, invigorate the spleen and resolve phlegm.

Prescription: Modified Da Buyuan Jian (Potent Decoction for Replenishing Primordial Qi) and Liujunzi Tang (Six Mild-Drug Decoction), composed of Dangshen (*Radix Codonopsis*) 10 g, Baizhu (*Rhizoma Atractylodis Macrocephalae*) 10 g, Fuling (*Poria*) 10 g, Chenpi (*Pericarpium Citri Reticulatae*) 10 g, Jiangbanxia (*Rhizoma Pinelliae*, ginger prepared) 10 g, Jiangzhuru (*Caulis Bambuswae in Taeniam*, ginger prepared) 10 g and Zhigancao (*Radix Glycyrrhizae*, roasted) 6 g.

Modifications: For lingered epilepsy with a dull look, add Fuxiaomai (*Fructus Tritici Levis*) 10 g and Dazao (*Fructus Jujubae*) 5 pcs; for nausea, vomiting and spitting foamy saliva due to excessive turbid phlegm, add Danxing (*Arisaema cum Bile*) 10 g, Gualou (*Fructus Trichosanthis*) 10 g, Shichangpu (*Rhizoma Acori Tatarinowii*) 10 g and Xuanfuhua (*Flos Inulae*, wrapped) 10 g; for loose stools, add Yiyiren (*Semen Coicis*) 20 g, Chaobiandou (*Semen Lablab Album*, stir-baked) 10 g and Paojiang (*Rhizoma Zingiberis*, roasted in hot cinders) 6 g.

5. Deficiency of Liver Yin and Kidney Yin

Chief Manifestations: Frequent recurrence, absent-mindedness, dizziness, dry eyes, dark complexion, dry and lusterless helix, amnesia, insomnia, soreness and weakness in the lumbar region and knees, dry and hard stool, red tongue, and thready, rapid pulse.

Therapeutic Methods: To nourish the liver and kidney, and suppress hyperactive yang to tranquilize the mind.

Prescription: Modified Zuogui Wan (Pill for Replenishing Kidney Yin), composed of Shudihuang (*Radix Rehmanniae Preparata*) 12 g, Shanyao (*Rhizoma Dioscoreae*) 10 g, Shanzhuyu (*Fructus Corni*) 10 g,

化痰。

方 药 大补元煎合六君子汤加减:党参10 g,白术10 g,茯苓10 g,陈皮10 g,姜半夏10 g,姜竹茹10 g,炙甘草6 g。

加 减 病变日久不愈,神情呆滞者,加浮小麦10 g,大枣 5 枚;痰浊盛而恶心呕吐痰涎者,加胆星10 g,瓜蒌10 g,石菖蒲10 g,旋覆花(包煎)10 g;大便溏薄者,加薏苡仁20 g,炒扁豆10 g,炮姜6 g。

5. 肝肾阴虚证

主要证候 痫病频发,神思恍惚,头晕目眩,两目干涩,面色晦暗,耳轮焦枯不泽,健忘失眠,腰膝酸软,大便干燥,舌质红,脉细数。

治 法 滋补肝肾,潜阳安神。

方 药 左归丸加减:熟地黄12 g,山药10 g,山茱萸10 g,枸杞子10 g,鹿角胶(烊化冲服)10 g,龟甲胶(烊化冲

Gouqizi (*Fructus Lycii*) 10 g, Lujiaojiao (*Colla Cornus Cervi*, to be melted and infused separately) 10 g, Guijiajiao (*Colla Carapacis et Plastri Testudinis*, to be melted and infused separately) 10 g, Tusizi (*Semen Cuscutae*) 10 g, Niuxi (*Radix Achyranthis Bidentatae*) 10 g, Yuanzhi (*Radix Polygalae*) 6 g and Zhigancao (*Radix Glycyrrhizae*, roasted) 6 g.

Modifications: For long-standing absent-mindedness, add Sheng Muli (*Concha Ostreae*, to be decocted first) 20 g, Biejia (*Carapax Trionycis*, to be decocted first) 15 g, Baiziren (*Semen Platycladi*) 10 g, Cishi (*Magnetitum*, to be decocted first) 30 g, Chuanbeimu (*Bulbus Fritillariae Cirrhosae*) 10 g, Tianzhuhuang (*Concretio Silicea Bambusae*) 10 g and Zhuru (*Caulis Bambuswae in taeniam*) 10 g; for restless fever, add Zhizi (*Fructus Gardeniae*) 10 g and Lianzixin (*Plumula Nelumbinis*) 10 g; for dry and hard stool, add Xuanshen (*Radix Scrophulariae*) 10 g, Tianhuafen (*Radix Trichosanthis*) 15 g, Huomaren (*Semen Cannabis*) 10 g and Yuliren (*Semen Pruni*) 10 g.

Other Treatments

1. Chinese Patent Drugs

(1) Zhenxian Pian (Tablet for Relieving Epilepsy): 10 tablets taken with warm boiled water each time, thrice daily; applicable to epilepsy and contraindicated in pregnant women. Abnormal emotions such as worry, pensiveness and angry should be avoided.

(2) Dianxianning Pian (Tablet for Curing Epilepsy): 4 - 6 tablets each time, taken with ginger soup or boiled water thrice daily; applicable to epilepsy due to phlegm-heat. Mutton, alcohol and pungent food are contraindicated. It is not suitable for deficient syndromes and should not be taken in heavy dose for a long time in excess syndromes.

服) 10 g, 菟丝子10 g, 牛膝 10 g, 远志6 g, 炙甘草6 g。

加 减 神思恍惚, 持续时间长者, 加生牡蛎 (先煎) 20 g, 鳖甲 (先煎) 15 g, 柏子仁 10 g, 磁石 (先煎) 30 g, 川贝母 10 g, 天竺黄10 g, 竹茹10 g; 心中烦热者, 加栀子10 g, 莲子心 10 g; 大便干燥者, 加玄参 10 g, 天花粉15 g, 火麻仁10 g, 郁李仁10 g。

【其他疗法】

1. 中成药

(1) 镇痫片 成人每服 10 片, 每日 3 次, 温开水送服。适用于痫证。忌忧思恼怒, 孕妇忌服。

(2) 癫痫宁片 每服4~6 片, 每日 3 次, 姜汤或白开水送服, 适用于痫证之痰热实火者。忌羊肉、酒辛。虚证勿用, 实证亦不宜长期超量服用。

(3) Renshen Guipi Wan (Ginseng Pill for Invigorating Spleen and Nourishing Heart): 1 bolus each time, twice daily; applicable to eilepsy with spleen deficiency at remission stage.

(4) Liuwei Dihuang Wan (Bolus of Six Drugs Containing Rehmanniae): 6 g each time, twice daily; applicable to epilepsy with kidney deficiency at remission stage.

(5) Yangxian Fengdian Wan (Pill for Arresting Epilepsy): 3 g each time, twice daily; applicable to epilepsy but used with caution for pregnant women.

2. Single-drug or Experiential Prescriptions

(1) Yujin (*Radix Curcumae*) 21 g, Baifan (*Alumen*) 9 g, Tianzhuhuang (*Concretio Silicea Bambusae*) 6 g, Hupo (*Succinum*) 6 g, Zhusha (*Cinnabaris*) 3 g and Bohe (*Herba Menthae*) 3 g. Dry and pulerize the drugs, screen the powder with a 100 - mesh sieve, fill the capsules with the powder. Take 3 g, thrice daily. Continue to use this prescription if it does work within 3 weeks. It is applicable to epilepsy with wind-phlegm.

(2) Danshen (*Radix Salviae Miltiorrhizae*) 30 g, Chishaoyao (*Radix Paeoniae Rubra*) 12 g, Honghua (*Flos Carthama*) 4.5 g, Yejiaoteng (*Caulis et Folium Polygoni Multiflori*) 30 g, Suanzaoren (*Semen Ziziphi Spinosae*) 15 g, Dilong (*Pheretima*) 9 g and Zhenzhumu (*Cincha Margaritifera Usta*, to be decocted first) 30 g. Decoct the drugs with water for oral use. It is applicable to epilepsy with restlessness due to blood stasis blockage.

(3) Bohe (*Herba Menthae*) 0.2 g, Fangfeng (*Radix Saposhnikoviae*) 0.3 g, Huanglian (*Rhizoma Coptidis*) 0.3 g, Jingjie (*Herba Schizonepetae*) 0.3 g, Danxing (*Arisaema cum Bile*) 0.3 g, Qingbanxia (*Rhizoma Pinelliae*) 0.3 g, Jinyinhua (*Flos Lonicerae*) 0.7 g and Badou (*Fructus Crotonis*, shelled and deoiled) 2 pcs.

（3）人参归脾丸　每服1丸,每日2次。适用于癫痫病缓解期以脾虚为主者。

（4）六味地黄丸　每服6 g,每日2次。适用于癫痫病缓解期以肾虚为主者。

（5）羊痫风癫丸　每服3 g,每日2次。适用于痫证。孕妇慎用。

2. 单验方

（1）郁金21 g,白矾9 g,天竺黄6 g,琥珀6 g,朱砂3 g,薄荷3 g。将上药晒干后研为细末,过100目筛,再将药粉装在空胶囊内备用。每服3粒,每日3次,用药3个星期有效者,可继续服用。适用于癫痫偏风痰者。

（2）丹参30 g,赤芍药12 g,红花4.5 g,夜交藤30 g,酸枣仁15 g,地龙9 g,珍珠母(先煎)30 g。水煎服。适用于癫痫瘀血阻滞,心神不宁者。

（3）薄荷0.2 g,防风0.3 g,黄连0.3 g,荆芥0.3 g,胆星0.3 g,清半夏0.3 g,金银花0.7 g,巴豆2粒(去壳去油)。上药共研细末,再和面粉400 g,芝麻120 g,烙成焦

Pulverize the drugs and mix the powder with 400 g of flour and 120 g of sesame, bake the mixture into cakes and take the cakes by three times in one day. It is applicable to epilepsy with excessive sputum and saliva.

(4) Danshen (*Radix Salviae Miltiorrhizae*) 30 g, Chuanxiong (*Rhizoma Chuanxiong*) 9 g, Honghua (*Flos Carthama*) 4.5 g, Zhibanxia (*Rhizoma Pinelliae Preparata*) 9 g, Danxing (*Arisaema cum Bile*) 6 g, Dilong (*Pheretima*) 9 g, Baijiangcan (*Bombyx Batryticatus*) 9 g, Yejiaoteng (*Caulis et Folium Polygoni Multiflori*) 30 g, Zhenzhumu (*Cincha Margaritifera Usta*, to be decocted first) 30 g. Decoct the drugs with water for oral use. The decoction is applicable to epilepsy due to obstruction of phlegm and blood stasis, and endogenous liver wind.

(5) Dangshen (*Radix Codonopsis*) 24g, Baizhu (*Rhizoma Atractylodis Macrocephalae*) 15 g, Fushen (*Sclerotium Poriae Circum Radicem Pini*) 9 g, Shanyao (*Rhizoma Dioscoreae*) 9 g, Yiyiren (*Semen Coicis*) 9 g, Zhibanxia (*Rhizoma Pinelliae Preparata*) 15 g, Guizhi (*Ramulus Cinnamomi*) 15 g and Zhifuzi (*Radix Aconiti Lateralis Preparata*) 15 g. Decoct the drugs with water for oral use, 1 dose daily. It is applicable to epilepsy with predominant spleen deficiency.

(6) Chantui (*Periostracum Cicadae*) 15 g, Gouteng (*Ramulus Uncariae cum Uncis*, to be decocted later) 30 g, Tianma (*Rhizoma Gastrodiae*) 15 g, Zhusha (*Cinnabaris*) 6 g, Yujin (*Radix Curcumae*) 15 g, Chuanxiong (*Rhizoma Chuanxiong*) 15 g, Mingfan (*Alumen*) 12 g and Zhiquanxie (*Scorpio Preparata*) 15 g. Pulverize the drugs and prepare the powder into gram-sized pills, 3 – 6 g each time, twice daily. It is applicable to epilepsy due to combination of phlegm and blood stasis.

(7) Mafeng Youchong (*Larva Scoliae*, still in the

饼,每日早、中、晚分 3 次服完。适用于痫证痰涎涌盛者。

(4) 丹参30 g,川芎9 g,红花4.5 g,制半夏9 g,胆星6 g,地龙9 g,白僵蚕9 g,夜交藤30 g,珍珠母(先煎)30 g。水煎服。适用于痰瘀交阻,肝风内动之癫痫。

(5) 党参24 g,白术15 g,茯神9 g,山药9 g,薏苡仁9 g,制半夏15 g,桂枝15 g,制附子15 g。水煎服,每日 1 剂。适用于癫痫偏脾虚者。

(6) 蝉蜕15 g,钩藤(后下)30 g,天麻15 g,朱砂6 g,郁金15 g,川芎15 g,明矾12 g,制全蝎15 g。以上各药共研细末,炼糊为丸,为绿豆大。每次服 3~6 g,早晚各 1 次。适用于癫痫痰瘀互结者。

(7) 马蜂幼虫(未出窝的)

comb) 7 –10 g. Deep fry the larvae with cottonseed oil and eat the fried larvae, once daily, 3 – 7 days as a treatment course. It is applicable to various kinds of epilepsy.

3. External Therapy

(1) Yuanhua (*Flos Genkwa*, soaked in vinegar for one day) 100 g, Xionghuang (*Realgar*) 12 g, Danxing (*Arisaema cum Bile*) 20 g and Baihujiao (*Fructus Piperis*) 10 g. Pulverize the drugs and fill the umbilicus fossa with a proper amount of the powder and fix it with adhesive plaster. It is applicable to various kinds of epilepsy.

(2) Adequate amount of Wuzhuyu (*Fructus Evodiae*). Pulverize the drug and fill the umbilical fossa with the powder, fix it with adhesive plaster and change the dressing every 7 – 10 days. It is applicable to frequent attack of epilepsy with sudden convulsions and unconsciousness.

(3) Shufuzi (*Radix Aconiti Lateralis Preparata*) 9 g. Pulverize the drug and mix it with a small amount of flour to make cakes. Put the cake onto Qihai (CV 6) and apply moxibustion with moxa cone on top of the cake for several times. It is applicable to the attack of epilepsy.

(4) Danshen (*Radix Salviae Miltiorrhizae*) 60 g, Maimendong (*Radix Ophiopogonis*) 60 g, Bohe (*Herba Menthae*) 60 g, Fushen (*Sclerotium Poriae Cirum Radicem Pini*) 30 g, Tianma (*Rhizoma Gastrodiae*) 30 g, Chuanbeimu (*Bulbus Fritillariae Cirrhosae*) 30 g, Zhibanxia (*Rhizoma Pinelliae Preparata*) 30 g, Danxing (*Arisaema cum Bile*) 30 g, Juhong (*Exocarpium Citri Rubrum*) 30 g, Yujin (*Radix Curcumae*) 45 g, Mingfan (*Alumen*) 24 g, Yuanzhi (*Radix Polygalae*) 21 g, Quanxie (*Scorpio*) 15 g, Baijiangcan (*Bombyx Batryticatus*) 15 g, Gancao (*Radix Glycyrrhizae*) 15 g, Yazao (*Fructus Gleditsiae*) 15 g, Zhusha (*Cinnabaris*) 15 g, Hupo (*Succinum*) 6 g, Xijiao (*Cornu Rhinocerotis*)

7～10 g,用棉子油炸焦食之,1次服用,连服 3～7 日。适用于癫痫各证型。

3. 外治法

(1) 芫花100 g(醋浸 1 日),雄黄12 g,胆星20 g,白胡椒10 g。取上药末适量纳入脐中,使之与脐平,胶布固定。适用于癫痫各证型。

(2) 吴茱萸适量,研为末,撒入脐窝内,外用胶布固定,7～10 日换药 1 次。适用于癫痫卒然抽搐、不省人事,发作频繁者。

(3) 熟附子9 g,研细末,用面粉少许合做成饼,把饼放在气海穴上。并用艾绒团灸数次。适用于癫痫发作期。

(4) 丹参60 g,麦门冬60 g,薄荷60 g,茯神30 g,天麻30 g,川贝母30 g,制半夏30 g,胆星30 g,橘红30 g,郁金45 g,明矾24 g,远志21 g,全蝎15 g,白僵蚕15 g,甘草 15 g,牙皂15 g,朱砂15 g,琥珀6 g,犀角6 g,雄黄6 g,石菖蒲90 g。上药共研为末,姜汁、竹沥为丸,如弹子大,临用时以姜汁化开,擦胸。适用于癫痫各证型。

6 g, Xionghuang (*Realgar*) 6 g and Shichangpu (*Rhizoma Acori Tatarinowii*) 90 g. Pulverize the drugs and mix the powder with ginger juice and Zhuli (*Succus Bambusae*) to make boluses. At the time of treatment, melt the bolus with ginger juice and rub the chest with it. It is applicable to various kinds of epilepsy.

2.2.6　Schizophrenia

General Description

Schizophrenia is the most commonly encountered psychonosema, characterized usually by thought and perception disorder, depersonalization, and disharmony between psychomotility and environment. Its manifestations mainly include hallucination, delusion, affective disorder and severe behavioral disorder. It may occur in all ages but mostly in young and middle-aged people, with half of the cases aged 21 – 30. Its incidence is about 0.3%-0.8%, higher in urban area than in rural area, and slightly higher in late spring and early summer, with a roughly equal ratio between males and females. It is estimated that about 2 million people suffer from this very harmful disease in the world every year.

No single and decisive cause of this disease has been found so far, but generally, it is related to genetic factors, psychologic and social factors, individual character, emotional irritation, infection, and neuroendocrine dysfunction.

This disease belongs to "dian kuang" (manic-depres-

第六节　精神分裂症

【概述】

精神分裂症系最常见的精神障碍。其基本特征是患者的思维和知觉异常、人格解体、精神活动与环境不协调。临床表现以听幻觉、妄想、情感异常及严重的行为紊乱为主。本病可发生于任何年龄，但多为青壮年，21~30岁发病者约占半数。男女两性发病率无明显差异。城市居民发病率略高于农村，春末夏初的发病率略高于其他季节。其患病率大致为0.3%~0.8%。据估计，全世界每年有新发病患者200万人左右，是一种危害很严重的疾病。

本病至今尚未找出单一的、决定性的致病因素。一般认为与遗传因素、心理社会因素、病前个性特征、情感刺激、感染、神经生化及内分泌紊乱等有关。

根据本病的临床表现，属

sive syndrome) in TCM in accordance with its clinical manifestations. Its causes are congenital defect, anger, fear and fright, or alternate grief and joy, or excessive anxiety. Its pathogenesis is disturbance of turbid phlegm in the heart causing confusion of the mind. Depressive syndrome is attributed to stagnation of phlegm qi while manic syndrome to excessive phlegm fire. In prolonged cases, deficiency of the heart and spleen or hyperactive fire impairing yin may appear.

Essentials for Diagnosis

(1) Presence of schizoid personality such as autism, introversion, sensitivity, abashment, dependence and fantasy in most cases and a family history of schizophrenia in some cases.

(2) Predisposing factors usually exist before the attack, but the clinical symptoms are not related to the factors.

(3) Among the symptoms such as disturbance of association, auditory hallucination, behavioral disorder, feeling of passivity, feeling of being revealed and thought insertion, at least 2 or 3 of them should be present.

Syndrome Differentiation and Treatment

At the initial stage, this disease usually belongs to excess syndrome mostly seen as stagnation of phlegm and qi, phlegm fire disturbing the mind, and blood stasis blocking the heart, while at the late stage, it usually pertains to deficiency syndrome manifested as deficiency of both heart and spleen, and excessive fire impairing yin. The therapeutic principle is to regulate qi and alleviate depression and to activate the mental function. According to the duration of the disease and its pathologic factors, methods such as regulating qi and alleviating depression, clearing heart fire and resolving phlegm, promoting blood circulation and removing blood stasis, invigorating the spleen

中医学"癫狂"范畴。其病因与禀赋不足,恼怒惊恐,或悲喜交加,或思虑不遂等有关。发病机理为痰浊蒙心,神志失常。癫证为痰气郁结,狂证为痰火炽盛;日久可致心脾两虚或火盛伤阴。

【诊断要点】

(1) 病前个性多属孤僻、内向、敏感、怕羞、好依赖、好幻想等分裂人格。部分病人有家族史。

(2) 起病前多有精神刺激诱发因素。起病后,临床症状远离精神刺激因素。

(3) 在联想障碍、幻听、行为障碍、被控制体验、被洞悉感、思维插入等症状中,至少具备2项或3项不典型症状。

【辨证论治】

本病初起多属实证,临床常见痰气郁结、痰火扰神和瘀血阻窍证,病久多虚,常见心脾两虚和火盛伤阴证。治疗以理气解郁,畅达神机为原则。根据其病程新久及病理因素,分别采用理气解郁、清心化痰、活血化瘀、补养心脾、滋阴降火之法。

and nourishing the heart, and nourishing yin and suppressing fire can be used.

1. Stagnation of Phlegm Qi

Chief Manifestations: Depression, apathetic expression, reticence, dementia, incoherent speech or muttering to oneself, changeable moods, no sense of hygiene, no desire for food, red tongue with greasy and white coating, and wiry and smooth pulse.

Therapeutic Methods: To regulate qi, alleviate depression, resolve phlegm and restore consciousness.

Prescription: Modified Shunqi Daotan Tang (Decoction for Regulating Qi and Resolving Phlegm), composed of Chenpi (*Pericarpium Citri Reticulatae*) 10 g, Zhibanxia (*Rhizoma Pinelliae Preparata*) 10 g, Fuling (*Poria*) 10 g, Danxing (*Arisaema cum Bile*) 10 g, Zhishi (*Fructus Aurantii Immaturus*) 10 g, Xiangfu (*Rhizoma Cyperi*) 10 g, Yuanzhi (*Radix Polygalae*) 10 g, Shichangpu (*Rhizoma Acori Tatarinowii*) 10 g, Yujin (*Radix Curcumae*) 10 g and Gancao (*Radix Glycyrrhizae*) 6 g.

Modifications: For frequent belching and feeling of oppression in the chest and abdomen, add Xuanfuhua (*Flos Inulae*, wrapped) 10 g, Daizheshi (*Haematitum*, wrapped) 15 g and Zisugeng (*Caulis Perillae*) 10 g; for restlessness, yellow and greasy tongue coating and smooth and rapid pulse due to phlegm stagnation turning into heat, add Huanglian (*Rhizoma Coptidis*) 5 g and Tianzhuhuang (*Concretio Silicea Bambusae*) 10 g.

2. Deficiency of Both Heart and Spleen

Chief Manifestations: Absent-mindedness, fantasy, palpitation, fright, grief, weeping, weak limbs, impaired appetite, pale tongue with greasy coating, and deep, thready and weak pulse.

Therapeutic Methods: To invigorate the spleen,

1. 痰气郁结证

主要证候　精神抑郁,表情淡漠,沉默痴呆,出言无序,或喃喃自语,喜怒无常,秽洁不分,不思饮食,舌质红,苔腻而白,脉弦滑。

治　法　理气解郁,化痰醒神。

方　药　顺气导痰汤加减:陈皮10 g,制半夏10 g,茯苓10 g,胆星10 g,枳实10 g,香附10 g,远志10 g,石菖蒲10 g,郁金10 g,甘草6 g。

加　减　嗳气频作,胸脘满闷者,加旋覆花(包煎)10 g,代赭石(包煎)15 g,紫苏梗10 g;痰郁化热,烦躁不安,舌苔黄腻,脉滑数者,加黄连5 g,天竺黄10 g。

2. 心脾两虚证

主要证候　神思恍惚,魂梦颠倒,心悸易惊,善悲欲哭,肢体困乏,饮食锐减,舌质淡,苔腻,脉沉细无力。

治　法　健脾养心,调节

nourish the heart and regulate the functional activity of qi.

Prescription: Modified Yangxin Tang (Decoction for Nourishing Heart), composed of Dangshen (*Radix Codonopsis*) 10 g, Huangqi (*Radix Astragali*) 10 g, Danggui (*Radix Angelicae Sinensis*) 10 g, Fushen (*Sclerotium Poriae Circum Radicem Pini*) 10 g, Yuanzhi (*Radix Polygalae*) 10 g, Suanzaoren (*Semen Ziziphi Spinosae*) 20 g, Wuweizi (*Fructus Schisandrae*) 10 g, Baiziren (*Semen Platycladi*) 10 g and Rougui (*Cortex Cinnamomi*, to de decocted later) 3 g.

Modifications: For palpitation and fright, add Cishi (*Magnetitum*, to be decocted first) 25 g and Longchi (*Dens Draconis*, to be decocted first) 25 g; for grief with susceptibility to weeping due to consumption of heart qi, add Zhigancao (*Radix Glycyrrhizae*, roasted) 10 g and Huaixiaomai (*Fructus Tritici Levis*) 10 g.

3. Phlegm Fire Disturbing the Mind

Chief Manifestations: Persistant restlessness, headache, insomnia, staring angrily, flushed complexion and congested eyes; followed by violent behavior like scolding and shouting, climbing over walls and houses, or smashing things and hitting people with extraordinary strength, refusing to eat and sleep, dark red tongue with yellow greasy or yellow dry and dirty coating, and wiry, large, smooth and rapid pulse.

Therapeutic Methods: To purge liver fire, eliminate phlegm and induce resuscitation.

Prescription: Modified Mengshi Guntan Wan (Chloriti Pill for Eliminating Phlegm), composed of Qingmengshi (*Lapis Chloriti*, to be decocted first) 15 g, Dahuang (*Radix et Rhizoma Rhei*, to be decocted later) 6 g, Huangqin (*Radix Scutellariae*) 10 g, Chenxiang (*Lignum Aquilariae Resinatum*) 3 g, Zhebeimu (*Bulbus*

气机。

方 药 养心汤加减:党参10 g,黄芪10 g,当归10 g,茯神10 g,远志10 g,酸枣仁20 g,五味子10 g,柏子仁10 g,肉桂(后下)3 g。

加 减 心悸易惊者,加磁石(先煎)25 g,龙齿(先煎)25 g;心气耗伤,喜悲伤欲哭者,加炙甘草10 g,淮小麦10 g。

3. 痰火扰神证

主要证候 素有性急易怒,头痛失眠,两目怒视,面红目赤,烦躁,突然狂乱无知,骂詈号叫,不避亲疏,逾垣上屋,或毁物伤人,气力逾常,不食不眠,舌质红绛,苔多黄腻或黄燥而垢,脉弦大滑数。

治 法 清泻肝火,涤痰醒神。

方 药 礞石滚痰丸加减:青礞石(先煎)15 g,大黄(后下)6 g,黄芩10 g,沉香3 g,浙贝母10 g,天竺黄10 g,胆星10 g,橘红10 g,连翘15 g,黄芩10 g,栀子10 g,龙胆草 6g。

Fritillariae) 10 g, Tianzhuhuang (*Concretio Silicea Bambusae*) 10 g, Danxing (*Arisaema cum Bile*) 10 g, Juhong (*Exocarpium Citri Rubrum*) 10 g, Lianqiao (*Fructus Forsythiae*) 15 g, Huangqin (*Radix Scutellariae*) 10 g, Zhizi (*Fructus Gardeniae*) 10 g and Longdancao (*Radix Gentianae*) 6 g.

Modifications: For restlessness and thirst with a desire to drink, add Shengshigao (*Gypsum Fibrosum*, to be decocted first) 30 g and Zhimu (*Rhizoma Anemarrhenae*) 10 g; for restlessness and insomnia due to lingered phlegm heat, add Huanglian (*Rhizoma Coptidis*) 5 g, Zhuru (*Caulis Bambuswae in Taeniam*) 10 g and Zhishi (*Fructus Aurantii Immaturus*) 10 g; for excessive yangming fire with constipation, yellow and coarse tongue coating, and solid and large pulse, add Mangxiao (*Natrii Sulfas*, to be infused) 5 g.

4. Excessive Fire Impairing Yin

Chief Manifestations: Prolonged manic state is gradually alleviated and crazy actions controllable by persuasion, but lassitude, polylogia, occasional restlessness, emaciation, flushed and dirty complexion may still exist. Red tongue with little or no coating, and thready and rapid pulse are present.

Therapeutic Methods: To nourish yin, suppress fire, tranquilize the mind and stabilize emotion.

Prescription: Modified Eryin Jian (Eryin Decoction), composed of Shendihuang (*Radix Rehmanniae*) 15 g, Maimendong (*Radix Ophiopogonis*) 15 g, Suanzaoren (*Semen Ziziphi Spinosae*) 15 g, Xuanshen (*Radix Scrophulariae*) 10 g, Fushen (*Sclerotium Poriae Circum Radicem Pini*) 15 g, Huanglian (*Rhizoma Coptidis*) 6 g, Mutong (*Caulis Akebiae*) 3 g and Zhigancao (*Radix Glycyrrhizae*, roasted) 5 g.

Modifications: For yellow and greasy tongue coa-

加 减 烦渴引饮者,加生石膏30 g(先煎),知母10 g;痰热未尽,心烦不寐者,加黄连5 g,竹茹10 g,枳实10 g;阳明热盛,大便秘结,舌苔黄糙,脉实大者,加芒硝(冲)5 g。

4. 火盛伤阴证

主要证候 狂病日久,其势渐减,呼之能自止,但形疲神倦,多言善惊,时而烦躁,形瘦面红而秽,舌红少苔或无苔,脉细数。

治 法 滋阴降火,安神定志。

方 药 二阴煎加减:生地黄15 g,麦门冬15 g,酸枣仁15 g,玄参10 g,茯神15 g,黄连6 g,木通3 g,炙甘草5 g。

加 减 痰火未平,舌苔

ting due to lingered phlegm fire, add Danxing (*Arisaema cum Bile*) 10 g and Zhuru (*Caulis Bambuswae in Taeniam*) 10 g; for amnesia, sore lower back and weak knees, add Guiban (*Plastrum Testudinis*, to be decocted first) 15 g, Gouqizi (*Fructus Lycii*) 10 g and Ejiao (*Colla Corii Asini*, to be melted and infused separately) 10 g.

5. Blood Stasis Blocking the Heart

Chief Manifestations: Insomnia, fright, suspiciousness, visual and auditory hallucination, incoherent speech, dark and lusterless complexion, purplish tongue with occasional ecchymosis, thin and smooth tongue coating, and small and wiry or thready and unsmooth pulse.

Therapeutic Methods: To remove blood stasis and cause resuscitation.

Prescription: Modified Diankuang Mengxing Tang (Decoction for Ceasing Mania and Depression), composed of Taoren (*Semen Persicae*) 10 g, Chishaoyao (*Radix Paeoniae Rubra*) 10 g, Chaihu (*Radix Bupleuri*) 6 g, Xiangfu (*Rhizoma Cyperi*) 10 g, Qingpi (*Pericarpium Citri Reticulatae Viride*) 10 g, Chenpi (*Pericarpium Citri Reticulatae*) 10 g, Dafupi (*Pericarpium Arecae*) 15 g, Sangbaipi (*Cortex Mori*) 15 g, Zisuzi (*Fructus Perillae*) 10 g, Zhibanxia (*Rhizoma Pinelliae Preparata*) 10 g, Gancao (*Radix Glycyrrhizae*) 6 g and Mutong (*Caulis Akebiae*) 5 g.

Modifications: For dry and bitter mouth and yellow and greasy tongue coating, add Huangqin (*Radix Scutellariae*) 10 g; for aversion to cold and cold limbs, add Ganjiang (*Rhizoma Zingiberis*) 6 g and Zhifuzi (*Radix Aconiti Lateralis Preparata*) 6 g; for dark purplish tongue, add Danshen (*Radix Salviae Miltiorrhizae*) 12 g and Honghua (*Flos Carthami*) 10 g.

黄腻者，加胆星 10 g，竹茹 10 g；健忘，腰膝酸软者，加龟版（先煎）15 g，枸杞子 10 g，阿胶（烊化冲服）10 g。

5. 瘀血阻窍证

主要证候　少寐易惊，疑虑丛生，妄见妄闻，言语支离，面色晦暗，舌青紫，或有瘀斑，苔薄滑，脉小弦或细涩。

治　法　疏瘀通窍。

方　药　癫狂梦醒汤加减：桃仁 10 g，赤芍药 10 g，柴胡 6 g，香附 10 g，青皮 10 g，陈皮 10 g，大腹皮 15 g，桑白皮 15 g，紫苏子 10 g，制半夏 10 g，甘草 6 g，木通 5 g。

加　减　口干口苦，舌苔黄腻者，加黄芩 10 g；畏寒肢冷者，加干姜 6 g，制附子 6 g；舌质紫暗者，加丹参 12 g，红花 10 g。

Other Treatments

1. Chinese Patent Drugs

（1）Angong Niuhuang Wan（Calculus Bovis Bolus for Resuscitation）：1 bolus each time, twice daily; applicable to various types of schizophrenia.

（2）Niuhuang Qingxin Wan（Calculus Bovis Bolus for Clearing Heart Fire）：6 g each time, twice daily; applicable to schizophrenia due to deficiency of qi and blood, and excessive endogenous phlegm fire.

（3）Dahuang Zhechong Wan（Pill of Rhei and Eupolyphaga seu Steleophaga）：3 - 6 g each time, twice daily; applicable to schizophrenia due to stagnation of blood stasis.

（4）Mengshi Guntan Wan（Chloriti Pill for Eliminating Phlegm）：6 g each time, twice daily; applicable to schizophrenia due to excessive heat and intractable phlegm.

（5）Suhexiang Wan（Styrax Bolus）：1 bolus each time, twice daily; applicable to schizophrenia due to phlegm obstructing the heart.

（6）Niuhuang Xingnao Pian（Calculus Bovis Tablet for Restoring Consciousness）：4 tablets each time, twice daily; applicable to schizophrenia due to heat invading pericardium and phlegm obstructing the heart.

2. Single-drug or Experiential Prescriptions

（1）Shuizhi（*Hirudo*）60 g, Mengchong（*Tabanus*）60 g, Taoren（*Semen Persicae*）60 g and Dahuang（*Radix et Rhizoma Rhei*）60 g. Pulverize the drugs, fill capsules with the powder and take 6 capsules, thrice daily. It is applicable to schizophrenia due to stagnation of qi and blood.

（2）Yuanhua（*Gemma Genkwa and Folium Genkwa*）. Pulverize the drugs and take 1.5 - 6 g of the powder before meals, 10 - 20 days as a treatment course. It is

【其他疗法】

1. 中成药

（1）安宫牛黄丸 每服1丸,每日2次。适用于精神分裂症各证型。

（2）牛黄清心丸 每服6 g,每日2次。适用于精神分裂症属气血不足,痰火内盛者。

（3）大黄䗪虫丸 每服3～6 g,每日2次。适用于精神分裂症属瘀血内结者。

（4）礞石滚痰丸 每服6 g,每日2次。适用于精神分裂症属实热顽痰者。

（5）苏合香丸 每服1丸,每日2次。适用于精神分裂症属痰迷心窍者。

（6）牛黄醒脑片 每服4片,每日2次。适用于精神分裂症属热入心包,痰迷心窍者。

2. 单验方

（1）水蛭60 g,虻虫60 g,桃仁60 g,大黄60 g,研末装胶囊,每服6个,每日3次。适用于精神分裂症属气滞血瘀证者。

（2）芫花,取花蕾及叶,研成面。每服1.5～6 g,饭前服,10～20日为1个疗程。适

applicable to schizophrenia due to phlegm fire disturbing the heart, but contraindicated in pregnant women, cases with weak constitution and those who have nausea, vomiting, diarrhea after administration of this drug.

(3) Danshen (*Radix Salviae Miltiorrhizae*) 60 g, Yejiaoteng (*Caulis et Folium Polygoni Multiflori*) 30 g, Lingzhi (*Ganoderma Lucidum seu Japonicum*) 10 g and Dazao (*Fructus Jujubae*) 10 pcs. Decoct the drugs, concentrate the decoction into 100 ml, and take the decoction in 3 divided doses daily. It is applicable to various types of schizophrenia.

3. External Therapy

(1) Gansui (*Radix Kansui*) 10 g, Daji (*Radix Euphorbiae Pekinensis*) 10 g, Dahuang (*Radix et Rhizoma Rhei*) 10 g, Baijiezi (*Semen Sinapis*) 6 g, Aiye (*Folium Artemisiae Argyi*) 10 g and Shichangpu (*Rhizoma Acori Tatarinowii*) 10 g. Pulverize the drugs, mix the powder with water into a paste. Apply a proper amount of the paste onto Shenque (CV 8), cover it with gauze and fix with adhesive plaster, once daily. This is applicable to various types of schizophrenia.

(2) Tougucao (*Herba Speranskiae Tuberculatae*) 20 g, Aiye (*Folium Artemisiae Argyi*) 10 g, Shichangpu (*Rhizoma Acori Tatarinowii*) 10 g, Mengshi (*Lapis Chloriti*) 20 g, Yuanzhi (*Radix Polygalae*) 10 g, Yujin (*Radix Curcumae*) 10 g, Danxing (*Arisaema cum Bile*) 10 g, Fuling (*Poria*) 10 g and Fabanxia (*Rhizoma Pinelliae Preparata*) 10 g. Decoct Mengshi first for 30 minutes, add the others and boil for another 30 minutes, remove the dregs, soak a piece of gauze in the decoction and get it wet thoroughly. Apply the warm medicated gauze to Shenque (CV 8), Qihai (CV 6) and Guanyuan (CV 4) for 15 minutes, then soak it again and apply it to Xinshu (BL 15) for 15 minutes, once daily. This is appli-

用于精神分裂症属痰火扰心者。服后有恶心、呕吐、腹泻、体弱者及孕妇忌用。

（3）丹参60 g，夜交藤30 g，灵芝10 g，大枣10 g。制成浓缩煎剂100 ml，每日 3 次口服。适用于精神分裂症各证型。

3. 外治法

（1）甘遂10 g，大戟10 g，大黄10 g，白芥子6 g，艾叶10 g，石菖蒲10 g。上药共研细末，洁净水调成糊状。取适量敷贴于神阙穴，盖以纱布，胶布固定，每日 1 次。适用于各型精神分裂症。

（2）透骨草20 g，艾叶10 g，石菖蒲10 g，礞石20 g，远志10 g，郁金10 g，胆星10 g，茯苓10 g，法半夏10 g。礞石先煎 30 分钟，再加入其余药物煎煮 30 分钟，去渣，将一块洁净纱布浸于药汁之中，使之湿透。取出温度适中后敷于者神阙、气海、关元穴处各 15 分钟。然后再浸泡于药汁中再敷于心俞 15 分钟，每日 1 次。适用于精神分裂症各证型。

cable to various types of schizophrenia.

(3) Aiye (*Folium Artemisiae Argyi*) 150 g, Shichangpu (*Rhizoma Acori Tatarinowii*) 150 g, Baizhi (*Radix Angelicae Dahuricae*) 60 g, Suanzaoren (*Semen Ziziphi Spinosae*) 50 g and Dazao (*Fructus Jujubae*) 60 g. Decoct the drugs first, then take a bath with the warm decoction in a bathtub, once every 3 - 4 days. This is applicable to schizophrenia.

(4) Gansui (*Radix Kansui*) 10 g, Ebushicao (*Herba Centipedae*) 10 g, Lilu (*Rhizoma et Radix Veratri*) 6 g, Baizhi (*Radix Angelicae Dahuricae*) 10 g and Bingpian (*Borneolum Syntheticum*) 5 g. Decoct the first four drugs and concentrate the decoction into 50 ml, then dissolve Bingpian (*Borneolum Syntheticum*) in the decoction and bottle the solution for later use. Fill the dropping bottle with the solution and put 4 - 5 drops in the nostrils, thrice daily. This is applicable to different types of schizophrenia.

(5) Shengtieluo (*Ferrum Squamae*) 20 g, Cishi (*Magnetitum*) 20 g, Danxing (*Arisaema cum Bile*) 10 g, Shichangpu (*Rhizoma Acori Tatarinowii*) 15 g, Baizhi (*Radix Angelicae Dahuricae*) 10 g, Gouteng (*Ramulus Uncariae cum Uncis*) 10 g and Lianqiao (*Fructus Forsythiae*) 10 g. Decoct Shengtieluo (*Squama Ferrum*) first for 30 minutes, remove the dregs, add in the others and decoct for 30 minutes and get the decoction. Soak the cloth waistbelt in the decoction until it is thoroughly wet and fasten it round the waist, change the belt once daily. This is applicable to schizophrenia due to disturbance of phlegm fire.

(6) Shengtieluo 30 g (*Ferrum Squamae*) 30 g, Muli (*Concha Ostreae*) 30 g, Shichangpu (*Rhizoma Acori Tatarinowii*) 15 g, Yujin (*Radix Curcumae*) 15 g, Danxing (*Arisaema cum Bile*) 20 g, Fabanxia (*Rhizo-*

（3）艾叶150 g，石菖蒲150 g，白芷60 g，酸枣仁50 g，大枣60 g。上药煎煮，在避风保暖处沐浴全身。有条件者可浸泡于浴池中，3～4 日 1 次。适用于精神分裂症。

（4）甘遂10 g，鹅不食草10 g，藜芦6 g，白芷10 g，冰片5 g。加水煎煮前 4 味药物50 ml，将冰片溶于药汁，盛入瓶中备用。使用时用小塑料瓶吸取，点滴于鼻腔中 4～5滴，每日 3 次。适用于各型精神分裂症。

（5）生铁落20 g，磁石20 g，胆星10 g，石菖蒲15 g，白芷10 g，钩藤10 g，连翘10 g。生铁落先煎 30 分钟，然后去渣加入其余药物煎煮 30 分钟，取汁。洁净布做成的腰带浸泡于药汁中，使之湿透，取出束于患者腰间。每日换 1次。适用于精神分裂症痰火上扰者。

（6）生铁落30 g，牡蛎30 g，石菖蒲15 g，郁金15 g，胆星20 g，法半夏10 g，礞石20 g，黄连9 g，竹叶10 g，灯心10 g，

ma Pinelliae Preparata) 10 g, Mengshi (*Lapis Chloriti*) 20 g, Huanglian (*Rhizoma Coptidis*) 9 g, Zhuye (*Herba Lophatheri*) 10 g, Dengxin (*Medulla Junci*) 10 g, Chishaoyao (*Radix Paeoniae Rubra*) 10 g, Taoren (*Semen Persicae*) 10 g and Honghua (*Flos Carthama*) 10 g. Decoct Shengtieluo (*Squama Ferrum*) and Mengshi (*Lapis Chloriti*) first for 30 minutes, remove the dregs, add in the others and decoct for another 30 minutes. Use the decoction for retention enema, once daily. This is applicable to schizophrenia due to stagnation of phlegm and qi.

赤芍药 10 g, 桃仁 10 g, 红花 10 g。生铁落、礞石先煎 30 分钟。去渣入余药煎 30 分钟, 取汁, 保留灌肠, 每日 1 次。适用于精神分裂症痰气郁结者。

2.3 Syndrome Patterns of the Spleen and Stomach

第三章　脾胃病证

2.3.1 Chronic Gastritis

第一节　慢性胃炎

General Description

【概述】

Chronic gastritis is the inflammatory lesion of the gastric mucosa caused by a variety of factors. Its clinical manifestations include epigastric discomfort or pain, anorexia, nausea, vomiting, belching, diarrhea, etc. Chronic gastritis has a high incidence with more than 20% of the adults affected and the incidence increases with age. According to the morphological change under the gastrofiberscope, this disease is classified into chronic superficial gastritis and chronic atrophic gastritis. The superficial layer of the gastric membrane is mainly affected in chronic superficial gastritis while chronic atrophic gastritis is characterized by the atrophy of the connatural glands of the gastric membrane, often accompanied with intestinal metaplasia and inflammatory reaction.

慢性胃炎是由各种原因引起的胃黏膜层的炎性病变,临床上多表现为上腹部不适或疼痛、食欲减退、恶心呕吐、嗳气、便溏等。本病的发病率甚高,成人的发病率一般在20%以上,且随年龄增长而增高。根据纤维胃镜下胃黏膜的形态变化,本病可分为慢性浅表性胃炎和慢性萎缩性胃炎两型。慢性浅表性胃炎炎性变主要累及胃黏膜的浅层,慢性萎缩性胃炎是以胃黏膜固有腺体萎缩为特征的病变,常伴有肠上皮化生及炎性反应。

Chronic gastritis belongs to the categories of "wei tong" (gastric pain), "pi man" (feeling of fullness), "ou tu" (vomiting), "cao za" (gastric discomfort) and "tun suan" (acid regurgitation) in TCM. It is believed that chronic gastritis is due to improper diet, irregular intake of food, or overeating of cold and raw food, irritating food, cigarette smoking and indulge in alcohol which dam-

本病属于中医学"胃痛"、"痞满"、"呕吐"、"嘈杂"、"吞酸"等病证范围。中医学认为,本病常由于饮食不节,饥饱无常,或过食生冷、刺激性食物,以及过度吸烟饮酒,损伤脾胃,以致胃失和降,气机

dage the spleen and stomach, causing undescending of stomach qi and qi stagnation; it may also be caused by emotional disturbance which results in stagnant liver qi attacking the stomach, or stagnant liver qi turning into fire which damages stomach yin; or long-term disorders causing qi and blood stagnation in the stomach channel.

Essentials for Diagnosis

(1) The main clinical manifestations include vague pain, burning pain, dull pain or distention in the epigastrium, especially after meals, frequently accompanied with belching, nausea, vomiting and anorexia. In general, there is no obvious physical sign, but slight tenderness appears sometimes.

(2) The secretion of the gastric juice is generally normal in chronic superficial gastritis, but its acidity is sometimes lower or higher. The secretion of gastric juice in a patient with atrophic gastritis is generally less than that in normal patients. The shortage of gastric juice depends on the location and scope of the atrophic area.

(3) The gastroscopy is the most reliable method to diagnose chronic gastritis. The pathological changes of chronic superficial gastritis is commonly seen in the gastric antrum manifested as congestion, edema, or bleeding and erosion of the mucous membrane. Chronic atrophic gastritis is mainly marked by glandular atrophy in the gastric mucosa or epithelial hyperplasia, the erosion and bleeding of the mucous membrane may also be present.

(4) The examination of the pylorus helical bacillus is generally positive, which may be done through gastric juice culture and smear, or urease test.

Syndrome Differentiation and Treatment

The differentiation of chronic gastritis is mainly to identify different syndromes in light of TCM theory. Is

阻滞;或因情志失调,肝失疏泄,横逆犯胃,或肝郁化火,火灼胃阴;或病久气滞血瘀,胃络阻滞等引起。

【诊断要点】

(1) 慢性胃炎临床主要表现有上腹部隐痛、灼痛、钝痛或饱胀,尤以食后为甚,常伴嗳气、恶心、呕吐、食欲不振等。一般无明显的体征,有时上腹部有轻度压痛。

(2) 慢性浅表性胃炎胃酸分泌一般正常,但有时酸度较低或较高。而萎缩性胃炎胃液分泌量一般较正常人为少。胃酸缺乏的程度根据萎缩病变部位和范围而定。

(3) 胃镜检查为诊断慢性胃炎最可靠的方法。慢性浅表性胃炎病变多见于胃窦部,表现为胃黏膜充血、水肿,或有出血和糜烂。慢性萎缩性胃炎主要是胃黏膜腺体的萎缩,或有上皮细胞增生,亦可有黏膜糜烂、出血现象。

(4) 慢性胃炎患者幽门螺杆菌检查多呈阳性。可通过培养、涂片、尿素酶测定等方法检查。

【辨证论治】

慢性胃炎的辨证主要是辨其寒热、虚实、气滞、血瘀的

the case caused by qi stagnation or by blood stagnation? Does the case pertain to cold syndrome or to heat syndrome, to deficiency syndrome or to excess syndrome? Generally, the case with a long course and manifested as cold pain, preference for hot food, vomiting of watery fluid belongs to cold syndrome. The case with a short course and manifested as burning pain, preference for cold food, vomiting of acid fluid belongs to heat syndrome. Deficiency syndrome has a long course with preference for pressure at the painful area, pain aggravated by hunger and alleviated by intake of food. Excess syndrome has a short course with pain aggravated by pressure and intake of food, alleviated by hunger. The case with a short course and manifested as paroxysmal painand distention is caused by qi stagnation. The case with a long course and manifested as continuous, fixed and pricking pain is caused by blood stagnation. The treatment should be based on the principle of regulating the flow of qi, normalizing the function of the stomach and relieving pain. For excess syndrome, cold accumulation, qi stagnation, stomach heat, blood stagnation should be identified and treated respectively by dispersing cold, relieving pain, soothing the liver, clearing liver and stomach heat and removing blood stasis in the channels. For deficiency syndrome, yang deficiency and yin deficiency should be identified and treated by warming the stomach and strengthening middle energizer or nourishing stomach yin.

1. Pathogenic Cold Attacking the Stomach

Chief Manifestations：Sudden onset of gastric pain which is aggravated by pressure and alleviated by hot compression, preference for warmth and aversion to cold, absence of thirst, preference for hot drinks, white tongue coating, wiry and tense pulse.

Therapeutic Methods：To disperse cold, warm the

不同。一般说来，凡病程较长，痛呈冷痛，饮食喜温，泛吐清水者，多属寒证；凡病程较短，痛呈灼痛，饮食喜凉，泛吐酸水者，多属热证。凡病程长，痛处喜按，饥时痛著，进食后痛减者，多属虚证；凡病程短，痛处拒按，饥时痛轻，进食后痛著者，多属实证。凡病程较短，痛呈阵发窜痛、胀痛者，多属气滞；病程较长，疼痛持续，固定不移、刺痛者，多属血瘀。治疗以理气和胃止痛为原则。实证者，应区别寒凝、气滞、胃热、血瘀，分别予以散寒止痛、疏肝解郁、清泄肝胃、通络化瘀之法；虚证者，当辨其虚寒与阴虚，分别治予温胃健中或滋阴养胃。

1. 寒邪犯胃证

主要证候　胃痛突然发生，脘部痛而拒急，痛处喜暖畏寒，温熨可使痛减，口不渴，喜热饮，舌苔白，脉弦紧。

治　法　散寒温胃，理气

stomach, regulate the flow of qi and relieve pain.

Prescription: Modified Liang Fu Wan (Pill of Alpiniae Officinarum and Cyperi) and Zhengqi Tianxiang San (Tianxiang Powder for Restoring Healthy Qi), composed of Gaoliangjiang (*Rhizoma Alpiniae Officinarum*) 5 g, Xiangfu (*Rhizoma Cyperi*) 10 g, Ganjiang (*Rhizoma Zingiberis*) 3 g, Zisuzi (*Herba Perillae*) 10 g, Wuyao (*Linderae*) 6 g, Chenpi (*Pericarpium Citri Reticulatae*) 6 g, Muxiang (*Radix Aucklandiae*) 6 g and Yanhusuo (*Rhizoma Corydalis*) 10 g.

Modifications: For more cold with severe pain, add Rougui (*Cortex Cinnamomi*) 3 g, Shufuzi (*Radix Aconiti Lateralis Preparata*) 6 g; for invasion of cold and dampness in summer with nausea, anorexia, thick and greasy tongue coating, add Huoxiang (*Herba Agastaches*) 10 g, Cangzhu (*Rhizoma Atractylodis*) 10 g and Baikouren (*Fructus Amomi Rotundus*, to be decocted later) 3 g.

2. Damp Heat in the Spleen and Stomach

Chief Manifestations: Fullness or distending pain in the gastric area, anorexia, bitter taste and stickiness in the mouth, heavy sensation in the head and body, dyschesia, feverish sensation in the anus, red tip and margin of the tongue, with yellow and greasy coating, wiry and smooth pulse.

Therapeutic Methods: To clear away heat, remove the turbidity, normalize the function of the stomach and relieve the distention.

Prescription: Modified Sanren Tang (Three-Seed Decoction), composed of Baikouren (*Fructus Amomi Rotundus*, to be decocted later) 3 g, Yiyiren (*Semen Coicis*) 12 g, Houpo (*Cortex Magnoliae Officinalis*) 10 g, Zhibanxia (*Rhizoma Pinelliae Preparata*) 10 g, Tongcao (*Medulla Tetrapanacis*) 5 g, Huashi (*Talcum*,

止痛。

方药 良附丸合正气天香散加减：高良姜5 g，香附10 g，干姜3 g，紫苏子10 g，乌药6 g，陈皮6 g，木香6 g，延胡索10 g。

加减 如寒重痛剧，加肉桂3 g，熟附子6 g；若夏月感受寒湿，伴恶心、纳呆，舌苔厚腻者，加藿香10 g，苍术10 g，白蔻仁（后下）3 g。

2. 脾胃湿热证

主要证候 胃脘痞满或胀痛，不思饮食，口苦口黏，头身困重，大便不爽，肛门灼热，舌边尖红，苔黄腻，脉弦滑。

治法 清热泄浊，和胃除痞。

方药 三仁汤加减：白蔻仁（后下）3 g，薏苡仁12 g，厚朴10 g，制半夏10 g，通草5 g，滑石（包煎）12 g，竹叶10 g，黄连3 g，茵陈12 g，丹参12 g。

wrapped) 12 g, Zhuye (*Herba Lophatheri*) 10 g, Huan-glian (*Rhizoma Copitdis*) 3 g, Yinchen (*Herba Artemisiae Scopariae*) 12 g and Danshen (*Radix Salviae Miltiorrhizae*) 12 g.

Modifications: For nausea and vomiting, add Zhuru (*Caulis Bambusae in Taeniam*) 10 g and Shengjiang (*Rhizoma Zingiberis Recens*) 3 g; for diarrhea and lassitude, add Dangshen (*Radix Codonopsis*) 10 g and Fuling (*Poria*) 12 g; for anorexia, add Jineijin (*Endothelium Corneum Gigeriae Galli*) 6 g, Shenqu (*Massa Medicata Fermentata*) 12 g and Maiya (*Fructus Hordei Germinatus*) 12 g.

3. Disharmony Between the Liver and Stomach

Chief Manifestations: Distending pain in the gastric area radiating to the hypochondriac area, fullness in the chest, belching, frequent sighing, vomiting, restlessness, irritability, dizziness, insomnia, dyschesia, or diarrhea or constipation, pale tongue with thin and yellow coating or thin and white coating, wiry pulse.

Therapeutic Methods: To soothe the liver, normalize the function of the stomach and relieve pain.

Prescription: Modified Chaihu Shugan San (Bupleuri Powder for Soothing Liver Qi), composed of Chaihu (*Radix Bupleuri*) 6 g, Zhike (*Fructus Aurantii*) 10 g, Zhixiangfu (*Rhizoma Cyperi Preparata*) 10 g, Chuanxiong (*Rhizoma Chuangxiong*) 6 g, Chenpi (*Pericarpium Citri Reticulatae*) 6 g, Baishaoyao (*Radix Paeoniae Alba*) 12 g, Shenggancao (*Radix Glycyrrhizae*) 3 g, Honghua (*Flos Carthama*) 10 g, Taoren (*Semen Persicae*) 10 g, Danshen (*Radix Salviae Miltiorrhizae*) 12 g and Ezhu (*Rhizoma Curcumae*) 10 g.

Modifications: For severe pain, add Yanhusuo (*Rhizoma Corydalis*) 10 g, Chuanlianzi (*Fructus Meliae Toosendan*) 10 g and Foshou (*Fructus Citri Sarco-*

加　减　恶心呕吐者,加竹茹10 g,生姜3 g;泄泻,倦怠者,加党参10 g,茯苓12 g;食欲不振明显者,加鸡内金6 g,神曲12 g,麦芽12 g。

3. 肝胃不和证

主要证候　胃脘胀满攻撑作痛,痛连两胁,胸闷嗳气,善太息,呕哕,心烦易怒,头昏寐差,大便不畅,或便溏或便秘,舌质淡红、苔薄黄或薄白,脉弦。

治　法　疏肝理气,和胃止痛。

方　药　柴胡疏肝散加减:柴胡6 g,枳壳10 g,制香附10 g,川芎6 g,陈皮6 g,白芍药12 g,生甘草3 g,红花10 g,桃仁10 g,丹参12 g,莪术10 g等。

加　减　痛甚者,加延胡索10 g,川楝子10 g,佛手6 g;嗳气较频者,加白豆蔻3 g,沉

dactylis） 6 g; for frequent belching, add Baikouren (*Fructus Amomi Rotundum*) 3 g, Chenxiang (*Lignum Aquilariae Resinatum*) 5 g and Xuanfuhua (*Flos Inulae*, wrapped) 6 g; for long-term liver qi stagnation turning into fire, stagnated heat in the liver and stomach with burning pain in gastric area, gastric discomfort and acid regurgitation, add Mudanpi (*Cortex Moutan Radicis*) 10 g, Zhizi (*Fructus Gardeniae*) 10 g, Huanglian (*Rhizoma Copitdis*) 3 g and Wuzhuyu (*Fructus Evodiae*) 3 g; for liver fire damaging yin, add Shengdihuang (*Radix Rehmanniae*) 12 g and Mudanpi (*Cortex Moutan Radicis*) 10 g; for liver qi and blood stagnation, add Danshen (*Radix Salviae Miltiorrhizae*) 12 g, Danggui (*Radix Angelicae Sinensis*) 10 g and Honghua (*Flos Carthami*) 6 g.

4. Blood Stasis Blocking the Collaterals

Chief Manifestations: Pricking or cutting epigastric pain, which is fixed and aggravated by pressure, or hematemesis, tarry stools, gloomy complexion, purple tongue or with purple spots, unsmooth pulse.

Therapeutic Methods: To invigorate blood circulation, remove blood stasis, activate the collaterals and relieve pain.

Prescription: Modified Shixiao San (Powder for Dissipating Blood Stasis), composed of Puhuang (*Pollen Typhae*, wrapped) 10 g, Wulingzhi (*Faeces Trogopterori*) 10 g, Yanhusuo (*Rhizoma Corydalis*) 10 g, Dilong (*Pheretima*) 6 g and Qingpi (*Pericarpium Citri Reticulatae Viride*) 6 g.

Modifications: For qi deficiency, add Huangqi (*Radix Astragali*) 12 g, Huangjing (*Rhizoma Polygonati*) 10 g, Baizhu (*Rhizoma Atractylodis Macrocephalae*) 10 g and Dangshen (*Radix Codonopsis*) 12 g; for qi and blood stagnation with severe pain, add Taoren (*Se-*

香5 g,旋覆花(包煎)6 g;肝气郁结日久化火,肝胃郁热,胃脘灼痛,嘈杂泛酸者,加牡丹皮10 g,栀子10 g,黄连3 g,吴茱萸3 g;肝火伤阴者,加生地黄12 g,牡丹皮10 g;肝郁气滞血瘀者,加丹参12 g,当归10 g,红花6 g。

4. 瘀血阻络证

主要证候 胃脘刺痛或刀割样痛,痛处固定,拒按,或见吐血、黑便,面色晦暗,舌质紫暗或有瘀斑,脉涩。

治 法 活血化瘀,通络止痛。

方 药 失笑散加味。蒲黄(包煎)10 g,五灵脂10 g,延胡索10 g,地龙6 g,青皮6 g。

加 减 兼有气虚者,加黄芪12 g,黄精10 g,白术10 g,党参12 g;血瘀气滞,疼痛剧者,可加桃仁10 g,红花10 g,赤芍药10 g。

men Persicae) 10 g, Honghua (*Flos Carthama*) 10 g and Chishaoyao (*Radix Paeoniae Rubra*) 10 g.

5. Qi Deficiency in the Spleen and Stomach

Chief Manifestations: Fullness in the gastric area, which is worse after intake of food, anorexia, lassitude, loose stools, pale and swollen tongue with thin and white coating, deep and weak pulse.

Therapeutic Methods: To tonify the spleen, nourish qi, strengthen middle energizer and stomach.

Prescription: Modified Buzhong Yiqi Tang (Decoction for Strengthening Middle Energizer and Benefiting Qi), composed of Dangshen (*Radix Codonopsis*) 10 g, Huangqi (*Radix Astragali*) 12 g, Baizhu (*Rhizoma Atractylodis Macrocephalae*) 10 g, Danggui (*Radix Angelicae Sinensis*) 10 g, Chenpi (*Pericarpium Citri Reticulatae*) 6 g, Zhigancao (*Radix Glycyrrhizae*, roasted) 5 g, Shengma (*Rhizoma Cimicifugae*) 6 g, Chaihu (*Radix Bupleuri*) 6 g and Sharen (*Fructus Amommi*, to be decocted later) 3 g.

Modifications: For food retention, add Laifuzi (*Semen Raphani*) 10 g and Maiya (*Fructus Hordei Germinatus*) 12 g; for qi and blood deficiency, add Gouqizi (*Fructus Lycii*) 10 g; for bleeding, add Shensanqifen (*Radix Notoginseng*, powdered and to be infused separately) 3 g and Baiji (*Rhizoma Bletillae*) 10 g.

6. Yang Deficiency in the Spleen and Stomach

Chief Manifestations: Continuous dull pain in the gastric area, which is relieved by warmth, pressure and intake of food, vomiting of clear fluid, anorexia, lassitude, cold limbs, loose stools, pale and swollen tongue with thin and white coating, thready and weak pulse.

Therapeutic Methods: To tonify qi, warm middle energizer, strengthen the spleen and stomach.

Prescription: Modified Huangqi Jianzhong Tang

5. 脾胃气虚证

主要证候 胃脘痞闷,似胀非胀,食少纳呆,食后胀甚,倦怠乏力,大便溏薄,舌质淡胖,苔薄白,脉沉弱。

治 法 补脾益气,健中和胃。

方 药 补中益气汤加减:党参10 g,黄芪12 g,白术10 g,当归10 g,陈皮6 g,炙甘草5 g,升麻6 g,柴胡6 g,砂仁(后下)3 g。

加 减 挟食滞者,加莱菔子10 g,麦芽12 g;气血两虚者,加枸杞子10 g;兼出血者,加参三七粉(另冲)3 g,白及10 g。

6. 脾胃虚寒证

主要证候 胃脘隐隐作痛,绵绵不断,喜暖喜按,得食则减,时吐清水,纳少,神疲乏力,手足欠温,大便溏薄,舌质淡胖,苔薄白,脉细弱。

治 法 益气温中,健脾和胃。

方 药 黄芪建中汤加

(Astragali Decoction for Warming Middle Energizer），composed of Huangqi（*Radix Astragali*）12 g, Guizhi（*Ramulus Cinnamomi*）6 g, Baishaoyao（*Radix Paeoniae Alba*）12 g, Zhigancao（*Radix Glycyrrhizae*, roasted）5 g, Shengjiang（*Rhizoma Zingiberis Recens*）3 g and Dazao（*Fructus Jujubae*）5 pcs.

Modifications：For vomiting of clear fluid, add Chenpi（*Pericarpium Citri Reticulatae*）6 g, Zhibanxia（*Rhizoma Pinelliae Preparata*）6 g and Fuling（*Poria*）12 g; for stomach cold with severe pain, add Gaoliangjiang（*Rhizoma Alpiniae Officinarum*）6 g and Xiangfu（*Rhizoma Cyperi*）10 g; for long-term pain with blood stasis blocking the channels, add Honghua（*Flos Carthama*）10 g, Puhuang（*Pollen Typhae*, wrapped）10 g Wulingzhi（*Faces Trogopterori*）10 g and Danshen（*Radix Salviae Miltiorrhizae*）12 g; for tarry stools, add Paojiangtan（*Rhizoma Zingiberis*, charred）3 g, Zaoxintu（*Terra Flava Usta*）10 g, Baiji（*Rhizoma Bletillae*）10 g and Diyutan（*Radix Sanguisorbae*, charred）12 g.

7. Yin Deficiency in the Spleen and Stomach

Chief Manifestations：Dull burning pain in the gastric area, restlessness and thirsty, dry mouth and throat, discomfort and feverish sensation in the gastric area, dry stools, dizziness, insomnia, poor appetite, or feverish sensation in the palms and soles, red tongue with little coating or cracks on the tongue, or peeling of the coating, thready and rapid pulse.

Therapeutic Methods：To nourish yin, clear away heat, strengthen the stomach and produce body fluid.

Prescription：Modified Yiwei Tang（Decoction for Nourishing Stomach）, composed of Beishashen（*Radix Glehniae*）10 g, Maimendong（*Radix Ophiopogonis*）10 g, Shengdihuang（*Radix Rehmanniae*）12 g, Yuzhu

减：黄芪12 g,桂枝6 g,白芍药12 g,炙甘草5 g,生姜3 g,大枣5 枚。

加　减　泛吐清水较多者,加陈皮6 g,制半夏6 g,茯苓12 g;胃寒痛甚者,加高良姜6 g,香附10 g;若久痛不止,瘀血阻络者,加红花10 g,蒲黄（包煎）10 g,五灵脂10 g,丹参12 g;便黑者,加炮姜炭3 g,灶心土10 g,白及10 g,地榆炭12 g。

7. 脾胃阴虚证

主要证候　胃脘隐隐灼痛,烦渴思饮,口干咽燥,胃中嘈杂灼热,大便干结,头昏寐差,食少纳呆,或有手足心热,舌红少苔或有裂纹,或花剥苔,脉细数。

治　法　养阴清热,益胃生津。

方　药　益胃汤加减：北沙参10 g,麦门冬10 g,生地黄12 g,玉竹10 g,柴胡6 g,地骨皮12 g,佛手6 g。

(*Rhizoma Polygonati Odorati*) 10 g, Chaihu (*Radix Bupleuri*) 6 g, Digupi (*Cortex Lycii*) 12 g and Foshou (*Fructus Citri Sarcodactylis*) 6 g.

Modifications: For stomach heat, add Huanglian (*Rhizoma Copitdis*) 3 g and Zhuye (*Herba Lophatheri*) 10 g; for poor appetite, add Chenpi (*Pericarpium Citri Reticulatae*) 6 g, Shenqu (*Massa Medicata Fermentata*) 12 g and Maiya (*Fructus Hordei Germinatus*) 12 g; for severe pain, add Baishaoyao (*Radix Paeoniae Alba*) 12 g and Zhigancao (*Radix Glycyrrhizae*, roasted) 3 g; for blood stasis, add Danshen (*Radix Salviae Miltiorrhizae*) 12 g and Taoren (*Semen Persicae*) 10 g.

Other Treatments

1. Chinese Patent Drugs

(1) Baohe Wan (Pill for Promoting Digestion): 6 - 9 g each time, twice daily; applicable to fullness and distention in the gastric and abdominal area, belching, anorexia and gastric discomfort.

(2) Shanzha Jianpi Wan (Crataegi Bolus for Invigorating Spleen): 2 boluses each time, twice daily; applicable to fullness and distention of the gastric and abdominal area caused by spleen deficiency and food retention.

(3) Kaixiong Shunqi Wan (Pill for Removing Stagnation in the chest): 3 - 6 g each time, twice daily; applicable to qi stagnation of the liver and stomach, food retention and distending pain in the gastric area.

(4) Liang Fu Wan (Pill of Alpiniae Officinarum and Cyperi): 3 - 6 g each time, twice daily; applicable to gastric pain and abdominal distention caused by cold accumulation and qi stagnation.

(5) Yanhu Zhitong Pian (Corydalis Tablet for Relieving Pain): 4 - 6 tablets each time, twice daily; applicable to gastric pain caused by qi stagnation and blood stasis.

加　减　胃热偏重者,加黄连3 g,竹叶10 g;纳差者,可加陈皮6 g,神曲12 g,麦芽12 g;疼痛较甚者,可加白芍药12 g,炙甘草3 g;兼有瘀滞者,加丹参12 g,桃仁10 g。

【其他疗法】

1.中成药

(1)保和丸　每服6~9 g,每日2次。适用于食滞引起的脘腹胀满,嗳腐厌食,嘈杂不适等症。

(2)山楂健脾丸　每服2丸,每日2次。适用于脾虚积滞内停引起的脘腹痞满胀痛等症。

(3)开胸顺气丸　每服3~6 g,每日2次。适用于肝胃气滞,饮食停滞,胃脘胀痛。

(4)良附丸　每服3~6 g,每日2次。适用于寒凝气滞引起的胃脘疼痛、腹胀喜暖。

(5)延胡止痛片　每服4~6片,每日2次。适用于气滞血瘀引起的胃痛。

(6) Xiang Sha Yangwei Wan (Pill of Aucklandiae and Amomi for Nourishing Stomach): 6 g each time, twice daily; applicable to spleen and stomach qi deficiency, with dull pain in the gastric area which is relieved after intake of food, lassitude and loose stools.

(7) Jianwei Pian (Tablet for Invigoratig Stomach): 3 tablets each time, twice daily; applicable to distending pain in the gastric area, belching and acid regurgitation caused by disharmony of the liver and stomach.

(8) Zuojin Wan (Zuojin Pill): 3 - 6 g each time, twice daily; applicable to pain in the gastric and hypochondriac area, gastric discomfort, bitter taste, nausea and vomiting caused by liver fire attacking the stomach.

(9) Fuzi Lizhong Wan (Aconiti Lateralis Bolus for Regulating Middle Energizer): 6 g each time, twice daily; applicable to yang deficiency of the spleen and stomach.

2. Single-drug or Experiential Prescriptions

(1) Ziwei Yin (Decoction for Nourishing Stomach): composed of Wumei (*Fructus Mume*) 6 g, Chaobaishaoyao (*Radix Paeoniae Alba*, stir-baked) 10 g, Shashen (*Radix Glehniae*) 10 g, Maimendong (*Radix Ophiopogonis*) 10 g, Shihu (*Herba Dendrobii*) 10 g, Danshen (*Radix Salviae Miltiorrhizae*) 10 g, Shengmaiya (*Fructus Hordei Germinatus*) 10 g, Zhijineijin (*Endothelium Corneum Gigeriae Galli*, roasted) 5 g, Meiguihua (*Flos Rosae Rugosae*) 5 g and Zhigancao (*Radix Glycyrrhizae*, roasted) 3 g. Decoct the drugs in water for oral administration, 1 dose daily. It is applicable to chronic superficial gastritis with stomach yin deficiency.

(2) Yizhong Huoxue Tang (Decoction for Benefiting Middle Energizer and Activating Blood): composed of Huangqi (*Radix Astragali*) 30 g, Rougui (*Cortex Cinnamomi*) 8 g, Wuzhuyu (*Fructus Evodiae*) 10 g, Ru-

（6）香砂养胃丸　每服 6g,每日2次。适用于脾胃气虚,胃脘隐痛不适,食后稍缓,伴有疲倦乏力,大便不实或溏薄等。

（7）健胃片　每服3片,每日2次。适用于肝胃不和引起的胃脘胀痛、嗳气、吞酸等。

（8）左金丸　每服3～6g,每日2次。适用于肝火犯胃所致的脘胁疼痛、嘈杂、口苦、泛恶呕吐等症。

（9）附子理中丸　每服 6g,每日2次。适用于脾胃虚寒之证。

2. 单验方

（1）滋胃饮　乌梅肉6g,炒白芍药10g,沙参10g,麦门冬10g,石斛10g,丹参10g,生麦芽10g,炙鸡内金5g,玫瑰花5g,炙甘草3g。水煎服,每日1剂。适用于慢性浅表性胃炎胃阴不足者。

（2）益中活血汤　黄芪30g,肉桂8g,吴茱萸10g,乳香8g,没药8g,生蒲黄(包煎)12g,三棱10g,莪术10g,川芎

xiang (*Olibanum*) 8 g, Moyao (*Myrrha*) 8 g, Shengpu-
huang (*Pollen Typhae*, wrapped) 12 g, Sanleng (*Rhizoma Sparganii*) 10 g, Ezhu (*Rhizoma Curcumae*) 10 g,
Chuanxiong (*Rhizoma Chuangxiong*) 12 g, Wuyao
(*Linderae*) 12 g and Danshen (*Radix Salviae Miltiorrhizae*) 15 g. Decoct the drugs in water for oral administration, one dose daily. It is applicable to chronic superficial gastritis with spleen deficiency and blood stasis.

(3) Wenwei Zhitong Tang (Decoction for Warming
Stomach and Relieving Pain): composed of Guizhi (*Ram-
ulus Cinnamomi*) 5 g, Baishaoyao (*Radix Paeoniae Alba*) 9 g, Wuzhuyu (*Fructus Evodiae*) 6 g, Dingxiang
(*Gemmma Caryophylli*) 3 g, Fuling (*Poria*) 6 g,
Sharen (*Fructus Amommi*, to be decocted later) 5 g,
Paojiang (*Rhizoma Zingiberis Recens*, roasted in hot
cinders) 5 g, Danggui (*Radix Angelicae Sinensis*) 9 g,
Yanhusuo (*Rhizoma Corydalis*) 9 g, Baizhu (*Rhizoma
Atractylodis Macrocephalae*) 12 g and Hongzao (*Fructus Jujubae*) 3 pcs. Decoct the above ingredients in water and take the decoction once daily. It is applicable to
chronic superficial gastritis with severe gastric pain due to
cold accumulation.

(4) Gancao Walengzi San (Powder of Glycyrrhizae
and Concha Arcae): composed of equal amount of Walengzi (*Concha Arcae*) and Gancao (*Radix Glycyrrhizae*).
Grind them into powder and take 5 - 15 g of the powder,
twice daily. It is applicable to chronic superficial gastritis
with excessive gastric juice.

(5) Lian Yu San (Copitdis and Evodiae Powder):
composed of Wuzhuyu (*Fructus Evodiae*) 20 g, Huanglian (*Rhizoma Copitdis*) 6 g, Haipiaoxiao (*Os Sepiae*)
15 g, Muli (*Concha Ostreae*) 15 g and Cangzhu (*Rhizoma Atractylodis*) 10 g. Grind them into powder and take
3 g of the powder, 3 times daily. It is applicable to chron-

12 g,乌药12 g,丹参15 g。水
煎服,每日1剂。适用于慢性
浅表性胃炎中虚血瘀者。

(3) 温胃止痛汤　桂枝
5 g,白芍药9 g,吴茱萸6 g,丁
香3 g,茯苓6 g,砂仁(后下)
5 g,炮姜5 g,当归9 g,延胡索
9 g,白术12 g,大枣3枚。水煎
服,每日1剂。适用于慢性浅
表性胃炎寒凝气滞,胃痛较
著者。

(4) 甘草瓦楞子散　瓦楞
子、甘草各等分,共研为细末,
每次服5~15 g,每日2次。适
用于慢性浅表性胃炎胃酸分
泌较多者。

(5) 连萸散　吴茱萸
20 g,黄连6 g,海螵蛸15 g,牡
蛎15 g,苍术10 g。上药研为
细末,每次服3 g,每日3次。
适用于慢性浅表性胃炎属寒
热错杂者。

ic superficial gastritis with intermingling cold and heat.

(6) Huang Pu Weiyan Tang (Astragali and Taraxaci Decoction for Gastritis): composed of Shenghuangqi (*Radix Astragali*) 30 g, Pugongying (*Herba Taraxaci*) 20 g, Baihe (*Bulbus Lilii*) 20 g, Wuyao (*Linderae*) 10 g, Baishaoyao (*Radix Paeoniae Alba*) 20 g, Gancao (*Radix Glycyrrhizae*) 10 g, Danshen (*Radix Salviae Miltiorrhizae*) 20 g, Chaoshenqu (*Massa Medicata Fermentata*, stir-baked) 10 g, Chaoshanzha (*Fructus Crataegi*, stir-baked) 10 g and Chaomaiya (*Fructus Hordei Germinatus*, stir-baked) 10 g. Decoct the above ingredients in water and take the decoction once daily. It is applicable to chronic atrophic gastritis with spleen and stomach deficiency, retention of food and internal heat accumulation.

(7) Shanzha Maiya Tang (Crataegi and Hordei Germinatus Decoction): composed of crystal sugar 20 g, Shanzha (*Fructus Crataegi*) 50 g and Maiya (*Fructus Hordei Germinatus*) 25 g. Decoct the above ingredients in water and take the decoction once daily. It is applicable to atrophic gastritis with less gastric juice.

(8) Shanzha Mitang Jiang (Crataegi and Honey Paste): composed of crystal sugar 20 g, Shanzha (*Fructus Crataegi*) 60 g and honey 30 g. Steam them in a non-iron container to prepare paste, take 2 - 4 spoons of the paste after meals. This can be taken for a long period of time and is applicable to atrophic gastritis with less gastric juice.

3. External Therapy

(1) Wuzhuyu (*Fructus Evodiae*) 50 g, Ganjiang (*Rhizoma Zingiberis*) 50 g, Dingxiang (*Gemmma Caryophylli*) 50 g, Xiaohuixiang (*Fructus Foeniculi*) 75 g, Rougui (*Cortex Cinnamomi*) 30 g, Shengliuhuang (*Sulfur*) 30 g, Zhizi (*Fructus Gardeniae*) 20 g, Hujiao

（6）黄蒲胃炎汤　生黄芪30 g,蒲公英20 g,百合20 g,乌药10 g,白芍药20 g,甘草10 g,丹参20 g,炒神曲10 g,炒山楂10 g,炒麦芽10 g。水煎服,每日1剂。适用于慢性萎缩性胃炎属脾胃虚弱,食滞不化,内有郁热者。

（7）山楂麦芽汤　冰糖20 g,山楂50 g,麦芽25 g。水煎服,每日1剂。适用于萎缩性胃炎胃酸低者。

（8）山楂蜜糖酱　冰糖20 g,山楂60 g,蜂蜜30 g。将上药放入非铁器皿中蒸熟如果酱,每次饭后食入2～4匙,可长期服用。适用于萎缩性胃炎胃酸低者。

3. 外治法

（1）吴茱萸50 g,干姜50 g,丁香50 g,小茴香75 g,肉桂30 g,生硫黄30 g,栀子20 g,胡椒5 g,荜茇25 g,共研粉末,密贮备用。治疗时取药末

(*Fructus Piperis*) 5 g and Biba (*Fructus Piperis Longi*) 25 g. Grind them into powder for later use. In the treatment, mix 25 g of the powder with 25 g of flour to prepare paste, apply the medicated paste at Shenque (CV8) and fix it with adhesive tape. Keep the application for 3 - 6 hours, once or twice daily. This treatment is applicable to cold in the stomach.

(2) Baizhu (*Rhizoma Atractylodis Macrocephalae*) 120 g, Fuling (*Poria*) 60 g, Baishaoyao (*Radix Paeoniae Alba*) 60 g, Shenqu (*Massa Medicata Fermentata*) 60 g, Maiya (*Fructus Hordei Germinatus*) 60 g, Xiangfu (*Rhizoma Cyperi*) 60 g, Danggui (*Radix Angelicae Sinensis*) 60 g, Zhike (*Fructus Aurantii*) 60 g, Zhibanxia (*Rhizoma Pinelliae Preparata*) 60 g, Chenpi (*Pericarpium Citri Reticulatae*) 20 g, Huanglian (*Rhizoma Copitdis*) 15 g, Wuzhuyu (*Fructus Evodiae*) 15 g, Shanzha (*Fructus Crataegi*) 15 g, Baikouren (*Fructus Amomi Rotundus*) 15 g, Yizhiren (*Fructus Alpiniae Oxyphyllae*) 15 g, Huangqi (*Radix Astragali*) 15 g, Shanyao (*Rhizoma Dioscoreae*) 15 g, Dangshen (*Radix Codonopsis*) 15 g, Muxiang (*Radix Aucklandiae*) 15 g and Gancao (*Radix Glycyrrhizae*) 15 g. Boil the sesame oil first, crush the above ingredients and put them in the oil until they become brownish-yellow, filtrate and remove the dregs, extract the oil into semifluid, then add red lead and stir them well into cream. Put the cream at the acupoints and change it every 3 days. It is applicable to deficiency of the spleen and stomach.

(3) Shengjiang (*Rhizoma Zingiberis Recens*) 500 g. Pound it and get the juice, add Niupijiao (*Colla Corium Bovis Seu Bubali*) 15 g, Ruxiangmo (*Olibanum*, powdered) 15 g and Moyaomo (*Myrrha*, powdered) 15 g. Decoct them in water until they are jellified. Make 3 big plasters, put one on the gastric pain area and

25 g,加入等量面糊调成糊状,贴神阙穴,外用胶布固定,每次敷贴 3～6 小时,每日 1～2 次。用于胃寒证。

(2) 白术120 g,茯苓60 g,白芍药60 g,神曲60 g,麦芽60 g,香附60 g,当归60 g,枳壳60 g,制半夏60 g,陈皮20 g,黄连15 g,吴茱萸15 g,山楂15 g,白蔻仁15 g,益智仁15 g,黄芪15 g,山药15 g,党参15 g,木香15 g,甘草15 g。将上药研碎,先将麻油加热至沸,再将上药放入炸枯,过滤去渣,再熬炼成稠膏状,至滴水成珠不散为度,再加入黄丹搅匀成膏,贴在穴位上,每 3 日更换 1 次。用于脾胃虚弱证。

(3) 生姜500 g,捣取汁,入牛皮胶15 g,乳香末15 g,没药末15 g,水煎,胶化离火,将药作 3 张大膏药,以 1 张贴胃脘痛处,并加热熨之。适用于慢性胃炎表现以胃脘不适,冷

warm it by hot compress. It is applicable to chronic gastritis with gastric discomfort, cold pain, vomiting of clear fluid.

（4） Shengjiang （*Rhizoma Zingiberis Recens*） 100 g, Chenpi （*Pericarpium Citri Reticulatae*） 100 g, Shichangpu （*Rhizoma Acori Tatarinowii*） 30 g, Congbai （*Bulbus Allii Fistulosi*） 60 g, Xiebai （*Bulbus Allii Macrostemi*） 60 g, Huoxiang （*Herba Agastaches*） 60 g, Baimaogen （*Rhizoma Imperatae*） 120 g, Sangye （*Folium Mori*） 120 g, Pipaye （*Folium Eriobotryae*） 120 g, Zhuye （*Herba Lophatheri*） 120 g, Huaizhi （*Ramulus Sophorae Juvenilis*） 240 g, Liuzhi （*Ramulus Salicis Balylonicae*） 240 g, Sangzhi （*Ramulus Mori*） 240 g, Juhua （*Flos Chrysanthemi*） 240 g and Wumei （*Fructus Mume*） 3 pcs. Stew the above the ingredients with sesame oil, prepare them with red lead into extract. Add Shengshigao （*Gypsum Fibrosum*） 240 g, Hanshuishi （*Mirabilitum*） 120 g, Qingdai （*Indigo Naturalis*） 30 g, Mulifen （*Concha Ostreae*, powdered） 100 g, Mangxiao （*Natrii Sulfas*） 100 g and Niupijiao （*Colla corium Bovis seu Bubali*） 120 g into the extract, prepare it with alcohol, apportion the extract to make plasters. Put the plasters at Shangwan （CV 13）, Zhongwan （CV 12）, Xiawan （CV 10） or the umbilicus, apply 1 - 2 plasters in each treatment and change them every seven days. It is applicable to gastritis with stomach heat.

（5） Maogen （*Herba Ranunculi Japonici*, fresh, leaves and stalks removed）. Wash the herbs clean, pound them with brown sugar （about 30% of the herbs） into a paste. Put the paste into the rubber caps of penicilline bottle and apply them at Weishu （BL21） and Shenshu （BL23） for about 15 minutes until feverish sensation appears. If the blisters appear, let them absorbed without breaking them. This is applicable to chronic superficial

痛,呕吐清涎为主者。

（4） 生姜100 g,陈皮100 g,石菖蒲30 g,葱白60 g,薤白60 g,藿香60 g,茅根120 g,桑叶120 g,枇杷叶120 g,竹叶120 g,槐枝240 g,柳枝240 g,桑枝240 g,菊花240 g,乌梅3个,麻油熬,铅丹收,再入生石膏240 g,寒水石120 g,青黛30 g,牡蛎粉100 g,芒硝100 g,牛皮胶120 g,酒蒸化下,分摊膏药。贴上、中、下三脘穴或脐,每次贴1～2张,每7日更换1张。适用于胃热型胃炎。

（5） 鲜毛茛,除去叶、茎,留下根须,清水洗净,然后切碎,加入红糖约30%,捣烂,装入青霉素瓶橡皮盖凹内,敷贴胃俞、肾俞穴,置15分钟左右,局部有烘热感时揭去。如发生水泡,不必刺破,让其自行吸收。本方主治慢性浅表

gastritis with gastric pain as the main manifestation.

(6) Congtou (*Bulbus Allii Fistulosi*, tassels reserved) 30 g and Shengjiang (*Rhizoma Zingiberis Recens*) 15 g. Pound the herbs and stir-bake them hot and fill the bag with them. Press the epigastric area with the bag and change it when it turns cool. Apply this treatment twice a day and 30 minutes for each time or keep the treatment until the pain is relieved. It is applicable to cold in the stomach.

(7) Biba (*Fructus Piperis Lonngi*) 15 g, Ganjiang (*Rhizoma Zingiberis*) 15 g, Gansong (*Radix et Rhizoma Nardostachyos*) 10 g, Shannai (*Rhizoma Kaempferiae*) 10 g, Rougui (*Cortex Cinnamomi*) 10 g, Wuzhuyu (*Fructus Evodiae*) 10 g, Baizhi (*Radix Angelicae Dahuricae*) 10 g, Huixiang (*Fructus Foeniculi*) 6 g and Aiye (*Folium Artemisiae Argyi*) 30 g. Grind them into powder. Make a 20 cm×20 cm square cloth pocket with a piece of soft cotton cloth, put a thin layer of cotton inside and sprinkle the powder on it evenly, sew the packet tight so as to prevent heaping up or leakage of the powder. Put the packet on the gastric area close to the skin and change the herbal powder every 1 - 2 months. It is applicable to gastric pain with deficiency of spleen and stomach yang.

2.3.2 Peptic Ulcer

General Description

Peptic ulcer refers to the benign ulcer in the stomach and duodenum. The clinical presentation includes periodic and rhythmic epigastric pain accompanied with dyspeptic symptoms: acid regurgitation, belching, nausea, vomiting, etc. The ulcer of the stomach, 0. 5 - 2. 5 cm in diameter, is generally larger than that of the duodenum.

性胃炎以胃痛为主症者。

(6) 连须葱头30 g,生姜15 g,两味共捣烂炒烫,热熨胃脘部,药袋冷即更换。每日 2 次,每次 30 分钟,或以疼痛缓解为度。适用于胃寒证。

(7) 荜茇15 g,干姜15 g,甘松10 g,山柰10 g,肉桂10 g,吴茱萸10 g,白芷10 g,茴香6 g,艾叶30 g。上药共研细末,用柔软的棉布40 cm折成20 cm见方的布兜,内铺一薄层棉花,将药均匀撒上,用线密密缝好,以防止药末堆积或漏出,将兜放在胃脘部,药兜内层紧贴皮肤,每 1~2 个月换药 1 次。适用于脾胃虚寒型胃痛。

第二节　消化性溃疡

【概述】

消化性溃疡主要指发生在胃和十二指肠的良性溃疡。临床特征为上腹部有周期性、节律性疼痛,并伴有泛酸、嗳气、恶心、呕吐等消化不良症候。胃溃疡一般比十二指肠

In most cases, there is only one ulcerative focus; in a few cases there may be two ulcerative foci simultaneously, which is called complex ulcer. Peptic ulcer is a frequently encountered disease and it may be found in 10% - 12% of the world's population. Most of the patients are young adults and there are more male patients than female ones. Duodenal ulcer is more common than gastric ulcer and both of them last a long period of 10 - 20 years or even longer. If large quantity of bleeding, perforation, pyloro-chesis and cancerization occur, it is indicative of a critical condition with poor prognosis.

It was thought that the formation of the ulcer is due to the autodigestion of the mucous membrane by the gastric acid and pepsin. In recent years, it has been considered that this disease is closely associated with the infection of helicobacter pylori (HP). In addition, it is also relevant to inheritance, geographic environmental factors, emotions, diet, cigarette smoking and some drugs.

This disease belongs to the scope of "wei wan tong" (epigastric pain), "tun suan" (acid regurgitation) and "cao za" (epigastric upset). It is due to long-term emotional disturbance, improper diet and over exertion. At the early stage, it presents as qi stagnation which is caused by spleen deficiency and liver qi stagnation. Qi stagnation may further turn into heat and cause retention of dampness and stagnation of blood.

Essentials for Diagnosis

(1) Repeated occurrence of chronic, periodic and rhymic epigastric burning, distending pain, dull pain, sharp pain and even colic. The attack is closely associated with food intake. Duodenal ulcer attacks between two meals and relieves after food intake. Gastric ulcer occurs

球部溃疡大，直径为 0.5～2.5 cm。一般溃疡病灶多为单个，少数可同时有 2 个，称为复合性溃疡。本病为全球性多发病，总发病率可能占人口的 10%～12%，以青壮年居多，男性多于女性，十二指肠溃疡比胃溃疡多见。其病程较长，有的可长达一二十年或更长，若并发大量出血、穿孔、幽门梗阻和癌变，则病情凶险，预后不佳。

以往认为溃疡的形成，主要是由于胃酸—胃蛋白酶对黏膜的自身消化作用引起。近年来，认为幽门螺杆菌（HP）感染与本病的发生密切相关。此外，还与遗传、地理环境、精神、饮食因素、吸烟及某些药品等有一定关系。

本病可归属于中医学"胃脘痛"、"吞酸"、"嘈杂"等范畴。多因长期情志失调、饮食不节、劳倦损伤所致。本病初起常呈气滞，多因脾虚或肝郁所致。气郁可化热，可致湿阻或留瘀。

【诊断要点】

（1）反复发作的慢性周期性节律性上腹部灼痛、胀痛、隐痛、刺痛甚至绞痛。节律性与进食关系密切，十二指肠溃疡多发于两餐之间，进食后缓

within the first hour after meal and relieves afterwards and occurs again after the next meal.

（2）Acid regurgitation, heartburn, uncomfortable feeling of hungry, fullness sensation in the epigastrium, belching, nausea, vomiting and increase of salivation.

（3）During the attack, localized tenderness usually occurs in the epigastrium, which locates right in the ulcerative focus. In gastric ulcer, tenderness is in the left side of the epigastric region, while in duodenal ulcer, it is in the right side of the epigastric region.

（4）The circular or elliptical ulcertive areas may be seen through fibergastroscope which is smooth margin and flat-bottom and covered with white coats. The mucous membranes around the ulcer areas are slightly swelling and red. The detection of HP for most of the patients is positive. Niche and irritation may be seen in X-ray with barium meal, or the local membrane folds centralize to the niche.

（5）The test of stools occult blood examination is always positive in active stage. In most of the cases, it will turn into negative through 1 - 2 weeks of active treatment. In gastric juice analysis, the secretion of gastric juice is normal or slightly low in patients with gastric ulcer and always increased in patients with duodenal ulcer.

Syndrome Differentiation and Treatment

The syndrome differentiation of this disease is to identify cold, heat, excess and deficiency. In general, most of the new and acute cases have excess and heat, while most of the chronic cases have deficiency and cold. Clinically, it is classified as syndromes of disharmony of liver and stomach, deficiency of spleen and stomach yang, deficiency of stomach yin, blood stagnation blocking stom-

解；胃溃疡多在进餐后 1 小时内发作，然后缓解，下一次进餐后再次出现。

（2）反酸烧心，有饥饿样不适感、上腹部饱胀感，嗳气、恶心、呕吐、唾液分泌增加等症状。

（3）发作期间常有上腹部局限性压痛，胃溃疡多在上腹部偏左，十二指肠溃疡多在上腹部偏右，与溃疡部位基本相符。

（4）纤维胃镜可见圆形或椭圆形溃疡面，边缘光滑，底部平整，上覆白苔，周围黏膜轻度红肿。幽门螺杆菌检测多数患者呈阳性。X线钡餐造影可见龛影、激惹现象，或局部黏膜皱襞向龛影集中。

（5）大便潜血检查，活动期大便潜血常为阳性，经积极治疗 1～2 个星期内多可转阴。胃液分析，胃溃疡患者胃液分泌正常或稍低，十二指肠溃疡患者多增加。

【辨证论治】

本病辨证主要是辨寒热虚实。一般新病、初病多实、多热，旧病、久病多虚、多寒。临床主要分为肝胃不和、脾胃虚寒、胃阴不足、瘀血阻胃和脾胃湿热证。治疗以健脾和胃，理气化瘀为主要大法，并

ach and damp-heat in spleen and stomach. The treatment principle is to strengthen the spleen and stomach, regulate the flow of qi and remove blood stasis. Depending on the differentiation of stagnated heat, yin deficiency, or yang deficiency, the methods of clearing stomach heat, nourishing stomach yin, warming middle energizer and dispersing cold are practiced.

1. Disharmony of the Liver and Stomach

Chief Manifestations: Fullness and pain in the epigastrium radiating to the hypochondriae regions, which are aggravated by emotional disturbance, frequent sighing, belching, acid regurgitation, red margin and tip of the tongue, thin and white coating, thready and wiry pulse.

Therapeutic Methods: To soothe the liver, normalize the function of the stomach, regulate the flow of qi and relieving stagnation.

Prescription: Modified Chaihu Shugan San (Bupleuri Powder for Soothing Liver Qi), composed of Chaihu (*Radix Bupleuri*) 6 g, Zhike (*Fructus Aurantii*) 10 g, Baishaoyao (*Radix Paeoniae Alba*) 10 g, Zhigancao (*Radix Glycyrrhizae*, roasted) 6 g, Chuanxiong (*Rhizoma Chuangxiong*) 10 g, Zhixiangfu (*Rhizoma Cyperi Preparata*) 10 g, Chuanlianzi (*Fructus Toosendan*) 10 g, Chenpi (*Pericarpium Citri Reticulatae*) 6 g and Yujin (*Radix Curcumae*) 10 g.

Modification: For patients with thirst and bitter taste, add Huanglian (*Rhizoma Copitdis*) 3 g and Zhizi (*Fructus Gardeniae*) 10 g.

2. Deficiency of Spleen Yang and Stomach Yang

Chief Manifestations: Persistent dull pain in the epigastrium which is relieved by warmth and pressure, poor appetite, fullness in the epigastrium, vomiting of watery fluid, cold body and limbs, lassitude, pale

根据郁热、阴虚、虚寒的不同，分别施以清胃热、滋胃阴和温中散寒法。

1. 肝胃不和证

主要证候　胃脘胀满疼痛，痛及两胁，逢情志不舒则加剧，善太息，嗳气，吐酸，舌边尖红，苔薄白，脉细弦。

治　法　疏肝和胃，理气解郁。

方　药　柴胡疏肝散加减：柴胡6 g，枳壳10 g，白芍药10 g，炙甘草6 g，川芎10 g，制香附10 g，川楝子10 g，陈皮6 g，郁金10 g。

加　减　若口干而苦者，加黄连3 g，栀子10 g。

2. 脾胃虚寒证

主要证候　胃脘隐痛，痛势缠绵，持续不已，喜温喜按，纳少脘痞，泛吐清水，手足不温，形寒肢冷，倦怠神疲，面色

complexion, loose stools, or diarrhea with undigested food in the stools, pale and tender tongue, white or watery, smooth coating, deep, thready and weak pulse or deep and slow pulse.

Therapeutic Methods: To warm the middle energizer, warm the stomach and disperse cold.

Prescription: Modified Huangqi Jianzhong Tang (Decoction of Astragali for Warming Middle Energizer) and Lizhong Tang (Decoction for Regulating Middle Energizer), composed of Dangshen (*Radix Codonopsis*) 10 g, Baizhu (*Rhizoma Atractylodis Macrocephalae*) 10 g, Huangqi (*Radix Astragali*) 10 g, Baishaoyao (*Radix Paeoniae Alba*) 10 g, Guizhi (*Ramulus Cinnamomi*) 6 g, Zhigancao (*Radix Glycyrrhizae*, roasted) 6 g, Ganjiang (*Rhizoma Zingiberis*) 3 g and Dazao (*Fructtus Jujubae*) 5 pcs.

Modifications: For patients with sallow complexion, add Danggui (*Radix Angelicae Sinensis*) 10 g; for severe epigastic pain, add Chaopuhuang (*Pollen Typhae*, stir-baked and wrapped) 10 g and Shensanqifen (*Radix Notoginseng*, powdered and to be infused separately) 3 g.

3. Deficiency of Stomach Yin

Chief Manifestations: Epigastric dull pain, gastric discomfort, hunger with no desire for eating, localized feverish sensation, especially in the afternoon and on empty stomach, dry mouth with reduced salivation, belching and retch, dry stools, red tongue with little coating, thready and rapid pulse.

Therapeutic Methods: To nourish stomach yin, promote salivation and clear away heat.

Prescription: Modified Yiwei Tang (Decoction for Nourishing Stomach), composed of Beishashen (*Radix Glehniae*) 12 g, Maimendong (*Radix Ophiopogonis*) 12 g, Shengdihuang (*Radix Rehmanniae*) 12 g, Yuzhu

苍白,大便溏薄,或下利清谷,舌质淡白而嫩,苔白或水滑,脉沉细无力,或沉迟。

治　法　温中健脾,暖胃散寒。

方　药　黄芪建中汤合理中汤加减:党参10 g,白术10 g,黄芪10 g,白芍药 10,桂枝6 g,炙甘草6 g,干姜3 g,大枣5枚。

加　减　面色萎黄者,加当归10 g;胃脘痛明显者,加炒蒲黄(包煎)10 g,参三七粉(另冲)3 g。

3. 胃阴不足证

主要证候　胃脘隐痛,嘈杂似饥,饥不欲食,局部有灼热感,多在午后、空腹时为重,口干少津,嗳气干呕,大便干结,舌质红,少苔,脉细数。

治　法　滋阴养胃,生津清热。

方　药　益胃汤加减:北沙参12 g,麦门冬12 g,生地黄12 g,玉竹10 g,冰糖10 g。

(*Rhizoma Polygonati Odorati*) 10 g and rock sugar 10 g.

Modifications: For blood stasis with severe epigastric pain, add Wulingzhi (*Faces Trogopterori*) 10 g, Shengpuhuan (*Pollen Typhae*, wrapped) 10 g; for patients with fullness sensation in the epigastrum, add Xiangyuan (*Fructus Citri*) 6 g, Foshou (*Fructus Citri Sarcodactylis*) 6 g, Daidaihua (*Flos Citri Amarae Immaturus*) 6 g, and Meiguihua (*Flos Rosae Rugosae*) 6 g.

4. Blood Stagnation Blocking the Stomach

Chief Manifestations: Pricking pain in the epigastrium especially at night, which is localized and aggravated by pressure, hunger with no desire for eating, belching, restlessness, insomnia, purple tongue or with purple spots on the tongue, varicosity under the tongue, deep and unsmooth pulse.

Therapeutic Methods: To regulate qi, activate blood, remove blood stagnation and relieve pain.

Prescription: Modified Shixiao San (Powder for Dissipating Blood Stasis) and Danshen Yin Jiawei (Decoction of Salviae Miltiorrhizae with Additions), composed of Puhuang (*Pollen Typhae*, wrapped) 10 g, Wu-lingzhi (*Faces Trogopterori*) 10 g, Danggui (*Radix Angelicae Sinensis*) 10 g, Chishaoyao (*Radix Paeoniae Rubra*) 10 g, Yanhusuo (*Rhizoma Corydalis*) 10 g, Danshen (*Radix Salviae Miltiorrhizae*) 12 g and Tan-xiang (*Lignum Santali Albi*) 5 g.

Modifications: For qi deficiency with poor appetite and lassitude, add Huangqi (*Radix Astragali*) 12 g and Huangjing (*Rhizoma Polygonati*) 10 g; for qi and blood stagnation with severe pain, add Wuyao (*Linderae*) 10 g and Xiangfu (*Rhizoma Cyperi*) 10 g.

5. Damp Heat in the Spleen and Stomach

Chief Manifestations: Fullness or pain in the

加 减 若挟瘀血,胃痛较剧者,加五灵脂10 g,生蒲黄(包煎)10 g;胃脘胀闷不适者,加香橼6 g,佛手6 g,玳玳花6 g,玫瑰花6 g。

4. 瘀血阻胃证

主要证候 胃脘疼痛,痛如针刺,夜间为甚,痛处固定,拒按,饥而不欲食,嗳气不爽,心烦少寐,舌质紫暗,或有瘀斑、瘀点,或舌下青筋暴露,脉沉涩。

治 法 理气活血,化瘀止痛。

方 药 失笑散合丹参饮加味:蒲黄(包煎)10 g,五灵脂10 g,当归10 g,赤芍药10 g,延胡索10 g,丹参12 g,檀香5 g。

加 减 若兼有气虚,食少神疲者,加黄芪12 g,黄精10 g;血瘀气滞,疼痛较剧者,加乌药10 g,香附10 g。

5. 脾胃湿热证

主要证候 胃脘痞满或

epigastrium, belching, nausea, epigastric upset, acid
regurgitation, foul smell, thirst and bitter taste, poor appetite, heavy sensation of the body, dizziness, insomnia,
thirst with no desire to drink, irregular bowl movement,
yellow and turbid urine, red tongue with yellow and
greasy coating, soft-superficial and rapid pulse or wiry and
smooth pulse.

Therapeutic Methods: To clear damp heat, regulate qi and normalize the function of the stomach.

Prescription: Modified Banxia Xiexin Tang (Decoction Pinelliae for Regulating Stomach), composed of
Huanglian (*Rhizoma Copitdis*) 5 g, Huangqin (*Radix
Scutellariae*) 10 g, Zhizi (*Fructus Gardeniae*) 10 g,
Chenpi (*Pericarpium Citri Reticulatae*) 6 g, Zhibanxia
(*Rhizoma Pinelliae Preparata*) 10 g, Fuling (*Poria*)
10 g, Houpo (*Cortex Magnoliae Officinalis*) 6 g, Huoxiang (*Herba Agastaches*) 10 g, Cangzhu (*Rhizoma Atractylodis*) 10 g and Gancao (*Radix Glycyrrhizae*) 5 g.

Modification: For poor appetite, add Jineijin (*Endothelium Corneum Gigeriae Galli*) 10 g, Shenqu
(*Massa Medicata Fermentata*) 10 g and Maiya (*Fructus Hordei Germinatus*) 12 g.

Other Treatments

1. Chinese Patent Drugs

(1) Qizhi Weitong Chongji (Granule for Qi Stagnancy
and Epigastric Pain): 10 g each time, 3 times daily; applicable to patients with peptic ulcer caused by liver qi
stagnation.

(2) Xuhan Weitong Chongji (Granule for Deficiency-
Cold Stomachache): 10 g each time, three times daily;
applicable to peptic ulcer caused by insufficient yang of the
spleen and stomach.

(3) Yinxu Weitong Chongji (Granule for Yin-Deficiency Stomachache): 10 g each time, 3 times daily;

疼痛,嗳气恶心,嘈杂泛酸,口
出浊气,口苦而干,纳少身困,
头晕寐差,渴不思饮,大便不
畅,小便黄浊,舌质红,苔黄
腻,脉濡数或弦滑。

治　法　清化湿热,理气
和胃。

方　药　半夏泻心汤加
减:黄连5g,黄芩10g,栀子
10g,陈皮6g,制半夏10g,茯
苓10g,厚朴6g,藿香10g,苍
术10g,甘草5g。

加　减　食欲不振明显
者,加鸡内金10g,神曲10g,
麦芽12g。

【其他疗法】
1. 中成药
(1) 气滞胃痛冲剂　每服
10g,每日3次。适用于消化
性溃疡肝气郁滞者。

(2) 虚寒胃痛冲剂　每服
10g,每日3次。适用于消化
性溃疡脾胃虚寒者。

(3) 阴虚胃痛冲剂　每服
10g,每日3次。适用于阴虚

applicable to epigastric pain caused by yin deficiency.

(4) Shugan Hewei Wan (Pill for Soothing Liver and Regulating Stomach): 3 - 6 g each time, twice daily; applicable to peptic ulcer caused by disharmony of the liver and stomach.

(5) Wu Bei Weitong Pian (Tablet of Os Sepiae and Fritillariae Thunbergii for Epigastric Pain): 2 - 4 tablets each time, 3 times daily; applicable to peptic ulcer with epigastric pain and hyperacidity.

(6) Jianwei Yuyang Pian (Tablet for Strengthening Stomach and Healing Ulcer): 1.2 - 1.8 g each time, 4 times daily; applicable to peptic ulcer caused by liver qi stagnation and spleen deficiency, epigastric pain caused by disharmony of the liver and stomach.

(7) Kuaiwei Pian (Tablet for Comforting Stomach): 4 - 6 g each time, 3 times daily; applicable to epigastric pain and hyperacidity.

(8) Liang Fu Wan (Pill of Alpiniae Officinarum and Cyperi): 3 - 6 g each time, twice daily; applicable to peptic ulcer with epigastric pain and abdominal distention alleviated by warmth.

2. Single-drug or Experiential Prescriptions

(1) Wu Bei San (Powder of Os Sepiae and Fritillariae Thunbergii): composed of 4 portions of Wuzeigu (*Os Sepiae*) and 1 portion of Xiangbeimu (*Bulbus Fritillariae Thunbergii*). Mix and grind them into power, take 3 - 6 g before meal, twice or thrice daily. It is applicable to peptic ulcer with heartburn and acid regurgitation.

(2) Danke Fen (Eggshell Powder): composed of Jidanke (*Chorion Ovi Galli*) 500 g, Chuanxiong (*Rhizoma Chuangxiong*) 15 g, Shengdahuang (*Radix et Rhizoma Rhei*) 15 g and Rougui (*Cortex Cinnamomi*) 15 g. Wash and dry the eggshells in the sun, grind them with

胃脘痛者。

（4）舒肝和胃丸　每服3~6g,每日2次。适用于消化性溃疡肝胃不和者。

（5）乌贝胃痛片　每服2~4片,每日3次。适用于消化性溃疡胃脘疼痛,胃酸过多者。

（6）健胃愈疡片　每服1.2~1.8g,每日4次。适用于消化性溃疡肝郁脾虚,肝胃不和之胃脘痛者。

（7）快胃片　每服4~6g,每日3次。适用于胃脘疼痛,胃酸较多者。

（8）良附丸　每服·3~6g,每日2次。适用于消化性溃疡胃脘疼痛,腹胀喜暖者。

2. 单验方

（1）乌贝散　乌贼骨4份,象贝母1份,共研细末,餐前每服3~6g,每日2~3次。适用于消化性溃疡伴明显烧心泛酸者。

（2）蛋壳粉　鸡蛋壳500g,川芎15g,生大黄15g,肉桂15g。先取鸡蛋壳洗净晒干,再与其他3味药共研细末。每服3g,每日3次。适用

the other herbs into powder. Take 3 g of the powder each time, 3 times daily. It is applicable to epigastric ulcer.

(3) Gancao Walengzi San (Powder of Glycyrrhizae and Concha Arcae): Grind equal amounts of Gancao (*Radix Glycyrrhizae*) and Walengzi (*Concha Arcae*) into powder, take 5 - 15 g of the powder each time, twice daily. It is applicable to peptic ulcer with hyperacidity.

(4) Lian Yu San (Powder of Copitdis and Evodiae): composed of Wuzhuyu (*Fructus Evodiae*) 20 g, Huanglian (*Rhizoma Copitdis*) 6 g, Haipiaoxiao (*Os Sepiae*) 15 g, Muli (*Concha Ostreae*) 15 g and Cangzhu (*Rhizoma Atractylodis*) 10 g. Grind the above ingredients into powder. Take 12 g of the powder each time, 3 times daily. It is applicable to peptic ulcer with intermingling of cold and heat.

(5) No. 1 Kuiyang Wan (No. 1 Bolus for Ulcer): composed of Wuzeigu (*Os Sepiae*) 18 g, Gancao (*Radix Glycyrrhizae*) 12 g, Ganjiang (*Rhizoma Zingiberis*) 15 g, Wuzhuyu (*Fructus Evodiae*) 10 g, Rougui (*Cortex Cinnamomi*) 3 g, Sharen (*Fructus Amommi*) 15 g, Wuyao (*Linderae*) 9 g and Yanhusuo (*Rhizoma Corydalis*) 9 g. Prepare the above ingredients with honey to make bolus, 6 g each. Take one bolus each time, twice or thrice daily. It is applicable to peptic ulcer with insufficient yang in spleen and stomach.

(6) No. 2 Kui Yang Wan (No. 2 Bolus for Ulcer): composed of Wuzeigu (*Os Sepiae*) 15 g, Gancao (*Radix Glycyrrhizae*) 15 g, Chuanlianzi (*Fructus Toosendan*) 9 g, Xiangfu (*Rhizoma Cyperi*) 6 g, Chenpi (*Pericarpium Citri Reticulatae*) 15 g, Baishaoyao (*Radix Paeoniae Alba*) 9 g and Walengzi (*Concha Arcae*) 15 g. Prepare the above ingredients with honey to make bolus, 6 g each. Take one bolus each time, twice or thrice daily. It is applicable to peptic ulcer with liver qi stagnation.

于胃溃疡。

（3）甘草瓦楞子散 瓦楞子、甘草各等分,共研细末,每服5～15 g,每日2次。适用于消化性溃疡胃酸分泌较多者。

（4）连萸散 吴茱萸20 g,黄连6 g,海螵蛸15 g,牡蛎15 g,苍术10 g。共研细末,每服12 g,每日3次。适用于消化性溃疡属寒热错杂者。

（5）溃疡丸1号 乌贼骨18 g,甘草12 g,干姜15 g,吴茱萸10 g,肉桂3 g,砂仁15 g,乌药9 g,延胡索9 g。上药炼蜜为丸,每丸重6 g,每服1丸,每日2～3次。适用于消化性溃疡脾胃虚寒者。

（6）溃疡丸2号 乌贼骨15 g,甘草15 g,川楝子9 g,香附6 g,陈皮15 g,白芍药9 g,瓦楞子15 g。上药炼蜜为丸,每丸重6 g,每服1丸,每日2～3次。适用于消化性溃疡肝郁气滞者。

(7) No. 3 Kui Yang Wan (No. 3 Bolus for Ulcer): composed of Wuzeigu (*Os Sepiae*) 15 g, Chuanlianzi (*Fructus Toosendan*) 9 g, Taoren (*Semen Persicae*) 6 g, Puhuang (*Pollen Typhae*) 3 g, Chishaoyao (*Radix Paeoniae Rubra*) 9 g and Yanhusuo (*Rhizoma Corydalis*) 9 g. Prepare the above ingredients with honey to make bolus, 6 g each. Take one bolus each time, twice or thrice daily. It is applicable to peptic ulcer and later stage of gastric perforation with qi and blood stagnation.

(8) Muli Danke San (Powder of Concha Ostreae and Eggshell): composed of equal amounts of Duanmuli (*Concha Ostreae Usta*) and calcined eggshells. Grind them into powder and take 4.5 g of the powder each time, 3 times daily. It is applicable to hyperacidity and gastric discomfort.

3. External Therapy

(1) Wuzhuyu (*Fructus Evodiae*) 50 g, Ganjiang (*Rhizoma Zingiberis*) 50 g, Dingxiang (*Gemma Caryophylli*) 50 g, Xiaohuixiang (*Fructus Foeniculi*) 75 g, Rougui (*Cortex Cinnamomi*) 30 g, Shengliuhuang (*Sulphur*) 30 g, Zhizi (*Fructus Gardeniae*) 20 g, Hujiao (*Fructus Piperis*) 5 g and Biba (*Fructus Piperis Lonngi*) 25 g. Grind them into powder and reserve them for use. In the treatment, mix 25 g of the powder with flour paste and put the paste at Shenque (CV 8) and fix it with adhesive tape. Keep the application for 3 - 6 hours, once or twice daily. This treatment is applicable to peptic ulcer with cold pain in the epigastrium.

(2) Chuanjiao (*Pericarpium Zanthoxyli*) 150 g, Paojiang (*Rhzioma Zingiberis*, roasted in hot cinders) 100 g, Shengfuzi (*Raw Radix Aconiti Lateralis*) 100 g, Tanxiang (*Lignum Santali Albi*) 100 g and Cangzhu (*Rhizoma Atractylodis*) 200 g. Grind them into powder and reserve for use. In the treatment, mix 30 g of the

（7）溃疡丸3号　乌贼骨15 g,川楝子9 g,桃仁6 g,蒲黄3 g,赤芍药9 g,延胡索9 g。上药炼蜜为丸,每丸重6 g,每服1丸,每日2～3次。适用于消化性溃疡及溃疡穿孔后期属血瘀气滞者。

（8）牡蛎蛋壳散　煅牡蛎、煅鸡蛋壳等分。共研细末,每服4.5 g,每日3次。适用于胃酸过多,嘈杂者。

3. 外治法

（1）吴茱萸50 g,干姜50 g,丁香50 g,小茴香75 g,肉桂30 g,生硫黄30 g,栀子20 g,胡椒5 g,荜茇25 g,共研粉末,密贮备用。治疗时取药末25 g,加入等量面糊调成糊状,贴神阙穴,外用胶布固定,每次敷贴3～6小时,每日1～2次。适用于消化性溃疡胃脘冷痛者。

（2）川椒150 g,炮姜100 g,生附子100 g,檀香100 g,苍术200 g,将上药共研细末,贮存备用,治疗时取药末30 g,用生姜汁调成糊状,敷于中脘、足三里、神阙、脾俞、

powder with ginger juice into paste and put at Zhongwan (CV 12), Zusanli (ST 36), Shenque (CV 8), Pishu (BL 20), Weishu (BL 21), one treatment every day. It is applicable to peptic ulcer with severe gastric pain.

(3) Equal amounts of Zhangnao (*Camphor*), Xuejie (*Resina Draconis*), Ruxiang (*Olibanum*), Moyao (*Myrrha*), Biba (*Fructus Piperis Lonngi*), Wuzhuyu (*Fructus Evodiae*), Xixin (*Herba Asari*), Muxiang (*Radix Aucklandiae*), Dingxiang (*Gemmma Caryophylli*) and Chaihu (*Radix Bupleuri*). Dry and grind the herbs into powder. Stir it with tea or vinegar into cream. Put the cream at Shangwan (CV 13), Zhongwan (CV 12), Xiawan (CV 10), Pishu (BL 20), Weishu (BL 21) and Liangmen (ST 21) for 8 hours as one treatment. One week makes up a treatment course. The prescription is applicable to peptic ulcer with epigastric pain, abdominal distention and belching and poor appetite.

(4) Maogen (*Herba Ranunculi Japonici*, fresh, leaves and stalks removed). Wash them with clean water. Cut them up and pound them with brown sugar (30% of the herb). Place them in the rubber caps of the penicillin container and apply them at Weishu (BL 21) and Shenshu (BL 23) for about 15 minutes until feverish sensation appears. If the blisters appear, let them absorbed without breaking them. This is applicable to peptic ulcer with gastric pain caused by insufficient yang.

(5) Congtou (*Bulbus Allii Fistulosi*, tassels reserved) 30 g and Shengjiang (*Rhizoma Zingiberis Recens*) 15 g. Pound them and stir-bake them hot, and fill the bag with the herbs. Iron the epigastric area with it and change it when it turns cool. Apply this treatment twice a day, 30 minutes for each time or keep the application until the pain is relieved. It is applicable to peptic ulcer with the gastric pain as the main manifestation.

胃俞等。每日 1 次。适用于消化性溃疡胃痛较甚者。

(3) 樟脑、血竭、乳香、没药、荜茇、吴茱萸、细辛、木香、丁香、柴胡各等分。上方烘干共研细末,以茶水或醋搅拌成膏,敷贴上、中、下三脘穴,脾、胃俞穴,梁门穴。每日 1 次,每次贴 8 小时后取下,1 个星期为 1 个疗程。本方适用于消化性溃疡,症见上腹疼痛、饱胀不适、嗳气纳少者。

(4) 取鲜毛茛,除去叶、茎,留下根须,清水洗净,然后切碎,加入红糖约 30%,捣烂,装入青霉素瓶橡皮盖凹内,敷贴胃俞、肾俞穴,置 15 分钟左右,局部有烘热感时揭去,如发生水泡,不必刺破,让其自行吸收。适用于消化性溃疡虚寒胃痛为主症者。

(5) 连须葱头 30 g,生姜 15 g,两味共捣烂炒烫,热熨胃脘部,药袋冷即更换。每日 2 次,每次 30 分钟,或以疼痛缓解为度。适用于消化性溃疡胃痛为主症者。

(6) Dahuang (*Radix et Rhizoma Rhei*, to be decocted later) 10 g, Rougui (*Cortex Cinnamomi*) 6 g, Wuzhuyu (*Fructus Evodiae*) 10 g, Huanglian (*Rhizoma Copitdis*) 10 g, Wuyao (*Linderae*) 20 g, Baishaoyao (*Radix Paeoniae Alba*) 30 g, Wumei (*Fructus Mume*) 20 g and Zhishi (*Fructus Aurantii Immaturus*) 15 g. Decoct them to make 200 ml of the decoction and fill the anus through the catheter. The retention enema lasts for 40 - 60 minutes, once every day, 7 days making up a treatment course. There is a 3 - day interval between treatment courses and generally 1 - 2 treatments are used. Stop the treatment when the pain is relieved. It is applicable to the epigastric pain caused by yin deficiency and blood stagnation.

2.3.3 Gastric Carcinoma

General Description

Gastric carcinoma is a commonly-seen malignant tumor, which accounts for 40%-50% of the tumors of digestive tract. The incidence and mortality of this disease remain the highest in different kinds of malignant tumors. Its clinical manifestations include epigastric discomfort and pain, vomiting, haematemesis, nausea and tarry stools and mass in the epigastric area. With no obvious symptoms at the early stage, it is often confused with gastritis, anorexia and gastric ulcer. And at the later stage, there appears epigastric mass and general cachexa, it is already the late stage of gastric carncinoma. This disease occurs in patients at any ages, but more common in patients between the ages of 40 - 60 and more common in males than in females.

The etiology and pathogenesis are not clear at present, but they are related to hypersaline diet, some

（6）大黄（后下）10 g, 肉桂6 g, 吴茱萸10 g, 黄连10 g, 乌药20 g, 白芍药30 g, 乌梅20 g, 枳实15 g。共煎取汁200 ml, 用导尿管经肛门灌入, 保留灌肠40～60分钟, 每日1次, 7日为1个疗程, 疗程间隔3日, 一般需1～2个疗程。痛止即停。适用于阴虚血瘀之胃痛。

第三节　胃癌

【概述】

胃癌是一种最常见恶性肿瘤, 约占消化道肿瘤的40%～50%。其发病率及死亡率均占各类恶性肿瘤之首位。临床主要表现为上腹部不适、疼痛, 呕吐, 呕血, 反胃, 黑便、上腹部出现包块等。早期患者症状不明显, 常易与胃炎、消化不良、胃溃疡的表现相混淆。至上腹部出现包块、全身出现恶病质时已为晚期。本病可发生于任何年龄, 但以40～60岁为多见, 男性较女性为多。

本病的病因和发病条件目前尚未完全明确, 多与过盐

carcinogenic substances like nitrosamine, polycyclic hydrocarbon, etc., chronic bacteria infection, post-gas-trectomy, some gastric diseases (such as gastric ulcer, chronic atrophic gastritis, gastric polyp, intestinal epithe-lial metaplasia), pernicious anemia and genetic factors.

According to its manifestations, the disease belongs to "fan wei" (regurgitation), "wei wan tong" (epigastric pain), "yi ge" (difficulty in swallowing), "xin fu pi" (fullness in the epigastrum) in traditional Chinese medi-cine. The causes of the disease are emotional disturbance, improper diet or long-term deficiency of the spleen and stomach. In terms of pathogenesis, the liver fails to main-tain free flow of qi, the stomach qi fails to descend, the viscera fail to function normally, and dampness, phlegm, toxic heat and blood stasis accumulate in the stomach, which may lead to gastric carcinoma.

Essentials for Diagnosis

(1) Over 30 years old patients suffering from gastric pain or flatulence for more than 1 year, recently with ag-gravation of the pain, changes of rhythm and slight tender in the gastric area, should be aware of the possibility of gastric carcinoma.

(2) The patient has no history of diagnosed gastric diseases, but suffers from emaciation with unknown cause, tarry stools and also anorexia, lassitude, reduced hematochrome, or frequent bleeding and stubborn pain.

(3) The patient has the history of gastric pain, transferring focus to the lung and liver, swelling of the supraclavicular lymph nodes or mass felt in the front wall of the rectum.

(4) Laboratory examination shows persistent positive occult blood in stools, deficiency or absence of gastric acid

饮食、亚硝胺、多环烃如 3－4 苯并芘等致癌物质、慢性细菌感染、胃大部切除术后、某些胃部疾患（如胃溃疡、慢性萎缩性胃炎、胃息肉、肠上皮化生、胃巨皱襞症）、恶性贫血及遗传因素等有关。

根据本病的临床表现，当属于中医学"反胃"、"胃脘痛"、"噎膈"、"心腹痞"范畴。其病因是忧思恼怒、饮食不节或久病脾胃虚弱。主要病机为肝失疏泄，胃失和降，气机郁滞，湿聚痰凝，热毒血瘀，阻结于胃腑而成癌肿。

【诊断要点】

（1）30 岁以上患者有胃痛或上腹部胀满史 1 年以上，近期疼痛加重，节律改变，上腹部轻压痛者，应警惕胃癌的发生。

（2）虽无胃病史，但出现原因不明的消瘦、黑便，伴有食欲不振、乏力、血色素降低，或多次出血、顽固性疼痛者。

（3）有胃痛史，且体检发现有肺、肝转移灶，锁骨上淋巴结肿大，或直肠前壁摸到肿块。

（4）实验室检查大便隐血持续阳性；胃液分析大多数胃

in gastric juice analysis, absence of free acid on empty stomach; biochemical examination indicates increased AFP content in the gastric juice, positive gastric carcinoma antigen, significant difference of akaline phosphatase and acid protease in biopsy sample of gastric membrane comparing with normal tissues and increase of CEA, CA19 - 9, CA242 in the blood.

(5) Barium meal X-ray examination indicates the ulcer larger than 2.5 cm with irregular shape of the niche, erect image in negative image, meniscus sign, irregular rough or vanishing membrane folds around the ulcer, nearby stomach wall rigid and disappearance of the movement. The size and location of the tumor or the surface of the tumor or ulcer, bleeding by touching can be observed under endoscope. To make clear diagnosis, biopsy or smear examination is recommended. The ultrasonic B and CT examination indicate the growth of the cancer inside and outside of the stomach cavity and the transference to the liver, pancreas, kidney, ovary or celiac lymph nodes.

Syndrome Differentiation and Treatment

At the early stage, most of the cases are characterized by excessive pathogenic factors, usually manifested as incoordination between the liver and the stomach, blockage of toxic stasis and stagnation of phlegm and dampness. Chronic cases are marked by deficient healthy qi, usually manifested as stomach heat damaging yin, yang deficiency of the spleen and deficiency of qi and blood. The treatment principle is to soothe the liver qi and strengthen the spleen, remove phlegm and blood stasis. At the late stage, the treatment principle is to nourish stomach qi and

酸偏低或缺酸,空腹时无游离酸;免疫学、生化学检查显示胃液中胎儿硫糖蛋白含量较高,胃癌抗原阳性,胃黏膜活检标本所含碱性磷酸酶及酸性蛋白酶均与正常组织间有显著差异,血中 CEA、CA19 - 9、CA242 升高等。

(5) X 钡餐检查提示溃疡大于 2.5 cm,龛影形状不规则,负影中有正影、有半月征,溃疡周围黏膜皱壁粗乱或消失,附近胃壁僵直,蠕动消失。内窥镜直视下可观察肿瘤大小、位置、肿物或溃疡表面情况、是否触之出血等。取活检行病理检查,或刷检细胞进行细胞涂片检查,可以明确诊断。B 超及 CT 检查显示胃癌累及胃壁向腔内和腔外生长的范围、邻近的解剖关系以及有无肝、胰、肾、卵巢及腹腔淋巴结等的转移。

【辨证论治】

本病初起以邪实为主,多见肝胃不和、瘀毒内阻和痰湿凝结证;久病则以正虚为主,多见胃热伤阴、脾胃虚寒和气血双亏证。治疗以疏肝健脾、化痰消瘀为原则,后期应养胃气及胃阴为主,且标本兼顾,扶正与祛邪并投。

stomach yin, treat the symptoms and the causes, strengthen the antipathogenic factors and expel the pathogenic factors simultaneusly.

1. Incoordination Between the Liver and Stomach

Chief Manifestations: Distention in the gastric area, intermittent dull pain radiating to the hypochondriac regions, belching with foul smell of undigested food, anorexia, or vomiting, nausea, pale tongue with thin and white coating, thready and wiry pulse.

Therapeutic Methods: To soothe the liver and regulate the function of the stomach, subdue the adverse flow of qi and relieve pain.

Prescription: Modified Xiaoyao San (Xiaoyao Powder) and Xuanfu Daizhe Tang (Inulae and Haematitum Decoction), composed of Chaihu (*Radix Bupleuri*) 6 g, Yujin (*Radix Curcumae*) 10 g, Zhibanxia (*Rhizoma Pinelliae Preparata*) 10 g, Zhike (*Fructus Aurantii*) 10 g, Danggui (*Radix Angelicae Sinensis*) 10 g, Xuanfuhua (*Flos Inulae*, wrapped) 10 g, Baishaoyao (*Radix Paeoniae Alba*) 15 g, Daizheshi (*Haematitum*, to be decocted first) 25 g, Chenpi (*Pericarpium Citri Reticulatae*) 6 g and Zhigancao (*Radix Glycyrrhizae*, roasted) 6 g.

Modifications: For distention in the gastric area, add Qingpi (*Pericarpium Citri Reticulatae Viride*) 6 g, Chenpi (*Pericarpium Citri Reticulatae*) 6 g, Zhixiangfu (*Rhizoma Cyperi Preparata*) 10 g and Chuanlianzi (*Fructus Toosendan*) 10 g; for severe pain, add Yanhusuo (*Rhizoma Corydalis*) 10 g and Muxiang (*Radix Aucklandiae*) 10 g; for poor appetite, add Jiaoshanzha (*Fructus Crataegi*, charred) 10 g, Shenqu (*Massa Medicata Fermentata*) 12 g, Maiya (*Fructus Hordei Germinatus*) 12 g and Jineijin (*Endothelium Corneum*

1. 肝胃不和证

主要证候 胃脘胀满,时时隐痛,串及两胁,嗳气陈腐,饮食少进,或呕吐反胃,舌质淡红,苔薄白,脉细弦。

治 法 疏肝和胃,降逆止痛。

方 药 逍遥散合旋覆代赭汤加减:柴胡6g,郁金10g,制半夏10g,枳壳10g,当归10g,旋覆花(包煎)10g,白芍药15g,代赭石(先煎)25g,陈皮6g,炙甘草6g。

加 减 胃脘胀满显著者,加青皮6g,陈皮6g,制香附10g,川楝子10g;胃脘痛甚者,加延胡索10g,木香10g;纳差食少者,加焦山楂10g,神曲12g,麦芽12g,鸡内金10g;口苦口黏,苔黄腻者,加藿香10g,佩兰10g,龙胆草6g;热结便秘者,加制大黄10g。

Gigeriae Galli) 10 g; for bitter taste and stickiness in the mouth and yellow greasy tongue coating, add Huoxiang (*Herba Agastaches*) 10 g, Peilan (*Herba Eupatorii*) 10 g and Longdancao (*Radix Gentianae*) 6 g; for heat constipation, add Zhidahuang (*Radix et Rhizoma Rhei Preparata*) 10 g.

2. Stomach Heat Damaging Yin

Chief Manifestations: Burning pain in the gastric area aggravated after meals, gastric discomfort, dryness in the mouth, feverish sensation in the soles, palms and chest, dry stools, anorexia, red tongue with little coating, thready and rapid pulse.

Therapeutic Methods: To nourish yin, clear away heat, regulate the stomach and remove toxic substance.

Prescription: Modified Yunü Jian (Jade Maid Decoction) and Zhengye Tang (Decoction for Increasing Fluid), composed of Shengdihuang (*Radix Rehmanniae*) 15 g, Shashen (*Radix Glehniae*) 15 g, Yuzhu (*Rhizoma Polygonati Odorati*) 15 g, Baishaoyao (*Radix Paeoniae Alba*) 15 g, Maimendong (*Radix Ophiopogonis*) 10 g, Zhimu (*Rhizoma Anemarrhenae*) 10 g, Tianhuafen (*Radix Trichosanthis*) 30 g and Baihuasheshecao (*Herba Hedyotis Diffusae*) 30 g.

Modifications: For distention in the gastric area, add Foshou (*Fructus Citri Sarcodactylis*) 10 g and Bayuezha (*Fructus Akebiae*) 10 g; for burning pain in the stomach, add Zhizi (*Fructus Gardeniae*) 10 g and Mudanpi (*Cortex Moutan Radicis*) 10 g; for restlessness and insomnia, add Lianzixin (*Plumula Nelumbinis*) 10 g.

3. Internal Stagnation of Blood and Toxic Substance

Chief Manifestations: Localized pricking pain in the gastric area and even cutting pain, abdominal mass with tenderness, or haematemesis, hematochezia,

2. 胃热伤阴证

主要证候 胃脘灼痛,嘈杂口干,食后痛甚,五心烦热,大便干结,食欲不振,舌红少苔,脉细数。

治 法 养阴清热,和胃解毒。

方 药 玉女煎合增液汤加减:生地黄15 g,沙参15 g,玉竹15 g,白芍药15 g,麦门冬10 g,知母10 g,天花粉30 g,白花蛇舌草30 g。

加 减 胃脘胀满不适者,加佛手10 g,八月札10 g;胃脘灼痛较著者,加栀子10 g,牡丹皮10 g;心烦少寐者,加莲子心10 g。

3. 瘀毒内阻证

主要证候 胃脘刺痛,甚如刀割,痛点固定,痞块拒按,或有呕血便血,肌肤甲错,舌

squamous and dry skin, purple tongue or dark spots on the tongue, deep, thready and unsmooth pulse.

Therapeutic Methods: To remove toxic substance and blood stasis, activate blood circulation and relieve pain.

Prescription: Modified Shixiao San (Powder for Dissipating Blood Stasis) and Gexia Zhuyu Tang (Decoction for Removing Blood Stasis Under Diaphram), composed of Taoren (*Semen Persicae*) 10 g, Puhuang (*Pollen Typhae, wrapped*) 10 g, Danggui (*Radix Angelicae Sinensis*) 10 g, Chishaoyao (*Radix Paeoniae Rubra*) 10 g, Baishaoyao (*Radix Paeoniae Alba*) 10 g, Wulingzhi (*Faces Trogopterori*) 10 g, Yanhusuo (*Rhizoma Corydalis*) 10 g, Longkui (*Herba Solani Nigri*) 30 g, Pugongying (*Herba Taraxaci*) 30 g, Xianhecao (*Herba Agrimoniae*) 30 g, Tengligen (*Radix Actinidiae Chinensis*) 30 g, Wuyao (*Linderae*) 10 g, Xuchangqing (*Radix Cynanchi Paniculati*) 10 g, Shetui (*Periostracum Serpentis*) 6 g and Lufengfang (*Nidus Pokistis Mandarini*) 6 g.

Modifications: For haematemesis and hematochezia, add Sanqifen (*Radix Notoginseng*, powdered and to be infused separately) 3 g, Baijifen (*Rhizoma Bletillae*, powdered and to be infused separately) 3 g, or Dahuangfen (*Radix et Rhizoma Rhei*, powdered and to be infused separately) 6–10 g; for abdominal mass with severe pain, add Shancigu (*Pseudobulbus Cremastrae seu Pleiones*) 10 g and Chuanlianzi (*Fructus Toosendan*) 10 g.

4. Accumulation of Phlegm and Dampness

Chief Manifestations: Fullness and pain in the chest, vomiting of phlegm, abdominal distention, diarrhea, swelling of the lymph nodes, pale tongue with smooth and greasy coating and deep, thready and soft-superficial

质紫暗或有瘀斑,脉沉细涩。

治　法　解毒祛瘀,活血止痛。

方　药　失笑散合膈下逐瘀汤加减:桃仁10 g,蒲黄(包煎)10 g,当归10 g,赤芍药10 g,白芍药10 g,五灵脂10 g,延胡索10 g,龙葵30 g,蒲公英30 g,仙鹤草30 g,藤梨根30 g,乌药10 g,徐长卿10 g,蛇蜕6 g,露蜂房6 g。

加　减　呕血便血者,加三七粉(冲服)3 g,白及粉(冲服)3 g,或大黄粉(冲服)6～10 g;伴肿块疼痛剧烈者,加山慈姑10 g,川楝子10 g。

4. 痰湿凝结证

主要证候　胸闷满痛,呕吐痰涎,腹胀便溏,痰核累累,舌淡白,苔滑腻,脉沉细濡。

pulse.

Therapeutic Methods: To strengthen the spleen, dry dampness, expel phlegm and disperse mass.

Prescription: Modified Kaiyu Erchen Tang (Erchen Decoction for Relieving Stagnation), composed of Cang-zhu (*Rhizoma Atractylodis*) 10 g, Fuling (*Poria*) 10 g, Zhibanxia (*Rhizoma Pinelliae Preparata*) 10 g, Xiaku-cao (*Spica Prunellae*) 10 g, Baizhu (*Rhizoma Atractylodis Macrocephalae*) 10 g, Haizao (*Sargassum*) 10 g, Zisuzi (*Fructus Perillae*) 10 g, Shengyiyiren (*Semen Coicis*) 30 g, Shengmuli (*Concha Ostreae*, to be decocted first) 30 g, Zhinanxing (*Arisaema cum Bile*) 6 g and Chenpi (*Pericarpium Citri Reticulatae*) 6 g.

Modification: For fullness in the gastric area with profuse sputum, add Quangualou (*Fructus Trichosanthis*) 20 g, Yujin (*Radix Curcumae*) 10 g and Zhuru (*Caulis Bambusae in Taeniam*) 10 g.

5. Yang Deficiency of the Spleen

Chief Manifestations: Dull gastric pain which is relieved by warmth and pressure, or vomiting of retained food, vomiting of clear fluid, pale complexion, lassitude, cold limbs, loose stools, edema, pale and swollen tongue with teeth marks and white, moist and smooth coating, deep and slow or deep, thready and soft-superficial pulse.

Therapeutic Methods: To warm the middle energizer and expel cold, strengthen the spleen and regulate the stomach.

Prescription: Modified Lizhong Tang (Decoction for Regulating Middle Energizer) and Huangqi Jianzhong Tang (Decoction of Astragali for Warming Middle Energizer), composed of Huangqi (*Radix Astragali*) 20 g, Dangshen (*Radix Codonopsis*) 15 g, Fuling (*Poria*) 15 g, Baishaoyao (*Radix Paeoniae Alba*) 15 g, Baizhu (*Rhizoma Atractylodis Macrocephalae*) 10 g, Zhibanxia

治　法　健脾燥湿,化痰散结。

方　药　开郁二陈汤加减:苍术10 g,茯苓10 g,制半夏10 g,夏枯草10 g,白术10 g,海藻10 g,紫苏子10 g,生薏苡仁30 g,生牡蛎(先煎)30 g,制南星6 g,陈皮6 g。

加　减　痰多脘闷明显者,加全瓜蒌20 g,郁金10 g,竹茹10 g。

5. 脾胃虚寒证

主要证候　胃脘隐痛,喜温喜按,或朝食暮吐,暮食朝吐,或食入经久仍复吐出,时呕清水,面色㿠白,神疲肢冷,便溏浮肿,舌质淡胖、有齿痕,苔白滑润,脉沉缓或沉细濡。

治　法　温中散寒,健脾和胃。

方　药　理中汤合黄芪健中汤加减:黄芪20 g,党参15 g,茯苓15 g,白芍药15 g,白术10 g,制半夏10 g,荜茇6 g,干姜5 g,桂枝6 g,炙甘草6 g。

(*Rhizoma Pinelliae Preparata*) 10 g, Biba (*Fructus Piperis Longi*) 6 g, Ganjiang (*Rhizoma Zingiberis*) 5 g, Guizhi (*Ramulus Cinnamomi*) 6 g and Zhigancao (*Radix Glycyrrhizae*, roasted) 6 g.

Modifications: For cold pain in the gastric area, add Zhifuzi (*Radix Aconiti Lateralis Preparata*) 6 g and Gaoliangjiang (*Rhizoma Alpiniae Officinarum*) 6 g; for palpitation, shortness of breath and lusterless complexion, add Danggui (*Radix Angelicae Sinensis*) 10 g, Shudihuang (*Radix Rehmanniae Preparata*) 12 g and Danshen (*Radix Salviae Miltiorrhizae*) 15 g; for anorexia, add Jiaoshanzha (*Fructus Crataegi*, charred) 12 g, Shenqu (*Massa Medicata Fermentata*) 10 g and Jineijin (*Endothelium Corneum Gigeriae Galli*) 10 g.

6. Deficiency of Qi and Blood

Chief Manifestations: Gastric carcinoma with severe anemia, lassitude, palpitation, shortness of breath, dizziness, lusterless complexion, restlessness, insomnia, spontaneous sweating, night sweating, anorexia, emaciation, pronounced mass in the epigastric area, pale and swollen tongue, thready and feeble pulse.

Therapeutic Methods: To nourish qi and blood, strengthen the spleen and kidney.

Prescription: Modified Shiquan Dabu Tang (Decoction of Ten Powerful Tonics), composed of Huangqi (*Radix Astragali*) 30 g, Dangshen (*Radix Codonopsis*) 10 g, Baizhu (*Rhizoma Atractylodis Macrocephalae*) 10 g, Danggui (*Radix Angelicae Sinensis*) 10 g, Ejiao (*Colla Corii Asini*, to be melted and taken with the decoction) 10 g, Yinyanghuo (*Herba Epimedii*) 10 g, Fuling (*Poria*) 15 g, Shudihuang (*Radix Rehmanniae Preparata*) 15 g, Baishaoyao (*Radix Paeoniae Alba*) 15 g, Heshouwu (*Radix Polygoni Multiflori*) 15 g, Huangjing (*Rhizoma Polygonati*) 15 g, Nüzhenzi

加　减　胃脘冷痛者,加制附子6 g,高良姜6 g;心悸气短,面色无华者,加当归10 g,熟地黄12 g,丹参15 g;食欲不振者,加焦山楂12 g,神曲10 g,鸡内金10 g。

6. 气血双亏证

主要证候　胃癌晚期,高度贫血,全身乏力,心悸气短,头晕目眩,面色无华,虚烦不寐,自汗盗汗,纳少乏味,形体羸瘦,上腹部包块明显,舌质淡胖,脉虚细无力。

治　法　补气养血,健脾益肾。

方　药　十全大补汤加减:黄芪30 g,党参10 g,白术10 g,当归10 g,阿胶(烊化冲服)10 g,淫羊藿10 g,茯苓15 g,熟地黄15 g,白芍药15 g,何首乌15 g,黄精15 g,女贞子15 g,炙甘草6 g。

(*Fructus Ligustri Lucidi*) 15 g and Zhigancao (*Prepared Radix Glycyrrhizaea*, roasted) 6 g.

Modifications: For severe shortness of breath and lassitude, add Xiyangshen (*Radix Panacis Quinquefolii*, to be decocted separately and taken at a draft) 3 - 6 g; for anorexia, add Guya (*Fructus Oryzae Germinatus*) 15 g and Maiya (*Fructus Hordei Germinatus*) 15 g.

Other Treatments

1. Chinese Patent Drugs

(1) Xi Huang Wan (Pills of Cornu Rhinocerotis Asiatici and Rehmanniae): 3 g each time, twice daily; applicable to gastric carcinoma with blockage of toxic stasis and masses.

(2) Fufang Tianxian Jiaonang (Compound Tianxian Capsule): 3 - 4 capsules each time, twice daily; applicable to gastric carcinoma with blockage of toxin stasis and masses.

(3) Shen Ling Baizhu Wan (Pill of Ginseng, Poria and Atractylodis Macrocephalae): 6 g each time, twice daily; applicable to gastric carcinoma with fullness and distention of the abdominal area, loose stools and lassitude.

(4) Yunnan Baiyao (Yunnan White Medicinal Powder): 2 - 3 g each time, twice daily and take the "safe pill" for the severe cases; applicable to gastric carcinoma with hematemesis, or other kinds of bleeding and blood stasis.

2. Single-drug or Experiential Prescriptions

(1) Fufang Langdu Tang (Compound Decoction of Euphorbiae Fischerianae): composed of Beilangdu (*Radix Euphorbiae Fischerianae*) 6 g, Banzhilian (*Herba Scutellariae Barbatae*) 30 g, Jixueteng (*Caulis Spatholobi*)30 g and Yiyiren (*Semen Coicis*) 30 g. Decoct the above drugs with water, one dose a day and take

加　减　气短乏力明显者,加西洋参(另煎顿服)3～6 g;纳少明显者,加谷芽15 g,麦芽15 g。

【其他疗法】

1. 中成药

(1) 犀黄丸　每服3 g,每日 2 次。适用于胃癌瘀毒内阻,百积凝结之证。

(2) 复方天仙胶囊　每服3～4 片,每日 2 次。适用于胃癌瘀毒内阻,百积凝结之证。

(3) 参苓白术丸　每服6 g,每日 2 次。适用于胃癌脘腹胀满,便溏乏力者。

(4) 云南白药　每服2～3 g,每日 2 次,重者可先将"保险子"服下。适用于胃癌呕血及其他出血、瘀血青紫等。

2. 单验方

(1) 复方狼毒汤　北狼毒6 g,半枝莲30 g,鸡血藤30 g,薏苡仁30 g。水煎服,每日 1 次,分 2 次服。适用于胃癌早期。

the decoction in two divided doses. It is applicable to the early gastric carcinoma.

(2) Teng Hu Tangjiang (Syrup of Actinidiae Chinensis and Polygoni Cuspidati): composed of Teng-ligen (*Radix Actinidiae Chinensis*) 500 g and Huzhang (*Rhizoma Polygoni Cuspidati*) 500 g. Decoct the above drugs and concentrate the decoction to get the extract (1 ml of the extract contains 1 g of crude drug each), add appropriate amount of honey and stir it well. Take 30 ml each time, twice daily. It is applicable to the early gastric carcinoma.

(3) Wushaoshe (*Zaocys*) 10 g, Zhechong (*Eupolyphaga seu Steleophaga*) 10 g, Chuanshanjia (*Squama Mantis*) 10 g, Shancigu (*Pseudobulbus Cremastrae seu Pleiones*) 10 g, Zicao (*Radix Arnebiae seu Lithospermi*) 10 g, Shidagonglaoye (*Folium Mahoniae*) 10 g, Huangbai (*Cortex Phellodendri*) 10 g, Wugong (*Scolopendra*) 2 pcs, Danshen (*Radix Salviae Miltiorrhizae*) 30 g, Yiyiren (*Semen Coicis*) 30 g, Dangshen (*Radix Codonopsis*) 30 g, Baizhu (*Rhizoma Atractylodis Macrocephalae*) 6 g and Qingdai (*Indigo Naturalis*, to be infused separately) 6 g. Decoct the drugs with water, 1 dose daily. It is applicable to gastric carcinoma with gastric distenting pain, vomiting after meals, progressing emaciation, sallow complexion, loose stools and dyschesia.

(4) Lixue Tang (Decoction for Benefiting Blood): composed of Shenghuangqi (*Radix Astragali*) 30 g, Jixueteng (*Caulis Spatholobi*) 15 g, Taizishen (*Radix Pseudostellariae*) 15 g, Baizhu (*Rhizoma Atractylodis Macrocephalae*) 15 g, Fuling (*Poria*) 15 g, Gouqizi (*Fructus Lycii*) 15 g, Nüzhenzi (*Fructus Ligustri Lucidi*) 15 g and Tusizi (*Semen Cuscutae*) 15 g. Decoct the drugs with water, 1 dose a day and take the decoction

（2）藤虎糖浆　藤梨根 500 g,虎杖500 g,水煎浓缩成每毫升含生药各1 g为度,加适量蜂蜜搅匀,每服 30 ml,每日 2 次。适用于胃癌早期。

（3）乌蛸蛇10 g,蟅虫10 g,穿山甲10 g,山慈姑10 g,紫草10 g,十大功劳叶10 g,黄柏10 g,蜈蚣 2 条,丹参30 g,薏苡仁30 g,党参30 g,白术6 g,青黛(另冲)6 g。水煎服,每日 1 剂。适用于胃癌伴上腹胀痛,饭后呕吐,进行性消瘦,面色萎黄,便溏不爽者。

（4）利血汤　生黄芪30 g,鸡血藤15 g,太子参15 g,白术15 g,茯苓15 g,枸杞子15 g,女贞子15 g,菟丝子15 g。每日 1 剂,水煎早晚分服,一般 6 个星期为 1 个疗程。适用于胃癌化疗者,可减轻其毒副反应。

in two divided doses, one in the morning and the other in the afternoon, six weeks making up a treatment course. This can relieve the toxic and side effects of chemiotherapy for gastric carcinoma.

(5) Xiangrikuigan (*Medulla Helianthi Annui Caulis*, *outer layer peeled*) 30 g. Decoct it with water to make a herbal tea, once daily. This may be used as the supplementary treatment for early gastric carcinoma.

3. External Therapy

(1) Sanqi (*Radix Notoginseng*) 10 g, Zaoxiu (*Rhizoma Paridis*) 10 g, Huangyaozi (*Tuber Dioscoreae Bulbiferae*) 10 g, Yanhusuo (*Rhizoma Corydalis*) 10 g, Lugen (*Rhizoma Phragmitis*) 20 g, Chuanwu (*Radix Aconiti*) 6 g, Bingpian (*Borneolum Syntheticum*) 8 g, garlic bulb 100 g and a proper amount of musk. Make some garlic juice, grind the herbs into fine powder and screen the powder with a 100 - mesh sieve, mix the herbal powder with garlic juice to make paste. Put the paste to the tender area or the tender point on the channels and change the paste every other day. This is applicable to carcinoma with severe pain.

(2) Chansu (*Venenum Bufonis*) 0.2 g, Shengchuanwu (*Radix Aconiti*) 5 g, Liangmianzhen (*Radix Zanthoxyli*) 30 g, Gongdingxiang (*Gemmma Caryophylli*) 10 g, Rougui (*Cortex Cinnamomi*) 10 g, Qiyeyizhihua (*Rhizoma Paridis*) 30 g and Honghua (*Flos Carthama*) 15 g. Grind them into powder and make a plaster, put the plaster on the painful area of the carcinoma and change the dressing every 24 hours, 7 days making up a treatment course. This is applicable to carcinoma with pain.

（5）向日葵秆,剥去外皮,取内白心,单味煎水代茶饮,每日30 g。适用于胃癌早期的辅助治疗。

3. 外治法

（1）三七10 g,蚤休10 g,黄药子10 g,延胡索10 g,芦根20 g,川乌6 g,冰片8 g,紫皮大蒜100 g,麝香适量。大蒜取汁,余药研为细粉过 100 目筛,用大蒜汁将药粉调成膏剂,贴于痛点,或经络压痛部位,隔日 2 贴。适用于胃癌疼痛显著者。

（2）蟾酥0.2 g,生川乌5 g,两面针30 g,公丁香10 g,肉桂10 g,七叶一枝花30 g,红花15 g。上药共研细末,制成橡皮膏,外贴于癌性疼痛处,24 小时换药 1 次,7 日为 1 个疗程。适用于胃癌肿痛为主者。

2.3.4 Chronic Colitis

General Description

Chronic colitis is an inflammatory disease of the intestines. The lesion is mainly in the rectal and sigmoidal mucosa and submucosal layer, but may also involve the whole colon. Most cases of chronic colitis result from acute enteritis which is not cured of and is apt to frequently recur, commonly seen in young adults. The main clinical manifestations include repeated attacks of abdominal pain, diarrhea and mucous stools or bloody stools.

This disease is included in the categories of "xie xie" (diarrhea), "li ji" (dysentery) and "fu tong" (abdominal pain) in traditional Chinese medicine. It is due to invasion of external pathogenic factors, improper diet, emotional disturbance and protracted illnesses causing weak constitution, which cause dysfunction of the spleen and stomach, the failure of the small intestine to receive food and the failure of the large intestine in transportation. In this case the pure and turbid substances mix together, running down to the intestines. The chief pathogenic factor is dampness and the pathogenesis is excessive dampness and the dysfunction of spleen with the involvemment in the spleen, stomach and intestines and the kidney and liver as well.

Essentials for Diagnosis

(1) Repeated attacks of abdominal pain, diarrhea, dyschesia with mucus and lassitude are the main symptoms of this disease. Diarrhea is predominant with blood, pus, mucus in the stools, accompanied with paroxysmal spastic colic pain. Different degrees of tenderness are present in the lower abdomen with hyperactive bowel sounds. Long-

第四节　慢性结肠炎

【概述】

慢性结肠炎是炎症性肠病，病变主要在直肠和乙状结肠的黏膜和黏膜下层，但也可遍及整个结肠。多由于急性肠炎治疗不彻底而成，有反复发作的趋势，多发于青壮年。临床主要表现为反复发作的腹痛、腹泻，黏液便或血便。

本病属于中医学"泄泻"、"痢疾"、"腹痛"等病证范畴。发病主要是由于感受外邪、饮食不节、情志失调、体虚久病等，导致脾胃运化失调，小肠受盛和大肠传导失常，清浊不分，相夹而下。病理因素主要是湿，发病的关键为脾病湿盛。病位在脾胃与大小肠，并可涉及肾和肝。

【诊断要点】

(1) 反复发作腹痛、腹泻，便下黏冻不爽，神疲乏力为本病中心证候。腹泻为主，排泄含有血、脓和黏液便，伴有阵发性结肠痉挛性疼痛，下腹部有不同程度的压痛，肠鸣音亢

term diarrhea will cause emaciation and anemia.

(2) Small amount of leucocytes appears in microscopic examination of the stools.

(3) Congestion and edema of the colic mucosa plica and mucous secretion may be seen under fibercoloscope.

(4) Derangement of the intestinal plica mucosa is present in X-ray examination with barium enema.

Syndrome Differentiation and Treatment

The syndromes of this disease include excess and deficiency. Excess syndromes are caused by cold and dampness blocking the middle energizer, damp heat damaging the middle energizer and liver qi attacking the spleen; deficiency syndromes are due to deficiency of the spleen and stomach, declination of kidney yang and deficiency of both qi and yin. The treatment principle is strengthening the spleen and expelling dampness, supplymented by the methods of warming the middle energizer and expelling cold, clearing heat and dampness, soothing liver qi stagnation and warming kidney yang. For persistent diarrhea, the method of relieving diarrhea with astringents is commonly used.

1. Cold and Dampness Blocking the Middle Energizer

Chief Manifestations: Loose or even watery stools, abdominal pain, borborygmus, gastric stuffiness, anorexia, chills and fever, nasal obstruction, headache, muscular soreness, thin and white or white and greasy tongue coating, soft-superficial and even-soft pulse.

Therapeutic Methods: To relieve superficies, expel cold and remove dampness with aromatic herbs.

Prescription: Modified Huoxiang Zhengqi San (Powder of Agastaches for Restoring Healthy Qi), composed of

进。长期腹泻可致消瘦、贫血。

(2) 大便镜检有少量的白血球。

(3) 纤维结肠镜检查可见结肠黏膜充血水肿,有黏液分泌物。

(4) 钡灌肠 X 线检查可见肠黏膜皱襞紊乱,粗细不一。

【辨证论治】

本病临床见证有虚有实,寒湿中阻、湿热伤中和肝气乘脾证属实;脾胃虚弱、肾阳虚衰和气阴两虚证属虚。治疗以健脾化湿为原则,同时采用散寒温中、清利湿热、疏肝解郁、温肾助阳等法。久泻不已者,还常用涩肠止泻的方法。

1. 寒湿中阻证

主要证候 大便清稀,甚至如水样,腹痛肠鸣,脘闷食少,恶寒发热,鼻塞头痛,肢体酸痛,苔薄白或白腻,脉濡缓。

治 法 解表散寒,芳香化湿。

方 药 藿香正气散加减:藿香10 g,厚朴6 g,紫苏叶

Huoxiang （*Herba Agastaches*） 10 g, Houpo （*Cortex Magnoliae Officinalis*） 6 g, Zisuye （*Folium Perillae*） 10 g, Chenpi （*Pericarpium Citri Reticulatae*） 6 g, Fuling（*Poria*） 10 g, Baizhu （*Rhizoma Atractylodis Macrocephalae*） 10 g, Dafupi （*Pericarpium Arecae*） 10 g, Banxiaqu （*Massa Fermentata Rhizomatis Pinelliae*） 10 g, Jiegeng （*Radix Platycodi*） 6 g, Baizhi （*Radix Angelicae Dahuricae*） 10 g and Zhigancao （*Radix Glycyrrhizae*, roasted) 3 g.

Modifications: For severe exterior syndromes, add Jingjie （*Herba Schizonepetae*） 6 g and Fangfeng （*Radix Saposhnikoviae*） 6 g; for fullness in the chest, abdominal distention, lassitude and white and greasy tongue coating, add Baikouren （*Fructus Amomi Rotundus*, to be decocted later) 3 g; for abdominal distenting pain and borborygmus, add Sharen （*Fructus Amommi*, to be decocted later) 3 g and Paojiang （*Rhzioma Zingiberis*, roasted in hot cinders) 5 g.

2. Damp Heat Damaging the Middle Energizer

Chief Manifestations: Urgent watery diarrhea, yellowish-brown stools with foul smell, abdominal pain, difficult defecation, feverish sensation in the anus, scanty deep yellow urine, restlessness, fever, thirsty, yellow and greasy tongue coating, soft-superficial and rapid pulse or smooth and rapid pulse.

Therapeutic Methods: To clear away heat and promote diuresis.

Prescription: Modified Gegen Qin Lian Tang （Decoction of Puerariae, Scutellariae and Rhizoma Coptidis）, composed of Gegen （*Radix Puerariae*） 15 g, Huangqin （*Radix Scutellariae*） 10 g, Huanglian （*Rhizoma Coptidis*） 6 g, Yiyiren （*Semen Coicis*） 20 g, Houpo （*Cortex Magnoliae Officinalis*） 10 g, Jinyinhua （*Flos Lonicerae*） 20 g, Pugongying （*Herba Taraxaci*） 20 g,

10 g,陈皮 6 g,茯苓 10 g,白术 10 g,大腹皮 10 g,半夏曲 10 g,桔梗 6 g,白芷 10 g,炙甘草 3 g。

加　减　表邪较重者,加荆芥 6 g,防风 6 g;胸闷腹胀、肢体倦怠,苔白腻者,加白蔻仁(后下) 3 g;腹部胀痛、肠鸣者,加砂仁(后下) 3 g,炮姜 5 g。

2. 湿热伤中证

主要证候　泻下急迫,势如水注,便色黄褐而臭,腹痛,泻下不爽,肛门灼热,小便短赤,烦热口渴,苔黄腻,脉濡数或滑数。

治　法　清热利湿。

方　药　葛根芩连汤加减:葛根 15 g,黄芩 10 g,黄连 6 g,薏苡仁 20 g,厚朴 10 g,金银花 20 g,蒲公英 20 g,连翘 15 g,甘草 6 g。

Lianqiao (*Fructus Forsythiae*) 15 g and Gancao (*Radix Glycyrrhizae*) 6 g.

Modifications: For predominent dampness with fullness in the chest and abdomen, add Shichangpu (*Rhizoma Acori Tatarinowii*) 10 g and Fuling (*Poria*) 15 g; for food retention, add Shenqu (*Massa Medicata Fermentata*) 12 g, Maiya (*Fructus Hordei Germinatus*) 12 g and Shanzha (*Fructus Crataegi*) 10 g; for severe abdominal pain, add Yanhusuo (*Rhizoma Corydalis*) 10 g and Zhishi (*Fructus Aurantii Immaturus*) 10 g; for bloody stools, add Diyu (*Radix Sanguisorbae*) 15 g and Cebaitan (*Cacumen Platycladi*, charred) 15 g.

3. Liver Qi Attacking the Spleen

Chief Manifestations: This syndrome is aggravated by depression, anger or stress and its symptoms include borborygmus, distending pain, abdominal pain before diarrhea with the pain relieved after diarrhea, stiffiness in the chest, distention of the hypochondrium, anorexia, belching, light red tongue, wiry pulse.

Therapeutic Methods: To depress the wood (liver) and strengthen the earth (spleen), regulate middle energizer and relieve diarrhea.

Prescription: Modified Tongxie Yaofang (Prescription for Diarrhea with Abdominal Pain), composed of Baishaoyao (*Radix Paeoniae Alba*) 10 g, Baizhu (*Rhizoma Atractylodis Macrocephalae*) 10 g, Chenpi (*Pericarpium Citri Reticulatae*) 6 g, Fangfeng (*Radix Saposhnikoviae*) 10 g, Chaihu (*Radix Bupleuri*) 6 g, Dangshen (*Radix Codonopsis*) 10 g, Yiyiren (*Semen Coicis*) 15 g, Jiaoshanzha (*Fructus Crataegi*, charred) 10 g and Wumei (*Fructus Mume*) 5 g.

Modifications: For spleen deficiency with lassitude and loose stools, add Fuling (*Poria*) 15 g and Shanyao (*Rhizoma Dioscoreae*) 10 g; for recurrent diarrhea, add

加　减　湿邪偏重,胸腹满闷者,加石菖蒲10 g,茯苓15 g;挟食滞,加神曲12 g,麦芽12 g,山楂10 g;腹痛甚者,加延胡索10 g,枳实10 g;血便者,加地榆15 g,侧柏炭15 g。

3. 肝气乘脾证

主要证候　肠鸣攻痛,腹痛即泻,泻后痛缓,胸胁胀闷,嗳气食少,每因抑郁恼怒或情绪紧张之时加重,舌淡红,脉弦。

治　法　抑木扶土,调中止泻。

方　药　痛泻要方加减:白芍药10 g,白术10 g,陈皮6 g,防风10 g,柴胡6 g,党参10 g,薏苡仁15 g,焦山楂10 g,乌梅5 g。

加　减　脾虚明显,神疲乏力,大便溏薄者,加茯苓15 g,山药10 g;泄泻反复不已

Mugua (*Fructus Chaenomelis*) 10 g and Hezi (*Fructus Chebulae*) 10 g.

4. Deficiency of the Spleen and Stomach

Chief Manifestations: Loose stools or diarrhea with undigested food, increase of bowl movements after intake of greasy food, reduced appetite, epigastric and abdominal flatulence, sallow complexion, lassitude, pale tongue with white coating, thready and weak pulse.

Therapeutic Methods: To invigorate the spleen and benefit qi, promote transportation and relieve diarrhea.

Prescription: Modified Shen Ling Baizhu San (Powder of Ginseng, Poria and Atractylodis Macrocephalae), composed of Dangshen (*Radix Codonopsis*) 10 g, Baizhu (*Rhizoma Atractylodis Macrocephalae*) 10 g, Fuling (*Poria*) 15 g, Shanyao (*Rhizoma Dioscoreae*) 10 g, Biandou (*Semen Dolichoris*) 10 g, Yiyiren (*Semen Coicis*) 15 g, Lianzirou (*Semen Nelumbinis*) 10 g, Sharen (*Fructus Amommi*, to be decocted later) 5 g, Chenpi (*Pericarpium Citri Reticulatae*) 6 g and Guya (*Fructus Oryzae Germinatus*) 15 g.

Modifications: For declination of spleen yang with cold pain in the abdomen and cold limbs, add Shufuzi (*Radix Aconiti Lateralis Preparata*) 6 g and Ganjiang (*Rhizoma Zingiberis*) 5 g; for long-term diarrhea, add Yingsuke (*Pericarpium Papaveris*) 10 g and Hezi (*Fructus Chebulae*) 10 g; for indigestion, add Maiya (*Fructus Hordei Germinatus*) 12 g and Jianqu (*Massa Medicata Fermentata*) 12 g.

5. Declination of Kidney Yang

Chief Manifestations: Abdominal pain and borborygmus at dawn followed by diarrhea, pain relieved after diarrhea, cold body and limbs, soreness of the waist and knees, pale tongue, deep and thready pulse.

Therapeutic Methods: To warm the kidney,

者,加木瓜10 g,诃子10 g。

4. 脾胃虚弱证

主要证候　大便时溏时泻,完谷不化,稍进油腻之物则大便次数增多,饮食减少,脘腹胀闷不舒,面色萎黄,肢倦乏力,舌淡,苔白,脉细弱。

治　法　健脾益气,运中止泻。

方　药　参苓白术散加减:党参10 g,白术10 g,茯苓15 g,山药10 g,扁豆10 g,薏苡仁15 g,莲子肉10 g,砂仁(后下)5 g,陈皮6 g,谷芽15 g。

加　减　脾阳虚衰,阴寒内盛,腹中冷痛,手足不温者,加熟附子6 g,干姜5 g;久泻不止者,加罂粟壳10 g,诃子10 g;纳运欠佳者,加麦芽12 g,建曲12 g。

5. 肾阳虚衰证

主要证候　黎明腹痛肠鸣即泻,泻后痛减,形寒肢冷,腰膝酸软,舌淡,脉沉细。

治　法　温肾健脾,固涩

strengthen the spleen, induce astringency and relieve diarrhea.

Prescription: Sishen Wan Jiawei (Pill of Four Miraculous Drugs with Additions), composed of Wuzhuyu (*Fructus Evodiae*) 6 g, Buguzhi (*Fructus Psoraleae*) 10 g, Wuweizi (*Fructus Schisandrae*) 5 g, Roudoukou (*Semen Myristicae*) 10 g, Shufuzi (*Radix Aconiti Lateralis Preparata*) 10 g, Chishizhi (*Halloysitum Rubrum*) 20 g, Dangshen (*Radix Codonopsis*) 10 g and Huangqi (*Radix Astragali*) 15 g.

Modification: For long-term diarrhea, add Yuyuliang (*Limonitum*) 10 g, Yingsuke (*Pericarpium Papaveris*) 10 g and Hezi (*Fructus Chebulae*) 10 g.

6. Deficiency of both Qi and Yin

Chief Manifestations: Long-term diarrhea with pus and bloody stools, dull pain in the abdomen, low fever in the afternoon, dizziness, insomnia, night sweating, restlessness, irritability, emaciation, red tongue with less coating, thready and rapid pulse.

Therapeutic Methods: To nourish yin, clear away heat, replenish qi and relieve diarrhea.

Prescription: Modified Shengmai San (Powder for Reinforcing Qi and Nourishing Yin) and Liujunzi Tang (Six Mild-Drug Decoction), composed of Dangshen (*Radix Codonopsis*) 10 g, Baizhu (*Rhizoma Atractylodis Macrocephalae*) 10 g, Fuling (*Poria*) 15 g, Chenpi (*Pericarpium Citri Reticulatae*) 6 g, Zhibanxia (*Rhizoma Pinelliae Preparata*) 10 g, Huangqi (*Radix Astragali*) 15 g, Wumei (*Fructus Mume*) 10 g, Wuweizi (*Fructus Schisandrae*) 5 g, Maimendong (*Radix Ophiopogonis*) 10 g, Qianshi (*Semen Euryales*) 15 g, Zhimu (*Rhizoma Anemarrhenae*) 12 g and Shanyao (*Rhizoma Dioscoreae*) 30 g.

Modifications: For feverish sensation in the chest,

止泻。

方　药　四神丸加味：吴茱萸6 g,补骨脂10 g,五味子5 g,肉豆蔻10 g,熟附子10 g,赤石脂20 g,党参10 g,黄芪15 g。

加　减　久泻滑脱者,加禹余粮10 g,罂粟壳10 g,诃子10 g。

6. 气阴两虚证

主要证候　久泻不止,便下脓血,腹中隐痛,午后低热,头晕目眩,失眠盗汗,心烦易怒,消瘦乏力,舌红少苔,脉细数。

治　法　养阴清热,益气固肠。

方　药　生脉散合六君子汤加减：党参10 g,白术10 g,茯苓15 g,陈皮6 g,制半夏10 g,黄芪15 g,乌梅10 g,五味子5 g,麦门冬10 g,芡实15 g,知母12 g,山药30 g。

加　减　五心烦热者,加

palms and soles, add Qinghao (*Herba Artemisiae Annuae*) 10 g and Yinchaihu (*Radix Stellaride*) 10 g; for restlessness and insomnia, add Chaosuanzaoren (*Semen Ziziphi Spinosae*, stir-baked) 15 g, Huanglian (*Rhizoma Copitdis*) 3 g and Danshen (*Radix Salviae Miltiorrhizae*) 15 g; for dizziness, add Tianma (*Rhizoma Gastrodiae*) 10 g and Zhenzhumu (*Concha Margaritifera Usta*, to be decocted first) 30 g; for severe diarrhea, add Chishizhi (*Halloysitum Rubrum*) 10 g and Yuyuliang (*Limonitum*) 10 g; for red and white mucus in the stools, add Baihuasheshecao (*Herba Hedyotis Diffusae*) 30 g and Machixian (*Herba Portulacae*) 30 g.

Other Treatments

1. Chinese Patent Drugs

（1）Huoxiang Zhengqi Ruanjiaonang (Agastaches Capsule for Restoring Healthy Qi): 2 - 4 capsules each time, 3 times daily; applicable to chronic colitis with invasion of wind and cold and internal dampness retention.

（2）Gegen Qin Lian Weiwan (Pill of Puerariae, Scutellariae and Coptidis): 3 g each time, 3 times daily; applicable to chronic colitis with viral and bacterial diarrhea, fever and restlessness.

（3）Jiawei Xiang Lian Wan (Pill of Aucklandiae and Coptidis with Additions): 6 g each time, 3 times daily; applicable to chronic colitis with diarrhea caused by damp heat.

（4）Xiang Sha Liujunzi Wan (Pill of Aucklanndiae and Amomi with Six Mild Drugs): 6 - 9 g each time, 2 - 3 times daily; applicable to chronic colitis with spleen deficiency and qi stagnation, indigestion, belching, reduced appetite, fullness in the chest and abdomen and diarrhea.

（5）Sishen Wan (Pill of Four Miraculous Drugs): 9 g each time, twice daily; applicable to chronic colitis with yang deficiency of the spleen and kidney, dawn diarrhea,

青蒿10 g,银柴胡10 g;虚烦少寐者,加炒酸枣仁15 g,黄连3 g,丹参15 g;眩晕明显者,加天麻10 g,珍珠母(先下)30 g;大便滑泻者加赤石脂10 g,禹余粮10 g;便下赤白黏冻者,加白花蛇舌草30 g,马齿苋30 g。

【其他疗法】

1. 中成药

（1）藿香正气软胶囊　每服2～4粒,每日3次。适用于慢性结肠炎外感风寒,内伤湿滞者。

（2）葛根芩连微丸　每服3 g,每日3次。适用于慢性结肠炎病毒性、细菌性腹泻,身热烦躁者。

（3）加味香连丸　每服6 g,每日3次。适用于慢性结肠炎表现为湿热腹泻者。

（4）香砂六君子丸　每服6～9 g,每日2～3次。适用于慢性结肠炎脾虚气滞,消化不良,嗳气食少,脘腹胀满,大便溏泻者。

（5）四神丸　每服9 g,每日2次。适用于慢性结肠炎脾肾虚寒,五更泄泻,食不消

indigestion, soreness in the waist and abdominal pain.

2. Single-drug or Experiential Prescriptions

(1) Wumei (*Fructus Mume*) 15 g. Decoct it with appropriate amount of water and take the decoction as normal drink. It is applicable to long-term diarrhea damaging yin.

(2) Cheqianzi (*Semen Plataginis*) 30 g, Machixian (*Herba Portulacae*) 30 g and Pugongying (*Herba Taraxaci*) 30 g. Decoct the drugs with water for oral administration, one dose every day. It is applicable to fever, chills, abdominal pain and diarrhea.

(3) Shengshanzha (*Fructus Crataegi*) 20 g and Jiaoshanzha (*Fructus Crataegi*, charred) 20 g. Decoct them with water for oral administration, one dose every day. It is applicable to dyspepsia.

(4) A handful of Chenai (*Folium Artemisiae Argyi*, long-stored) and a block of ginger. Decoct them with water for oral administration, one dose every day. It is applicable to acute attack of chronic colitis.

(5) Five blocks of garlic bulbs and 100 g of white turnip. Decoct them with water and drink the decoction. It is applicable to cold diarrhea.

(6) Gegen (*Radix Puerariae*) 9 g, Huanglian (*Rhizoma Copitdis*) 6 g, Huangqin (*Radix Scutellariae*) 6 g, Mutong (*Caulis Akebiae*) 9 g and Gancao (*Radix Glycyrrhizae*) 3 g. Decoct the drugs with water for oral administration, 2 doses daily for 3 consecutive days. It is applicable to damp-heat diarrhea.

(7) Chaoshanzha (*Fructus Crataegi*, stir-baked) 12 g, Jianqu (*Massa Medicata Fermentata*) 9 g, Cangzhu (*Scolopendra*) 6 g, Houpo (*Cortex Magnoliae Officinalis*) 6 g and Chenpi (*Pericarpium Citri Reticulatae*) 6 g. Decoct them with water for oral administration, 2 doses daily for 3 consecutive days. It is applicable to

化,腰酸腹痛者。

2. 单验方

(1) 乌梅15 g,加水适量煎汤,代茶饮服。适用于久泻及伤阴者。

(2) 车前子30 g,马齿苋30 g,蒲公英30 g,水煎服,每日1剂。适用于发热恶寒,腹痛泄泻者。

(3) 生山楂20 g,焦山楂20 g,水煎服,每日1剂。适用于伤食者。

(4) 陈艾1把,生姜1块,水煎服,每日1剂。适用于慢性结肠炎急性发作者。

(5) 大蒜头5个,白萝卜100 g,加水同煮饮水。适用于寒泻者。

(6) 葛根9 g,黄连6 g,黄芩6 g,木通9 g,甘草3 g。水煎服,每日2次,连服3日。适用于湿热泄泻者。

(7) 炒山楂12 g,建曲9 g,苍术6 g,厚朴6 g,陈皮6 g。水煎服,每日2次,连服3日。适用于食滞泄泻者。

food-retention diarrhea.

(8) Shiliupi (*Pericarpium Granati*) 1 piece and 30 g of brown sugar. Decoct them with water for oral administration, 2 doses daily for consecutive 10 days. It is applicable to long-term diarrhea.

(9) Lianzirou (*Semen Nelumbinis*) 100 g, Shanyao (*Rhizoma Dioscoreae*) 100 g, Yiyiren (*Semen Coicis*) 100 g and Qianshi (*Semen Euryales*) 100 g. Stir-bake and grind them into powder, take 6 g every day for 15 consecutive days. It is applicable to long-term diarrhea due to deficiency of the spleen and stomach.

3. External Therapy

(1) Wubeizi (*Galla Chinensis*) 10 g. Grind it into powder, mix it with vinegar to make paste, put the paste into the umbilicus, cover it with gauze and fix it with adhesive tape. It is applicable to long-term diarrhea.

(2) Roudoukou (*Semen Myristicae*) 90 g, Mutong (*Caulis Akebiae*) 200 g, Zexie (*Rhizoma Alismatis*) 100 g, Zhuling (*Polyporus*) 100 g, Cangzhu (*Rhizoma Atractylodis*) 100 g, Gaoliangjiang (*Rhizoma Alpiniae Officinarum*) 100 g, Houpo (*Cortex Magnoliae Officinalis*) 100 g and Rougui (*Cortex Cinnamomi*) 100 g. Fry the herbs with 2,500 ml of sesame oil. Remove the dregs and add Zhangdan (*Minium*) to make plaster. Put the plaster in the umbilicus and change it every other days. It is applicable to cold-damp diarrhea.

(3) Gegen (*Radix Puerariae*) 5 g, Huanglian (*Rhizoma Copitdis*) 5 g, Huangqin (*Radix Scutellariae*) 10 g, Muxiang (*Radix Aucklandiae*) 10 g and Machixian (*Herba Portulacae*) 30 g. Decoct them with water twice until an extract was made. Add 3% - 5% sodium Benzoate in every 100 ml of the extract. Take proper amount of the extract for retention enema, twice daily until recovery. It is applicable to damp-heat diarrhea.

（8）石榴皮 1 个,红糖 30 g。水煎服,每日 2 次,连服 10 日。适用于久泻不止者。

（9）莲子肉100 g,山药 100 g,薏 苡 仁 100 g,芡实 100 g。共炒研末,每次6 g,不拘时服,连服 15 日。适用于脾胃虚弱之久泻者。

3. 外治法

（1）五倍子10 g,研末,醋调为糊状,敷脐中,外以纱布敷盖,胶布固定。适用于久泻不止。

（2）肉豆蔻90 g,木通 200 g,泽泻100 g,猪苓100 g,苍术100 g,高良姜100 g,厚朴 100 g,肉桂100 g,上药以香油 2 500 ml,炸枯去渣,入章丹收膏。贴脐,隔日更换 1 张。适用于寒湿泄泻者。

（3）葛根5 g,黄连5 g,黄芩10 g,木香10 g,马齿苋30 g。上药水煎 2 次,取药汁混合浓煎瓶贮,每100 ml加入 3% ～ 5%苯甲酸纳1 ml备用。取药适重,保留灌肠,每日 2 次,治愈为度。适用于湿热型泄泻者。

(4) Qingpi (*Pericarpium Citri Reticulatae Viride*) 12 g, Chenpi (*Pericarpium Citri Reticulatae*) 12 g, Baishaoyao (*Radix Paeoniae Alba*) 12 g, Fangfeng (*Radix Saposhnikoviae*) 10 g, Chaihu (*Radix Bupleuri*) 10 g, Fuling (*Poria*) 20 g, Chaoyiyiren (*Semen Coicis*, stir-baked) 15 g and Baizhu (*Rhizoma Atractylodis Macrocephalae*) 15 g. Decoct the drugs with water and concentrate the decoction for enema, twice daily until recovery. It is applicable to diarrhea due to liver-stagnation.

(5) Lücao (*Herba Humuli Scandentis*, *fresh*) 500 g. Decoct it with 2,000 ml of water for 20 minutes, one dose a day. Put the decoction into a basin for washing and soaking the feet for 30 minutes, twice daily, 15 days making up a treatment course. It is applicable to ulcerative colitis.

(6) A piece of 20 - 30 cm Ejiao (*Colla Corii Asini*). Steam it until it is soft and cut it into 1.5 - 2 cm sections. Put the sections into boiling water and soften them thoroughly, take them out with forceps, mould them into elliptic suppositories for later use. Soften them in hot water before inserting them into the annus. The depth and dosage of the suppository depends on the depth and size of the focus. Use them once every day after bowl movement with 7 - 10 days as a treatment course. It is applicable to ulcerative colitis.

2.3.5 Constipation

General Description

Constipation refers to a disorder of prolonged defecation or difficult defecation.

This disorder is mainly caused by improper diet,

（4）青皮12 g,陈皮12 g, 白芍药 12,防风10 g,柴胡 10 g,茯苓20 g,炒薏苡仁15 g, 白术15 g。浓煎取药汁灌肠, 每日 2 次,治愈为度。适用于 肝郁型泄泻者。

（5）鲜葎草500 g,洗净加 水2 000 ml,煎沸 20 分钟,去渣 取药液,倒入盆内待药液温后, 浸泡洗浴双足,每日 1 剂,每日 2 次,每次 30 分钟,15 日为 1 个 疗程。适用于溃疡性结肠炎。

（6）取20～30 cm阿胶 1 块,隔水加热使之软化,取出 剪成1.5～2 cm的小段,将小 段投入沸水中使其充分软化 后,用镊子摄出,捏成光滑的 椭圆形栓备用。用时将其投 入热水软化,塞入肛门,送入 的深度和枚数,视病位高低和 病变范围而定。每日大便后 上药 1 次,7～10 日为 1 个疗 程。适用于溃疡性结肠炎。

第五节　便秘

【概述】

便秘指大便秘结不通,排 便时间延长,或欲解大便而艰 涩不畅的一种病证。

本病主要因饮食不当、思

excessive anxiety, lack of physical exercise, constitutional yang preponderance and weak constitution after an illness. The pathogenesis of constipation is mainly due to the dysfunction of the large intestine in transmission and also related to the dysfunction of the spleen, stomach, liver and kidney. Pathologically it can be divided into excess type and deficiency type. The excess type includes heat accumulation in the intestine and stomach and qi stagnation; while the deficiency type includes yang qi deficiency and yin-blood deficiency.

The disorder can be seen in functional constipation, intestinal neurosis and constipation due to the side effect of drugs in western medicine.

Essentials for Diagnosis

(1) Reduced bowel movements, prolonged circle of defecation, or hard stools and difficulty in emptying the bowels.

(2) Accompanied symptoms include abdominal distention, abdominal pain, poor appetite, dizziness, halitosis, anal fissure, hemorrhoid, bloody stools, sweating, shortness of breath, dizziness and palpitation.

(3) The occurrence is related to invasion of cold and heat, diet, emotions, dysfunction of zang and fu organs, lack of physical exercise, aging and weak constitution. The onset and the development are slow.

(4) Fibercoloscope and other laboratory examinations are usually helpful to the diagnosis.

Syndrome Differentiation and Treatment

Constipation may be excessive or deficient. The excess syndromes include heat accumulation in the intestine and stomach, qi stagnation in the intestine and retention of yin cold; the deficiency syndromes include spleen

虑少动、素体阳盛及病后体虚所致。病机总属肠腑传导失常。病在大肠,与脾胃肝肾相关。病理性质有虚实之分。因肠胃积热、气机郁滞者属实,因阳气不足、阴血亏虚者属虚。

本病可见于西医学中的功能性便秘、肠神经官能症及药物所致的便秘。

【诊断要点】

(1) 排便次数减少,排便周期延长;或粪质坚硬,便下困难,或排出无力,出而不畅。

(2) 常兼有腹胀、腹痛、纳呆、头晕、口臭、肛裂、痔疮、排便带血以及汗出气短、头晕心悸等兼杂证。

(3) 发病常与外感寒热、饮食情志、脏腑失调、坐卧少动、年老体弱等因素有关。起病缓慢,多表现为慢性病变过程。

(4) 实验室检查如纤维结肠镜等有关检查,常有助于部分便秘的诊断。

【辨证论治】

便秘一证有虚有实,实证包括肠胃积热、肠道气滞、阴寒积滞证,虚证包括脾气虚弱、血虚津少、脾肾阳虚证。

qi deficiency, deficiency of blood and body fluid and deficiency of spleen and kidney yang. The treatment principle is chiefly the purgation, but clinically purgation should be combined with other treatments according to the differentiation of the syndrome. For excess syndromes, clearing heat and purging fire, regulating qi and expelling stagnation, expelling cold and warming the middle energizer are adopted; for deficiecy syndromes, tonifying spleen qi, nourishing blood and moistening the intestine and warming yang and relieving constipation are often used.

1. Heat Accumulation in the Intestines and Stomach

Chief Manifestations: Dry stools, abdominal distention, abdominal pain, red complexion, fever, thirsty, bad breath, restlessness, scanty deep yellow urine, red tongue with yellow and dry coating, smooth and rapid pulse.

Therapeutic Methods: To clear away heat, relieve stagnation, moisten intestines and promote defecation.

Prescription: Modified Maziren Wan (Cannabis Pill), composed of Huomaren (*Semen Cannabis*) 15 g, Baishaoyao (*Radix Paeoniae Alba*) 10 g, Zhishi (*Fructus Aurantii Immaturus*) 10 g, Houpo (*Cortex Magnoliae Officinalis*) 10 g, Dahuang (*Radix et Rhizoma Rhei*, to be decocted later) 10 g, Xingren (*Semen Armeniacae Amarum*) 10 g and white honey 10 ml.

Modifications: For damage of body fluid, add Shengdihuang (*Radix Rehmanniae*) 10 g, Xuanshen (*Radix Scrophulariae*) 10 g, Maimendong (*Radix Ophiopogonis*) 10 g; for irritability and red eyes, add Mudanpi (*Cortex Moutan Radicis*) 10 g and Zhizi (*Fructus Gardeniae*) 10 g; for bloody stools caused by heat, add Huaihua (*Flos Sophorae*) 10 g and Diyu (*Radix Sanguisorbae*) 10 g.

治疗以通下为原则,但决不可单纯用泻下药,需结合其病变性质而施以相应的治法。实证常用清热泻火、理气导滞、散寒温中法,虚证常用补益脾气、养血润肠、温阳开秘法。

1. 肠胃积热证

主要证候 大便干结,腹胀腹痛,面红身热,口干口臭,心烦不安,小便短赤,舌质红,苔黄燥,脉滑数。

治 法 泻热导滞,润肠通便。

方 药 麻子仁丸加减:火麻仁15 g,白芍药10 g,枳实10 g,厚朴10 g,大黄(后下)10 g,杏仁10 g,白蜜 10 ml。

加 减 津液已伤,可加生地黄10 g,玄参10 g,麦门冬10 g;易怒目赤者,加牡丹皮10 g,栀子10 g;热甚便血者,加槐花10 g,地榆10 g。

2. Qi Stagnation in the Intestines

Chief Manifestations: Dry or not very dry stools, urgency to defecate but having difficulty in passing stools, borborygmus, passing gas, distending pain in the abdomen, fullness in the chest and hypochondriac area, frequent belching, poor appetite, thin and greasy tongue coating, wiry pulse.

Therapeutic Methods: To restore the free flow of qi and relieve stagnation.

Prescription: Modified Liumo Tang (Liumo Decoction), composed of Binglang (*Semen Arecae*) 10 g, Wuyao (*Linderae*) 15 g, Guangmuxiang (*Radix Aucklandiae*) 10 g, Zhishi (*Fructus Aurantii Immaturus*) 10 g, Chenxiangfen (*Lignum Aquilariae Resinatum*, powdered and to be taken with the decoction) 3 g, Dahuang (*Radix et Rhizoma Rhei*, to be decocted later) 6 g and Yuliren (*Semen Pruni*) 10 g.

Modifications: For qi stagnation turning into fire with bitter mouth and dry throat, add Huangqin (*Radix Scutellariae*) 10 g, Zhizi (*Fructus Gardeniae*) 10 g and Longdancao (*Radix Gentianae*) 6 g; for vomiting with adverseness of qi, add Zhibanxia (*Rhizoma Pinelliae Preparata*) 10 g, Xuanfuhua (*Flos Inulae*, wrapped) 10 g and Daizheshi (*Haematitum*, to be decocted first) 30 g; for emotional disturbance and silence, add Baishaoyao (*Radix Paeoniae Alba*) 10 g, Chaihu (*Radix Bupleuri*) 6 g and Hehuanpi (*Cortex Albiziae*) 10 g; for constipation after trauma or abdominal surgery with qi and blood stagnation, add Taoren (*Semen Persicae*) 10 g, Honghua (*Flos Carthami*) 10 g and Chishaoyao (*Radix Paeoniae Rubra*) 10 g.

3. Retention of Yin cold

Chief Manifestations: Difficult defecation, abdominal pain and distention aggravated by pressure, pain in

2. 肠道气滞证

主要证候 大便干结,或不甚干结,欲便不得出,或便而不爽,肠鸣矢气,腹中胀痛,胸胁满闷,嗳气频作,食少纳呆,舌苔薄腻,脉弦。

治 法 顺气导滞。

方 药 六磨汤加减:槟榔10 g,乌药15 g,广木香10 g,枳实10 g,沉香粉(冲服)3 g,大黄(后下)6 g,郁李仁10 g。

加 减 气郁化火,口苦咽干者,加黄芩10 g,栀子10 g,龙胆草6 g;气逆呕吐者,加制半夏10 g,旋覆花(包煎)10 g,代赭石(先煎)30 g;七情郁结,忧郁寡言者,加白芍药10 g,柴胡6 g,合欢皮10 g;跌仆损伤,腹部术后,便秘不通,属气滞血瘀者,加桃仁10 g,红花10 g,赤芍药10 g。

3. 阴寒积滞证

主要证候 大便艰涩,腹痛拘急,胀满拒按,胁下偏痛,

the hypochondriac area, cold limbs, hiccup and vomiting, white and greasy tongue coating, wiry and tense pulse.

Therapeutic Methods: To warm the interior, expel cold, promote bowel movement and relieve pain.

Prescription: Modified Dahuang Fuzi Tang (Rhei and Aconiti Lateralis Decoction), composed of Shufuzi (*Radix Aconiti Lateralis Preparata*) 10 g, Dahuang (*Radix et Rhizoma Rhei*, to be decocted later) 5 - 10 g, Xixin (*Herba Asari*) 3 g, Zhishi (*Fructus Aurantii Immaturus*) 10 g, Houpo (*Cortex Magnoliae Officinalis*) 6 g, Muxiang (*Radix Aucklandiae*) 6 g, Ganjiang (*Rhizoma Zingiberis*) 5 g and Xiaohuixiang (*Fructus Foeniculi*) 4 g.

Modification: For cold pain in the abdomen, add Rougui (*Cortex Cinnamomi*) 3 g and Wuyao (*Linderae*) 6 g.

4. Spleen Qi Deficiency

Chief Manifestations: Neither dry nor hard stools, urgency to defecate with difficulty in passing stools, sweating, shortness of breath, fatigue after bowl movement, pale complexion and lassitude, tiredness of the limbs, dislike of speaking, pale tongue with white coating, weak pulse.

Therapeutic Methods: To tonify qi and lubricate the intestines.

Prescription: Modified Huangqi Tang (*Astragali Decoction*), composed of Zhihuangqi (*Radix Astragali*, roasted) 15 g, Dangshen (*Radix Codonopsis*) 10 g, Chenpi (*Pericarpium Citri Reticulatae*) 10 g, Huomaren (*Semen Cannabis*) 10 g, Danggui (*Radix Angelicae Sinensis*) 10 g and white honey 10 ml.

Modifications: For severe qi deficiency, add Dangshen (*Radix Codonopsis*) 10 g and Baizhu (*Rhizoma Atractylodis Macrocephalae*) 10 g; for prolapse of the anus

手足不温,呃逆呕吐,舌苔白腻,脉弦紧。

治 法 温里散寒,通便止痛。

方 药 大黄附子汤加减:熟附子10 g,生大黄(后下)5～10 g,细辛3 g,枳实10 g,厚朴6 g,木香6 g,干姜5 g,小茴香4 g。

加 减 腹部冷痛者,加肉桂3 g,乌药6 g。

4. 脾气虚弱证

主要证候 粪质并不干硬,虽有便意,但临厕努挣乏力,便难排出,汗出气短,便后乏力,面白神疲,肢倦懒言,舌质淡,苔白,脉弱。

治 法 补气润肠。

方 药 黄芪汤加减:炙黄芪15 g,党参10 g,陈皮10 g,火麻仁10 g,当归10 g,白蜜10 ml。

加 减 气虚较甚者,加党参10 g,白术10 g;气虚下陷脱肛者,加升麻10 g,柴胡

caused by sinking of qi, add Shengma (*Rhizoma Cimicifugae*) 10 g, Chaihu (*Radix Bupleuri*) 10 g and Jiegeng (*Radix Platycodi*) 6 g; for dry stools and difficult defecation, add Yuliren (*Semen Pruni*) 10 g, Xingren (*Semen Armeniacae Amarum*) 10 g and Roucongrong (*Herba Cistanchis*) 10 g; for dizziness and pale finger nails, add Shengheshouwu (*Radix Polygoni Multiflori*) 10 g, Shengdihuang (*Radix Rehmanniae*) 10 g; for shortness of breath, add Gejiefen (*Gecko*, powdered and to be taken with the decoction) 2 g; for poor appetite, add Chaomaiya (*Fructus Hordei Germinatus*, stir-baked) 15 g.

5. Deficiency of Blood and Body Fluid

Chief Manifestations: Dry stools, lusterless complexion, palpitation, shortness of breath, insomnia, dream-disturbed sleeping, poor memory, pale lips, pale tongue with white coating, thready pulse.

Therapeutic Methods: To nourish blood and moisten the dryness.

Prescription: Modified Zunsheng Runchang Wan (*Zunsheng* Pill for Lubricating Intestine), composed of Zhidahuang (*Radix et Rhizoma Rhei Preparata*) 10 g, Danggui (*Radix Angelicae Sinensis*) 12 g, Shengdihuang (*Radix Rehmanniae*) 10 g, Huomaren (*Semen Cannabis*) 10 g, Taoren (*Semen Persicae*) 10 g, Zhike (*Fructus Aurantii*) 10 g, Shengheshouwu (*Radix Polygoni Multiflori*) 10 g and Baiziren (*Semen Platycladi*) 10 g.

Modifications: For blood deficiency and internal heat, add Zhimu (*Rhizoma Anemarrhenae*) 10 g and Huhuanglian (*Rhizoma Copitdis*) 5 g; for recovery of the blood and fluid and dry stools, add Yuliren (*Semen Pruni*) 10 g and Songziren (*Semen Pini Koraiensis*) 10 g.

10 g,桔梗 6 g；大便燥结难下者,加郁李仁 10 g,杏仁 10 g,肉苁蓉 10 g；头昏,爪甲淡白者,加生何首乌 10 g,生地黄 10 g；喘促甚者,加蛤蚧粉(冲) 2 g；纳谷不香者,加炒麦芽 15 g。

5. 血虚津少证

主要证候　大便干结,面色无华,心悸气短,失眠多梦,健忘,口唇色淡,舌质淡,苔白,脉细。

治　法　养血润燥。

方　药　《尊生》润肠丸加减：制大黄 10 g,当归 12 g,生地黄 10 g,火麻仁 10 g,桃仁 10 g,枳壳 10 g,生何首乌 10 g,柏子仁 10 g。

加　减　血虚内热者,可加知母 10 g,胡黄连 5 g；阴血已复,大便仍干燥者,加郁李仁 10 g,松子仁 10 g。

6. Deficiency of Spleen Yang and Kidney Yang

Chief Manifestations: Dry or not dry stools, difficult bowl movement, large quantity of clear urine, cold limbs, cold pain in the abdomen relieved by warmth, cold pain in the waist and knees, pale tongue with white coating, deep and slow pulse.

Therapeutic Methods: To warm yang and promote bowel movement.

Prescription: Modified Jichuan Jian (Jichuan Decoction), composed of Danggui (*Radix Angelicae Sinensis*) 12 g, Huainiuxi (*Radix Achyranthis Bidentatae*) 10 g, Rousongrong (*Herba Cistanchis*) 15 g, Shengma (*Rhizoma Cimicifugae*) 3 g, Zhike (*Fructus Aurantii*) 10 g, Ganjiang (*Rhizoma Zingiberis*) 5 g, Zhifupian (*Radix Aconiti Lateralis Preparata*, to be decocted first) 6 g and Rougui (*Cortex Cinnamomi*) 3 g.

Modifications: For nocturnal polyuria, add Jinyingzi (*Fructus Rosae Laevigatae*) 15 g, Wuyao (*Linderae*) 10 g and Shanyao (*Rhizoma Dioscoreae*) 15 g; for severe abdominal pain, add Muxiang (*Radix Aucklandiae*) 10 g and Yanhusuo (*Rhizoma Corydalis*) 10 g.

Other Treatments

1. Chinese Patent Drugs

(1) Huanglian Shangqing Wan (Copitdis Pill for Clearing away Heat in Upper Energizer): 6 g each time, twice daily; applicable to constipation with red eyes, toothache and boils of the lip and tongue.

(2) Maren Jiaonang (Cannabis Capsule): 0.7-1.4 g each time, twice daily; applicable to weak bowl movement in elderly people and habitual constipation caused by dry and heat agglomeration.

(3) Congrong Tongbian Koufuye (Oral Liquid of Cistanches for Constipation): 10-20 ml each time, once

6. 脾肾阳虚证

主要证候 大便干或不干,排出困难,小便清长,四肢不温,腹中冷痛,得热则减,腰膝冷痛,舌质淡,苔白,脉沉迟。

治 法 温阳通便。

方 药 济川煎加减:当归12 g,怀牛膝10 g,肉苁蓉15 g,升麻3 g,枳壳10 g,干姜5 g,炙附片(先煎)6 g,肉桂3 g。

加 减 夜尿多,加金樱子15 g,乌药10 g,山药15 g;腹痛明显者,加木香10 g,延胡索10 g。

【其他疗法】

1. 中成药

(1)黄连上清丸 每服6 g,每日2次。适用于大便秘结,目赤齿痛,口舌生疮者。

(2)麻仁胶囊 每粒3.5 g,每次0.7~1.4 g,每日2次。适用于老年人无力性便秘、习惯性便秘属燥热内结者。

(3)苁蓉通便口服液 每服10~20 ml,每日1次。适用

daily; applicable to deficiency type constipation after ill-ness in middle-aged and elderly people or in post-partum women or deficiency type habitual constipation. It should be used with caution to treat pregnant women.

(4) Gengyi Pian (Tablet for Constipation): 4 tablets each time, thrice daily; applicable to constipation with de-ficiency of yin fluid and excessive liver fire and given cau-tiously to pregnant women.

(5) Muxiang Binlang Wan (Aucklandiae and Arecae Pill): 3 - 6 g each time, twice or thrice daily; applicable to constipation with abdominal distention and pain.

(6) Qinglin Wan (Qinglin Pill): 3 - 6 g each time, twice daily; applicable to constipation caused by heat ag-glomeration.

2. Single-drug or Experiential Prescriptions

(1) Fanxieye (*Folium Sennae*) 6 g. Put it in boiling water to make tea, one dose a day. It is applicable to con-stipation caused by heat accumulation in the intestines.

(2) Shengdahuang (*Radix et Rhizoma Rhei*) 6 g. Put it in boiling water to make tea, one dose a day. It is applicable to constipation caused by heat accumulation in the intestines.

(3) Gualoupi (*Pericarpium Trichosanthis*) 6 g, Gua-louren (*Semen Trichosanthis*) 6 g, Qingpi (*Pericarpi-um Citri Reticulatae Viride*) 6 g and Xingren (*Semen Armeniacae Amarum*) 6 g. Decoct them with water and take the decoction, twice daily. It is applicable to consti-pation caused by intestinal qi stagnation.

(4) Shengheshouwu (*Radix Polygoni Multiflori*) 30 g. Decoct it with water, one dose daily and take the decoction in 3 - 4 divided doses. It is applicable to constipa-tion caused by dryness of the intestine and blood deficiency.

(5) Shufuzi (*Radix Aconiti Lateralis Preparata*) 6 g, Shengjiang (*Rhizoma Zingiberis Recens*) 3 g and

于中老年病后、产后虚型便秘及虚型习惯性便秘。孕妇慎用。

(4) 更衣片 每服 4 片，每日 3 次。适用于阴津亏虚、肝火内炽之便秘。孕妇慎用。

(5) 木香槟榔丸 每服3～6 g，每日 2～3 次。适用于脘腹胀痛，大便不通者。

(6) 青麟丸 每服 3～6 g，每日 2 次。适用于热结便秘。

2. 单验方

(1) 番泻叶6 g，开水泡服，每日 1 剂。适用于肠道积热之便秘者。

(2) 生大黄6 g，开水泡服，每日 1 剂。适用于肠道积热之便秘者。

(3) 瓜蒌皮6 g，瓜蒌仁6 g，青皮 6 g，杏仁6 g。水煎服，每日 2 次。适宜用于肠道气滞便秘者。

(4) 生何首乌30 g，水煎服，每日 1 剂，分 3～4 次温服。适用于血亏肠燥便秘者。

(5) 熟附子6 g，生姜3 g，大黄6 g。水煎服，每日 1 剂。

Dahuang (*Radix et Rhizoma Rhei*) 6 g. Decoct them with water for oral administration, one dose daily. It is applicable to constipation caused by cold agglomeration.

3. External Therapy

(1) Dacong (*Bulbus Allii Fistulosi*) 250 g, pound and shape it into a cake and put it on the umbilicus, then put a hot water bag on the cake for 30 minutes, once daily, 3 days making up a treatment course. It is applicable to constipation caused by yang deficiency and cold agglomeration.

(2) Zhishi (*Fructus Aurantii Immaturus*) 30 g, Qingpi (*Pericarpium Citri Reticulatae Viride*) 15 g, Binglang (*Semen Arecae*) 15 g and salt 30 g. Grind them into rough powder, stir-bake them hot in the pan, wrap them up with a piece of cloth and foment the umbilicus with the cloth bag, stir-bake the powder again when it becomes cool and foment the umbilicus again, Apply this treatment for 40 minutes each time, twice or thrice daily. It is applicable to constipation caused by qi stagnation in the intestine.

(3) Zhuye (*Folium Phyllostachydis Henonis*) 200 g, Lüfan (*Melanteritum*) 30 g and Luoboye (*Folium Raphani*) 200 g. Decoct Zhuye and Luoboye with water for 20 minutes, put them into the bucket and add Lüfan when they are still hot. Fumigate the anus with the steam in a sedentary posture, once daily, 3 days making up a treatment course. It is applicable to constipation caused by qi stagnation in the intestine and heat accumulation.

(4) Prepare 50 - 100 ml of suds with a proper amount of soap for enema. It is applicable to various kinds of constipation.

(5) Zhudan (*Fel Suillus*) 2 pcs. Get the bile and steam it for sterilization, then add boiled water to prepare

适用于寒气凝结之便秘者。

3. 外治法

（1）大葱250 g，捣成饼敷脐上，用热水袋熨葱饼上，每日1次，每次30分钟，3日为1个疗程。适用于阳虚阴寒凝结之便秘者。

（2）枳实30 g，青皮15 g，槟榔15 g，食盐30 g。将4味药混合共研成粗末，在锅内炒热，用布包裹，将药包放于患者脐部熨之，冷后再炒再熨，持续40分钟，每日2～3次。适用于肠道气滞便秘者。

（3）竹叶200 g，绿矾30 g，萝卜叶200 g。竹叶及萝卜叶水煎20分钟，趁热并倒入桶内，撒入绿矾，坐薰。每日1次，3日为1个疗程。适用于肠道气滞便秘及积热便秘者。

（4）肥皂适量，制成肥皂水，取50～100 ml灌肠。适用于各种便秘。

（5）大猪胆2枚。取猪胆汁隔水炖透消毒，用时加开

50% solution and take 40 ml for enema each time. It is applicable to constipation caused by excessive heat in the intestine.

(6) Zhuyazao (*Fructus Gleditsiae*) 12 g and Xixin (*Herba Asari*) 3 g. Grind them into fine powder, mix it with hot honey and make suppositories. Put the suppositories into the anus, twice daily, 3 days making up a treatment course. It is applicable to constipation caused by yang deficiency and cold agglomeration.

(7) Huomaren (*Semen Cannabis*) 60 g, Dahuang (*Radix et Rhizoma Rhei*) 15 g and Yuliren (*Semen Pruni*) 30 g. Grind them into fine powder and decoct the powder with water on a slow fire until it becomes very thick and make suppositories about 3 cm long. Put one into the anus each time, twice daily. It is applicable to constipation caused by consumption of the body fluid.

(8) Dahuang (*Radix et Rhizoma Rhei*) 15 g, Mangxiao (*Natrii Sulfas*) 15 g and Zaojiao (*Fructus Gleditsiae*) 15 g. Decoct them with water to get 200 ml of the decoction. Dip the gauze or cotton ball into the decoction and embrocate the umbilicus and the abdomen, once or twice daily. It is applicable to constipation caused by heat accumulation.

2.3.6　Large Intestinal Carcinoma

General Description

Large intestinal carcinoma, one of the commonly encountered malignant tumors, refers to carcinoma of colon and rectum. It is also called anal carcinoma when the lesion is at the anus. The incidence and mortality rank the 4th~6th in the malignant tumors. There are more male patients than female patients with a ratio of 1.1~3.4 : 1.

水,调成 50% 胆汁液,每次 40 ml灌肠。适用于肠道实热便秘者。

(6) 猪牙皂12 g,细辛3 g。共研细末,以热蜂蜜调匀制成柱状,塞入肛门内。每日 2 次,3 日为 1 个疗程。适用于阳虚寒凝之便秘者。

(7) 火麻仁60 g,大黄 15 g,郁李仁30 g。共研细末,水煎,文火炼稠,制成柱形,长约3 cm,每次用 1 颗塞入肛门内,每日 2 次。适用于津枯便秘者。

(8) 大黄15 g,芒硝15 g,皂角15 g,加水煎取200 ml,用纱布或棉球蘸药液,涂搽脐腹部,每日 1～2 次。适用于热结便秘者。

第六节　大肠癌

【概述】

大肠癌包括结肠癌和直肠癌,病变位于肛门者又称肛门癌,是常见的恶性肿瘤之一。其发病率和死亡率在恶性肿瘤中处于第 4～6 位。男性多于女性,男女之比为

It mainly affects the patients aged 30 - 50, mostly around 45, but it is also common in patients younger than 30. The cancer is most commonly found in rectum and sigmoid colon which occupies a percentage of 77.8%, followed by the tumors in the cecum and ascending colon and less common in hepatic flexure and splenic flexure of the descending colon. The growth of the large intestinal carcinoma is slow and the metastasis of the cancer occurs late. Most of the metastasis occur at the anal canal, rectum and the junction of rectum and sigmoid colon. At present, it is still difficult to make an early diagnosis of the disease. The post-operative survival rate of 5 years is rather low.

The pathogenesis of this disease is complicated. It is believed to be related to the chronic inflammation, polyp and adenoma of the large intestine, diet and environmental factors.

According to its clinical manifestations, the disease belongs to the categories of "zang du" (visceral toxin), "chang feng" (intestinal wind), "chang xun" (intestinal fungus) and "ji ju" (masses) in traditional Chinese medicine. The pathogenesis of this disease is that the constitutional asthenic spleen and kidney or improper diet causes deficiency of the spleen and stomach; moreover, accumulation of toxic heat, fire and dampness flow downwards to the intestines, and in the course of time, the mass is formed. Damp heat, toxic heat and blood stagnation are the secondary aspect of the disease; spleen deficiency, kidney deficiency and deficiency of healthy qi are the principal aspect. However, the principal and secondary aspects interact as both cause and effect and most of the cases are characterized by principal deficiency and secondary excess.

Essentials for Diagnosis

(1) Patients with chronic colitis, colon adenomatous

1.1～3.4∶1,多发于30～50岁,发病高峰在45岁左右,但30岁以下者也不少见。癌肿部位最常发生于直肠和乙状结肠,约占77.8%,其次为盲肠和升结肠,再次为降结肠的肝曲及脾曲。大肠癌生长较慢,转移较晚,且大多发生在肛管、直肠及直肠乙状结肠交界处。目前早期诊断仍有困难,手术后5年存活率较低。

本病的病因较复杂,一般认为与大肠的慢性炎症、息肉、大肠腺瘤,饮食和环境等因素有关。

根据本病的临床表现,当属于中医学"脏毒"、"肠风"、"肠蕈"、"积聚"的范畴。其产生是由于素体脾肾不足,或饮食不当,致脾胃虚弱,复因热毒蕴结,火热湿毒下注肠道,日久积结而成。湿热、火毒、瘀滞属病之标;脾虚、肾亏、正气不足乃病之本,二者互为因果,故大多属本虚标实之证。

【诊断要点】

(1) 有慢性结肠炎、结肠

polyp, especially those with a familial history of intestinal polyposis have changes of bowel evacuation habit recently, such as diarrhea, alternate appearance of constipation and diarrhea, abdominal discomfort and hematochezia.

(2) Iron-deficiency anemia with unknown causes, emaciation, lassitude, or intestinal obstruction, abdominal mass, abdominal pain are highly suspected as intestinal cancer.

(3) There appears positive occult blood in stools, reduced ferrohemoglobin in routine blood test and increased carcinoembryonic antigen (CEA).

(4) The tumor can be felt by digital examination of rectum, and those 'that can not be touched by digital examination of rectum can be found by rectoscope, romanoscope or fiberenteroscope. The biopsy may be done when necessary. Barium enema or double contrast radiograph may find filling defect in the cancer area with damage of the mucosa, stiffness of the intestinal wall and narrow intestinal cavity.

Syndrome Differentiation and Treatment

This disease is characterized by principal deficiency and secondary excess. The cases with agglomeration of dampness and heat or stagnation of toxic materials and blood stasis belong to excess; those with deficiency of liver yin and stomach yin, deficiency of qi and blood, deficiency of spleen yang and kidney yang or deficiency of liver yin and kidney yin belong to deficiency. Excess complicated with deficiency is usually seen during the progress of the diseases. Therefore eliminating pathogenic factors and supporting healthy qi is the treatment principle. Damp heat and excess of blood stasis are common at the early stage and the treatment principle should be expelling pathogenic factors. Deficiencies of the spleen, kidney, yin,

腺瘤性息肉,特别是家族性结肠息肉病患者,近期出现原因不明的排便习惯改变,如腹泻,便秘与腹泻交替出现,腹部不适,便血。

(2) 有原因不明的缺铁性贫血、消瘦、乏力,或肠梗阻、腹部肿块、腹痛等,应高度疑及肠癌。

(3) 实验室检查大便隐血阳性,血常规中血红蛋白明显降低,癌胚抗原(CEA)升高。

(4) 直肠指诊可触及肿块,直肠镜、乙状结肠镜或纤维肠镜可发现指诊无法摸到的肿块,并可取组织活检。钡灌肠或气钡双重造影可见癌肿部位充盈缺损、黏膜破坏、肠壁僵硬、肠腔狭窄等改变。

【辨证论治】

本病大多属本虚标实之证。湿热蕴结和瘀毒交阻证属实;肝胃阴虚、气血亏虚、脾肾阳虚和肝肾阴虚证属虚。病程中每见虚实夹杂之证,治疗当以祛邪扶正为原则,早期多以湿热、瘀毒偏盛,治以祛邪为主,晚期则脾肾阴阳气血俱虚,治以扶正固本为主。

yang, qi and blood are common at the late stage and the treatment principle should be supporting healthy qi.

1. Agglomeration of Dampness and Heat

Chief Manifestations: Paroxysmal abdominal pain, bloody stools, or rectal tenesmus, burning sensation in the anus, or fever, fullness in the chest, restlessness, thirst, nausea, poor appetite, frequent bowel movements, heaviness and distention of the abdomen, red tongue, with yellow and greasy coating, smooth and rapid pulse.

Therapeutic Methods: To clear away heat and promote diuresis.

Prescription: Modified Huaihua Diyu Tang (Sophorae and Sanguisorbae Decoction) and Gegen Qin Lian Tang (Decoction of Puerariae, Scutellariae and Coptidis), composed of Huaijiao (*Fructus Sophorae*) 10 g, Diyu (*Radix Sanguisorbae*) 10 g, Huangqin (*Radix scutellariae*) 10 g, Zhike (*Fructus Aurantii*) 10 g, Fangfeng (*Radix Saposhnikoviae*) 10 g, Huanglian (*Rhizoma Copitdis*) 5 g, Danggui (*Radix Angelicae Sinensis*) 15 g, Qinpi (*Cortex Fraxini*) 15 g, Longkui (*Herba Solanni Nigri*) 15 g, Fuling (*Poria*) 15 g, Gegen (*Radix Puerariae*) 15 g, Baijiangcao (*Herba Patrinniae cum Radice*) 30 g, Banzhilian (*Herba Scutellariae Barbatae*) 30 g, Yiyiren (*Semen Coicis*) 30 g, Shancigu (*Pseudobulbus Cremastrae seu Pleiones*) 30 g and Baihuasheshecao (*Herba Hedyotis Diffusae*) 30 g.

Modifications: For severe abdominal pain, add Yingsuke (*Pericarpium Papaveris*) 6 g and Yanhusuo (*Rhizoma Corydalis*) 12 g; for bloody stools, add Xueyutan (*Crinis Carbonisatus*) 10 g, Qiancao (*Radix Rubiae*) 10 g, Shensanqifen (*Radix Notoginseng*, powdered and to be infused separately) 5 g; for constipation caused by heat agglomeration, add Zhidahuang (*Radix et*

1. 湿热蕴结证

主要证候　腹部阵痛,便中夹血,或里急后重,肛门灼热,或有发热,胸闷烦渴,恶心纳呆,大便次频,小腹坠胀,舌质红,苔黄腻,脉滑数。

治　法　清热利湿。

方　药　槐花地榆汤合葛根芩连汤加减:槐角10 g,地榆10 g,黄芩10 g,枳壳10 g,防风10 g,黄连5 g,当归15 g,秦皮15 g,龙葵15 g,茯苓15 g,葛根15 g,败酱草30 g,半枝莲30 g,薏苡仁30 g,山慈姑30 g,白花蛇舌草30 g。

加　减　腹痛较剧者,加罂粟壳6 g,延胡索12 g;大便下血者,加血余炭10 g,茜草10 g,参三七粉(另冲)5 g;热结便秘者,加制大黄(后下)6 g,枳实10 g,厚朴10 g;腹泻明显者,加马齿苋30 g,白头翁

Rhizoma Rhei Preparata, to be decocted later) 6 g, Zhishi (*Fructus Aurantii Immaturus*) 10 g and Houpo (*Cortex Magnoliae Officinalis*) 10 g; for severe diarrhea, add Machixian (*Herba Portulacae*) 30 g and Baitouweng (*Radix Pulsatillae*) 30 g; for abdominal mass, add Xiakucao (*Spica Prunellae*) 30 g, Haizao (*Sargassum*) 15 g and Kunbu (*Thallus Laminariae et Eckloniae*) 15 g.

2. Stagnation of Toxic Materials and Blood Stasis

Chief Manifestations: Feverish sensation with restlessness, thirst, diarrhea with profuse pus and blood in purple color, rectal tenesmus, pricking pain in the abdomen, purple tongue with dark spots and yellow coating, thready and unsmooth or thready and rapid pulse.

Therapeutic Method: To remove blood stasis and toxic materials.

Prescription: Modified Gexia Zhuyu Tang (Decoction for Removing Blood Stasis Under Diaphram) and Tao Hong Siwu Tang (Four-Ingredient Decoction with Pericae and Carthami), composed of Taoren (*Semen Persicae*) 10 g, Honghua (*Flos Carthami*) 10 g, Chuan-xiong (*Rhizoma Chuanxiong*) 10 g, Danggui (*Radix Angelicae Sinensis*) 10 g, Wuyao (*Linderae*) 10 g, Zhike (*Fructus Aurantii*) 10 g, Mudanpi (*Cortex Moutan Radicis*) 12 g, Chishaoyao (*Radix Paeoniae Rubra*) 12 g, Baishaoyao (*Radix Paeoniae Alba*) 12 g, Yanhusuo (*Rhizoma Corydalis*) 15 g, Wulingzhi (*Faces Trogopterori*) 15 g, Liujinu (*Herba Artemisiae Anomalae*) 20 g, Shiliupi (*Pericarpium Granati*) 20 g, Baijiangcao (*Herba Patriniae cum Radice*) 30 g, Banzhilian (*Herba Scutellariae Barbatae*) 30 g, Shancigu (*Pseudobulbus Cremastrae seu Pleiones*) 30 g and Baihuasheshecao (*Herba Hedyotis Diffusae*) 30 g.

30 g;腹部肿块者,加夏枯草30 g,海藻15 g,昆布15 g。

2. 瘀毒交阻证

主要证候　烦热口渴,泻下脓血,色紫暗而量多,里急后重,腹部刺痛,舌质紫暗或有瘀点,苔黄,脉细涩或细数。

治　法　化瘀解毒。

方　药　膈下逐瘀汤合桃红四物汤加减:桃仁10 g,红花10 g,川芎10 g,当归10 g,乌药10 g,枳壳10 g,牡丹皮12 g,赤芍药12 g,白芍药12 g,延胡索15 g,五灵脂15 g,刘寄奴20 g,石榴皮20 g,败酱草30 g,半枝莲30 g,山慈姑30 g,白花蛇舌草30 g。

Modifications: For stiffness and fullness of the abdomen with pain, add Chuanlianzi (*Fructus Meliae Toosendan*) 15 g, Paochuanshanjia (*Squama Manitis* , roasted in hot cinders and to be decocted first) 15 g and Danshen (*Radix Salviae Miltiorrhizae*) 15 g; for rectal tenesmus, add Muxiang (*Radix Aucklandiae*) 10 g and Tengligen (*Radix Actinidiae Chinensis*) 30 g; for hard mass in the abdomen, add Sanleng (*Rhizoma Sparganii*) 10 g and Ezhu (*Rhizoma Curcumae*) 10 g; for deficient diathesis with constipation, add Huomaren (*Semen Cannabis*) 10 g, Yuliren (*Semen Pruni*) 10 g and Baiziren (*Semen Platycladi*) 10 g; for excessive diathesis with constipation, add Shengdahuang (*Radix et Rhizoma Rhei* , to be decocted later) 10 g, Zhishi (*Fructus Aurantii Immaturus*) 10 g and Mangxiao (*Natrii Sulfas* , to be infused separately) 10 g; for poor appetite, shortness of breath and lassitude, add Baizhu (*Rhizoma Atractylodis Macrocephalae*) 10 g and Fuling (*Poria*) 15 g.

3. Deficiency of Liver Yin and Stomach Yin

Chief Manifestations: Dull pain in the abdomen, constipation, or vomiting, thirst, bitter taste, preference for cold, aversion to heat, red and dry tongue, thready and rapid pulse.

Therapeutic Methods: To nourish yin and clean the intestines.

Prescription: Modified Shaoyao Gancao Tang (Paeoniae and Glycyrrhizae Decoction) and Qingchang Tang (Decoction for Clearing Intestines), composed of Jinyinhua (*Flos Lonicerae*) 10 g, Xuanshen (*Radix Scrophulariae*) 10 g, Huangqin (*Radix Scutellariae*) 10 g, Maimendong (*Radix Ophiopogonis*) 10 g, Diyu (*Radix Sanguisorbae*) 10 g, Gancao (*Radix Glycyrrhizae*) 10 g, Danggui (*Radix Angelicae Sinensis*) 15 g, Shihu

加　减　腹硬满而痛者，加川楝子15 g，炮穿山甲（先煎）15 g，丹参15 g；里急后重者，加木香10 g，藤梨根30 g；腹内结块而体实者，加三棱10 g，莪术10 g；大便秘结属体虚者，加火麻仁10 g，郁李仁10 g，柏子仁10 g；体实便秘者，加生大黄（后下）10 g，枳实10 g，芒硝（另冲）10 g；纳呆，气短乏力者，加白术10 g，茯苓15 g。

3. 肝胃阴虚证

主要证候　腹痛隐隐，大便秘结，或有呕吐，口干口苦，喜冷恶热，舌质红而干，脉细数。

治　法　养阴清肠。

方　药　芍药甘草汤合清肠汤加减：金银花10 g，玄参10 g，黄芩10 g，麦门冬10 g，地榆10 g，甘草10 g，当归15 g，石斛15 g，白芍药15 g，天花粉30 g，薏苡仁30 g。

(*Herba Dendrobii*) 15 g, Baishaoyao (*Radix Paeoniae Alba*) 15 g, Tianhuafen (*Radix Trichosanthis*) 30 g and Yiyiren (*Semen Coicis*) 30 g.

Modifications: For pus and blood in the stools, add Diyutan (*Radix Sanguisorbae*, charred) 15 g, Cebaiye (*Cacumen Platycladi*) 15 g, Huaijiao (*Fructus Sophorae*) 15 g, Shensanqifen (*Radix Notoginseng*, powdered and to be infused separately) 3 g and Qiancao (*Radix Rubiae*) 10 g; for yin deficiency with fever, add Qinghao (*Herba Artemisiae Annuae*) 15 g, Baiwei (*Radix Cynanchi Atrati*) 15 g and Digupi (*Cortex Lycii*) 15 g; for pricking pain in the abdomen with purple tongue, add Taoren (*Semen Persicae*) 15 g, Honghua (*Flos Carthama*) 15 g, Chuanxiong (*Rhizoma Chuangxiong*) 15 g and Lufengfang (*Nidus Polistis Mandarini*) 15 g.

4. Deficiency of Qi and Blood

Chief Manifestations: Pale complexion, pale lips and nails, shortness of breath and lassitude, dislike of speaking, prolapse of the anus, pale tongue with thin and white coating, weak and thready pulse.

Therapeutic Method: To nourish qi and blood.

Prescription: Modified Bazhen Tang (Decoction of Eight Precious Drugs) and Danggui Buxue Tang (Angelicae Sinensis Decoction for Tonifying Blood), composed of Huangqi (*Radix Astragali*) 30 g, Dangshen (*Radix Codonopsis*) 15 g, Danggui (*Radix Angelicae Sinensis*) 15 g, Fuling (*Poria*) 10 g, Baizhu (*Rhizoma Atractylodis Macrocephalae*) 10 g, Chuanxiong (*Rhizoma Chuanxiong*) 10 g, Baishaoyao (*Radix Paeoniae Alba*) 10 g, Gancao (*Radix Glycyrrhizae*) 10 g and Dazao (*Fructus Jujubae*) 5 pcs.

Modifications: For palpitation and insomnia, add Chaosuanzaoren (*Semen Ziziphi Spinosae*, stir-baked) 10 g, Baiziren (*Semen Platycladi*) 10 g and Yuanzhi

加　减　大便脓血者,加地榆炭15 g,侧柏叶15 g,槐角15 g,参三七粉(另冲)3 g,茜草10 g;阴虚发热者,加青蒿15 g,白薇15 g,地骨皮15 g;腹部刺痛,舌质紫暗者,加桃仁15 g,红花15 g,川芎15 g,露蜂房15 g。

4. 气血亏虚证

主要证候　面色苍白,唇甲不华,少气乏力,神疲懒言,脱肛下坠,舌质淡,苔薄白,脉细弱。

治　法　益气养血。

方　药　八珍汤合当归补血汤加减:黄芪30 g,党参15 g,当归15 g,茯苓10 g,白术10 g,川芎10 g,白芍药10 g,甘草10 g,大枣5枚。

加　减　心悸失眠者,加炒酸枣仁10 g,柏子仁10 g,远志10 g;脱肛下坠,大便频繁

(*Radix Polygalae*) 10 g; for prolapse of anus and frequent bowl movements, add Shengma (*Rhizoma Cimicifugae*) 5 g, Chaihu (*Radix Bupleuri*) 5 g and Hezi (*Fructus Chebulae*) 10 g; for bloody stools, add Aiye (*Folium Artemisiae Argyi*) 10 g, Shensanqifen (*Radix Notoginseng*, powdered and to be infused separately) 3 g and Zaoxintu (*Terra Flava Usta*) 30 g.

5. Deficiency of Spleen Yang and Kidney Yang

Chief Manifestations: Abdominal pain relieved by pressing, cold limbs and loose stools, shortness of breath and lassitude, or dawn diarrhea, pale and swollen tongue with teeth marks, deep and slow pulse or deep, thready and forceless pulse.

Therapeutic Method: To warm and tonify the spleen and kidney.

Prescription: Modified Fuzi Lizhong Tang (Aconti Lateralis Decoction for Regulating Middle Energizer) and Sishen Wan (Pill of Four Miraculous Drugs), composed of Shufuzi (*Radix Aconiti Lateralis Preparata*) 10 g, Ganjiang (*Rhizoma Zingiberis*) 6 g, Dangshen (*Radix Codonopsis*) 10 g, Baizhu (*Rhizoma Atractylodis Macrocephalae*) 10 g, Roudoukou (*Semen Myristicae*) 5 g, Buguzhi (*Fructus Psoraleae*) 15 g and Yiyiren (*Semen Coicis*) 30 g.

Modifications: For soreness of the lower back and aversion to cold, add Yinyanghuo (*Herba Epimedii*) 10 g, Bajitian (*Radix Morindae Officinalis*) 10 g and Rougui (*Cortex Cinnamomi*) 5 g; for large quantity of blood in the stools, add Aiye (*Folium Artemisiae Argyi*) 15 g and Zaoxintu (*Terra Flava Usta*) 30 g; for frequent bowl movements, add Hezi (*Fructus Chebulae*) 20 g, Yingsuke (*Pericarpium Papaveris*) 15 g and Baijinhua (*Flos Hibisci Syriaci*) 15 g; for ascites with scanty urine, add Baimaogen (*Rhizoma Imperatae*) 30 g, Dafu-

者,加升麻5 g,柴胡5 g,诃子10 g;大便带血者,加艾叶10 g,参三七粉(另吞)3 g,灶心土30 g。

5. 脾肾阳虚证

主要证候 腹痛喜按,肢冷便溏,气短乏力,或见五更泄泻,舌质淡有齿痕,舌体胖大,脉沉迟或沉细无力。

治　法 温补脾肾。

方　药 附子理中汤合四神丸加减:熟附子10 g,干姜6 g,党参10 g,白术10 g,肉豆蔻5 g,补骨脂15 g,薏苡仁30 g。

加　减 腰酸怕冷明显者,加淫羊藿10 g,巴戟天10 g,肉桂5 g;便血量多者,加艾叶15 g,灶心土30 g;大便无度者,加诃子20 g,罂粟壳15 g,白槿花15 g;腹水、尿少者,加白茅根30 g,大腹皮30 g,茯苓皮30 g。

pi (*Pericarpium Arecae*) 30 g and Fulingpi (*Cortex Sclerotii Poriae*) 30 g.

6. Deficiency of Liver Yin and Kidney Yin

Chief Manifestations: Emaciation, feverish sensation in soles, palms and the chest, dizziness, tinnitus, soreness of the lower back and knees, night sweating, seminal emission, leukorrhea, deep red tongue with less coating, wiry and thready pulse.

Therapeutic Method: To nourish kidney yin.

Prescription: Modified Zhi Bai Dihuang Tang (Decoction of Anemarrhenae, Phellodendri and Rehmanniae), composed of Zhimu (*Rhizoma Anemarrhenae*) 10 g, Huangbai (*Cortex Phellodendri*) 10 g, Mudanpi (*Cortex Moutan Radicis*) 10 g, Shengdihuang (*Radix Rehmanniae*) 10 g, Fuling (*Poria*) 10 g, Shanyao (*Rhizoma Dioscoreae*) 10 g, Shanzhuyu (*Fructus Corni*) 10 g, Zexie (*Rhizoma Alismatis*) 15 g, Banzhilian (*Herba Scutellariae Barbatae*) 30 g, Baihuasheshecao (*Herba Hedyotis Diffusae*) 30 g and Baimaoteng (*Herba Solani*) 30 g.

Modifications: For thirst with desire for drinking, add Tianhuafen (*Radix Trichosanthis*) 30 g; for feverish sensation in soles, palms and the chest, tidal fever and night sweating, add Digupi (*Cortex Lycii*) 15 g, Baiwei (*Radix Cynanchi Atrati*) 15 g, Huangbai (*Cortex Phellodendri*) 10 g and Zhimu (*Rhizoma Anemarrhenae*) 10 g; for dizziness, add Juhua (*Flos Chrysanthemi*) 10 g and Gouqizi (*Fructus Lycii*) 10 g; for constipation, add Xuanshen (*Radix Scrophulariae*) 10 g, Maimendong (*Radix Ophiopogonis*) 10 g and Huomaren (*Semen Cannabis*) 10 g; for goiter and tumor, add Tubeimu (*Rhizoma Bolbostemmae*) 15 g, Xiakucao (*Spica Prunellae*) 30 g, Kunbu (*Thallus Laminariae et Eckloniae*) 30 g and Shancigu (*Pseudobulbus Cremastrae*

6. 肝肾阴虚证

主要证候 形体消瘦,五心烦热,头昏耳鸣,腰膝酸软,盗汗,遗精,带下,舌质红绛而少苔,脉弦细。

治 法 滋补肾阴。

方 药 知柏地黄汤加减:知母10 g,黄柏10 g,牡丹皮10 g,生地黄10 g,茯苓10 g,山药10 g,山茱萸10 g,泽泻15 g,半枝莲30 g,白花蛇舌草30 g,白毛藤30 g。

加 减 口干喜饮者,加天花粉30 g;五心烦热,潮热盗汗者,加地骨皮15 g,白薇15 g,黄柏10 g,知母10 g;头晕目眩者,加菊花10 g,枸杞子10 g;便秘者,加玄参10 g,麦门冬10 g,火麻仁10 g;兼见瘿瘤者,加土贝母15 g,夏枯草30 g,昆布30 g,山慈姑30 g;兼有腹痛,腹内积块者,加鳖甲(先煎)30 g,乳香10 g,没药10 g。

seu Pleiones) 30 g; for abdominal pain and mass in the abdomen, add Biejia (*Carapax Trionycis*, to be decocted first) 30 g, Ruxiang (*Olibanum*) 10 g and Moyao (*Myrrha*) 10 g.

Other Treatments

1. Chinese Patent Drugs

(1) Kangliu Xiaoyan Jiaonang (Antineoplastic and Anti-inflammatory Capsule): 2 - 3 capsules each time, three times daily; applicable to different stages of large intestinal carcinoma.

(2) Xiaoliu Pian (Tablet for Removing Tumor): 4 tablets each time, three times daily; applicable to large intestinal carcinoma of excess syndrome in middle and late stages.

(3) Muxiang Shunqi Wan (Aucklandiae Pill for Soothing Qi): 6 g each time, three times daily, applicable to severe abdominal distention in large intestinal carcinoma combined with intestinal obstruction.

(4) Fuzheng Jiedu Chongji (Granule for Strengthing Healthy Qi and Detoxification): 1 sachet each time, twice daily; applicable to patients receiving radiotherapy and chemotherapy.

(5) Shen Ling Baizhu Wan (Pill of Ginseng, Poria and Atractylodis Macrocephalae): 6 g each time, twice daily; applicable to abdominal distension, diarrhea and lassitude in large intestinal carcinoma.

2. Single-drug or Experiential Prescriptions

(1) Seventy percent of Niubanggen (*Radix Arctii*) and 30% of Chixiaodou San (*Phaseoli Powder*), a mixture composed of equal amounts of Chixiaodou (*Semen Phaseoli*), Danggui (*Radix Angelicae Sinensis*), Dahuang (*Radix et Rhizoma Rhei*) and Pugongying (*Herba Taraxaci*). Grind them into powder for infusion and take 3 - 6 g each time, 3 times daily. It is applicable

【其他疗法】

1. 中成药

(1) 抗瘤消炎胶囊　每服 2~3 粒,每日 3 次。适用于大肠癌各期。

(2) 消瘤片　每服 4 片, 每日 3 次。适用于各种中、晚期大肠癌属实证者。

(3) 木香顺气丸　每服 6 g,每日 3 次。适用于大肠癌合并肠梗阻致腹胀甚者。

(4) 扶正解毒冲剂　每服 1 袋,每日 2 次。适用于大肠癌放疗、化疗者。

(5) 参苓白术丸　每服 6 g,每日 2 次。适用于大肠癌腹部胀满,便溏乏力者。

2. 单验方

(1) 牛蒡根 70%,赤小豆散(赤小豆、当归、大黄、蒲公英各等分)30%,共为细末,调匀冲服,每服 3~6 g,每日 3 次。适用于直肠癌患者。

to rectum cancer.

（2）Cook Shishangbai (*Herba Selaginellae*) with salt water first, then with fresh water, bake it dry and grind it into powder for infusion. Take 15 g each time, twice daily for oral administration. It is applicable to large intestinal carcinoma.

（3）Shuizhi Zao Yaosan (*Powder of Hirudo and Sargassum*), composed of Shuizhi (*Hirudo*) 15 g and Haizao (*Sargassum*) 30 g. Bake them dry and grind them into powder, divide the powder into 10 portions and take 1－2 portions each time with yellow rice wine, twice daily. It is applicable to stagnation of blood stasis and toxin in large intestinal carcinoma.

（4）Jinniu Jian (*Decoction of Lonicerae and Cornu Bubali*), composed of Jinyinhua (*Flos Lonicerae*) 15 g, Shuiniujiao (*Cornu Bubali*) 40 g, Shancigu (*Pseudobulbus Cremastrae seu Pleiones*) 30 g, Daqingye (*Folium Isatidis*) 30 g and Ganchanpi (*Periostracum Bufonis, dried*) 12 g. Decoct them with water, one dose daily, 7 days making up a treatment course. It is applicable to intestinal cancer and other cancers of late stage with fever.

（5）Hongshen (*Radix Ginseng Rubra*) 10 g and Baishen (*Radix Ginseng*) 10 g. Decoct them with water or make tea, 1 dose daily. It is applicable to decreased leukocyte after radiotherapy and chemotherapy for intestinal cancer or other cancers.

3. External Therapy

（1）Chansu (*Venenum Bufonis*, powdered) and vaseline with the proportion of 1∶10. Warm up the vaseline, mix it with Chansu powder and place the mixture to the painful area. It is applicable to intestinal cancer and other late cancers with severe pain.

（2）Qingdai (*Indigo Naturalis*) 15 g, Chanyi (*Periostracum Cicadae*) 30 g and Bingpian (*Borneolum*

（2）石上柏全草，先用盐水煮，后用开水煮，再焙干研末，每服取15 g，每日 2 次，开水泡服。适用于大肠癌患者。

（3）水蛭藻药散　水蛭15 g，海藻30 g，焙干研细末，分10包，每日1～2包，黄酒冲服，每日 2 次。适用于大肠癌瘀毒交阻者。

（4）金牛煎　金银花15 g，水牛角40 g，山慈姑30 g，大青叶30 g，干蟾皮12 g，水煎服，每日 1 剂，7 日为 1 个疗程。适用于肠癌及其他晚期肿瘤发热者。

（5）红参10 g，白参10 g，每日 1 剂，水煎服或泡茶服。适用于肠癌及其他恶性肿瘤放疗、化疗引起白细胞减少者。

3. 外治法

（1）取蟾酥和凡士林按1∶10比例调制，将凡士林加温，按比例与蟾酥粉混合即成，外涂痛处。适用于肠癌及其他晚期肿瘤疼痛剧烈者。

（2）青黛15 g，蝉衣30 g，冰片3 g，研细末，撒绵纸上贴

Syntheticum) 3 g. Grind them into powder, sprinkle the powder on tissue paper and apply it on the affected area. It is applicable to rectum cancer and anus cancer with watery pus, pain and itching.

(3) Shechuangzi (*Fructus Cnidii*) 30 g, Kushen (*Radix Sophorae Flavescentis*) 30 g and Bohe (*Herba Menthae*) 10 g. Boil the drugs with 1,000 ml of water, add Shengdahuang (*Radix et Rhizoma Rhei*) 10 g to boil for another 2 minutes. Put Xionghuang (*Realgar*) 10 g and Mangxiao (*Natrii Sulfas*) 10 g in the basin, then pour the boiling decoction in and stir the decoction. Squat over the basin and fumigate the anus, then immerse the anus in the basin when the decoction turns warm, once every night. It is applicable to anus cancer.

(4) Yadanzi (*Fructus Bruceae*) 15 g, Huaihua (*Flos Sophorae*) 15 g, Zaojiaoci (*Spina Gleditsiae*) 10 g, Xuejie (*Resina Draconnis*) 10 g, Baihuasheshecao (*Herba Hedyotis Diffusae*) 40 g, Shengdahuang (*Radix et Rhizoma Rhei*) 40 g and Baijiangcao (*Herba Patriniae cum Radice*) 40 g. Boil the drugs with 1,000 ml of water into 200 ml of the decoction and use it for retention enema for 1 - 2 hours. It is applicable to rectum cancer.

(5) Naosha (*Sal Ammoniac*) 3 g, Yadanzi (*Fructus Bruceae*) 9 g, Wumeirou (*Fructus Mume*, stones removed) 15 g and Bingpian (*Borneolum Syntheticum*) 1.5 g. Make 3 suppositories of the same size with the above drugs and put one suppository into the anus, once or twice daily. It is applicable to narrow intestinal cavity and constipation in rectum cancer. This medicine is corrosive and should be used cautiously to avoid bleeding in defecation.

患处。适用于直肠癌、肛门癌脓水淋漓且痛痒者。

(3) 蛇床子30 g, 苦参30 g, 薄荷10 g, 加水1 000 ml, 煮沸后加入生大黄10 g, 煎 2 分钟, 将雄黄10 g, 芒硝10 g放入盆中, 将煮沸的汤药倒入盆内搅拌, 乘热气上蒸之际蹲于盆上, 薰蒸肛门, 待水变温后则改为坐浴, 每晚 1 次。适用于肛管癌。

(4) 鸦胆子15 g, 槐花15 g, 皂角刺10 g, 血竭10 g, 白花蛇舌草40 g, 生大黄40 g, 败酱草40 g, 加水1 000 ml, 煎至200 ml, 灌肠保留 1～2 小时。适用于直肠癌者。

(5) 硇砂3 g, 鸦胆子9 g, 乌梅肉15 g, 冰片1.5 g, 制成 3 个等量栓子, 每日 1～2 次, 每次 1 粒, 塞肛。适用于直肠癌肠腔狭窄, 大便困难者。该药有腐蚀作用, 用时慎防大便出血。

2.4 Syndrome Patterns of the Liver and Gallbladder

第四章　肝胆病证

2.4.1 Headache

第一节　头痛

General Description

Headache refers to a disease with pain in the head as the major symptom, which is caused by exogenous factors or by internal disorders. Exogenous factors causing headache are chiefly wind, usually accompanied with cold, heat and dampness; internal disorders include emotional stress, improper diet, deuteropathic debility, postpartum, blood loss and excessive sexual intercourse. Its location is the head, with the spleen, liver and kidney involved. Wind, fire, phlegm, blood stagnation and deficiency are the major pathogenic factors and its pathogenesis is obstruction of the meridians and failure of lucid yang to ascend.

This disease is attributive to periodic migraine, overstrain headache, cluster headache and chronic paroxysmal migraine in western medicine.

【概述】

头痛是指以头部疼痛为主症的一类病证。其病因有外感与内伤两方面。外感以风为主，多挟寒、热、湿邪；内伤与情志、饮食、病后、产后、失血、劳欲有关。病位在头，涉及脾、肝、肾等脏腑，风、火、痰、瘀、虚为致病之主要因素，脉络阻闭，清窍不利为其病机。

本病相当于西医学周期性偏头痛、紧张性头痛、丛集性头痛及慢性阵发性偏头痛等。

Essentials for Diagnosis

(1) The chief complaint is headache, which may involve the entire head or the forehead, the frontotemple, the vertex and the occiput. Headache may be manifested as a throbbing pain, a stabbing pain, a distending pain, a dizzy pain and a dull pain. It may have a sudden onset with a splitting and ceaseless pain or an intermittent pain,

【诊断要点】

(1) 以头痛为主症，或前额、额颞、巅顶、顶枕部或全头部疼痛，头痛性质多为跳痛、刺痛、胀痛、昏痛、隐痛等。有突然而作，其痛如破而无休止者；也有反复发作，久治不愈，

which is irresponsible to treatment. The attack of the pain may last for minutes, hours, days or weeks.

(2) Headache caused by exogenous factors or internal disorders is manifested as a sudden onset or repeated attacks.

(3) A routine check on blood and blood pressure, and CSF examination and electroencephalography if necessary. Doppler cranial detector and craniocerebral CT or MRI may help to establish the diagnosis.

Syndrome Differentiation and Treatment

It is essential to differentiate whether the headache is caused by exogenous factors or by internal disorders. Headache due to exogenous factors is characterized by an abrupt onset and a short course, or accompanied with exterior syndrome; while headache due to internal disorders has a long course with frequent attacks and intermittent pain. The former is usually of the excess type while the latter, of the deficiency-excess type. The treatment for the former is to disperse and expel exogenous factors; for the latter, it is to nourish both blood and yin.

1. Wind-cold Headache

Chief Manifestations: Abrupt onset with a splitting pain radiating to the neck and the back which is aggravated by exposure to wind, aversion to wind and cold, absence of thirst, thin and white tongue coating, and superficial and tense pulse.

Therapeutic Methods: To eliminate wind and disperse cold.

Prescription: Modified Chuanxiong Chatiao San (Chuanxiong Powder Mixed with Camelliae Sinensis), composed of Chuanxiong (*Rhizoma Chuanxiong*) 10 g, Qianghuo (*Rhizoma et Radix Notopterygii*) 10 g, Jingjie (*Herba Schizonepetae*) 6 g, Baizhi (*Radix Angelicae*

时痛时止者；头痛每次发作可持续数分钟、数小时、数天或数星期不等。

（2）因外感、内伤等因素，突然而病或有反复发作的病史。

（3）血常规、血压,必要时做脑脊液、脑电图检查,有条件时作经颅多普勒、颅脑 CT 和 MRI 检查,以明确诊断。

【辨证论治】

本病在辨证上主要辨外感与内伤。外感头痛,起病急,病程短,或伴表证;内伤头痛,病程较长,头痛反复发作,时轻时重。外感头痛多属实,内伤头痛多虚实夹杂。外感头痛治宜疏散祛邪为主,内伤头痛治当滋阴养血为要。

1. 风寒证

主要证候　头痛起病较急,其痛如裂,连及项背,恶风畏寒,遇风尤剧,口不渴,苔薄白,脉多浮紧。

治　法　疏风散寒。

方　药　川芎茶调散加减:川芎10 g,羌活10 g,荆芥6 g,白芷6 g,蔓荆子6 g,细辛3 g,藁本8 g。

Dahuricae) 6 g, Manjingzi (*Fructus Viticis*) 6 g, Xixin (*Herba Asari*) 3 g and Gaoben (*Rhizoma Ligustici*) 8 g.

Modifications: For pathogenic cold invading Jueyin meridian which results in headache in the vertex, retching and salivation, add Wuzhuyu (*Fructus Evodiae*) 3 g and Zhibanxia (*Rhizoma Pinelliae Preparata*) 10 g; for a feeling that the head is tightly wrapped and heavy sensation in the limbs, add Duhuo (*Radix Angelicae Pubescents*) 10 g, Cangzhu (*Rhizoma Atractylodis*) 10 g and Cang'erzi (*Fructus Xanthii*) 10 g.

2. Wind-heat Headache

Chief Manifestations: Distending pain, or even splitting pain in the head, fever or aversion to wind, thirst with a desire to drink, flushed face, red eyes, constipation, deep yellow urine, red tongue with yellow coating, and superficial and rapid pulse.

Therapeutic Methods: To eliminate wind and clear away heat.

Prescription: Modified Xiong Zhi Shigao Tang (Decoction of Chuanxiong, Angelicae Dahuricae and Gypsum Fibrosum), composed of Sangye (*Folium Mori*) 10 g, Juhua (*Flos Chrysanthemi*) 10 g, Baijili (*Fructus Tribuli*) 10 g, Chuanxiong (*Rhizoma Chuanxiong*) 10 g, Baizhi (*Radix Angelicae Dahuricae*) 6 g, Manjingzi (*Fructus Viticis*) 6 g, Shigao (*Gypsum Fibrosum*, to be decocted first) 30 g, Zhizi (*Fructus Gardeniae*) 10 g and Huangqin (*Radix Scutellariae*) 10 g.

Modification: For constipation, presence of boils in the mouth and nose, and blockage of qi of the bowels, add Zhidahuang (*Radix et Rhizoma Rhei Preparata*) 8 g.

3. Wind-dampness Headache

Chief Manifestations: Headache with a feeling that the head is tightly wrapped, heavy sensation in the limbs,

加　减　若寒犯厥阴,巅顶头痛,干呕,吐涎,加吴茱萸3 g,制半夏10 g;头痛如裹,肢体困重,加独活10 g,苍术10 g,苍耳子10 g。

2. 风热证

主要证候　头痛而胀,甚则头痛如裂,发热或恶风,口渴欲饮,面红目赤,便秘溲黄,舌质红,苔黄,脉浮数。

治　法　疏风清热。

方　药　芎芷石膏汤加减:桑叶10 g,菊花10 g,白蒺藜10 g,川芎10 g,白芷6 g,蔓荆子6 g,石膏(先煎)30 g,栀子10 g,黄芩10 g。

加　减　若大便秘结,口鼻生疮,腑气不通者,可加制大黄8 g。

3. 风湿证

主要证候　头痛如裹,肢体困重,胸闷纳呆,小便不利,

feeling of oppression of the chest, loss of appetite, dysuria, loose stools, white and greasy tongue coating, and soft-superficial and smooth pulse.

Therapeutic Methods: To expel wind and eliminate dampness.

Prescription: Modified Qianghuo Shengshi Tang (Notopterygii Decoction for Eliminating Dampness), composed of Qianghuo (*Rhizoma et Radix Notopterygii*) 10 g, Duhuo (*Radix Angelicae Pubescentis*) 10 g, Chuanxiong (*Rhizoma Chuanxiong*) 8 g, Fangfeng (*Radix Saposhnikoviae*) 6 g, Manjingzi (*Fructus Viticis*) 6 g and Gaoben (*Rhizoma Ligustici*) 6 g.

Modifications: For retention of dampness in the middle energizer, manifested as chest oppression, loss of appetite and loose stools, add Cangzhu (*Rhizoma Atractylodis*) 10 g, Houpo (*Cortex Magnoliae Officinalis*) 10 g and Chenpi (*Pericarpium Citri Reticulatae*) 6 g; for nausea and vomiting, add Shengjiang (*Rhizoma Zingiberis Recens*) 3 g, Zhibanxia (*Rhizoma Pinelliae Preparata*) 10 g and Huoxiang (*Herba Agastaches*) 10 g.

4. Headache due to Hyperactivity of Liver Yang

Chief Manifestations: Distending pain in the head, dizziness, restlessness, irritability, hypochondriac pain, insomnia, bitter taste in the mouth, red tongue with thin and yellow coating, and deep, wiry and forceful pulse.

Therapeutic Methods: To calm the liver and suppress hyperactivity of liver yang.

Prescription: Modified Tianma Gouteng Yin (Gastrodiae and Uncariae Decoction), composed of Tianma (*Rhizoma Gastrodiae*) 10 g, Gouteng (*Ramulus Uncariae cum Uncis*) 10 g, Shijueming (*Concha Haliotidis*, to be decocted first) 20 g, Cishi (*Magnetitum*, to be decocted first) 20 g, Huangqin (*Radix Scutellariae*)

大便或溏,苔白腻,脉濡滑。

治　法　祛风胜湿。

方　药　羌活胜湿汤加减:羌活10 g,独活10 g,川芎8 g,防风6 g,蔓荆子6 g,藁本6 g。

加　减　若湿浊中阻,症见胸闷纳呆、便溏,可加苍术10 g,厚朴10 g,陈皮6 g;若恶心呕吐者,可加生姜3 g,制半夏10 g,藿香10 g。

4. 肝阳证

主要证候　头胀痛而眩,心烦易怒,胁痛,夜眠不宁,口苦,舌红,苔薄黄,脉沉弦有力。

治　法　平肝潜阳。

方　药　天麻钩藤饮加减:天麻10 g,钩藤10 g,石决明(先煎)20 g,磁石(先煎)20 g,黄芩10 g,菊花10 g,桑叶10 g。

10 g, Juhua (*Flos Chrysanthemi*) 10 g and Sangye (*Folium Mori*) 10 g.

Modification: For headache caused by deficiency of liver yin and kidney yin which is slight in early morning and severe in late afternoon, or aggravated by overstrain, dry mouth, red tongue with thin coating, and wiry and thready pulse, add Shengdihuang (*Radix Rehmanniae*) 10 g, Heshouwu (*Radix Polygoni Multiflori*) 10 g, Nüzhenzi (*Fructus Ligustri Lucidi*) 10 g, Gouqizi (*Fructus Lycii*) 10 g and Hanliancao (*Herba Ecliptae*) 10 g.

加 减 若见肝肾阴虚而头痛,朝轻暮重,或遇劳而剧,脉弦细,舌红苔薄少津者,可加生地黄10 g,何首乌10 g,女贞子10 g,枸杞子10 g,旱莲草10 g。

5. Headache due to Kidney Deficiency

Chief Manifestations: Headache with an empty feeling, vertigo, soreness and weakness in the loins and knees, lassitude, seminal emission, leukorrhea, tinnitus, insomnia, red tongue with little coating, deep, thready and forceless pulse.

Therapeutic Methods: To replenish yin and nourish the kidney.

Prescription: Modified Da Buyuan Jian (Potent Decoction for Replenishing Primordial Qi), composed of Shudihuang (*Radix Rehmanniae Preparata*) 12 g, Shanzhuyu (*Fructus Corni*) 10 g, Shanyao (*Rhizoma Dioscoreae*) 10 g, Gouqizi (*Fructus Lycii*) 10 g, Dangshen (*Radix Codonopsis*) 10 g, Danggui (*Radix Angelicae Sinensis*) 10 g and Duzhong (*Cortex Eucommiae*) 10 g.

Modifications: For insufficiency of kidney yang, add Shufuzi (*Radix Aconiti Lateralis Preparata*) 8 g and Rougui (*Cortex Cinnamomi*) 3 g; for that attacked by exogenous cold, add Mahuang (*Herba Ephedrae*) 5 g, Shufuzi (*Radix Aconiti Lateralis Preparata*) 8 g and Xixin (*Herba Asari*) 3 g.

6. Headache due to Deficiency of Qi and Blood

Chief Manifestations: Headache, dizziness and

5. 肾虚证

主要证候 头痛而空,每兼眩晕,腰痛酸软,神疲乏力,遗精,带下,耳鸣少寐,舌红少苔,脉沉细无力。

治 法 补肾养阴。

方 药 大补元煎加减:熟地黄12 g,山茱萸10 g,山药10 g,枸杞子10 g,党参10 g,当归10 g,杜仲10 g。

加 减 若肾阳不足者,加熟附子8 g,肉桂3 g;若兼见外感寒邪者,可加麻黄5 g,熟附子8 g,细辛3 g。

6. 气血虚证

主要证候 头痛而晕,心

palpitation which are aggravated by overstrain, spontaneous sweating, shortness of breath, aversion to wind, lassitude, pale complexion, pale tongue with thin and white
coating, and deep, thready and weak pulse.

Therapeutic Methods: To replenish qi and nourish
blood.

Prescription: Modified Bazhen Tang (Decoction of
Eight Precious Drugs), composed of Dangshen (*Radix
Codonopsis*) 10 g, Shanyao (*Rhizoma Dioscoreae*) 10 g,
Fuling (*Poria*) 10 g, Baizhu (*Rhizoma Atractylodis
Macrocephalae*) 10 g, Baishaoyao (*Radix Paeoniae Al-
ba*) 10 g, Danggui (*Radix Angelicae Sinensis*) 10 g,
Chuanxiong (*Rhizoma Chuanxiong*) 10 g and Shudihuang
(*Radix Rehmanniae Preparata*) 10 g.

Modification: For sweating, shortness of breath
and lassitude, add Huangqi (*Radix Astragali*) 12 g.

7. Headache due to Retention of Phlegm

Chief Manifestations: Headache, dizziness, fullness and stuffiness in the chest and epigastrium, vomiting
and nausea with sputum, swollen tongue with teeth marks
on the margins, white and greasy coating, deep and wiry
or deep and smooth pulse.

Therapeutic Methods: To invigorate the spleen,
resolve phlegm to make the adverse-rising qi descend and
relieve headache.

Prescription: Modified Banxia Baizhu Tianma Tang
(Decoction of Pinelliae, Atractylodis Macrocephalae and
Gastrodiae), composed of Zhibanxia (*Rhizoma Pinelliae
Preparata*) 10 g, Baizhu (*Rhizoma Atractylodis Macro-
cephalae*) 10 g, Tianma (*Rhizoma Gastrodiae*) 10 g,
Fuling (*Poria*) 12 g, Chenpi (*Pericarpium Citri Retic-
ulatae*) 6 g and Shengjiang (*Rhizoma Zingiberis Recens*)
3 g.

Modification: For heat transformation from phl-

悸不宁,遇劳则重,自汗,气
短,畏风,神疲乏力,面色㿠
白,舌淡,苔薄白,脉沉细
而弱。

治　法　气血双补。

方　药　八珍汤加减:
党参10 g,山药10 g,茯苓10 g,
白术10 g,白芍药10 g,当归
10 g,川芎10 g,熟地黄10 g。

加　减　汗出气短,乏力
神疲者,加黄芪12 g。

7. 痰浊证

主要证候　头痛昏蒙,胸
脘满闷,呕恶痰涎,舌胖大有
齿痕,苔白腻,脉沉弦或沉滑。

治　法　健脾化痰,降逆
止痛。

方　药　半夏白术天麻
汤加减:制半夏10 g,白术
10 g,天麻10 g,茯苓12 g,陈皮
6 g,生姜3 g。

加　减　若痰郁化热显

egm, add Zhuru (*Caulis Bambusae in Taeniam*) 10 g, Zhi-shi (*Fructus Aurantii Immaturus*) 10 g and Huangqin (*Radix Scutellariae*) 10 g.

8. Headache due to Blood Stasis

Chief Manifestions: Persistent headache with a stabbing and fixed pain, or trauma in the head, purple tongue with occasional ecchymosis and petechiae, thin and white coating, deep and thready or thready and unsmooth pulse.

Therapeutic Methods: To dredge the orifices, activate the meridians and resolve blood stasis.

Prescription: Modified Tongqiao Huoxue Tang (Decoction for Activating Blood Circulation), composed of Baizhi (*Radix Angelicae Dahuricae*) 6 g, Congbai (*Bolbus Allii Fistulosi*) 5 g, Taoren (*Semen Persicae*) 10 g, Honghua (*Flos Carthami*) 6 g, Chuanxiong (*Rhizoma Chuanxiong*) 6 g, Chishaoyao (*Radix Paeoniae Rubra*) 10 g and Shengjiang (*Rhizoma Zingiberis Recens*) 3 g.

Modification: For severe headache, add Quanxie (*Scorpio*) 3 g and Wugong (*Scolopendra*) 3 g.

Other Treatments

1. Chinese Patent Drugs

(1) Qi Ju Dihuang Wan (Rehmanniae Pill with Lycii and Chrysanthemi): 6 g each time, twice a day; applicable to headache caused by deficiency of kidney yin and failure of the water to nourish the wood.

(2) Quan Tianma Jiaonang (Gastrodiae Capsule): 4 capsules each time, 3 times a day; suitable for headache caused by hyperactivity of liver yang and upward invasion of liver wind.

(3) Tianma Shouwu Pian (Tablet of Gastrodiae and Polygoni Multiflori): 6 tablets each time, 3 times a day; suitable for headache due to deficiency of liver yin and kidney yin.

著者,可加竹茹 10 g,枳实 10 g,黄芩10 g。

8. 瘀血证

主要证候　头痛经久不愈,其痛如刺,固定不移,或头部有外伤史,舌紫或有瘀斑、瘀点,苔薄白,脉沉细或细涩。

治　法　通窍活络化瘀。

方　药　通窍活血汤加减:白芷6 g,葱白5 g,桃仁10 g,红花6 g,川芎6 g,赤芍药10 g,生姜3 g。

加　减　疼痛明显者,加全蝎3 g,蜈蚣3 g。

【其他疗法】

1. 中成药

(1)杞菊地黄丸　每服6 g,每日2次。适用于肾阴亏虚,水不涵木所致的头痛。

(2)全天麻胶囊　每服4粒,每日3次。适用于肝阳上亢、肝风上扰之头痛。

(3)天麻首乌片　每服6片,每日3次。适用于肝肾阴虚之头痛。

2. Single-drug or Experiential Prescriptions

（1）Chuanxiong (*Rhizoma Chuanxiong*) 10 g and Manjingzi (*Fructus Viticis*) 10 g. Decoct the drugs in water for oral administration. It is applicable to headache caused by exogenous wind.

（2）Ganjuhua (*Flos Chrysanthemi*) 6 g. Infuse the drug in boiling water to make tea. It is applicable to headache caused by hyperactive liver yang.

（3）Danggui (*Radix Angelicae Sinensis*) 10 g and Chuanxiong (*Rhizoma chuanxiong*) 6 g. Decoct the herbs in water for oral administration. It is applicable to headache caused by deficiency of blood.

（4）Quanxie (*Scorpio*), Dilong (*Pheretima*) and Gancao (*Radix Glycyrrhizae*) in equal proportions. Grind the drugs into powder and then infuse in green tea for oral taking, 3 g each time, twice a day. It is suitable for intractable headache due to liver wind entering the meridians.

（5）Zhichuanwu (*Radix Aconiti Preparata*) 3 g, Zhicaowu (*Radix Aconiti Kusnezoffii Preparata*) 3 g, Baizhi (*Radix Angelicae Dahuricae*) 18 g, Baijiangcan (*Bombyx Batrycatus*) 18 g and Shenggancao (*Radix Glycyrrhizae*) 10 g. Grind the above drugs into powder, divide it into 6 portions and take one portion a day with green tea in 3 divided dose. It is suitable for intractable headache due to wind cold.

3. External Therapy

（1）Slice Shengfupian (*Radix Aconiti Lateralis*) and stir-bake it with salt, then apply it to the pain spot when it is hot. It is suitable for headache due to kidney yang deficiency.

（2）Apply small magnetic Sheets to Quchi (LI11) and Zusanli (ST36) for headache due to hyperactivity of liver yang.

2. 单验方

（1）川芎10 g，蔓荆子10 g，水煎服。适用于外感风邪头痛。

（2）甘菊花6 g，开水泡茶。适用于肝阳头痛。

（3）当归10 g，川芎6 g，水煎服。适用于血虚头痛。

（4）全蝎、地龙、甘草各等分，研粉，每服3 g，每日2次，用绿茶冲服。适用于顽固性头痛，偏于肝风入络者。

（5）制川乌3 g，制草乌3 g，白芷18 g，白僵蚕18 g，生甘草10 g，研细，分成6包，每日1包，分3次，用绿茶送服。适用于顽固性头痛，偏于风寒者。

3. 外治法

（1）生附片切成薄片，和盐同炒，热熨痛处。适用于肾阳虚头痛。

（2）用小块磁片贴于曲池、足三里穴。适用于肝阳头痛。

(3) Tianma (*Rhizoma Gastrodiae*) 15 g, Chuanwu (*Radix Aconiti*) 15 g, Caowu (*Radix Aconiti Kusnezoffii*) 15 g, Xixin (*Herba Asari*) 15 g, Baifuzi (*Rhizoma Typhonii*) 15 g, Xionghuang (*Realgar*) 15 g, Quanxie (*Scorpio*) 15 g, Chuanxiong (*Rhizoma Chuanxiong*) 15 g, Cangzhu (*Rhizoma Atractylodis*) 15 g, Bohe (*Herba Menthae*) 15 g, Gansong (*Radix et Rhizoma Nardostachyos*) 15 g, Fangfeng (*Radix Saposhnikoviae*) 15 g, Baizhi (*Radix Angelicae Dahuricae*) 15 g and Gancao (*Radix Glycyrrhizae*) 15 g. Grind the above drugs into powder and make paste with the fistular onion juice. Apply the paste to Taiyang (EX – HN5) for migraine of various types.

(4) Chuanxiong (*Rhizoma Chuanxiong*), Baizhi (*Radix Angelicae Dahuricae*), Ruxiang (*Olibanum*), Moyao (*Myrrha*) and Mangxiao (*Natrii Sulfas*) in equal proportions. Grind the drugs into fine powder and put the powder into the nostril. This is suitable for persistent headache.

（3）天麻15 g，川乌15 g，草乌15 g，细辛15 g，白附子15 g，雄黄15 g，全蝎15 g，川芎15 g，苍术15 g，薄荷15 g，甘松15 g，防风15 g，白芷15 g，甘草15 g。上药共研末，加大葱汁调成膏敷贴太阳穴。适用于各种偏头痛。

（4）川芎、白芷、乳香、没药、芒硝各等分，研细末塞鼻。适用于头痛日久不愈者。

2.4.2 Vertigo

General Description

Vertigo is chiefly manifested as dizziness and blurred vision, which usually occur simultaneously. The mild case can be relieved by closing one's eyes; while the serious one has a rotatary sensation like sitting in a sailing boat or moving car, difficulty in standing steadly and accompanying symptoms such as nausea, vomiting, sweating and pale complexion.

Emotional depression, anger, improper diet, debility due to prolonged illness and excessive sexual intercourse may cause vertigo. The pathogenesis of the excess type is stagnation of turbid phlegm in the middle energizer resul-

第二节　眩晕

【概述】

眩晕是以头晕、眼花为主症的一类病证。眩即眼花，晕是头晕，两者常同时并见，故统称为"眩晕"。轻者闭目可止，重者如坐车船，旋转不定，不能站立，或伴有恶心、呕吐、汗出、面色苍白等症状。

眩晕的病因有忧郁恼怒、饮食不节、久病体虚及房室劳倦等。病变机理实者为痰浊中阻，清阳不升，或肝阳上亢，

ting in failure of lucid yang to ascend, or hyperactivity of liver yang disturbing the head; while that of the deficiency type is deficiency of both blood and qi or insufficiency of kidney essence leading to failure of qi to ascend to the head. In fact, most of the cases are of deficiency type. As for its location, vertigo involves the head and is closely related to the liver, spleen and kidney.

Vertigo may be found in hypertension, hypotension, hypoglycemia, anemia, Meniere's disease, cerebral arteriosclerosis, vertebrobasilar ischemia and neurasthenia.

Essentials for Diagnosis

(1) The chief manifestations are dizziness and blurred vision. The mild case can be relieved by closing one's eyes; the severe case is characterized by a rotatary feeling like sitting in a sailing boat or moving car, even fainting.

(2) There may be accompanying symptoms such as nausea, vomiting, nystagmus, tinnitus, deafness, sweating and pale complexion.

(3) Slow onset, gradual aggravation, or repeated attacks.

(4) To make a clear diagnosis, hemoglobin, red cell count, blood pressure, electrocardiogram, cervical vertabrae X-ray radiography, Doppler transcranial ultrasonic examination, CT and MRI examinations may be done.

Syndrome Differentiation

It is essential to differentiate vertigo of excess type from that of deficiency type. The excess type is usually caused by both hyperactivity of liver yang and retention of turbid phlegm and induced by emotional depression and anger; it is characterized by a short course or intermittent episodes, severe dizziness with a rotatory feeling accompanied by nausea, vomiting and salivation and often found

上扰清空;虚者为气血亏虚,或肾精不足,不能上承清窍。但病性以虚者居多。本病的病位在清窍,与肝、脾、肾三脏关系密切。

本病可见于高血压病、低血压、低血糖、贫血、梅尼埃病、脑动脉硬化、椎-基底动脉供血不足、神经衰弱等病。

【诊断要点】

(1) 以头晕目眩为主症。轻者闭目即止,重者视物旋转,或如坐车船,甚至仆倒。

(2) 可伴有恶心呕吐,眼球震颤,耳鸣耳聋,汗出,面色苍白等。

(3) 慢性起病,逐渐加重,或反复发作。

(4) 血红蛋白、红细胞计数、血压、心电图、颈椎 X 线摄片、经颅多普勒、CT、MRI 等检查,有助于明确诊断。

【辨证论治】

眩晕的辨证以辨虚实为主,凡病程短,或呈发作性,易因情志郁怒诱发,眩晕重而视物旋转,伴有呕恶痰涎,外观形体壮实者,常由肝阳兼痰浊所致,属于实证;如病程长,反复或持续不解,每遇烦劳发作

in those with strong physique. Deficiency of blood or insufficiency of kidney essence often contributes to deficiency type which is characterized by a long course, intermittent or persistent occurrence and is induced or aggravated by overstrain; it is also manifested as dizziness and heavy sensation in the head with no rotatory feeling, and general debility as well. The treatment for the excess type is to calm the liver to stop wind, eliminate fire and resolve phlegm; for deficiency one, to replenish qi and blood and nourish the liver and kidney.

1. Upward Disturbance of Wind Yang

Chief Manifestations: Vertigo, tinnitus and headache with a distending feeling which are aggravated by overstrain or anger, numbness and tremor of the limbs, insomnia, dreamfulness, soreness and weakness in the loins and knees, or flushed face, red tongue with yellow coating, and wiry thready and rapid pulse.

Therapeutic Methods: To calm the liver, suppress hyperactive liver yang and nourish the liver and kidney.

Prescription: Modified Tianma Gouteng Yin (Gastrodiae and Uncariae Decoction), composed of Tianma (*Rhizoma Gastrodiae*) 10 g, Gouteng (*Ramulus Uncariae cum Uncis*) 10 g, Shijueming (*Concha Haliotidis*, to be decocted first) 20 g, Cishi (*Magnetitum*, to be decocted first) 20 g, Huangqin (*Radix Scutellariae*) 10 g, Juhua (*Flos Chrysanthemi*) 10 g and Sangye (*Folium Mori*) 10 g.

Modifications: For pronounced deficiency of yin with red tongue, little coating, and wiry, thready and rapid pulse, add Shengdihuang (*Radix Rehmanniae*) 10 g, Maimendong (*Radix Ophiopogonis*) 10 g, Xuanshen (*Radix Scrophulariae*) 10 g, Heshouwu (*Radix Polygoni Multiflori*) 10 g and Shengbaishaoyao (*Radix Paeoniae Alba*) 10 g; for hyperactive liver fire, manifested

或加重,头目昏晕,但无眩转感,并有全身虚弱见证者,常因血虚或肾精不足所致,多属虚证。实证治予平肝熄风,清火化痰;虚证宜补益气血,滋养肝肾。

1. 风阳上扰证

主要证候　眩晕耳鸣,头痛且胀,遇劳或恼怒加重,肢麻震颤,失眠多梦,腰膝酸软,或颜面潮红,舌红,苔黄,脉弦细数。

治　法　平肝潜阳,滋养肝肾。

方　药　天麻钩藤饮加减:天麻10 g,钩藤10 g,石决明(先煎)20 g,磁石(先煎)20 g,黄芩10 g,菊花10 g,桑叶10 g。

加　减　若阴虚较甚,舌红,少苔,脉弦细数者,可加生地黄10 g,麦门冬10 g,玄参10 g,何首乌10 g,生白芍药10 g;若肝火亢盛,眩晕、头痛较甚,耳鸣、耳聋暴作,目赤,口苦,舌红,苔黄燥,脉弦数

as severe vertigo and headache, sudden occurrence of tinnitus and deafness, red eyes, bitter taste in the mouth, red tongue with yellow and dry coating, and wiry and rapid pulse, add Longdancao (*Radix Gentianae*) 6 g, Mudanpi (*Cortex Moutan Radicis*) 10 g, Juhua (*Flos Chrysanthemi*) 10 g and Xiakucao (*Spica Prunellae*) 10 g; for the case with transformation of liver-yang hyperactivity into wind, manifested as severe vertigo, nausea, vomiting, and numbness or tremor of the limbs, add Zhenzhumu (*Concha Margaritifera Usta*, to be decocted first) 30 g, Shenglonggu (*Os Draconis*, to be decocted first) 30 g and Shengmuli (*Concha Ostreae*, to be decocted first) 30 g.

2. Flaring-up of Liver Fire

Chief Manifestations: Dizziness, headache, red eyes, bitter taste in the mouth, distending pain in the hypochondrium, restlessness, irritability, poor sleep, dreamfulness, red tongue with yellow and greasy coating, and wiry and rapid pulse.

Therapeutic Methods: To reduce liver fire and eliminate damp heat.

Prescription: Modified Longdan Xiegan Tang (Gentianae Decoction for Purging Liver Fire), composed of Longdancao (*Radix Gentianae*) 6 g, Zhizi (*Fructus Gardeniae*) 10 g, Huangqin (*Radix Scutellariae*) 10 g, Chaihu (*Radix Bupleuri*) 6 g, Gancao (*Radix Glycyrrhizae*) 3 g, Mutong (*Caulis Akebiae*) 5 g, Zexie (*Rhizoma Alismatis*) 10 g, Cheqianzi (*Semen Plantaginis*, wrapped) 10 g, Shengdihuang (*Radix Rehmanniae*) 12 g and Danggui (*Radix Angelicae Sinensis*) 10 g.

Modifications: For disturbance of the mind by liver fire with insomnia and restlessness, add Cishi (*Magnetitum*, to be decocted first) 30 g, Longchi (*Dens Draconis*) 15 g, Zhenzhumu (*Concha Margaritifera Usta*, to

者,可加用龙胆草6 g,牡丹皮10 g,菊花10 g,夏枯草10 g;眩晕剧烈,呕恶,手足麻木或震颤者,有阳动化风之势,加珍珠母(先煎)30 g,生龙骨(先煎)30 g,生牡蛎(先煎)30 g。

2. 肝火上炎证

主要证候 头晕且痛,目赤口苦,胸胁胀痛,烦躁易怒,寐少多梦,舌红苔黄腻,脉弦数。

治 法 清肝泻火,清利湿热。

方 药 龙胆泻肝汤加减:龙胆草6 g,栀子10 g,黄芩10 g,柴胡6 g,甘草3 g,木通5 g,泽泻10 g,车前子(包煎)10 g,生地黄12 g,当归10 g。

加 减 若肝火扰动心神,失眠、烦躁者,加磁石(先煎)30 g,龙齿15 g,珍珠母(先煎)30 g,琥珀粉(另冲)1 g;肝

be decocted first) 30 g and Hupofen (*Succinum*, to be powdered and infused separately) 1 g; for transformation of liver fire into wind and internal stirring of liver wind manifested as numbness or tremor of the limbs and premonitory symptom of stroke, add Quanxie (*Scorpio*) 3 g, Wugong (*Scolopendra*) 3 g, Dilong (*Pheretima*) 10 g and Baijiangcan (*Bombyx Batrycatus*) 10 g.

3. Upward Disturbance of Turbid Phlegm

Chief Manifestations: Dizziness accompanied by a heavy sensation and a rotatory feeling in the head, chest oppression, nausea, vomiting of sputum, white and greasy tongue coating, and wiry and smooth pulse.

Therapeutic Methods: To dry up dampness, resolve phlegm, invigorate the spleen and harmonize the stomach.

Prescription: Modified Banxia Baizhu Tianma Tang (Decoction of Pinelliae, Atractylodis Macrocephalae and Gastrodiae), composed of Zhibanxia (*Rhizoma Pinelliae Preparata*) 10 g, Baizhu (*Rhizoma Atractylodis Macrocephalae*) 10 g, Fuling (*Poria*) 10 g, Chenpi (*Pericarpium Citri Retitculatae*) 6 g, Shengjiang (*Rhizoma Zingiberis Recens*) 3 g, Tianma (*Rhizoma Gastrodiae*) 10 g, Gouteng (*Ramulus Uncariae cum Uncis*) 10 g and Baijili (*Fructus Tribuli*) 10 g.

Modifications: For frequent vomiting, add Daizheshi (*Haematitum*, to be decocted first) 30 g and Zhuru (*Caulis Bambusae in Taeniam*) 6 g; for epigastric distress and abdominal distension, add Baikouren (*Fructus Amomi Rotundus*, to be decocted later) 3 g and Sharen (*Fructus Amomi*, to be decocted later) 3 g; for heavy sensation in the limbs and greasy tongue coating, add Huoxiang (*Herba Agastaches*) 10 g, Peilan (*Herba Eupatorii*) 10 g and Shichangpu (*Rhizoma Acori Tatarinowii*) 6 g; for tinnitus and hypoacusis, add Cong-

火化风,肝风内动,肢体麻木、震颤,欲发中风者,加全蝎3 g,蜈蚣3 g,地龙10 g,白僵蚕10 g。

3. 痰浊上蒙证

主要证候　头重如蒙,视物旋转,胸闷作恶,呕吐痰涎,苔白腻,脉弦滑。

治　法　燥湿祛痰,健脾和胃。

方　药　半夏白术天麻汤加减:制半夏10 g,白术10 g,茯苓10 g,陈皮6 g,生姜3 g,天麻10 g,钩藤10 g,白蒺藜10 g。

加　减　若呕吐频繁,加代赭石(先煎)30 g,竹茹6 g;脘闷、腹胀者,加白蔻仁(后下)3 g,砂仁(后下)3 g;肢体沉重,苔腻者,加藿香10 g,佩兰10 g,石菖蒲6 g;耳鸣、重听者,加葱白6 g,郁金10 g,石菖蒲6 g;痰浊郁而化热,痰火上扰清窍,眩晕,苔黄腻,脉弦滑者,加黄连3 g,竹茹10 g。

bai (*Bolbus Allii Fistulosi*) 6 g, Yujin (*Radix Curcum-ae*) 10 g and Shichangpu (*Rhizoma Acori Tatarinowii*) 6 g; for retained turbid phlegm transforming into heat and phlegm fire disturbing the clear orifices, manifested as vertigo, yellow and greasy tongue coating, and wiry and smooth pulse, add Huanglian (*Rhizoma Coptidis*) 3 g and Zhuru (*Caulis Bambusae in Taeniam*) 10 g.

4. Deficiency of Qi and Blood

Chief Manifestations: Dizziness and blurred vision which are aggravated by exertion and induced by over-strain, pale complexion, lassitude, palpitation, poor sleep, pale tongue with thin and white coating, and thready and weak pulse.

Therapeutic Methods: To replenish qi, nourish blood, invigorate the spleen and regulate the stomach.

Prescription: Modified Guipi Tang (Decoction for Invigorating Spleen and Nourishing Heart), composed of Dangshen (*Radix Codonopsis*) 10 g, Baizhu (*Rhizoma Atractylodis Macrocephalae*) 10 g, Huangqi (*Radix As-tragali*) 12 g, Danggui (*Radix Angelicae Sinensis*) 10 g, Baishaoyao (*Radix Paeoniae Alba*) 10 g, Guiyuanrou (*Arillus Longan*) 10 g, Yuanzhi (*Radix Po-lygalae*) 6 g, Fushen (*Sclerotium Poriae circum Radi-cem Pini*) 10 g, Yejiaoteng (*Caulis et Folium Polygoni Multiflori*) 10 g, Chenpi (*Pericarpium Citri Reticula-tae*) 6 g, Dazao (*Fructus Jujubae*) 5 pcs and Zhigancao (*Radix Glycyrrhizae*, roasted) 3 g.

Modifications: For frequent spontaneous sweating due to qi deficiency and weakened yang qi in weifen, in-crease Huangqi (*Radix Astragali*) to 30 g, and add Fang-feng (*Radix Saposhnikoviae*) 6 g and Fuxiaomai (*Fructus Tritici Levis*) 12 g; for diarrhea or loose stools due to deficiency of qi and excess of dampness, add Yiyiren (*Semen Coicis*) 15 g, Zexie (*Rhizoma Alismatis*) 10 g,

4. 气血亏虚证

主要证候 头晕目眩,动则加剧,遇劳则发,面色㿠白,神疲乏力,心悸少寐,舌淡,苔薄白,脉细弱。

治 法 补养气血,健运脾胃。

方 药 归脾汤加减:党参10 g,白术10 g,黄芪12 g,当归10 g,白芍药10 g,桂圆肉10 g,远志6 g,茯神10 g,夜交藤10 g,陈皮6 g,大枣5枚,炙甘草3 g。

加 减 若气虚卫阳不固,自汗时出,重用黄芪30 g,加防风6 g,浮小麦12 g;气虚湿盛,泄泻或便溏者,加薏苡仁15 g,泽泻10 g,炒扁豆10 g,炒当归10 g;兼见畏寒肢冷,腹中隐痛等阳虚症状,加桂枝

Chaobiandou (*Semen Dolichoris*, stir-baked) 10 g and Chaodanggui (*Radix Angelicae Sinensis*, stir-baked) 10 g; for vertigo accompanied by such yang-deficiency symptoms as aversion to cold, cold limbs and dull pain in the abdomen, add Guizhi (*Ramulus Cinnamomi*) 6 g and Ganjiang (*Rhizoma Zingiberis*) 3 g; for palpitation and insomnia, add Baiziren (*Semen Platycladi*) 10 g and Cishi (*Magnetitum*, to be decocted first) 20 g; for pronounced deficiency of blood with sallow and lusterless complexion, add Shudihuang (*Radix Rehmanniae Preparata*) 12 g and Ejiao (*Colla Corii Asini*, to be melted and infused in the finished decoction) 10 g.

5. Deficiency of Liver Yin and Kidney Yin

Chief Manifestations: Prolonged vertigo, hypopsia, dryness and pain of eyes, poor sleep, amnesia, restlessness, dry mouth, tinnitus, lassitude, soreness and weakness in the loins and knees, red tongue with thin coating, and wiry and thready pulse.

Therapeutic Methods: To nourish the liver and kidney, and replenish kidney essence.

Prescription: Modified Zuogui Wan (Bolus for Replenishing Kidney Yin), composed of Shudihuang (*Radix Rehmanniae Preparata*) 12 g, Shanyao (*Rhizoma Dioscoreae*) 10 g, Shanzhuyu (*Fructus Corni*) 10 g, Gouqizi (*Fructus Lycii*) 10 g, Heshouwu (*Radix Polygoni Multiflori*) 10 g, Sangjisheng (*Herba Taxilli*) 10 g, Cishi (*Magnetitum*, to be decocted first) 30 g and Hutaorou (*Semen Juglandis*) 15 g.

Modifications: For deficiency of yin producing internal heat, manifested as dysphoria with feverish sensation in the chest, palms and soles, red tongue, and wiry, thready and rapid pulse, add Zhibiejia (*Carapax Trionycis*, roasted, to be decocted first) 15 g, Zhimu (*Rhizoma Anemarrhenae*) 10 g, Huangbai (*Cortex Phellodendri*)

6 g,干姜3 g;心悸怔忡、不寐者,加柏子仁10 g,磁石(先煎)20 g;血虚较甚,面色萎黄无华,加熟地黄12 g,阿胶(烊化冲服)10 g。

5. 肝肾阴虚证

主要证候 眩晕久发不已,视力减退,两目干涩,少寐健忘,心烦口干,耳鸣,神疲乏力,腰酸膝软,舌红,苔薄,脉弦细。

治 法 滋养肝肾,养阴填精。

方 药 左归丸加减:熟地黄12 g,山药10 g,山茱萸10 g,枸杞子10 g,何首乌10 g,桑寄生10 g,磁石(先煎)30 g,胡桃肉15 g。

加 减 若阴虚生内热,表现五心烦热,舌红,脉弦细数者,加炙鳖甲(先煎)15 g,知母10 g,黄柏10 g,牡丹皮10 g;心肾不交,失眠,多梦,健忘者,加酸枣仁10 g,柏子仁

10 g and Mudanpi (*Cortex Moutan Radicis*) 10 g; for disharmony between the heart and kidney manifested as insomnia, dreamfulness and amnesia, add Suanzaoren (*Semen Ziziphi Spinosae*) 10 g and Baiziren (*Semen Platycladi*) 10 g; for child-organ disorder involving its mother-organ and deficiency of lung yin and kidney yin, add Beishashen (*Radix Glehniae*) 10 g, Maimendong (*Radix Ophiopogonis*) 10 g and Yuzhu (*Rhizoma Polygonati Odorati*) 10 g.

6. Retention of Blood Stasis in the Orifices

Chief Manifestations: Vertigo and headache with accompanying symptoms such as amnesia, insomnia, palpitation, listlessness, tinnitus, deafness, dark purple complexion and lips, petechiae or ecchymosis on the tongue, wiry and unsmooth pulse or thready and unsmooth pulse.

Therapeutic Methods: To eliminate blood stasis, promote blood circulation and activate the collaterals.

Prescription: Modified Tongqiao Huoxue Tang (Decoction for Activating Blood Circulation), composed of Chishaoyao (*Radix Paeoniae Rubra*) 10 g, Chuanxiong (*Rhizoma Chuanxiong*) 10 g, Taoren (*Semen Persicae*) 10 g, Honghua (*Flos Carthami*) 10 g, Danshen (*Radix Salviae Miltiorrhizae*) 10 g, Baizhi (*Radix Angelicae Dahuricae*) 6 g, Congbai (*Bulbus Allii Fistulosi*) 6 g and Xixin (*Herba Asari*) 3 g.

Modifications: For qi deficiency cases with lassitude, shortness of breath and spontaneous sweating, add Huangqi (*Radix Astragali*) 12 g; for those accompanied with aversion to cold and cold limbs and aggravated by pathogenic cold, add Zhifuzi (*Radix Aconiti Lateralis Preparata*) 6 g and Guizhi (*Ramulus Cinnamomi*) 6 g; for those aggravated by changes of weather or induced by exposure to wind, increase Chuanxiong (*Rhizoma*

10 g;若子盗母气,肺肾阴虚,加北沙参10 g,麦门冬10 g,玉竹10 g。

6. 瘀血阻窍证

主要证候 眩晕头痛,兼见健忘,失眠,心悸,精神不振,耳鸣耳聋,面唇紫暗,舌有瘀点或瘀斑,脉弦涩或细涩。

治 法 祛瘀生新,通窍活络。

方 药 通窍活血汤加减:赤芍药10 g,川芎10 g,桃仁10 g,红花10 g,丹参10 g,白芷6 g,葱白6 g,细辛3 g。

加 减 若见神疲乏力,少气自汗等气虚证者,加黄芪12 g;若兼有畏寒肢冷,感寒加重者,加制附子6 g,桂枝6 g;若天气变化加重,或当风而发,可重用川芎15 g,加防风6 g,白芷 6 g,荆芥6 g,天麻10 g。

Chuanxiong) to 15 g, and add Fangfeng (*Radix Saposh-nikoviae*) 6 g, Baizhi (*Radix Angelicae Dahuricae*) 6 g, Jingjie (*Herba Schizonepetae*) 6 g and Tianma (*Rhizoma Gastrodiae*) 10 g.

Other Treatments

1. Chinese Patent Drugs

(1) Niuhuang Qingxin Wan (Calculus Bovis Bolus for Clearing Heart Fire): 1 bolus each time, twice daily; applicable to vertigo caused by hyperactivity of liver yang and excess of phlegm fire.

(2) Quan Tianma Jiaonang (Gastrodiae Capsule): 4 capsules each time, thrice daily; applicable to vertigo caused by hyperactivity of liver yang and upward disturbance of liver wind.

(3) Qi Ju Dihuang Ye (Oral Liquid of Rehmanniae with Lycii and Chrysanthemi): 1 vial each time, thrice daily; applicable to vertigo due to deficiency of liver yin and kidney yin.

(4) Tianma Shouwu Pian (Tablet of Gastrodiae and Polygoni Multiflori): 6 tablets each time, thrice daily; applicable to vertigo due to deficiency of liver yin and kidney yin.

2. Single-drug or Experiential Prescriptions

(1) Cheqiancao (*Herba Plantaginis*) 30 g and Xi-xiancao (*Herba Siegesgeckiae*) 30 g. Decoct the herbs in water for oral administration, 1 dose a day. It is applicable to vertigo caused by hyperactivity of liver yang.

(2) Zexie (*Rhizoma Alismatis*) 30 g, Chaobaizhu (*Rhizoma Atractylodis Macrocephalae*, *stir-baked*) 15 g and Huainiuxi (*Radix Achyranthis Bidentatae*) 10 g. Decoct the herbs in water for oral administration, 1 dose a day. It is suitable for vertigo caused by turbid phlegm.

(3) Sangshenzi (*Fructus Mori*) 15 g and Heidadou

【其他疗法】

1. 中成药

(1) 牛黄清心丸　每服 1 丸,每日 2 次。适用于肝阳上亢及痰火壅盛所致的眩晕。

(2) 全天麻胶囊　每服 4 粒,每日 3 次。适用于眩晕属于肝阳上亢,肝风上扰者。

(3) 杞菊地黄液　每服 1 支,每日 3 次。适用于肝肾阴虚型眩晕。

(4) 天麻首乌片　每服 6 片,每日 3 次。适用于眩晕属于肝肾阴虚者。

2. 单验方

(1) 车前草 30 g,豨莶草 30 g,水煎服,每日 1 剂。适用于肝阳上亢之眩晕。

(2) 泽泻 30 g,炒白术 15 g,怀牛膝 10 g,水煎服,每日 1 剂。适用于痰浊眩晕。

(3) 桑椹子 15 g,黑大豆

(*Semen Sojae*) 15 g. Decoct the drugs in water for oral administration, 1 dose a day. It is applicable to vertigo caused by yin and blood deficiency of the liver and kidney.

(4) Shengdihuang (*Radix Rehmanniae*) 30 g, Gouteng (*Ramulus Uncariae cum Uncis*) 30 g, Yimucao (*Herba Leonuri*) 60 g, Xiaoji (*Herba Cirsii*) 30 g, Baimaogen (*Rhizoma Imperatae*) 30 g, Xiakucao (*Spica Prunellae*) 60 g, Shanzha (*Fructus Crataegi*) 30 g, Honghua (*Flos Carthami*) 9 g, Dilong (*Pheretima*) 30 g and Caojueming (*Semen Casslae*) 30 g. Decoct the drugs in water and concentrate into 160 ml for oral administration, 40 ml each time, twice a day. It is applicable to vertigo due to blood stasis.

(5) Shengmingfan (*Alumen*) and Lüdou (*Semen Phaseoli Radiati*) in equal proportions. Grind them into powder and then mix with rice to make bolus, 5 boluses each time, twice a day. It is suitable for phlegm-retention vertigo.

3. External Therapy

(1) Gouteng (*Ramulus Uncariae cum Uncis, cut into small pieces*) 30 g and a little Bingpian (*Borneolum Syntheticum, wrapped in a piece of cloth*). Put them in warm water to bathe feet, twice a day after getting up and before going to bed, 30 - 45 minutes each time and 10 days as a treatment course. It is applicable to vertigo caused by liver-yang hyperactivity.

(2) Juhua (*Flos Chrysanthemi*) 500 g, Sangye (*Folium Mori*) 500 g, Xinyi (*Flos Magnoliae*) 500 g, Bohe (*Herba Menthae*) 200 g, Honghua (*Flos Carthami*) 100 g and Bingpian (*Borneolum Syntheticum*) 50 g. Pound the above ingredients into small pieces and then put them into a cloth bag to make a medicated pillow. One pillow may be used for 3 - 6 months. It is applicable to vertigo with liver-yang hyperactivity.

15 g,水煎服,每日 1 剂。适用于肝肾阴血亏虚之眩晕。

（4）生地黄 30 g,钩藤 30 g,益母草60 g,小蓟30 g,白茅根 30 g,夏枯草 60 g,山楂 30 g,红花9 g,地龙30 g,草决明30 g,浓煎成160 ml,每次服40 ml,每日 2 次。适用于瘀血眩晕。

（5）生明矾、绿豆粉各等分研末,用饭和丸如梧桐子大。每日早、晚各服5 丸。适用于痰饮眩晕。

3. 外治法

（1）钩藤30 g,剪碎,布包冰片少许,于每日晨起和临睡前放入盆内并加温水浴脚,每次 30～45 分钟,10 日为 1 个疗程。适用于肝阳上亢之眩晕。

（2）菊花 500 g,桑叶 500 g,辛夷500 g,薄荷200 g,红花100 g,冰片50 g。上药研碎后装入布袋作药枕用,每个药枕可用 3～6 个月。适用于肝阳偏旺之眩晕。

2.4.3　Viral Hepatitis

General Description

Viral hepatitis is an infectious disease caused by various hepatitis viruses. It is clinically manifested as fatigue, impaired appetite, nausea, vomiting, hepatosplenomegaly and impaired function of the liver, and jaundice and fever in some cases.

Viral hepatitis can be divided into five types — Type A, Type B, Type C, Type D and Type E; and two types in terms of its onset — acute and chronic. Hepatitis A and E are mostly manifested as acute type and may recover within 6 months. Hepatitis B, C and D are liable to become chronic, but seldom serious, and only a few cases develop to cirrhosis. Chronic hepatitis B and C have a close relation to hepatocellular carcinoma.

In TCM, "huang dan" (jaundice), "xie tong" (hypochondriac pain) and "gan wen" (fulminant hepatitis) may manifest similar symptoms of hepatitis. Exogenous factors of this disease are pathogenic damp heat. Its pathogenesis is chiefly retention of damp heat in the interior and incoordination between the liver and spleen, and the diseased location is the spleen, stomach, liver and gallbladder.

Essentials for Diagnosis

(1) It is clinically manifested as general debility, poor appetite, nausea, vomiting, fullness in the epigastrium, and dull pain in the hepatic region.

第三节　病毒性肝炎

【概述】

病毒性肝炎是由多种肝炎病毒引起的传染病。临床主要表现为乏力,食欲减退,恶心,呕吐,肝脾肿大及肝功能损害等,部分患者可有黄疸和发热。

病毒性肝炎根据病毒的类型主要分为甲型、乙型、丙型、丁型和戊型肝炎,按照起病方式可分为急性和慢性病毒性肝炎。甲型、戊型肝炎多为急性肝炎,患者大多在 6 个月内恢复,乙型、丙型和丁型肝炎易转为慢性,少数可发展为肝硬化,极少数呈重症经过。慢性乙型和丙型肝炎与肝细胞癌的发生有密切关系。

根据本病的临床表现,与中医学"黄疸"、"胁痛"、"肝瘟"等病证颇相类似。本病的主要病因是外感湿热邪毒,病机以湿热内蕴、肝脾失和为主,病位主要在脾胃肝胆。

【诊断要点】

(1) 本病临床主要表现为全身无力,食欲不振,恶心呕吐,上腹部饱胀不适,肝区隐痛。

(2) Various degrees of jaundice may be found in the skin and sclera. The liver becomes slightly enlarged with tenderness and percussion pain. Hepatic face, vascular spiders, liver palms and hepatosplenomegaly with slightly hard texture may be present in chronic active hepatitis.

(3) An increase of direct bilirubin in blood, gradual deepening color of urine and an apparent rise of serum aminotransferase may occur.

(4) Hepatitis virus or antigen can be detected in etiological examination; and specific antibody of hepatitis virus in serological examination.

(5) Rapid deepening of jaundice, frequent vomiting, abdominal distension, anorexia, hiccup, extreme fatigue, an inclination of bleeding, or mental disturbance occur, and progressive shrinking of the liver with impaired function of the liver is manifested in severe cases. Prothrombin time is prolonged and cholinesterase activity is reduced.

Syndrome Differentiation and Treatment

Clinically there is excess-type and deficiency-type hepatitis. The cases with damp-heat retention, dampness stagnation in the spleen, liver qi stagnation, and blood stagnation blocking the meridians are of excess type; those with deficiency of the liver and spleen, deficiency of liver yin and kidney yin, and deficiency of spleen yang and kidney yang belong to deficiency type. The treatment is primarily to clear damp heat, remove dampness to restore the splenic function, soothe the liver and regulate the circulation of qi, activate blood to remove blood stasis, invigorate the spleen and nourish the liver, nourish the liver and kidney, and invigorate the spleen and warm the kidney.

1. Damp-heat Retention

Chief Manifestations: Bright yellow coloration of

（2）皮肤巩膜不同程度黄染，肝脏稍肿大及有叩痛和压痛。慢性活动性肝炎可出现慢性肝病面容、蜘蛛痣及肝掌，肝、脾肿大，质地中等偏硬。

（3）血中直接胆红素量增加，尿色逐渐加深，血清转氨酶明显升高。

（4）病原学检查可检测到肝炎病毒或抗原；血清学可检查到肝炎病毒的特异性抗体。

（5）重症型患者黄疸迅速加深，频繁呕吐，腹胀，厌食，呃逆，极度乏力，出血倾向，或有神志障碍。肝脏进行性缩小。肝功能严重损害，凝血酶原时间明显延长，胆碱酯酶活力明显降低。

【辨证论治】

本病临床见证有实有虚。湿热薰蒸、湿困脾运、肝郁气滞、瘀血阻络者属实；肝脾不足、肝肾阴虚、脾肾阳虚者属虚。治疗以清利湿热、化湿运脾、疏肝理气、活血化瘀、健脾养肝、滋养肝肾、健脾温肾为主。

1. 湿热薰蒸证

主要证候 面目肌肤俱

the face, sclera and skin, fever, thirst, lassitude, poor appetite, dark yellow urine, constipation, yellow and greasy tongue coating, wiry and rapid or soft-superficial and rapid pulse.

Therapeutic Methods: To clear away heat, remove the toxic substance, promote diuresis and relieve jaundice.

Prescription: Modified Yinchenhao Tang (Artemisiae Scopariae Decoction), composed of Yinchen (*Herba Artemisiae Scopariae*) 30 g, Shengdahuang (*Radix et Rhizoma Rhei*, to be decocted later) 5 - 10 g, Pugongying (*Herba Taraxaci*) 15 g, Chifuling (*Poria Rubra*) 15 g, Cheqianzi (*Semen Plantaginis*, wrapped) 15 g, Shengzhizi (*Fructus Gardeniae*) 10 g, Huangqin (*Radix Scutellariae*) 10 g, Guangyujin (*Radix Curcumae*) 10 g, Chenpi (*Pericarpium Citri Reticulatae*) 10 g and Gancao (*Radix Glycyrrhizae*) 5 g.

Modifications: For cases accompanied by exterior syndrome at the onset, manifested as aversion to cold, fever, headache, fatigue, thin and yellow tongue coating, and superficial pulse, use Mahuang (*Herba Ephedrae*) 8 g, Lianqiao (*Fructus Forsythiae*) 12 g, Cheqiancao (*Herba Plantaginis*) 15 g, Yiyiren (*Semen Coicis*) 15 g, Chixiaodou (*Semen Phaseoli*) 30 g, Banlangen (*Radix Isatidis*) 30 g and Gancao (*Radix Glycyrrhizae*) 5 g; for stagnation of damp heat, adverse rising of stomach qi, nausea, vomiting and impaired appetite, add Jiangbanxia (*Rhizoma Pinelliae*, ginger prepared) 10 g, Jupi (*Pericarpium Citri Reticulatae*) 10 g, Danzhuru (*Caulis Bambusae in Taeniam*) 10 g and Shenqu (*Massa Medicata Fermentata*) 10 g.

2. Dampness Stagnation in the Spleen

Chief Manifestations: Epigastric oppression, abdominal distension, nausea, vomiting, poor appetite, fa-

黄,其色鲜明如橘,发热口渴,倦怠纳少,小便黄赤,大便秘结,舌苔黄腻,脉象弦数或濡数。

治　法　清热解毒,利湿退黄。

方　药　茵陈蒿汤加减:茵陈30 g,生大黄(后下)5～10 g,蒲公英15 g,赤茯苓15 g,车前子(包煎)15 g,生栀子10 g,黄芩10 g,广郁金10 g,陈皮10 g,甘草5 g。

加　减　初起挟有表证,恶寒发热,头痛身困,苔薄黄,脉浮者,用麻黄8 g,连翘12 g,车前草15 g,薏苡仁15 g,赤小豆30 g,板蓝根30 g,甘草5 g;湿热蕴阻,胃气上逆,恶心呕吐,纳食减少,加姜半夏10 g,橘皮10 g,淡竹茹10 g,神曲10 g。

2. 湿困脾运证

主要证候　脘闷腹胀,恶心呕吐,胃纳不佳,肢体困倦,

tigue, hypochondriac pain, or jaundice in the face, sclera and skin, loose stools, tastelessness or stickiness in the mouth, greasy, white and yellowish tongue coating, and soft-superficial and smooth pulse.

Therapeutic Methods: To invigorate the spleen, remove dampness and regulate qi and middle energizer.

Prescription: Modified Yinchen Weiling Tang (Poria Decoction for Regulating Stomach with Artemisiae Scopariae), composed of Yinchen (*Herba Artemisiae Scopariae*) 15 g, Cangzhu (*Rhizoma Atractylodis*) 10 g, Houpo (*Cortex Magnoliae Officinalis*) 10 g, Chenpi (*Pericarpium Citri Reticulatae*) 6 g, Zhuling (*Polyporus*) 12 g, Zexie (*Rhizoma Alismatis*) 12 g, Huangqin (*Radix Scutellariae*) 10 g, Jiaoshanzha (*Fructus Crataegi*, charred) 10 g, Shenqu (*Massa Medicata Fermentata*) 10 g, Baikouren (*Fructus Amomi Rotundus*, to be decocted later) 4 g and Gancao (*Radix Glycyrrhizae*) 3 g.

Modifications: For thick and greasy tongue coating, pronounced abdominal distension and epigastric stuffiness, add Huoxiang (*Herba Agastaches*) 10 g and Peilan (*Herba Eupatorii*) 10 g; for cold-dampness retention in the spleen, abdominal distension and epigastric stuffiness, dark yellow coloration of the skin and sclera, lassitude, aversion to cold, cold limbs, tastelessness in the mouth, no desire to drink, pale tongue with white greasy coating, soft-superficial and even-soft or deep and slow pulse, use Yinchen (*Herba Artemisiae Scopariae*) 30 g, Zhifupian (*Radix Aconiti Lateralis*) 6 g, Ganjiang (*Rhizoma Zingiberis*) 6 g, Gancao (*Radix Glycyrrhizae*) 6 g, Baizhu (*Rhizoma Atractylodis Macrocephalae*) 10 g, Baishaoyao (*Radix Paeoniae Alba*) 10 g, Fuling (*Poria*) 20 g and Yiyiren (*Semen Coicis*) 20 g.

胁肋疼痛,或面目皮肤发黄,大便稀溏,口淡或黏,苔白腻微黄,脉濡滑。

治　法　健脾化湿,理气和中。

方　药　茵陈胃苓汤加减:茵陈15 g,苍术10 g,厚朴10 g,陈皮6 g,猪苓12 g,泽泻12 g,黄芩10 g,焦山楂10 g,神曲10 g,白蔻仁(后下)4 g,甘草3 g。

加　减　舌苔厚腻,腹胀脘痞明显者,加藿香10 g,佩兰10 g;寒湿困脾,腹胀脘痞,身目发黄,黄色晦暗,犹如烟薰,神疲畏寒,四肢不温,口淡不渴,舌质淡,苔白腻,脉濡缓或沉迟者,用茵陈30 g,制附片6 g,干姜6 g,甘草6 g,白术10 g,白芍药10 g,茯苓20 g,薏苡仁20 g。

3. Stagnation of Liver Qi

Chief Manifestations: Distension, oppression and pain in the chest and hypochondrium, epigastric fullness, abdominal distension, frequent belching and wind from the bowels, poor appetite, bitter taste in the mouth, thin, white or yellow tongue coating, and wiry pulse.

Therapeutic Methods: To disperse stagnant liver qi, and regulate qi to stop pain.

Prescription: Modified Chaihu Shugan San (Bupleuri Powder for Soothing Liver Qi), composed of Chaihu (*Radix Bupleuri*) 8 g, Zhike (*Fructus Aurantii*) 10 g, Baishaoyao (*Radix Paeoniae Alba*) 10 g, Zhi-xiangfu (*Rhizoma Cyperi Preparata*) 10 g, Yujin (*Radix Curcumae*) 10 g, Yanhusuo (*Rhizoma Corydalis*) 10 g, Chuanlianzi (*Fructus Meliae Toosendan*) 10 g, Jinjuye (*Folium Fortunellae*) 10 g, Pugongying (*Herba Taraxaci*) 15 g and Gancao (*Radix Glycyrrhizae*) 5 g.

Modifications: For liver qi stagnation, deficiency of the spleen, hypochondriac distension and pain, belching, oppression in the chest, tastelessness in the mouth, fatigue, impaired appetite, abdominal distension and loose stools, use Chaihu (*Radix Bupleuri*, stir-baked with vinegar) 6 g, Danggui (*Radix Angelicae Sinensis*) 10 g, Baishaoyao (*Radix Paeoniae Alba*) 10 g, Fuling (*Poria*) 12 g, Guangyujin (*Radix Curcumae*) 10 g, Chaobaizhu (*Rhizoma Atractylodis Macrocephalae*, stir-baked) 10 g, Chaoyiyiren (*Semen Coicis*, stir-baked) 15 g, Chaoguya (*Fructus Oryzae Germinatus*, stir-baked) 15 g and Chaomaiya (*Fructus Hordei Germinatus*, stir-baked) 15 g.

4. Obstruction of the Collaterals by Blood Stasis

Chief Manifestations: Dark dusty complexion or vascular spiders, hepatosplenomegaly with hard texture, stabbing pain in the hypochondria, bright red palms, fre-

3. 肝郁气滞证

主要证候　胸胁胀闷疼痛,脘痞腹胀,嗳气、矢气频作,食欲不振,口苦,苔薄白或黄,脉弦。

治　法　疏肝解郁,理气止痛。

方　药　柴胡疏肝散加减:柴胡8 g,枳壳10 g,白芍药10 g,制香附10 g,郁金10 g,延胡索10 g,川楝子10 g,金橘叶10 g,蒲公英15 g,甘草5 g。

加　减　肝郁脾虚,胁肋胀痛,嗳气胸闷,口淡乏力,纳食减少,腹胀便溏者,用醋炒柴胡6 g,当归10 g,白芍药10 g,茯苓12 g,广郁金10 g,炒白术10 g,炒薏苡仁15 g,炒谷芽15 g,炒麦芽15 g。

4. 瘀血阻络证

主要证候　面色晦暗,或见赤缕红痣,肝脾肿大,质地较硬,两胁刺痛,手掌殷红,时

quent nasal and gingival hemorrhage, low fever aggravated at night, dysmenorrhea with dark-colored clots in female patients, dark purple tongue with ecchymoses, deep, thready and unsmooth pulse.

Therapeutic Methods: To activate blood, remove stasis, eliminate stagnation and dredge the collaterals.

Prescription: Modified Gexia Zhuyu Tang (Decoction for Removing Blood Stasis under Diaphragm), composed of Chaihu (*Radix Bupleuri*) 6 g, Zhike (*Fructus Aurantii*) 10 g, Chishaoyao (*Radix Paeoniae Rubra*) 10 g, Danggui (*Radix Angelicae Sinensis*) 10 g, Taoren (*Semen Persicae*) 10 g, Honghua (*Flos Carthami*) 8 g, Shengdihuang (*Radix Rehmanniae*) 20 g, Danshen (*Radix Salviae Miltiorrhizae*) 12 g, Chuanxiong (*Rhizoma Chuanxiong*) 12 g, Zhibiejia (*Carapax Trionycis*, roasted and to be decocted first) 15 g and Gancao (*Radix Glycyrrhizae*) 5 g.

Modifications: For heat retention, fixed stabbing pain in the hypochondrium, palpable masses in the hypochondriac region, and nasal and gingival hemorrhage, use Shuiniujiao (*Cornu Bubali*, to be decocted first) 15 g, Sheng Dihuang (*Radix Rehmanniae*) 12 g, Chishaoyao (*Radix Paeoniae Rubra*) 20 g, Baihuasheshecao (*Herba Hedyotis Diffusae*) 30 g, Huzhang (*Rhizoma Polygoni Cuspidati*) 30 g, Mudanpi (*Cortex Moutan Radicis*) 10 g, Chaihu (*Radix Bupleuri*) 10 g, Fuling (*Poria*) 10 g and Gouqizi (*Fructus Lycii*) 10 g.

5. Deficiency of the Liver and Spleen

Chief Manifestations: Shortness of breath, dislike of speaking, lassitude, lusterless complexion, impaired appetite, abdominal distension after intake of food, dull pain in the hypochondrium, dizziness, dryness and pain of eyes, emaciation or puffy face, occasional loose stools, pale tongue with white coating, and thready and weak

时鼻齿衄血,低热夜甚,女子行经腹痛,经血色暗有块,舌质紫暗有瘀斑,脉沉细涩。

治　法　活血化瘀,消积通络。

方　药　膈下逐瘀汤加减:柴胡6g,枳壳10g,赤芍药10g,当归10g,桃仁10g,红花8g,生地黄20g,丹参12g,川芎12g,炙鳖甲(先煎)15g,甘草5g。

加　减　瘀热内阻,胁痛如刺,痛处固定,胁下癥积,齿鼻衄血,用水牛角(先煎)15g,生地黄12g,赤芍药20g,白花蛇舌草30g,虎杖30g,牡丹皮10g,柴胡10g,茯苓10g,枸杞子10g。

5. 肝脾不足证

主要证候　气短懒言,倦怠乏力,面色无华,食欲不振,纳后腹胀,胁肋隐痛,头昏目涩,形体消瘦或面部虚浮,大便时溏,舌淡苔白,脉细而弱。

pulse.

Therapeutic Methods: To invigorate the liver to support the spleen.

Prescription: Modified Gui Shao Liujunzi Tang (Six-Mild-Drug Decoction with Angelicae Sinensis and Paeoniae Alba), composed of Fuling (*Poria*) 12 g, Chaodangshen (*Radix Codonopsis*, stir-baked) 10 g, Chaobaizhu (*Rhizoma Atractulodis Macrocephalae*, *stir-baked*) 10 g, Baishaoyao (*Radix Paeoniae Alba*) 10 g, Shanyao (*Rhizoma Dioscoreae*) 15 g, Muxiang (*Radix Aucklandiae*) 6 g, Sharen (*Fructus Amomi*, to be decocted later) 4 g, Chenpi (*Pericarpium Citri Reticulatae*) 8 g and Zhigancao (*Radix Glycyrrhizae*, roasted) 5 g.

Modification: For dull pain in the hypochondrium, distension in the epigastrium and abdomen, and wiry and thready pulse, add Chaihu (*Radix Bupleuri*) 8 g and Chaozhike (*Fructus Aurantii*, stir-baked) 10 g.

6. Deficiency of Liver Yin and Kidney Yin

Chief Manifestations: Dull pain in the hypochondrium which is aggravated by exertion, dizziness, tinnitus, dryness and pain of eyes, dry mouth and throat, insomnia, dreamfulness, feverish sensation in the chest, palms and soles, soreness and weakness in the loins and knees, hypomenorrhea or amenorrhea in female patients, red small tongue with little saliva or with cracks, thin coating, thready and rapid pulse.

Therapeutic Methods: To nourish blood, soothe the liver, nourish yin and tonify the kidney.

Prescription: Modified Yiguan Jian (Ever-effective Decoction for Nourishing Liver and Kidney), composed of Shengdihuang (*Radix Rehmanniae*) 20 g, Shashen (*Radix Glehniae*) 10 g, Gouqizi (*Fructus Lycii*) 10 g, Huzhang (*Rhizoma Polygoni Cuspidati*) 10 g, Maimendong (*Radix Ophiopogonis*) 10 g, Danggui (*Radix*

治　法　补肝扶脾。

方　药　归芍六君子汤加减：茯苓12 g，炒党参10 g，炒白术10 g，白芍药10 g，山药15 g，木香6 g，砂仁(后下)4 g，陈皮8 g，炙甘草5 g。

加　减　胁肋隐痛，脘痞腹胀，脉细弦者，加柴胡8 g，炒枳壳10 g。

6. 肝肾阴虚证

主要证候　胁痛隐隐，劳累尤甚，头晕耳鸣，两目干涩，口燥咽干，失眠多梦，五心烦热，腰膝酸软，女子经少经闭，舌红体瘦少津，或有裂纹，苔少，脉细数。

治　法　养血柔肝，滋阴补肾。

方　药　一贯煎加减：生地黄20 g，沙参10 g，枸杞子10 g，虎杖10 g，麦门冬10 g，当归10 g，玄参10 g，川楝子10 g，牡丹皮10 g，酸枣仁10 g，五味子6 g，甘草6 g。

Angelicae Sinensis) 10 g, Xuanshen (*Radix Scrophulariae*) 10 g, Chuanlianzi (*Fructus Meliae Toosendan*) 10 g, Mudanpi (*Cortex Moutan Radicis*) 10 g, Suanzaoren (*Semen Ziziphi Spinosae*) 10 g, Wuweizi (*Fructus Schisandrae*) 6 g and Gancao (*Radix Glycyrrhizae*) 6 g.

Modifications: For deficiency of qi and yin, emaciation, restlessness, dry mouth, sweating on exertion, dizziness, and dryness and pain of eyes, use Taizishen (*Radix Pseudostellariae*) 15 g, Maimendong (*Radix Ophiopogonis*) 12 g, Baishaoyao (*Radix Paeoniae Alba*) 12 g, Gouqizi (*Fructus Lycii*) 12 g and Shanyao (*Rhizoma Dioscoreae*) 12 g; for nasal and gingival hemorrhage, add Baimaogen (*Rhizoma Imperatae*) 15 g and Hanliancao (*Herba Ecliptae*) 12 g.

7. Deficiency of Spleen Yang and Kidney Yang

Chief Manifestations: Intolerance of cold and preference for warmth, cold limbs, cold pain in the lower abdomen, loins and knees, lassitude, dull pain in the hypochondrium, impaired appetite, loose stools with undigested food, even frequent diarrheas or fecal incontinence, abdominal fullness, scanty urine, no edema of the lower limbs, pale and swollen tongue, deep, thready and forceless pulse, or deep and slow pulse.

Therapeutic Methods: To invigorate the spleen, replenish qi, warm the kidney and nourish yang.

Prescription: Modified Fuzi Lizhong Wan (Aconiti Lateralis Bolus for Regulating Middle Energizer) and Jingui Shenqi Wan (Pill for Invigorating Kidney Qi from *Golden Cabinet*), composed of Dangshen (*Radix Codonopsis*) 15 g, Zhihuangqi (*Radix Astragali*, roasted) 15 g, Baizhu (*Rhizoma Atractylodis Macrocephalae*) 10 g, Fuling (*Poria*) 12 g, Shudihuang (*Radix Rehmanniae Preparata*) 15 g, Shanyao (*Rhizoma*

加 减　气阴两虚,形体消瘦,心烦口干,动则汗出,头晕目涩者,用太子参15 g,麦门冬12 g,白芍药12 g,枸杞子12 g,山药12 g;齿鼻衄血者,加白茅根15 g,旱莲草12 g。

7. 脾肾阳虚证
主要证候　畏寒喜暖,四肢不温,少腹腰膝冷痛,精神疲惫,胁肋隐痛,食少便溏,完谷不化,甚则滑泄失禁,腹满尿少,下肢不肿,舌质淡胖,脉沉细无力或沉迟。

治　法　健脾益气,温肾补阳。

方　药　附子理中丸合《金匮》肾气丸加减:党参15 g,炙黄芪15 g,白术10 g,茯苓12 g,熟地黄15 g,山药15 g,牡丹皮12 g,炮附子6 g,肉桂3 g,干姜6 g,炙甘草6 g,补骨脂10 g,丹参12 g,泽泻10 g,陈皮5 g。

Dioscoreae）15 g, Mudanpi（*Cortex Moutan Radicis*）12 g, Paofuzi（*Radix Aconiti Lateralis*, roasted in hot cinders）6 g, Rougui（*Cortex Cinnamomi*）3 g, Ganjiang（*Rhizoma Zingiberis*）6 g, Zhigancao（*Radix Glycyrrhizae*, roasted）6 g, Buguzhi（*Fructus Psoraleae*）10 g, Danshen（*Radix Salviae Miltiorrhizae*）12 g, Zexie（*Rhizoma Alismatis*）10 g and Chenpi（*Pericarpium Citri Reticulatae*）5 g.

Modifications: For pronounced kidney-yang deficiency, cold and sore loins and knees, deep, thready and weak pulse, add Yinyanghuo（*Herba Epimedii*）10 g, Xianmao（*Rhizoma Curculiginis*）10 g, Bajitian（*Radix Morindae Officinalis*）10 g and Buguzhi（*Fructus Psoraleae*）10 g; for abdominal distension, edema of the limbs and scanty urine, add Cheqianzi（*Semen Plantaginis*, wrapped）12 g and Zexie（*Rhizoma Alismatis*）10 g.

Other Treatments

1. Chinese Patent Drugs

（1）Aotaile Chongji（Aotaile Granule）: 15 g each time, 3 times a day, infused with warm water, taken after meals, and 30 days as a treatment course; applicable to hepatitis A and B, with retention of damp heat in the liver and gallbladder or incoordination between the liver and spleen.

（2）Jianganle（Granule for Invigorating Liver）: 15 g each time, twice a day, infused with warm water for oral administration; applicable to all types of acute or chronic viral hepatitis.

（3）Yizhou Qingkailing（Yizhou Oral Liquid for Clearing away Heat and Inducing Rescuscition）: 3 - 6 g each time, 3 times a day; applicable to acute icterohepatitis.

（4）Wuweizi San（Schisandrae Powder）: 3 g each time, 3 times a day, infused with warm water for oral administration, 2 - 4 consecutive weeks as a treatment

加 减　肾阳虚明显,腰膝酸冷,脉沉细而弱者,加淫羊藿10 g,仙茅10 g,巴戟天10 g,补骨脂10 g;腹胀肢胀,小便量少者,加车前子(包煎)12 g,泽泻10 g。

【其他疗法】

1. 中成药

（1）澳泰乐冲剂　每服15 g,每日 3 次,饭后温水冲服,30 日为 1 个疗程。适用于甲型及乙型肝炎肝胆湿热、肝脾不和证。

（2）健肝乐　每次15 g,每日 2 次,温水冲服。适用于各型急慢性病毒性肝炎。

（3）一洲清开灵　每服3~6 g,每日 3 次。适用于急性黄疸型肝炎。

（4）五味子散　每次3 g,每日 3 次,温水冲服。连服2~4 个星期为 1 个疗程。适

course; applicable to hepatitis with increased aminotrans-ferase and indistinct damp heat.

(5) Yunzhi Duotang Jiaonang (Ganoderma Polysac-charide Capsule): 1 - 2 capsules each time, 3 times a day; applicable to chronic hepatitis B and immunologic hypo-function.

(6) Jigucao Jiaonang (Abri Capsule): 4 capsules each time, 3 times a day; applicable to acute or chronic hepati-tis.

(7) Yin Zhi Huang Zhusheye (Injection of Artemisiae Scoparime, Gardeniae and Scutellariae): 2 - 4 ml for in-tramuscular injection each time, once a day, or 10 - 20 ml with 250 - 500 ml of 10% glucose solution for intravenous drip; applicable to acute, chronic active or persistent hepatitis.

(8) Ganyanling Zhusheye (Injection for Hepatitis): 4 ml for intramuscular injection, which should be done everyday until ALT turns to normal and for a period of time afterwards, then every other day in case of rebound of ALT. This is suitable for all types of viral hepatitis.

2. Single-drug or Experiential Prescriptions

(1) Yinchenhao (*Herba Artemisiae Scopariae*) 30 g. Decoct the herb in water for oral administration, one dose a day. It is applicable to jaundice of various cau-ses.

(2) Banlangen (*Radix Isatidis*) 30 g. Decoct the herb in water for oral administration, one dose a day. It is applicable to acute viral hepatitis.

(3) Chuipencao (*Herba Sedi*) 30 g. Decoct the herb in water for oral administration, once or twice a day, 2 - 4 weeks in succession as a course. It is applicable to viral hepatitis with an increase of ALT.

用于肝炎转氨酶升高而湿热不明显者。

（5）云芝多糖胶囊　每服1～2粒，每日3次。适用于慢性乙型肝炎、免疫功能低下者。

（6）鸡骨草胶囊　每服4粒，每日3次。适用于急、慢性肝炎。

（7）茵栀黄注射液　肌肉注射，每日1次，每次2～4 ml；或静脉滴注，每日1次，10～20 ml加于10%葡萄糖溶液250～500 ml内使用。适用于急性肝炎、慢性活动性肝炎及迁延性肝炎。

（8）肝炎灵注射液　每日肌注1次4 ml，连续注射到ALT正常后再使用一段时间，然后改为隔日肌注1次，以免ALT反跳。适用于各型病毒性肝炎。

2.　单验方

（1）茵陈蒿30 g，水煎服，每日1剂。适用于各种原因引起的黄疸。

（2）板蓝根30 g，水煎服，每日1剂。适用于急性病毒性肝炎。

（3）垂盆草30 g，水煎服，每日1～2次，连服2～4个星期为1个疗程。适用于病毒性肝炎ALT升高者。

(4) Tianjihuang (*Herba Hyperici Japonici*) 30 g and Pangqiju (*Herba seu Radix Wedeliae Chinensis*) 30 g. Decoct the herbs in water for oral administration, 1 dose a day. It is applicable to acute hepatitis and chronic active hepatitis.

(5) Qingre Jiedu Huoxue Tang (Decoction for Clearing away Heat, Removing Toxic Substance and Activating Blood Circulation): composed of Yinchen (*Herba Artemisiae Scopariae*) 15 g, Guanzhong (*Rhizoma Dryopteris Crassirhizomae*) 15 g, Huzhang (*Rhizoma Polygoni Cuspidati*) 30 g, Banzhilian (*Herba Scutellariae Barbatae*) 30 g, Chaihu (*Radix Bupleuri*) 10 g, Zicao (*Radix Arnebiae seu Lithospermi*) 10 g, Tufuling (*Rhizoma Smilacis Glabrae*) 10 g and Shenggancao (*Radix Glycyrrhizae*) 6 g. Decoct the herbs in water for oral administration, 1 dose a day. It is applicable to chronic active hepatitis B and hepatitis B virus carriers with toxic heat and blood stagnation.

(6) Fuzheng Fugan Tang (Decoction for Supporting Healthy Qi and Restoring Liver Function): composed of Dangshen (*Radix Codonopsis*) 10 g, Baizhu (*Rhizoma Atractylodis Macrocephalae*) 10 g, Gouqizi (*Fructus Lycii*) 10 g, Gancao (*Radix Glycyrrhizae*) 6 g, Pingdimu (*Caulis et Folium Ardisiae Japonicae*) 15 g, Fuling (*Poria*) 15 g, Banzhilian (*Herba Scutellariae Barbatae*) 15 g, Huzhang (*Rhizoma Polygoni Cuspidati*) 30 g, Baihuasheshecao (*Herba Hedyotis Diffusae*) 30 g and Beidougen (*Rhizoma Menispermi*) 6 g. Decoct the herbs in water for oral administration, 1 dose a day. It is applicable to chronic hepatitis B and hepatitis B virus carriers with qi deficiency and toxin stagnation.

(7) Wenyang Huoxue Jiedu Tang (Decoction for Warming Yang, Activating Blood and Removing Toxic Substance): composed of Paofuzi (*Radix Aconiti Lateralis*,

（4）田基黄30 g,蟛蜞菊30 g,水煎服,每日1剂。适用于急性肝炎、慢性活动性肝炎。

（5）清热解毒活血汤　茵陈15 g,贯众15 g,虎杖30 g,半枝莲30 g,柴胡10 g,紫草10 g,土茯苓10 g,生甘草6 g。水煎服,每日1剂。适用于慢性乙型肝炎活动期及乙肝病毒携带者热毒血瘀证。

（6）扶正复肝汤　党参10 g,白术10 g,枸杞子10 g,甘草6 g,平地木15 g,茯苓15 g,半枝莲15 g,虎杖30 g,白花蛇舌草30 g,北豆根6 g。水煎服,每日1剂。适用于慢性乙型肝炎和乙肝病毒携带者气虚瘀毒证。

（7）温阳活血解毒汤　炮附子10 g,赤芍药60 g,生大黄30 g,丹参30 g,茵陈30 g,金钱

roasted in hot cinders) 10 g, Chishaoyao (*Radix Paeoni-ae Rubra*) 60 g, Shengdahuang (*Radix et Rhizoma Rhei*) 30 g, Danshen (*Radix Salviae Miltiorrhizae*) 30 g, Yinchen (*Herba Artemisiae Scopariae*) 30 g, Jin-qiancao (*Herba Lysimachiae*) 15 g and Haijinsha (*Spora Lygodii*, wrapped) 15 g. Decoct the herbs in water for oral administration, 1 dose a day. It is applicable to chronic hepatitis B with refractory severe jaundice.

(8) Huoxue Jiedu Tang (Decoction for Activating Blood and Removing Toxic Substance): composed of Yinchen (*Herba Artemisiae Scopariae*) 30 g, Huzhang (*Rhizoma Polygoni Cuspidati*) 30 g, Chishaoyao (*Radix Paeoniae Rubra*) 30 g, Huangqin (*Radix Scutellariae*) 10 g and Beidougen (*Rhizoma Menispermi*) 6 g. Decoct the herbs in water for oral administration, 1 dose a day. It is applicable to acute hepatitis C or chronic hepatitis C with pronounced symptoms.

(9) Dahuang Kushen Yin (Decoction of Rhei and Sophorae Flavescentis): composed of Zhidahuang (*Radix et Rhizoma Rhei Preparata*) 15 g, Shengdahuang (*Radix et Rhizoma Rhei*) 15 g, Kushen (*Radix Sophorae Flavescentis*) 30 g, Yinchen (*Herba Artemisiae Scopariae*) 30 g, Chaozhizi (*Fructus Gardeniae*, stir-baked) 10 g, Danshen (*Radix Salviae Miltiorrhizae*) 20 g and Chenpi (*Pericarpium Citri Reticulatae*) 12 g. Decoct the herbs in water for oral administration, 1 dose a day. It is applicable to chronic hepatitis C with jaundice due to stagnation of heat.

3. External Therapy

(1) Huangbai (*Cortex Phellodendri*), Huangqin (*Radix Scutellariae*) and Dahuang (*Radix et Rhizoma Rhei*) in equal proportions and Qingdai (*Indigo Naturalis*) in half proportion. Grind the drugs into fine powder and mix thoroughly with equal amount of water and honey into paste. Then spread the paste on oilpaper, and apply it

草15 g,海金沙(包煎)15 g。水煎服,每日1剂。适用于慢性乙型肝炎难治型高度黄疸患者。

(8)活血解毒汤 茵陈30 g,虎杖30 g,赤芍药30 g,黄芩10 g,北豆根6 g。水煎服,每日1剂。适用于急性丙型肝炎,或慢性丙型肝炎症状显著者。

(9) 大黄苦参饮 制大黄15 g,生大黄15 g,苦参30 g,茵陈30 g,炒栀子10 g,丹参20 g,陈皮12 g。水煎服,每日1剂。适用于慢性丙型肝炎瘀热发黄者。

3. 外治法

(1)黄柏、黄芩、大黄等量,青黛半量,研成细末和匀,以水蜜各半调成膏,摊于油纸敷右胁期门穴,每日1贴,20日为1个疗程。适用于急性病毒性肝炎。

to Qimen point (LR 14) on the right hypochondrium, 1 piece a day, 20 days as a treatment course. It is applicable to acute viral hepatitis.

(2) Guadi (*Pedicellus Melo Fructus*), Baihujiao (*Fructus Piperis*) and Baidingxiang (*Faeces Passeris*) in equal proportions. Grind them into fine powder for later use. Insufflate a small amount of the powder into the nostrils until the yellow fluid flows out, once every other day, 10 times being a treatment course. This is suitable for acute icterohepatitis.

(3) Maogen (*Herba Ranunculi Japonici*, fresh) 50 g and salt 5 g. Crush them into a mash and apply to the area below the navel or the gluteal region. When vesicles appear, remove the mash, clean with normal saline, prick the vesicles with a sterilized needle to release the yellow fluid, then bandage with antiseptic gauze. This is suitable for hepatitis with marked jaundice.

(4) Taoren (*Semen Persicae*) 15 g, Xingren (*Semen Armeniacae Amarum*) 15 g and Sangshenzi (*Fructus Mori*) 15 g. Bake the herbs dry, grind them into fine powder, mix the powder with vinegar and wrap the paste with gauze, then apply the paste to the navel and change the dressing every 2 days. This is suitable for chronic hepatitis with healthy qi deficiency and blood stagnation.

2.4.4　Hepatocirrhosis

General Description

Hepatocirrhosis is a chronic, progressive or diffuse hepatic disease induced by one or various causes. Its pathological features are extensive necrosis and degeneration of the hepatic cells, diffuse proliferation of fibrous tissue and formation of regenerated nodule, structural destruction of hepatic lobules and blood vessels, leading to gradu-

（2）瓜蒂、白胡椒、白丁香各等分，研为细末，装瓶备用。用时取少许，吹入鼻中，以流出黄水为度，隔日1次，10次为1个疗程，病愈停用。适用于急性黄疸型肝炎。

（3）新鲜毛茛50 g，加食盐5 g捣烂，敷于脐下或臀部，局部起泡后，将药渣取下，用生理盐水洗净，所起的泡用消毒针头轻轻挑破，让泡内黄水畅流，最后用消毒纱布包扎好。适用于肝炎黄疸较重者。

（4）桃仁15 g，杏仁15 g，桑椹子15 g，烘干共研为细末，醋调成糊状，纱布包贴肚脐中，每2日换药1次。适用于慢性肝炎正虚血瘀证。

第四节　肝硬化

【概述】

肝硬化是由一种或多种原因引起的慢性、进行性、弥漫性肝病。其病理特点表现为广泛的肝细胞坏死和变性，纤维组织弥漫性增生，并有再生小结形成，正常肝小叶结构

al degeneration and cirrhosis of the liver, i.e., hepatocirrhosis. At the early stage, the disease may be symptomless; while at the later stage, hypofunction of the liver, portal hypertension and involvement of various systems may be manifested.

This disease usually occurs in young adults between the age of 20–50, and is more common in males. Infectious hepatitis and parasitization in some districts are common causes of this disease. Chronic alcoholism, malnutrition, chemicals and toxic substance, hereditary and metabolic diseases are also responsible. Moreover, the cause is unknown in some cases.

Clinically, the cases during compensatory phase of hepatic function may be included in the categories of "xie tong" (hypochondriac pain) and "ji ju" (abdominal mass) in TCM; while those during decompensatory phase are similar to "gu zhang" (tympanites) in TCM. The pathogenesis is invasion of exogenous seasonal pathogens, excessive drinking, contaminated food or emotional upset, resulting in damage of the liver and spleen and stagnation of qi and blood. The kidney is also involved in longstanding cases, causing failure of qi to discharge water and retention of water in the interior.

Essentials for Diagnosis

(1) Mild symptoms are manifested during compensatory phase as fatigue, poor appetite, nausea, vomiting, discomfort in the epigastrium, dull pain in the right epigastrium, abdominal distension and diarrhea. The chief manifestations of decompensatory phase are poor appetite, emaciation, lassitude, diarrhea, epigastric pain, low fever, abdominal distension, hemorrhage and neuropsychic symptoms.

(2) During compensatory phase, There are no obvi-

和血管解剖的破坏,导致肝脏逐渐变性变硬而成为肝硬化。临床上早期可无症状,后期可出现肝功能减退、门脉高压和多系统受累的各种表现。

肝硬化患者以20～50岁的青壮年较为多见,男性多于女性;病因多与传染性肝炎及某些地区寄生虫感染有关。其他病因如慢性酒精中毒、营养不良、化学药物和毒物的损害、遗传和代谢疾病等,尚有部分病例原因不明。

根据本病的临床表现,肝功能代偿期患者,多可归属于中医学"胁痛"、"积聚"的范畴;而失代偿期患者,则与中医学中的"鼓胀"类似。其病因病机,主要是外感时邪病毒,或嗜酒过度,或饮食不洁,或情志不遂,致肝脾受损,气血瘀滞。病久及肾,气不化水,水湿内停。

【诊断要点】

(1) 本病代偿期症状较轻,有时可有乏力、纳差、恶心、呕吐、上腹不适、右上腹隐痛、腹胀、腹泻等。失代偿期主要表现为纳差、消瘦、疲倦乏力、腹泻、上腹疼痛、低热、腹胀、出血以及神经精神症状。

(2) 代偿期体征不明显,

ous physical signs but hepatomegaly may be present. Some patients may also suffer from splenomegaly accompanied by vascular spider and liver palms. But during decompensatory phase, there are manifestations as darker complexion, jaundice, fever, varicose veins of abdominal wall, ascites, hydrothorax, moderate splenomegaly, enlargement or shrinkage of the liver, gynecomastia and sparsity of pubic hair in males, scanty menstruation or amenorrhea in females, bleeding of skin and mucosa, emaciation, anemia, edema and angular stomatitis.

(3) Anemia, decrease in white blood cell and blood platelet count can be found in blood routine examination; in liver function test, increase in aminotransferase, serum bilirubin and globulin, and decrease in albumin can be found.

(4) Ultrasonography B shows that hepatic echo grows stronger, coarser and uneven. Hepatomegaly is manifested at the early stage of the disease and hepatic shrinkage at the later stage. The surface of the liver is rough, serrate and wavy. Splenic shadow becomes larger; splenic veins thicker and curved; and portal vein thickened.

(5) Hepatic biopsy shows the histological type of hepatocirrhosis, as well as the degree of hepatic cells damage and formation of connective tissue.

Syndrome Differentiation and Treatment

It is clinically essential to differentiate excess types from deficiency ones. Excess types include liver qi stagnation and spleen deficiency, blood stagnation in the liver and spleen, accumulation of damp heat and obstruction of meridians by blood stasis. The treatment for such types is chiefly to soothe the liver and invigorate the spleen, regulate qi circulation and activate blood, and eliminate damp

肝脏常肿大,部分患者伴有脾肿大,并可出现蜘蛛痣和肝掌。失代偿期面容较病前黝黑,黄疸,发热,腹壁静脉怒张,腹水征,胸水征,脾脏中度肿大,肝肿大或缩小,男性乳房发育和阴毛稀少,女性月经过少和闭经,皮肤和黏膜出血,消瘦,贫血,水肿,口角炎等。

(3) 血常规检查可见贫血、血白细胞及血小板均见降低;肝功能试验可见转氨酶升高,血清胆红素升高,白蛋白减少,球蛋白增高。

(4) B型超声波检查可见肝内回声增强、增粗、不均匀。早期肝肿大,晚期肝缩小,肝表面不平,呈锯齿状,波浪状。脾影增大,脾静脉增粗、弯曲,门脉增粗。

(5) 肝活组织检查可了解肝硬化的组织学类型,肝细胞损害和结缔组织形成的程度。

【辨证论治】

本病临床主要辨其虚实。实证有肝郁脾虚、肝脾血瘀、湿热蕴结、瘀血阻络等证,治疗以疏肝健脾、理气活血、清利湿热为主;虚证有肝肾阴虚、脾肾阳虚等证,治疗则以滋养肝肾或健脾温肾为要。

heat. Deficiency types include deficiency of liver yin and kidney yin, and deficiency of spleen yang and kidney yang, which should be treated by nourishing the liver and kidney, invigorating the spleen and warming the kidney.

1. Liver qi Stagnation and Spleen Deficiency

Chief Manifestations: Abdominal distension which is mild in early morning and severe in late afternoon and is aggravated after intake of food, lassitude, emotional depression, yellow and lusterless complexion, impaired appetite, swollen tongue with white greasy coating, and wiry, even-soft and forceless pulse.

Therapeutic Methods: To soothe the liver, regulate qi circulation, activate the spleen and eliminate dampness.

Prescription: Modified Chaihu Shugan San (Bupleuri Powder for Soothing Liver Qi) and Weiling Tang (Poria Decoction for Regulating Stomach), composed of Chaochaihu (*Radix Bupleuri*, stir-baked) 6 g, Chao-zhike (*Fructus Aurantii*, stir-baked) 10 g, Baishaoyao (*Radix Paeoniae Alba*) 10 g, Chuanxiong (*Rhizoma Chuanxiong*) 10 g, Zhixiangfu (*Rhizoma Cyperi Preparata*) 10 g, Chenpi (*Pericarpium Citri Reticulatae*) 6 g, Foshou (*Fructus Citri Sarcodactylis*) 6 g, Chaocangzhu (*Rhizoma Atractylodis*, stir-baked) 10 g, Houpo (*Cortex Magnoliae Officinalis*) 10 g, Fuling (*Poria*) 12 g, Zexie (*Rhizoma Alismatis*) 12 g, Baizhu (*Rhizoma Atractylodis Macrocephalae*) 10 g and Zhigancao (*Radix Glycyrrhizae*, roasted) 3 g.

Modifications: For dysfunction of the spleen in transport, add Dangshen (*Radix Codonopsis*) 10 g and Sharen (*Fructus Amomi*, to be decocted later) 3 g; for liver qi stagnation, add Yujin (*Radix Curcumae*) 10 g and Chao Laifuzi (*Semen Raphani*, stir-baked) 10 g; for dampness retention, add Dafupi (*Pericarpium*

1. 肝郁脾虚证

主要证候 腹胀,朝宽暮急,纳后胀甚,疲倦乏力,精神抑郁,面黄无华,食量减少,舌胖,苔白腻,脉弦缓无力。

治 法 疏肝理气,运脾化湿。

方 药 柴胡疏肝散合胃苓汤加减:炒柴胡6 g,炒枳壳10 g,白芍药10 g,川芎10 g,制香附10 g,陈皮6 g,佛手6 g,炒苍术10 g,厚朴10 g,茯苓12 g,泽泻12 g,白术10 g,炙甘草3 g。

加 减 偏脾虚运滞者,加党参10 g,砂仁(后下)3 g;偏肝气郁滞者,加郁金10 g,炒莱菔子10 g;偏水湿阻滞者,加大腹皮10 g,车前子(包煎)12 g。

Arecae) 10 g and Cheqianzi (*Semen Plantaginis*, wrapped) 12 g.

2. Blood Stagnation in the Liver and Spleen

Chief Manifestations: Papable mass in the left hypochondrium, red threads on the cheeks, red marks on the thenar eminence, red nevi on the arms, dark and lusterless complexion, occasional stabbing and distending pain in the hypochondrium, dark purple tongue or with ecchymosis, and deep, wiry and unsmooth pulse.

Therapeutic Methods: To regulate qi circulation, activate blood, and remove blood stasis to resolve masses.

Prescription: Modified Gexia Zhuyu Tang (Decoction for Removing Blood Stasis under Diaphragm), composed of Wulingzhi (*Faeces Trogopterori*) 10 g, Danggui (*Radix Angelicae Sinensis*) 10 g, Chuanxiong (*Rhizoma Chuanxiong*) 10 g, Taoren (*Semen Persicae*) 10 g, Mudanpi (*Cortex Moutan Radicis*) 10 g, Chishaoyao (*Radix Paeoniae Rubra*) 10 g, Wuyao (*Radix Linderae*) 6 g, Chaoyanhusuo (*Rhizoma Corydalis*, stir-baked) 10 g, Zhixiangfu (*Rhizoma Cyperi Preparata*) 10 g, Honghua (*Flos Carthami*) 10 g, Chaozhike (*Fructus Aurantii*, stir-baked) 10 g and Zhigancao (*Radix Glycyrrhizae*, roasted) 3 g.

Modifications: For severe pain, add Yujin (*Radix Curcumae*) 10 g; for cases with phlegm retention, add Fabanxia (*Rhizoma Pinelliae*) 6 g and Baijiezi (*Semen Sinapis Albae*) 6 g; for those accompanied by dampness, add Zexie (*Rhizoma Alismatis*) 12 g and Zelan (*Herba Lycopi*) 12 g; for severe blood stagnation, add Zhibiejia (*Carapax Trionycis*, roasted and to be decocted first) 15 g and Muli (*Concha Ostreae*, to be decocted first) 15 g.

2. 肝脾血瘀证

主要证候 左胁下可触及明显积块，颧有红纹，鱼际有红斑，膺臂有红痣，面色晦暗，两胁时见刺痛、胀痛，舌质紫暗或有瘀斑，脉沉弦而涩。

治 法 理气活血，消积散结。

方 药 膈下逐瘀汤加减：五灵脂10 g，当归10 g，川芎10 g，桃仁10 g，牡丹皮10 g，赤芍药10 g，乌药6 g，炒延胡索10 g，制香附10 g，红花10 g，炒枳壳10 g，炙甘草3 g。

加 减 疼痛明显者，加郁金10 g；挟痰浊者，加法半夏6 g，白芥子6 g；兼水湿者，加泽泻12 g，泽兰12 g；血瘀明显者，加炙鳖甲(先煎)15 g，牡蛎(先煎)15 g。

3. Accumulation of Damp Heat

Chief Manifestations: A large, hard and full abdomen, abdominal distension and tenderness, protruding umbilicus in severe cases, hot sensation, jaundice in the skin and sclera, feverish sensation with restlessness, bitter taste and foul breath, thirst with a desire to drink, constipation or loose stools, red tongue with yellow and greasy coating, smooth and rapid pulse.

Therapeutic Methods: To clear away heat, eliminate dampness and remove toxic substance.

Prescription: Modified Yinchenhao Tang (Artemisiae Scopariae Decoction) and Ganlu Xiaodu Dan (Sweet Dew Detoxication Pill), composed of Yinchen (*Herba Artemisiae Scopariae*) 12 g, Zhizi (*Fructus Gardeniae*) 10 g, Zhidahuang (*Radix et Rhizoma Rhei Preparata*) 6 g, Huashi (*Talcum*, wrapped) 12 g, Huangqin (*Radix Scutellariae*) 10 g, Shichangpu (*Rhizoma Acori Tatarinowii*) 6 g, Beimu (*Bulbus Fritillariae*) 10 g, Mutong (*Caulis Akebiae*) 6 g, Lianqiao (*Fructus Forsythiae*) 15 g and Bohe (*Herba Menthae*) 6 g.

Modifications: For excessive toxic heat, add Mabiancao (*Herba Verbenae*) 15 g, Banzhilian (*Herba Scutellariae Barbatae*) 12 g and Longdancao (*Radix Gentianae*) 6 g; for abdominal distension and constipation, add Shengdahuang (*Radix et Rhizoma Rhei*, to be decocted later) 6 g and Zhishi (*Fructus Aurantii Immaturus*) 10 g; for dampness stagnation, add Peilan (*Herba Eupatorii*) 10 g, Zelan (*Herba Lycopi*) 10 g and Zisuye (*Folium Periliae*) 6 g; for yin deficiency with dampness retention, add Yimucao (*Herba Leonuri*) 12 g, Hanliancao (*Herba Ecliptae*) 10 g, Nüzhenzi (*Fructus Ligustri Lucidi*) 10 g and Cheqianzi (*Semen Plantaginis*, wrapped) 10 g.

3. 湿热蕴结证

主要证候 腹大坚满,腹胀拒按,甚则脐尖高突,身热,肤目黄染,烦热,口苦口臭,口渴欲饮,腹胀便秘或大便垢溏,苔黄腻,质红,脉滑数。

治 法 清热化湿解毒。

方 药 茵陈蒿汤合甘露消毒丹加减:茵陈12 g,栀子10 g,制大黄6 g,滑石(包煎)12 g,黄芩10 g,石菖蒲6 g,贝母10 g,木通6 g,连翘15 g,薄荷6 g。

加 减 热毒炽盛者,加马鞭草15 g,半枝莲12 g,龙胆草6 g;腹胀便秘者,加生大黄(后下)6 g,枳实10 g;湿浊阻滞者,加佩兰10 g,泽兰10 g,紫苏叶6 g;阴虚湿停者,加益母草12 g,旱莲草10 g,女贞子10 g,车前子(包煎)10 g。

4. Obstruction of Meridians by Blood Stasis

Chief Manifestations: A large, hard and full abdomen, varicose veins of abdominal wall, severe pain in the abdomen and hypochondrium, dimish black or darkish grey complexion, red spots or threads on the head, neck, chest and abdomen, dark purple lips, tarry stools, scanty and dark yellow urine, purple-red tongue or with petechia and ecchymosis, hypoglossal varicose veins, thin yellow and greasy tongue coating, and thready and unsmooth pulse.

Therapeutic Methods: To remove blood stasis, dredge the collaterals, activate blood and promote diuresis.

Prescription: Modified Gexia Zhuyu Tang (Decoction for Removing Blood Stasis under Diaphragm), composed of Wulingzhi (*Faeces Trogopterori*) 10 g, Danggui (*Radix Angelicae Sinensis*) 10 g, Chuanxiong (*Rhizoma Chuanxiong*) 10 g, Taoren (*Semen Persicae*) 10 g, Mudanpi (*Cortex Moutan Radicis*) 10 g, Chishaoyao (*Radix Paeoniae Rubra*) 10 g, Wuyao (*Radix Linderae*) 6 g, Yanhusuo (*Rhizoma Corydalis*) 10 g, Zhixiangfu (*Rhizoma Cyperi Preparata*) 10 g, Honghua (*Flos Carthami*) 10 g, Chaozhike (*Fructus Aurantii*, stir-baked) 10 g and Zhigancao (*Radix Glycyrrhizae*, roasted) 3 g.

Modifications: For severe abdominal distension and fullness, add Chenxiang (*Lignum Aquilariae Resinatum*) 5 g, Jiangxiang (*Lignum Dalbergiae Odoriferae*) 5 g and Laifuzi (*Semen Raphani*) 10 g; for constipation, add Zhishi (*Fructus Aurantii Immaturus*) 10 g and Shengdahuang (*Radix et Rhizoma Rhei*, to be decocted later) 6 g; for skin ecchymosis, nasal and gingival hemorrhage, add Shensanqifen (*Radix Notoginseng*, to be powdered and infused separately) 3 g, Baiji (*Rhizoma Bletillae*) 10 g and Xianhecao (*Herba Agrimoniae*) 12 g.

4. 瘀血阻络证

主要证候　腹大坚满,腹壁青筋暴露,胁腹攻痛,面色黧黑或晦暗,头颈胸腹红点赤缕,唇色紫褐,大便色黑,小便短赤,舌质暗红或有瘀点、瘀斑,舌下脉络迂曲,舌苔薄黄腻,脉细涩。

治　法　祛瘀通络,活血利水。

方　药　膈下逐瘀汤加减:五灵脂10 g,当归10 g,川芎10 g,桃仁10 g,牡丹皮10 g,赤芍药10 g,乌药6 g,延胡索10 g,制香附10 g,红花10 g,炒枳壳10 g,炙甘草3 g。

加　减　腹胀满甚者,加沉香5 g,降香5 g,莱服子10 g;大便秘结者,加枳实10 g,生大黄(后下)6 g;皮肤瘀斑、鼻衄、齿衄者,加参三七粉(另冲)3 g,白及10 g,仙鹤草12 g。

5. Deficiency of Liver Yin and Kidney Yin

Chief Manifestations: A large, distended and full abdomen with the skin tightly stretched, thin limbs, dimish black complexion, afternoon fever, restlessness, dry lips and mouth, insomnia, dreamfulness, nasal bleeding, atrophy of the gum, red tongue with little coating, and wiry, thready and rapid pulse.

Therapeutic Methods: To nourish yin, reinforce the kidney, cool blood and clear away heat.

Prescription: Modified Yiguan Jian (Ever-effective Decoction for Nourishing Liver and Kidney), composed of Shashen (*Radix Glehniae*) 10 g, Maimendong (*Radix Ophiopogonis*) 10 g, Chuanlianzi (*Fructus Meliae Toosendan*) 10 g, Danggui (*Radix Angelicae Sinensis*) 10 g, Shengdihuang (*Radix Rehmanniae*) 12 g, Gouqizi (*Fructus Lycii*) 10 g, Nüzhenzi (*Fructus Ligustri Lucidi*) 10 g and Hanliancao (*Herba Ecliptae*) 10 g.

Modifications: For abnormal mentality, add Shichangpu (*Rhizoma Acori Tatarinowii*) 6 g and Yujin (*Radix Curcumae*) 10 g; for hectic fever, add Yinchaihu (*Radix Stellariae*) 6 g, Digupi (*Cortex Lycii*) 10 g and Baiwei (*Radix seu Folium Millettiae Bonatianae*) 10 g; for prolonged cases with collaterals involved, add Zhibiejia (*Carapax Trionycis*, roasted and to be decocted first) 15 g, Zhiguiban (*Plastrum Testudinis*, roasted and to be decocted first) 15 g and Lulutong (*Fructus Liquidambaris*) 10 g.

6. Deficiency of Spleen Yang and Kidney Yang

Chief Manifestations: Distended and full abdomen which feels like a bag full of water and looks like the abdomen of a frog in a supine position, edema of the lower limbs, cold limbs, lusterless complexion, stuffiness in the epigastrium, impaired appetite, pale tongue, and thready pulse.

5. 肝肾阴虚证

主要证候　腹大中满,腹皮紧,四肢瘦,面色黧黑,午后发热,心烦,唇干口燥,失眠多梦,鼻衄牙宣,舌红少苔,脉弦细数。

治　法　养阴益肾,凉血清热。

方　药　一贯煎加减:沙参10 g,麦门冬10 g,川楝子10 g,当归10 g,生地黄12 g,枸杞子10 g,女贞子10 g,旱莲草10 g。

加　减　神志异常者,加石菖蒲6 g,郁金10 g;潮热起伏者,加银柴胡6 g,地骨皮10 g,白薇10 g;久病入络者,加炙鳖甲(先煎)15 g,炙龟版(先煎)15 g,路路通10 g。

6. 脾肾阳虚证

主要证候　脘腹胀大,如囊裹水,仰卧似蛙腹,下肢浮肿,四肢不温,面色无华,脘闷纳差,舌淡,脉细。

Therapeutic Methods: To warm and nourish the spleen and kidney, remove dampness and promote diuresis.

Prescription: Modified Fuzi Lizhong Tang (Aconiti Lateralis Decoction for Regulating Middle Energizer) and Wuling San (Powder of Five Drugs Containing Poria), composed of Zhifuzi (*Radix Aconiti Lateralis Preparata*) 6 g, Dangshen (*Radix Codonopsis*) 10 g, Baizhu (*Rhizoma Atractylodis Macrocephalae*) 10 g, Ganjiang (*Rhizoma Zingiberis*) 3 g, Zhigancao (*Radix Glycyrrhizae, roasted*) 3 g, Guizhi (*Ramulus Cinnamomi*) 6 g, Zhuling (*Polyporus*) 10 g, Fuling (*Poria*) 10 g and Zexie (*Rhizoma Alismatis*) 12 g.

Modifications: For deficiency of spleen yang, add Huangqi (*Radix Astragali*) 12 g and Gaoliangjiang (*Rhizoma Alpiniae Officinarum*) 5 g; for deficiency of kidney yang, add Buguzhi (*Fructus Psoraleae*) 10 g and Yinyanghuo (*Herba Epimedii*) 10 g; for yang deficiency and cold excess, add Biba (*Fructus Piperis Longi*) 3 g and Wuzhuyu (*Fructus Evodiae*) 3 g.

Other Treatments

1. Chinese Patent Drugs

(1) Biejia Jianwan (Carapax Trionycis Pill): 5 – 6 g each time, twice a day; suitable for stagnation of qi and blood resulting in hepatosplenomegaly with hard texture, especially for splenomegaly.

(2) Zhouju Wan (Zhouche Pill): 3 g each time, taken on empty stomach in the morning for 2 – 3 days in succession; applicable to severe hepatocirrhotic ascites when the pathogenic factor is hyperactive and the healthy qi is not too deficient.

2. Single-drug or Experiential Prescriptions

(1) Baimaogen (*Rhizoma Imperatae*, fresh) 250 g. Clean and then decoct it in water for 10 minutes, and take

治　法　温补脾肾,化湿利水。

方　药　附子理中汤合五苓散加减:制附子6 g,党参10 g,白术10 g,干姜3 g,炙甘草3 g,桂枝6 g,猪苓10 g,茯苓10 g,泽泻12 g。

加　减　偏脾阳虚者,加黄芪12 g,高良姜5 g;偏肾阳虚者,加补骨脂10 g,淫羊藿10 g;阳虚寒盛者,加荜茇3 g,吴茱萸3 g。

【其他疗法】

1. 中成药

(1) 鳖甲煎丸　每服5～6 g,每日 2 次。适用于气滞血瘀,肝脾肿大,质硬,而以脾肿大为主者。

(2) 舟车丸　每服3 g,早晨空腹服下,可连用2～3 日。适用于肝硬化高度腹水,邪实而正气不过虚者。

2. 单验方

(1) 鲜白茅根250 g,洗净,水煎 10 分钟,当茶饮,连

the decoction as tea for 1 – 2 months in succession. It is applicable to hepatocirrhotic ascites accompanied by dysuria.

（2）Biandoujiao（*Semen Dolichoris*, fresh）100 g. Take it as a dish for 1 month in succession. It is applicable to hepatocirrhotic ascites with pronounced abdominal distension.

（3）Cangzhu（*Rhizoma Atractylodis*）10 g, Baizhu（*Rhizoma Atractylodis Macrocephalae*）10 g, Qingpi（*Pericarpium Citri Reticulatae Viride*）6 g, Chenpi（*Pericarpium Citri Reticulatae*）6 g, Houpo（*Cortex Magnoliae Officinalis*）9 g, Chaozhishi（*Fructus Aurantii Immaturus*, stir-baked）9 g, Zhixiangfu（*Rhizoma Cyperi Preparata*）6 g, Muxiang（*Radix Aucklandiae*）6 g, Sharen（*Fructus Amomi*, to be decocted later）3 g, Zhuling（*Polyporus*）10 g, Fuling（*Poria*）15 g, Dafupi（*Pericarpium Arecae*）15 g, Zexie（*Rhizoma Alismatis*）15 g, Dengxincao（*Medulla Junci*）6 g and Shengjiang（*Rhizoma Zingiberis Recens*）3 pcs. Decoct the drugs in water for oral administration, 1 dose a day; take the decoction in two divided doses. It is applicable to hepatocirrhotic ascites.

（4）Chuanshanjia（*Squama Manitis*）10 g, Sanleng（*Rhizoma Sparganii*）10 g, Ezhu（*Rhizoma Curcumae*）10 g, Zhechong（*Eupolyphaga seu Steleophaga*）10 g, Biejia（*Carapax Trionycis*）30 g, Danggui（*Radix Angelicae Sinensis*）10 g, Huangqi（*Radix Astragali*）15 g, Baizhu（*Rhizoma Atractylodis Macrocephalae*）10 g, Zhibanxia（*Rhizoma Pinelliae Preparata*）10 g, Shensanqifen（*Radix Notoginseng*, to be powdered and infused separately）3 g, Yujin（*Radix Curcumae*）15 g, Dangshen（*Radix Codonopsis*）15 g, Fuling（*Poria*）24 g, Zhigancao（*Radix Glycyrrhizae*, roasted）3 g, Ganjiang（*Rhizoma Zingiberis*）3 g and Taoren（*Semen*

用1~2个月。适用于肝硬化腹水伴小便不利者。

（2）新鲜扁豆角100 g,当菜食用,连续 1 个月。适用于肝硬化腹水脘腹胀满明显者。

（3）苍术10 g,白术10 g,青皮6 g,陈皮6 g,厚朴9 g,炒枳实9 g,制香附6 g,木香6 g,砂仁（后下）3 g,猪苓10 g,茯苓15 g,大腹皮15 g,泽泻15 g,灯心草6 g,生姜 3 片。水煎服,每日 1 剂,早晚分服。适用于肝硬化腹水。

（4）穿山甲10 g,三棱10 g,莪术10 g,䗪虫10 g,鳖甲30 g,当归10 g,黄芪15 g,白术10 g,制半夏10 g,参三七粉（另冲）3 g,郁金15 g,党参15 g,茯苓24 g,炙甘草3 g,干姜3 g,桃仁12 g。用水 5 碗,先煎鳖甲、穿山甲,纳诸药煎成 2 碗半,分 2 次冲服。

Persicae) 12 g. Decoct Biejia and Chuanshanjia first with 5 bowls of water, put the remaining herbs in the decoction and boil it into two and a half bowls, then take the decoction in two divided doses.

(5) Haizao (*Sargassum*) 40 g, Heichou (*Semen Pharbitidis Nigrum*) 30 g, Baichou (*Semen Pharbitidis Alba*) 30 g, Muxiang (*Radix Aucklandiae*) 15 g, Chuanhoupo (*Cortex Magnoliae Officinalis*) 50 g, Shengjiang (*Rhizoma Zingiberis Recens*) 25 g, Binglang (*Semen Arecae*) 20 g, Baizhu (*Rhizoma Atractylodis Macrocephalae*) 25 g, Renshen (*Radix Ginseng*) 15 g and Fuling (*Poria*) 50 g. Decoct the herbs in water and take the decoction in divided doses. It is applicable to hepatocirrhotic ascites.

3. External Therapy

(1) Shexiang (*Moschus*, artificial) 0.6 g, Weilingxian (*Radix Clematidis*) 30 g, Baigefen (*Faeces Columbae*) 30 g, Ximutong (*Caulis Akebiae*) 9 g, Baizhi (*Radix Angelicae Dahuricae*) 9 g and Xixin (*Herba Asari*) 9 g. Grind the above drugs into fine powder for use. Put the powder into Zhufu (Vesica Urinaria Suillus) together with Baijiu (*Vinum*) 250 ml, tie the opening and place it with the opening close to the navel, then wrap a bandage around the waist. This is applicable to hepatocirrhotic ascites.

(2) Gansui (*Radix Kansui*, powdered) 3 g and Shengjiang (*Rhizoma Zingiberis Recens*, mashed) 9 g. Mix them thoroughly and spread the mixture over a gauze. Apply the mixture to the navel and wrap a bandage around the waist. This is applicable to hepatocirrhotic ascites.

(3) Shexiang (*Moschus*, artificial) 0.3 g and Gansui (*Radix Kansui*) 9 g. Grind them into fine powder, mix it thoroughly with Shengjiang (*Rhizoma Zingiberis*

（5）海藻40 g，黑丑30 g，白丑30 g，木香15 g，川厚朴50 g，生姜25 g，槟榔20 g，白术25 g，人参15 g，茯苓50 g。水煎分次口服。适用于肝硬化腹水。

3. 外治法

（1）麝香0.6 g，威灵仙30 g，白鸽粪30 g，细木通9 g，白芷9 g，细辛9 g。上药共研细粉备用，白酒 250 ml。将药粉及白酒装入猪脬内，将猪脬口扎紧，将脬口对准肚脐，以纱布扎到腰里。适用于肝硬化腹水者。

（2）甘遂（研末）3 g，生姜（捣泥）9 g，两者调匀摊于纱布之上，敷于脐部，以纱布裹之。适用于肝硬化腹水者。

（3）麝香0.3 g，甘遂9 g，共研细末，生姜捣泥调匀，摊于纱布之上，敷脐，外以纱布

Recens, mashed), spread the mixture over a gauze, then apply it to the navel and wrap a bandage around the waist, once every 3 days.

裹之,每3日重复1次。

2.4.5　Liver Cancer

General Description

Liver cancer or hepatocarcinoma is either primary or metastatic in origin. Those originating in hepatic cells or intrahepatic duct are recognized as primary hepatocarcinoma; while those originating in other regions and moving to the liver are known as metastatic hepatocarcinoma. Generally speaking, liver cancer refers to primary hepatocarcinoma. It is chiefly manifested as pain in the right espigastrium, emaciation, anorexia, lassitude and progressive hepatomegaly. It is one of the most common malignant tumors. According to epidemiological data, its morbidity and mortality in China come in third, next to stomach and lung cancer.

In TCM, liver cancer is included in the categories of "zheng ji" (abdominal mass) and "huang dan" (jaundice). It is the result of a blending disorder of qi, blood, dampness, heat, blood stasis and toxic substance, which is caused by deficiency of qi and blood in zang-fu organs, spleen deficiency with accumulation of dampness, phlegm stagnation and blood stasis, invasion and retention of exogenous pathogenic factors as well as impairment by emotional upsets with mental depression. The diseased location is the liver, with the spleen, gallbladder and stomach involved. Deficiency of visceral qi and blood is the principal aspect; a blending disorder of qi, blood, dampness,

第五节　肝癌

【概述】

肝癌是指发生于肝脏的恶性肿瘤。肝癌分原发性和转移性两种,源于肝细胞或肝内胆管细胞的癌肿称为原发性肝癌,其他部位的癌肿转移至肝脏的称为转移性肝癌。一般所说的肝癌指的是原发性肝癌。本病临床以右上腹疼痛、消瘦、食欲不振、乏力、肝脏进行性肿大为主要表现。本病是目前临床常见的恶性肿瘤之一,根据流行病学资料,中国肝癌的发病率和死亡率占全部恶性肿瘤的第三位,仅次于胃癌、肺癌。

本病属于中医学"癥积"、"黄疸"等病证范畴。脏腑气血亏虚,脾虚湿聚,痰凝血瘀,或邪毒凝结,七情内伤等,可使气、血、湿、热、瘀、毒互结而成肝癌。其病位在肝,与脾、胆、胃密切相关。主要病机以脏腑气血亏虚为本,气、血、湿、热、瘀、毒互结为标。

heat, blood stasis and toxic substance is the secondary aspect.

Essentials for Diagnosis

(1) Liver cancer is clinically manifested as pain in the liver or espigastrium, abdominal distension, lassitude, poor appetite, emaciation, or diarrhea and fever. Progressive hepatomegaly is present, with tenderness, hard texture and nodular protrusion on its surface.

(2) A history of chronic viral hepatitis and hepatocirrhosis.

(3) A rise in γ - GT and positive AFP in serological examination.

(4) Ultrasonography B, CT scanning and MRI suggest a space occupying lesion in the liver.

Syndrome Differentiation and Treatment

This disease is characterized by principal deficiency and secondary excess. Principal deficiency is manifested as lassitude, rapidly progressive emaciation, and even sallow complexion and indolence of speaking; hard lump in the right espigastrium with tenderness, or accompanied by jaundice, ascites, edema, distension and fullness and oppression of the abdomen are the manifestations of secondary excess. For severe cases, it is advisable to focus the treatment on the secondary aspect, chiefly to eliminate pathogenic factors with the methods of activating blood to remove stasis, eliminating mass, purging retained fluid and dissipating stagnant qi. But generally, purging therapy and tonifying therapy should be used at the same time to strengthen healthy qi and eliminate pathogenic factors, and corresponding methods are invigorating the spleen, replenishing qi, nourishing yin and blood, soothing the liver, activating blood to remove stasis, regulating qi and dissipating stagnant qi, purging retained

【诊断要点】

(1) 本病临床主要表现为肝区或上腹部疼痛、腹胀、乏力、食少、消瘦,或有腹泻、发热等。肝脏进行性肿大,压痛,质地坚硬,表面有结节隆起。

(2) 有慢性病毒性肝炎和肝硬化病史。

(3) 血清学检查,γ - GT增高,AFP 阳性。

(4) B 超、CT 扫描、MRI提示肝脏占位性改变。

【辨证论治】

本病患者本虚标实极为明显,本虚表现为乏力倦怠,形体急骤消瘦,甚至面色萎黄,懒言等;而右上腹有坚硬肿物而拒按,甚至伴黄疸、腹水、浮肿、脘腹胀满而闷等,则属标实的表现。治疗当急则治其标,以祛邪为主,常用活血化瘀、消积散结、逐水破气等为法;一般宜攻补兼施,扶正祛邪,常用健脾益气、养血柔肝、滋补阴液、活血化瘀、理气破气、逐水消肿等法。

fluid and alleviating edema.

1. Liver Qi Stagnation

Chief Manifestations: Distending pain in the right hypochondrium, chest oppression, frequent sighing, impaired appetite, occasional diarrhea, mass in the right lower hypochondrium, thin and greasy tongue coating, and wiry pulse.

Therapeutic Methods: To soothe the liver, invigorate the spleen, activate blood and remove stasis.

Prescription: Modified Chaihu Shugan San (Bupleuri Powder for Soothing Liver Qi), composed of Chaihu (*Radix Bupleuri*) 6 g, Chenpi (*Pericarpium Citri Reticulatae*) 6 g, Zhike (*Fructus Aurantii*) 10 g, Xiangfu (*Rhizoma Cyperi*) 10 g, Chuanxiong (*Rhizoma Chuanxiong*) 10 g, Yujin (*Radix Curcumae*) 10 g, Shengyiyiren (*Semen Coicis*) 12 g, Baizhu (*Rhizoma Atractylodis Macrocephalae*) 10 g and Huangqi (*Radix Astragali*) 12 g.

Modifications: For anorexia and loose stools, add Fuling (*Poria*) 12 g and Shanyao (*Rhizoma Dioscoreae*) 10 g; for pronounced abdominal distension and frequent belching, add Houpo (*Cortex Magnoliae Officinalis*) 6 g and Binglang (*Semen Arecae*) 10 g.

2. Qi Stagnation and Blood Stasis

Chief Manifestations: Huge mass in the hypochondrium, hypochondric pain radiating to the back, which is aggravated at night, tenderness, abdominal distension and fullness, impaired appetite, loose stools sometimes and dry stools at other times, lassitude, dark purple tongue with petechia and ecchymosis, deep and thready or wiry and unsmooth pulse.

Therapeutic Methods: To promote circulation of qi, activate blood, remove stasis and eliminate mass.

Prescription: Modified Fuyuan Huoxue Tang (De-

1. 肝气郁结证

主要证候　右胁部胀痛，胸闷不舒，善太息，纳呆食少，时有腹泻，右胁下肿块，舌苔薄腻，脉弦。

治　法　疏肝健脾，活血化瘀。

方　药　柴胡疏肝散加减：柴胡6 g，陈皮6 g，枳壳10 g，香附10 g，川芎10 g，郁金10 g，生薏苡仁12 g，白术10 g，黄芪12 g。

加　减　食少，便溏者，加茯苓12 g，山药10 g；腹胀明显，嗳气频频，加厚朴6 g，槟榔10 g。

2. 气滞血瘀证

主要证候　胁下痞块巨大，胁痛引背，拒按，入夜更甚，脘腹胀满，食欲不振，大便溏结不调，倦怠乏力，舌质紫暗有瘀点瘀斑，脉沉细或弦涩。

治　法　行气活血，化瘀消积。

方　药　复元活血汤加

coction for Restoration and Blood Activation), composed of Danggui (*Radix Angelicae Sinensis*) 10 g, Taoren (*Semen Persicae*) 10 g, Honghua (*Flos Carthami*) 10 g, Chuanshanjia (*Squama Manitis*, to be decocted first) 15 g, Tianhuafen (*Radix Trichosanthis*) 12 g, Sanleng (*Rhizoma Sparganii*) 10 g, Ezhu (*Rhizoma Curcumae*) 10 g, Yanhusuo (*Rhizoma Corydalis*) 10 g and Yujin (*Radix Curcumae*) 10 g.

Modification: For blood stagnation, add Shuizhi (*Hirudo*) 6 g and Zhechong (*Eupolyphaga seu Steleophaga*) 6 g.

3. Damp-heat Accumulation

Chief Manifestations: Restlessness, irritability, yellowish skin and sclera, dryness and bitterness in the mouth, abdominal distension and fullness, impaired appetite, stabbing pain in the hypochondrium, deep yellow urine, dry stools, dark purple tongue with yellow coating, wiry and smooth or smooth and rapid pulse.

Therapeutic Methods: To clear away heat, normalize the function of gallbladder and purge fire to remove toxic substance.

Prescription: Modified Yinchenhao Tang (Artemisiae Scopariae Decoction), composed of Yinchen (*Herba Artemisiae Scopariae*) 12 g, Zhizi (*Fructus Gardeniae*) 10 g, Shengdahuang (*Radix et Rhizoma Rhei*, to be decocted later) 10 g, Houpo (*Cortex Magnoliae Officinalis*) 10 g, Shuihonghuazi (*Fructus Polygoni Orientalis*) 6 g and Banzhilian (*Herba Scutellariae Barbatae*) 12 g.

Modifications: For fever and thirst, add Qinghao (*Herba Artemisiae Annuae*) 12 g and Huzhang (*Rhizoma Polygoni Cuspidati*) 15 g; for marked jaundice, add Zexie (*Rhizoma Alismatis*) 12 g and Fuling (*Poria*) 10 g.

4. Liver-yin Deficiency

Chief Manifestations: Hypochondriac pain, dys-

减：当归10 g,桃仁10 g,红花10 g,穿山甲(先煎)15 g,天花粉12 g,三棱10 g,莪术10 g,延胡索10 g,郁金10 g。

加　减　血瘀明显者,加水蛭6 g,蛰虫6 g。

3. 湿热聚毒证

主要证候 心烦易怒,身黄目黄,口干口苦,食少,腹胀满,胁肋刺痛,溲赤便干,舌质紫暗,苔黄,脉弦滑或滑数。

治　法 清热利胆,泻火解毒。

方　药 茵陈蒿汤加减：茵陈12 g,栀子10 g,生大黄(后下)10 g,厚朴10 g,水红花子6 g,半枝莲12 g。

加　减 发热,口渴者,加青蒿12 g,虎杖15 g;黄疸明显者,加泽泻12 g,茯苓10 g。

4. 肝阴亏虚证

主要证候 胁肋疼痛,五

phoria with feverish sensation in the chest, palms and soles, vertigo, impaired appetite, distended abdomen with varicose veins, or hematemesis, hemafecia and subcutaneous hemorrhage in severe case, red tongue with little coating, and thready and rapid pulse.

Therapeutic Methods: To nourish blood, soothe the liver and cool blood to remove toxic substance.

Prescription: Modified Yiguan Jian (Ever-effective Decoction for Nourishing Liver and Kidney), composed of Shengdihuang (*Radix Rehmanniae*) 12 g, Shashen (*Radix Glehniae*) 12 g, Maimendong (*Radix Ophiopogonis*) 10 g, Danggui (*Radix Angelicae Sinensis*) 10 g, Gouqizi (*Fructus Lycii*) 10 g, Biejia (*Carapax Trionycis*, to be decocted first) 15 g, Guiban (*Plastrum Testudinis*, to be decocted first) 15 g and Nüzhenzi (*Fructus Ligustri Lucidi*) 10 g.

Modifications: For yin deficiency and blood heat, add Mudanpi (*Cortex Moutan Radicis*)10 g and Banbianlian (*Herba Lobeliae Chinensis*) 15 g; for severe hemorrhage, add Hanliancao (*Herba Ecliptae*) 12 g and Baimaogen (*Rhizoma Imperatae*) 20 g.

Other Treatments

1. Chinese Patent Drugs

(1) Dahuang Zhechong Wan (Bolus of Rhei and Eupolyphaga seu Steleophaga): 1 bolus each time, once or twice a day; suitable for liver cancer with blood stagnation.

(2) Shugan Zhitong Wan (Pill for Soothing Liver and Relieving Pain): 4 - 4.5 g each time, twice or thrice daily; suitable for early liver cancer with pronounced distending pain in the abdomen due to incoordination between the liver and stomach.

(3) Xiaozheng Yigan Pian (Tablet for Removing Mass and Reinforcing Liver): 6 - 8 tablets each time,

心烦热,头晕目眩,食少,腹胀大,青筋暴露,甚则呕血、便血、皮下出血,舌红少苔,脉细而数。

治　法　养血柔肝,凉血解毒。

方　药　一贯煎加减:生地黄12 g,沙参12 g,麦门冬10 g,当归10 g,枸杞子10 g,鳖甲(先煎)15 g,龟版(先煎)15 g,女贞子10 g。

加　减　阴虚血热者,加牡丹皮10 g,半边莲15 g;出血明显者,加旱莲草12 g,白茅根20 g。

【其他疗法】

1. 中成药

(1) 大黄䗪虫丸　每服1丸,每日1～2次。适用于瘀血毒结之证。

(2) 舒肝止痛丸　每服4～4.5 g,每日2～3次。适用于肝癌早期,肝胃不和,脘腹胀痛明显者。

(3) 消癥益肝片　每服6～8片,每日2次。适用于

twice a day; applicable to intermediate and late stages of primary liver cancer.

（4）Shen Lian Jiaonang（Ginseng and Nelumbinis Capsule）：6 capsules, 3 times a day, taken with warm water half an hour after meals, 42 days making up a course.

2. Single-drug or Experiential Prescriptions

（1）Daimao（*Carapax Exetmochelydis*）15 g, Lufengfang（*Nidus Polistis Mandarini*）15 g, Guiban（*Plastrum Testudinis*）25 g, Yadanzi（*Fructus Bruceae*）15 g and Chansu（*Venenum Bufonis*）1 g. Grind the drugs into fine powder and take 1 - 2 g each time, twice daily. It is used as auxiliary treatment for liver cancer.

（2）Yinchen（*Herba Artemisiae Scopariae*）15 g, Zhizi（*Fructus Gardeniae*）10 g, Shenqu（*Massa Medicata Fermentata*）12 g, Maiya（*Fructus Hordei Germinatus*）12 g, Fuling（*Poria*）12 g, Cheqianzi（*Semen Plantaginis*, wrapped）12 g, Banzhilian（*Herba Scutellariae Barbatae*）15 g and Tianjihuang（*Herba Hyperici Japonici*）15 g. Decoct the drugs in water for oral administration, 1 dose a day. It is applicable to liver cancer with jaundice.

（3）Chishaoyao（*Radix Paeoniae Rubra*）10 g, Danshen（*Radix Salviae Miltiorrhizae*）12 g, Sanleng（*Rhizoma Sparganii*）10 g, Ezhu（*Rhizoma Curcumae*）10 g, Zhechong（*Eupolyphage seu Steleophaga*）5 g, Yujin（*Radix Curcumae*）10 g, Cheqianzi（*Semen Plantaginis*, wrapped）12 g, Banzhilian（*Herba Scutellariae Barbatae*）15 g, Chenhulu（*Pericarpium Lagenariae*）15 g and Zhuling（*Polyporus*）10 g. Decoct the drugs in water for oral administration, 1 dose a day. It is applicable to hepatocarcinoma with ascites.

3. External Therapy

（1）Zhiruxiang（*Olibanum Preparata*）30 g, Zhi-

中、晚期原发性肝癌。

（4）参莲胶囊　每服 6 粒,每日 3 次,饭后半小时温开水送服,42 日为 1 个疗程。

2. 单验方

（1）玳瑁15 g,露蜂房15 g,龟版25 g,鸦胆子15 g,蟾酥 1 g,共研细末。每次服 1~2 g,每日早晚各服 1 次。适用于肝癌的辅助治疗。

（2）茵陈15 g,栀子10 g,神曲12 g,麦芽12 g,茯苓12 g,车前子（包煎）12 g,半枝莲15 g,田基黄15 g。水煎服,每日 1 剂。适用于肝癌出现黄疸者。

（3）赤芍药10 g,丹参12 g,三棱10 g,莪术10 g,䗪虫5 g,郁金10 g,车前子（包煎）12 g,半枝莲15 g,陈葫芦15 g,猪苓10 g。水煎服,每日 1 剂。适用于肝癌出现腹水者。

3. 外治法

（1）制乳香30 g,制没药

moyao (*Myrrha Preparata*) 30 g, Mituoseng (*Litharg-yrum*) 30 g, Ganchanpi (*Cutis Bufonis, dried*) 30 g, Longdancao (*Radix Gentianae*) 15 g, Qiandan (*Mini-um*) 15 g, Bingpian (*Borneolum Syntheticum*) 15 g, Gongdingxiang (*Gemma Caryophylli*) 15 g, Xixin (*Her-ba Asari*) 15 g, Duanhanshuishi (*Mirabilitum Usta, calcined*) 60 g, Dahuang (*Radix et Rhizoma Rhei*) 50 g, Jianghuang (*Rhizoma Curcumae Longae*) 50 g and Shengdanxing (*Arisaema cum Bile*) 20 g. Grind the above drugs into fine powder and mix them thoroughly. Then mix proper amount of the powder with vaseline, spread the mixture onto a gauze, apply it to the tumor ar-ea and change it every other day. Suspend the treatment if local papule or blister occurs until the skin recovers. This is suitable for liver cancer with severe pain.

(2) Shannai (*Rhizoma Kaempferiae*) 20 g, Ruxiang (*Olibanum*) 20 g, Moyao (*Myrrha*) 20 g, Dahuang (*Radix et Rhizoma Rhei*) 20 g, Jianghuang (*Rhizoma Curcumae Longae*) 20 g, Zhizi (*Fructus Gardeniae*) 20 g, Baizhi (*Radix Angelicae Dahuricae*) 20 g, Huang-qin (*Radix Scutellariae*) 20 g, Xiaohuixiang (*Fructus Foeniculi*) 15 g, Dingxiang (*Gemma Caryophylli*) 15 g, Chishaoyao (*Radix Paeoniae Rubra*) 15 g, Muxiang (*Radix Aucklandiae*) 15 g, Huangbai (*Cortex Phello-dendri*) 15 g and Bimaren (*Semen Ricini*) 20 pcs. Grind the above drugs into fine powder, mix them thoroughly with proper amount of egg white into paste, then apply it to Qimen (LR 14) in the right espigastrium, cover the paste with a gauze or wax paper and fix it with adhesive plaster. For intense pain, change the dressing every 6 hours; for less severe pain, change the dressing every 12 hours. This method can be used in succession until the pain is alleviated or relieved and is applicable to liver cancer with pain.

30 g,密陀僧30 g,干蟾皮30 g,龙胆草15 g,铅丹15 g,冰片15 g,公丁香15 g,细辛15 g,煅寒水石60 g,大黄50 g,姜黄50 g,生胆星20 g,各为细末和匀。用适量药粉调入凡士林内,摊于纱布,贴敷肿块部位,隔日1换。如局部出现丘疹或水疱则停止使用,待皮肤正常后再用。适用于肝癌疼痛明显者。

(2) 山柰20 g,乳香20 g,没药20 g,大黄20 g,姜黄20 g,栀子20 g,白芷20 g,黄芩20 g,小茴香15 g,丁香15 g,赤芍药15 g,木香15 g,黄柏15 g,蓖麻仁20粒。上药共研细末,取鸡蛋清适量,混合,搅拌均匀成糊状,外敷右上腹期门穴处。敷药后用纱布或蜡纸覆盖,胶布固定。疼痛剧烈者,6小时换药1次;疼痛较轻者,12小时更换1次。可连续用至疼痛缓解或消失为止。适用于肝癌疼痛。

2.4.6 Cholecystitis

General Description

Cholecystitis is the inflammation of gallbladder, caused by biliary stone, bacterial infection and other factors. It may be acute or chronic, clinically manifested as various severity of pain in the right middle or upper abdomen and nausea and vomiting as well. Acute cholecystitis is characterized by high fever and chill, or by jaundice. It is more often found in people aged 40 - 65 and in fat persons, more common in females than in males. Besides, the disease is related to diet constitution.

In TCM, cholecystitis belongs to the categories of "xie tong" (hypochondriac pain), "dan zhang" (biliary distension) and "huang dan" (jaundice). It is chiefly induced by disorder of qi in ascending and descending. The causes of this disease may be prolonged stagnation of liver qi due to worry, pensiveness and anger; disorder of the gallbladder due to stagnation of damp heat; deficiency with impairment and overstrain followed by cold invasion; stagnant qi causing blood stagnation blocking the meridians. It is closely related to the liver, spleen and stomach; and its location is in the gallbladder. As for its pathogenesis, qi stagnation, heat accumulation, blood stasis, gallstones and dampness retention cause stagnation of liver qi and gallbladder qi and failure of gallbladder qi to ascend and descend; prolonged qi stagnation causes blood stagnation or transforms into fire. Furthermore, recurrence of the disease leads to deficiency of healthy qi, and retained phlegm and damp heat in the gallbladder eventually result in the

第六节　胆囊炎

【概述】

胆囊炎系由胆道系统的结石、细菌感染及其他原因引起的胆囊炎症性疾病。胆囊炎包括急性胆囊炎和慢性胆囊炎。临床主要表现为不同程度的右上腹或中上腹部疼痛,伴恶心呕吐。急性胆囊炎常有高热、寒战,或有黄疸。本病年龄多发生在 40~65 岁年龄组,女性高于男性,而且偏肥胖体型为多见。另外与人们的饮食结构变化有关。

本病属于中医学"胁痛"、"胆胀"、"黄疸"等范畴。胆囊炎的发生,主要在于胆腑气机通降失常。其因或为忧思气恼,肝气久郁;或为湿热内蕴,胆腑不通;或为虚损劳倦,继而感寒;或为气滞及血,瘀血阻络。病位在胆腑,与肝、脾、胃关系最为密切。其病机为气滞、热郁、瘀血、砂石、湿阻致使肝胆气郁、胆失通降,久而气滞及血或郁而化火。日久不愈,反复发作,正气渐虚,邪恋不去,痰浊湿热,久酿成石,胆腑通降受阻,脾胃生化不足,进一步耗伤正气,最后致肝肾阴亏或脾肾阳虚。

formation of gallstones. In this case, the ability of the gallbladder to promote the flow of qi is impaired and disorder of the spleen and stomach further consumes healthy qi, consequently deficiency of liver yin and kidney yin or deficiency of spleen yang and kidney yang ensues.

Essentials for Diagnosis

(1) The chief clinical manifestation is frequent recurrence of pain in the epigastrium, usually on the right or in the middle, radiating to the right infrascapular region. The pain usually attacks at night or after heavy meals. During the intermission of attacks, there may be stuffiness and discomfort sensation in the right epigastrium accompanied by burning sensation in the stomach, nausea, belching, acid regurgitation and impaired appetite, which are usually aggravated by intake of greasy food.

(2) The chief physical signs are tenderness in the right epigastrium and positive Murphy's sign. A cystic mass is palpable in the right epigastrium.

(3) Cholesterol crystal, sediment of calcium bilirubinate and a large number of white blood cells, especially bile-stained pus cells can be found in the bile by duodenal biliary drainage examination. Pathogens may be found in the bacterial culture of the bile.

(4) Ultrasonography B is helpful in detecting the size of gallbladder, the thickness of gallbladder wall and the existence of gallstone.

(5) X-ray plain film reveals radiopaque calculus, calcification, and enlargement of gallbladder. Intravenous cholecystography shows radiopaque stone, enlarged or shrinked or deformed gallbladder, ill concentrating and contracting function of the gallbladder, and undeveloped

【诊断要点】

(1) 临床症状以反复发作性上腹部疼痛为主,多发生于右上腹或中上腹部,并向右侧肩胛下区放射。疼痛常发生于夜间或饱餐后。发作间歇期可有右上腹胀闷不适,常伴有胃灼热感、恶心、嗳气、泛酸、食欲减退等胃肠道症状。进食油腻多脂食物后往往加重。

(2) 体征主要是右上腹部压痛,墨菲(Murphy)征阳性。当胆囊增大时,右上腹可扪及囊性包块。

(3) 十二指肠引流胆汁检查可发现胆汁内有胆固醇结晶,胆红素钙沉淀,大量白细胞,特别是被胆汁黄染的脓细胞等。胆汁细菌培养可有致病菌。

(4) B型超声波检查可了解胆囊的大小、囊壁的厚度,及有无胆石存在。

(5) 腹部X线平片可见阳性结石、胆囊钙化及胆囊膨胀等。静脉胆囊造影可显示透X线的胆石、胆囊胀大、缩小或变形,胆囊浓缩与收缩功能不

or underdeveloped opacity of the gallbladder.

Syndrome Differentiation and Treatment

It is clinically essential to differentiate excess type from deficiency one. Stagnation of liver qi and gallbladder qi, blood stasis caused by qi stagnation, heat accumulation in the gallbladder, and damp heat in the liver and gallbladder are of the excess type; deficiency of liver yin and kidney yin, and deficiency of spleen yang and kidney yang belong to the deficiency type. Concerning the treatment principle, it is to soothe the liver, increase bile secretion, promote descending and dredge fu-organs. For the excess type, it is to purge fu-organs to eliminate heat, while for the deficiency type, tonic therapy and purgative therapy should be used at the same time.

1. Stagnation of Liver Qi and Gallbladder Qi

Chief Manifestations: Distension, fullness and pain in the right hypochondrium radiating to the right shoulder or aggravated by anger, chest oppression, frequent sighing and belching, acid regurgitation, eructation with foul odor, white and greasy tongue coating, and wiry and large pulse.

Therapeutic Methods: To soothe the liver, increase bile secretion, regulate qi and promote descending.

Prescription: Modified Chaihu Shugan San (Bupleuri Powder for Soothing Liver Qi), composed of Chaihu (*Radix Bupleuri*) 10 g, Zhike (*Fructus Aurantii*) 10 g, Chuanxiong (*Rhizoma Chuanxiong*) 10 g, Xiangfu (*Rhizoma Cyperi*) 10 g, Chenpi (*Pericarpium Citri Reticulatae*) 6 g, Yujin (*Radix Curcumae*) 10 g, Baishaoyao (*Radix Paeoniae Alba*) 15 g and Gancao (*Radix Glycyrrhizae*) 6 g.

Modifications: For dry stools, add Zhidahuang (*Radix et Rhizoma Rhei Preparata*) 6 g and Binglang

良,胆囊显影淡或不显影等征象。

【辨证论治】

本病临床辨证以辨虚实为要点。肝胆气郁、气滞血瘀、胆腑郁热、肝胆湿热者属实,肝肾阴亏、脾肾阳虚者属虚。治疗以疏肝利胆、和降通腑为原则。实者宜泻中通降,虚者宜补中寓通。

1. 肝胆气郁证

主要证候 右胁胀满疼痛,连及右肩,遇怒加重,胸闷善太息,嗳气频作,吞酸嗳腐,苔白腻,脉弦大。

治 法 疏肝利胆,理气通降。

方 药 柴胡疏肝散加减:柴胡10 g,枳壳10 g,川芎10 g,香附10 g,陈皮6 g,郁金10 g,白芍药15 g,甘草6 g。

加 减 若大便干燥者,加制大黄6 g,槟榔10 g;腹部

(*Semen Arecae*) 10 g; for abdominal distension and full-ness, add Houpo (*Cortex Magnoliae Officinalis*) 10 g and Caokouren (*Semen Alpiniae Katsumadai*, to be de-cocted later) 3 g; for bitter taste in the mouth and rest-lessness, add Huangqin (*Radix Scutellariae*) 10 g and Zhizi (*Fructus Gardeniae*) 10 g; for belching and vomi-ting, add Daizheshi (*Haematitum*, to be decocted first) 15 g and Chaolaifuzi (*Semen Raphani*, stir-baked) 10 g; for liver qi stagnation impairing the spleen, impaired ap-petite and loose stools, add Fuling (*Poria*) 10 g, Baizhu (*Rhizoma Atractylodis Macrocephalae*) 10 g and Shan-yao (*Rhizoma Dioscoreae*) 12 g.

2. Qi Stagnation and Blood Stasis

Chief Manifestations: Severe localized stabbing pain and tenderness in the right hypochondrium, sallow complexion, dry mouth with bitter taste, dark purple tongue or with ecchymosis on the margin, wiry, thready and unsmooth pulse.

Therapeutic Methods: To soothe the liver, regu-late qi, and activate blood to stop pain.

Prescription: Modified Chaihu Shugan San (Bupleuri Powder for Soothing Liver Qi) and Shixiao San (*Powder for Dissipating Blood Stasis*), composed of Chaihu (*Ra-dix Bupleuri*) 10 g, Zhike (*Fructus Aurantii*) 10 g, Chuanxiong (*Rhizoma Chuanxiong*) 10 g, Xiangfu (*Rhizoma Cyperi*) 10 g, Wulingzhi (*Faeces Trogoptero-ri*) 10 g, Puhuang (*Pollen Typhae*, wrapped) 10 g, Baishaoyao (*Radix Paeoniae Alba*) 15 g and Gancao (*Radix Glycyrrhizae*) 6 g.

Modifications: For intense pain in the right hypo-chondrium, add Yanhusuo (*Rhizoma Corydalis*) 10 g; for nausea and vomiting, add Zhuru (*Caulis Bambusai in Taeniam*) 10 g; for constipation, add Shengdahuang (*Radix et Rhizoma Rhei*, to be decocted later) 6 g; for

胀满,加厚朴10 g,草蔻仁(后下)3 g;口苦、心烦,加黄芩10 g,栀子10 g;嗳气、呕吐,加代赭石(先煎)15 g,炒莱菔子10 g;肝郁侮脾,食少,便溏者,加茯苓10 g,白术10 g,山药12 g。

2. 气滞血瘀证

主要证候 右胁部刺痛较剧,痛有定处而拒按,面色晦暗,口干口苦,舌质紫暗或舌边有瘀斑,脉弦细涩。

治 法 疏肝理气,活血止痛。

方 药 柴胡疏肝散合失笑散加减:柴胡10 g,枳壳10 g,川芎10 g,香附10 g,五灵脂10 g,蒲黄(包煎)10 g,白芍药15 g,甘草6 g。

加 减 右胁痛甚,加延胡索10 g;泛恶作呕者,加竹茹10 g;大便秘结,加生大黄(后下)6 g;兼挟湿热者,加茵陈15 g,栀子10 g;脾胃虚弱,加

cases accompanied by damp heat, add Yinchen (*Herba Artemisiae Scopariae*) 15 g and Zhizi (*Fructus Gardeniae*) 10 g; for deficiency of the spleen and stomach, add Dangshen (*Radix Codonopsis*) 10 g and Shanyao (*Rhizoma Dioscoreae*) 10 g; for gallstone, add Haijinsha (*Spora Lygodii*, wrapped) 15 g and Jineijin (*Endothelium Corneum Gigeriae Galli*) 10 g.

3. Heat Accumulation in the Gallbladder

Chief Manifestations: Burning pain in the right hypochondrium, bitter taste in the mouth, dry throat, flushed face with red eyes, constipation, scanty and deep-yellow urine, restlessness, insomnia, irritability, red tongue with yellow, thick and dry coating, and wiry and rapid pulse.

Therapeutic Methods: To clear away heat in the liver and gallbladder, and relieve stagnation to stop pain.

Prescription: Modified Qingdan Tang (Decoction for Clearing away Heat in Gallbladder), composed of Shengdahuang (*Radix et Rhizoma Rhei*, to be decocted later) 10 g, Zhizi (*Fructus Gardeniae*) 10 g, Huanglian (*Rhizoma Coptidis*) 5 g, Chaihu (*Radix Bupleuri*) 10 g, Baishaoyao (*Radix Paeoniae Alba*) 12 g, Pugongying (*Herba Taraxaci*) 15 g, Jinqiancao (*Herba Lysimachiae*) 15 g, Gualou (*Fructus Trichosanthis*) 10 g, Yujin (*Radix Curcumae*) 10 g, Yanhusuo (*Rhizoma Corydalis*) 10 g and Chuanlianzi (*Fructus Meliae Toosendan*) 10 g.

Modifications: For restlessness and insomnia, add Danshen (*Radix Salviae Miltiorrhizae*) 12 g and Chaosuanzaoren (*Semen Ziziphi Spinosae*, stir-baked) 10 g; for jaundice, add Yinchen (*Herba Artemisiae Scopariae*) 15 g and Zhike (*Fructus Aurantii*) 10 g; for thirst with a desire to drink, add Tianhuafen (*Radix Trichosanthis*) 15 g and Maimendong (*Radix Ophiopogonis*) 10 g; for

党参10 g，山药10 g；有胆石者，加海金沙（包煎）15 g，鸡内金10 g。

3. 胆腑郁热证

主要证候 右胁部灼热疼痛，口苦咽干，面红目赤，大便秘结，小溲短赤，心烦失眠易怒，舌质红，苔黄厚而干，脉弦数。

治 法 清泻肝胆，解郁止痛。

方 药 清胆汤加减：生大黄（后下）10 g，栀子10 g，黄连5 g，柴胡10 g，白芍药12 g，蒲公英15 g，金钱草15 g，瓜蒌10 g，郁金10 g，延胡索10 g，川楝子10 g。

加 减 若心烦失眠者，加丹参12 g，炒酸枣仁10 g；有黄疸者，加茵陈15 g，枳壳10 g；口渴喜饮，加天花粉15 g，麦门冬10 g；恶心欲吐者，加制半夏6 g，竹茹10 g。

nausea, add Zhibanxia (*Rhizoma Pinelliae Preparata*) 6 g and Zhuru (*Caulis Bambusae in Taeniam*) 10 g.

4. Damp Heat in the Liver and Gallbladder

Chief Manifestations: Distension, fullness and pain in the right hypochondrium, chest oppression, impaired appetite, bitter taste in the mouth, restlessness, mucous stools, or jaundice, red tongue with yellow and greasy coating, and wiry and smooth pulse.

Therapeutic Methods: To soothe the liver, increase bile secretion and clear away damp heat.

Prescription: Modified Da Chaihu Tang (Major Bupleuri Decoction) and Yinchenhao Tang (Artemisiae Scopariae Decoction), composed of Chaihu (*Radix Bupleuri*) 10 g, Yinchen (*Herba Artemisiae Scopariae*) 15 g, Zhizi (*Fructus Gardeniae*) 10 g, Huangqin (*Radix Scutellariae*) 10 g, Zhishi (*Fructus Aurantii Immaturus*) 10 g, Shengdahuang (*Radix et Rhizoma Rhei*, to be decocted later) 6 g, Zhibanxia (*Rhizoma Pinelliae Preparata*) 10 g and Baishaoyao (*Radix Paeoniae Alba*) 15 g.

Modifications: For palpable mass in the right hypochondrium with tenderness, add Chuanxiong (*Rhizoma Chuanxiong*) 10 g and Danshen (*Radix Salviae Miltiorrhizae*) 30 g; for severe qi stagnation, add Xiangfu (*Rhizoma Cyperi*) 10 g and Chuanlianzi (*Fructus Meliae Toosendan*) 10 g; for cases accompanied by dry mouth and feverish feeling due to yin deficiency, add Shihu (*Herba Dendrobii*) 10 g and Shashen (*Radix Glehniae*) 15 g; for gallstone, add Jineijin (*Endothelium Corneum Gigeriae Galli*) 10 g, Chuanshanjia (*Squama Manitis*, to be decocted first) 12 g, Haijinsha (*Spora Lygodii*, wrapped) 12 g and Jinqiancao (*Herba Lysimachiae*) 15 g; for deep yellow urine, add Huashi (*Talcum*, wrapped) 10 g, Cheqianzi (*Semen Plantaginis*,

4. 肝胆湿热证

主要证候 右胁胀满疼痛,胸闷纳呆,恶心呕吐,口苦心烦,大便黏滞,或见黄疸,舌质红,苔黄腻,脉弦滑。

治 法 疏肝利胆,清利湿热。

方 药 大柴胡汤合茵陈蒿汤加减:柴胡10 g,茵陈15 g,栀子10 g,黄芩10 g,枳实10 g,生大黄(后下)6 g,制半夏10 g,白芍药15 g。

加 减 若右胁下触及包块,疼痛拒按者,加川芎10 g,丹参30 g;气滞甚者,加香附10 g,川楝子10 g;若兼阴虚口干烦热者,加石斛10 g,沙参15 g。有胆石者,加鸡内金10 g,穿山甲(先煎)12 g,海金沙(包煎)12 g,金钱草15 g;小便黄赤者,加滑石(包煎)10 g,车前子(包煎)10 g,通草6 g;苔白腻而湿重者,去大黄、栀子,加茯苓10 g,白蔻仁(后下)3 g,砂仁(后下)3 g。

wrapped) 10 g and Tongcao (*Medulla Tetrapanacis*) 6 g; for severe dampness with white greasy tongue coating, remove Dahuang (*Radix et Rhizoma Rhei*) and Zhizi (*Fructus Gardeniae*), add Fuling (*Poria*) 10 g, Baikouren (*Fructus Amomi Rotundus*, to be decocted later) 3 g and Sharen (*Fructus Amomi*, to be decocted later) 3 g.

5. Yin Deficiency and Liver-qi Stagnation

Chief Manifestations: Dull pain or slight burning sensation in the right hypochondrium, dryness in the mouth and throat, irritability, feverish sensation in the chest, vertigo, low fever in the afternoon, red tongue with little coating, and thready and rapid pulse.

Therapeutic Methods: To nourish yin, clear away heat, soothe the liver and increase bile secretion.

Prescription: Modified Yiguan Jian (Ever-effective Decoction for Nourishing Liver and Kidney), composed of Shengdihuang (*Radix Rehmanniae*) 12 g, Shashen (*Radix Glehniae*) 10 g, Maimendong (*Radix Ophiopogonis*) 10 g, Danggui (*Radix Angelicae Sinensis*) 10 g, Gouqizi (*Fructus Lycii*) 10 g and Chuanlianzi (*Fructus Meliae Toosendan*) 10 g.

Modifications: For restlessness and insomnia, add Suanzaoren (*Semen Ziziphi Spinosae*) 10 g, Baiziren (*Semen Platycladi*) 10 g and Yejiaoteng (*Caulis et Folium Polygoni Multiflori*) 12 g; for burning pain in the right epigastrium, add Baishaoyao (*Radix Paeoniae Alba*) 12 g and Gancao (*Radix Glycyrrhizae*) 3 g; for irritability, add Zhizi (*Fructus Gardeniae*) 10 g, Qingpi (*Pericarpium Citri Reticulatae Viride*) 6 g and Zhenzhumu (*Concha Margaritifera Usta*, to be decocted first) 20 g.

6. Yang Deficiency and Liver-qi Stagnation

Chief Manifestations: Intermittent dull pain in the

5. 阴虚郁滞证

主要证候　右胁隐隐作痛,或略有灼热感,口燥咽干,急躁易怒,胸中烦热,头晕目眩,午后低热,舌红,少苔,脉细数。

治　法　滋阴清热,疏肝利胆。

方　药　一贯煎加减:生地黄12 g,沙参10 g,麦门冬10 g,当归10 g,枸杞子10 g,川楝子10 g。

加　减　心烦失眠者,加酸枣仁10 g,柏子仁10 g,夜交藤12 g;右上腹灼痛者,加白芍药12 g,甘草3 g;急躁易怒者,加栀子10 g,青皮6 g,珍珠母(先煎)20 g。

6. 阳虚郁滞证

主要证候　右胁隐隐胀

right hypochondrium, distension and fullness in the abdomen, vomiting of saliva, aversion to cold, cold limbs, lassitude, shortness of breath, pale tongue with white greasy coating, and wiry and weak pulse.

Therapeutic Methods: To warm yang, replenish qi, regulate the liver and increase bile secretion.

Prescription: Lizhong Tang Jiawei (Decoction for Regulating Middle Energizer with Additions), composed of Dangshen (*Radix Codonopsis*) 10 g, Baizhu (*Rhizoma Atractylodis Macrocephalae*) 10 g, Fuling (*Poria*) 12 g, Ganjiang (*Rhizoma Zingiberis*) 3 g, Paofuzi (*Radix Aconiti Lateralis*, roasted in hot cinders) 6 g, Chaihu (*Radix Bupleuri*) 6 g, Baishaoyao (*Radix Paeoniae Alba*) 12 g, Muxiang (*Radix Aucklandiae*) 10 g, Sharen (*Fructus Amomi*, to be decocted later) 3 g, Zhibanxia (*Rhizoma Pinelliae Preparata*) 10 g and Chenpi (*Pericarpium Citri Reticulatae*) 6 g.

Modifications: For cold pain in the abdomen, add Wuzhuyu (*Fructus Evodiae*) 3 g and Wuyao (*Radix Linderae*) 10 g; for gallstone, add Jinqiancao (*Herba Lysimachiae*) 15 g and Jineijin (*Endothelium Corneum Gigeriae Galli*) 10 g.

Other Treatments

1. Chinese Patent Drugs

(1) Shugan Zhitong Wan (Bolus for Soothing Liver and Relieving Pain): 1 bolus each time, 3 times a day; applicable to hypochondriac pain caused by liver qi stagnation.

(2) Danshitong Jiaonang (Capsule for Discharging Gallstone): 4 - 6 capsules each time, 3 times a day; applicable to cholecystitis with gallstone.

(3) Jiawei Xiaoyao Wan (Xiaoyao Pill with Additions): 6 g each time, twice or thrice daily; applicable to cholecystitis due to liver qi stagnation and spleen deficiency.

痛,时作时止,脘腹胀满,呕吐清涎,畏寒肢凉,神疲气短,乏力倦怠,舌质淡,苔白腻,脉弦弱无力。

治　法　温阳益气,调肝利胆。

方　药　理中汤加味:党参10 g,白术10 g,茯苓12 g,干姜3 g,炮附子6 g,柴胡6 g,白芍药12 g,木香10 g,砂仁(后下)3 g,制半夏10 g,陈皮6 g。

加　减　脘腹冷痛者,加吴茱萸3 g,乌药10 g;有结石者,加金钱草15 g,鸡内金10 g。

【其他疗法】

1. 中成药

(1) 舒肝止痛丸　每服1丸,每日3次。适用于肝郁气滞胁痛。

(2) 胆石通胶囊　每服4~6粒,每日3次。适用于胆囊炎及伴胆石者。

(3) 加味逍遥丸　每服6 g,每日2~3次。适用于肝郁脾虚型胆囊炎。

(4) Longdan Xiegan Wan (Gentianae Pill for Purging Liver Fire): 6 g each time, twice or thrice daily; applicable to cholecystitis due to damp heat in the liver and gallbladder.

2. Single-drug or Experiential Prescriptions

(1) Yumixu (*Stylus Zeae Maydis*) 30 g, Pugongying (*Herba Taraxaci*) 15 g and Yinchenhao (*Herba Artemisiae Scopariae*) 15 g. Decoct the herbs in water for oral administration. It is applicable to damp-heat type cholecystitis.

(2) Ludangshen (*Radix Codonopsis*) 15 g, Chaobaizhu (*Rhizoma Atractylodis Macrocephalae*, stir-baked) 12 g, Chenpi (*Pericarpium Citri Reticulatae*) 6 g, Fuling (*Poria*) 12 g, Gancao (*Radix Glycyrrhizae*) 5 g, Muxiang (*Radix Aucklandiae*) 5 g, Yujin (*Radix Curcumae*) 10 g, Chenxiangyuan (*Fructus Citri*) 6 g, Hehuanpi (*Cortex Albiziae*) 10 g, Chuanlianzi (*Fructus Meliae Toosendan*) 12 g and Shensanqi (*Radix Notoginseng*) 10 g. Decoct the above herbs in water for oral administration, 1 dose daily.

3. External Therapy

(1) Grind Qingpi (*Pericarpium Citri Reticulatae Viride*) 15 g into powder, stir-bake it with vinegar and apply to the affected part when it is still hot. This is applicable to cholecystitis caused by stagnation of liver qi and gallbladder qi.

(2) Mix equal amounts of Zhizifen (*Fructus Gardeniae*, to be powdered) and Dahuangfen (*Radix et Rhizoma Rhei*, to be powdered) with ricini oil, or paraffin oil and several drops of 75% alcohol to make paste. Apply the paste to the pain spot, cover it with a gauze and fix it with adhesive plaster, once a day. This is applicable to acute cholecystitis or episodes of chronic cholecystitis.

(3) Dahuang (*Radix et Rhizoma Rhei*) 50 g, Mu-

（4）龙胆泻肝丸　每服6 g,每日2～3次。适用于肝胆湿热型胆囊炎。

2. 单验方

（1）玉米须30 g,蒲公英15 g,茵陈蒿15 g,水煎服。适用于胆囊炎湿热证。

（2）潞党参15 g,炒白术12 g,陈皮6 g,茯苓12 g,甘草5 g,木香5 g,郁金10 g,陈香橼6 g,合欢皮10 g,川楝子12 g,参三七10 g,水煎服,每日1剂。

3. 外治法

（1）青皮15 g,研末,醋炒后趁热熨患处。适用于胆囊炎肝胆气滞证。

（2）栀子粉、大黄粉各等分。用蓖麻子油或液体石蜡油加数滴75%酒精调和成糊状,敷于痛处,纱布覆盖,胶布固定,每次保持1日。适用于急性胆囊炎或慢性胆囊炎急性发作。

（3）大黄50 g,木香30 g,

xiang (*Radix Aucklandiae*) 30 g, Ruxiang (*Olibanum*) 20 g, Baijiezi (*Semen Sinapis Albae*) 20 g and Bingpian (*Borneolum Syntheticum*) 5 g. Grind the drugs into powder and mix them thoroughly. Then mix 10 - 15 g of the powder with proper amount of boiled vinegar into paste, and spread the paste on a 15 cm × 10 cm dressing. Apply it to the tender point and fix it with adhesive plaster. This is applicable to episodes of cholecystitis with pronounced pain.

乳香 20 g, 白芥子 20 g, 冰片 5 g。共研细末和匀,每次取药末 10～15 g,用适量煮沸食醋拌成糊状,涂于 15 cm × 10 cm 的敷料上,贴敷胆囊压痛点,四周用胶布固定。适用于胆囊炎急性发作腹痛明显者。

2.5 Syndrome Patterns of the Kidney

2.5.1 Chronic Nephritis

General Description

Chronic nephritis is a short form of chronic glomerular nephritis. It is an immune inflammatory disease involving glomerulus and caused by multiple etiological factors. It is usually lingering, in most cases, slowly progressive. Proteinuria, hematuria and cylindruria can be found in routine uronoscopy. Edema, high blood pressure and impairment of renal function can also be found in most patients.

There is no such term as nephritis in ancient Chinese medical literature. By its clinic manifestations, it falls into the category of "shui zhong"(edema), "niao xue"(hematuria) and "xu lao"(consumptive disease) in TCM. The causes can be either endogenous or exogenous. Exogenous causes refer to six exogenous pathogenic factors or pyogenic infection of skin, while endogenous causes are mainly dysfunction of the lung, spleen and kidneys, and also involvement of the heart and liver. At the advanced stage, those cases with deficient healthy qi and excessive pathogenic factors are manifested as vomiting, edema, anuresis, convulsion, bleeding and coma.

Essentials for Diagnosis

(1) The disease develops slowly with sustained symptoms which wax and wan from time to time. The

第五章 肾系病证

第一节 慢性肾炎

【概述】

慢性肾炎是慢性肾小球肾炎的简称,是由多种原因引起的原发于肾小球的一组免疫性炎症性疾病。临床特点为病程长,多为缓慢进行性;尿常规检查有程度不等的蛋白尿、血尿和管型尿;大多数患者有不同程度的浮肿、高血压及肾功能损害。

在中医古典医学文献中虽无肾炎病名,但根据肾炎的临床表现可归属于中医学"水肿"、"尿血"、"虚劳"等病证范畴。其发病原因有内外之分,外因是六淫外邪或皮肤疮毒内侵,内因以肺、脾、肾三脏功能失调为主,病变脏器也可累及心、肝。病至晚期正虚邪实者,可见呕逆、水肿、尿闭、抽搐、出血、昏迷等多种危重证候。

【诊断要点】

(1)起病缓慢,病情迁延,时轻时重,肾功能逐步减退,

function of the kidneys decreases gradually, and anemia, retinal degeneration, urinaemia occur at the late stage.

(2) It is manifested as various degrees of proteinuria, hematuria, edema and high blood pressure.

(3) Symptoms like those of acute nephritis may be induced by respiratory tract infection during the course of the disease. Some cases can have a spontaneous remission stage.

(4) General chronic nephritis is the most common type with various symptoms of chronic nephritis, which is not serious, without pronounced manifestations. The disease is usually protracted, sometimes lasts for years, possibly with impairment of renal function at the late stage.

(5) The nephrotoid type is characterized by proteinuria, hypoproteinemia, edema and hyperlipemia, often complicated with high blood pressure, hematuria and renal insufficiency.

(6) High blood pressure type, apart from common symptoms of chronic nephritis, is also marked by prolonged and at least moderate high blood pressure, cardiovascular injuries and ocular fundus changes. Renal function deteriorates rapidly with unfavorable prognosis.

(7) If possible, renopuncture biopsy is recommended to confirm the diagnosis.

Syndrome Differentiation and Treatment

Chronic nephritis is normally classified into the category of principal deficiency and secondary excess. Principal deficiency refers to the impaired function of the spleen and kidneys as well as deficiency of yin, yang, qi and blood. Secondary excess is usually marked by retention of water, damp heat and blood stasis within the body. The treatment principles for secondary-excess lie in eliminating

后期可出现贫血、视网膜病变及尿毒症。

（2）有不同程度的蛋白尿、血尿、水肿及高血压等表现，轻重不一。

（3）病程中可因呼吸道感染等原因诱发，出现类似急性肾炎的表现。部分病例有自动缓解期。

（4）慢性肾炎普通型是慢性肾炎最常见的一种类型。有慢性肾炎的多种症状，但无突出表现，一般均不严重。病程进展缓慢，可持续多年，后期可有肾功能损害。

（5）类肾病型主要表现为大量蛋白尿、低蛋白血症、明显水肿和高脂血症。常伴有高血压、血尿或肾功能不全。

（6）高血压型除一般慢性肾炎症状外，突出表现为持续性中度以上的高血压及心血管损害，常引起眼底病变。肾功能恶化较快，预后不良。

（7）有条件者应作肾穿刺活组织检查，以明确诊断。

【辨证论治】

慢性肾炎辨证多属本虚标实之证。本虚主要是指脾肾功能不足，阴阳气血亏虚；标实以水湿、湿热、血瘀为常见。本病的治标之法主要在于祛除外邪，疏理气血，常用疏风宣肺、清热解毒、利湿消

exogenous pathogens, regulating qi and blood. Often employed are the treatments such as dispelling wind and releasing the lung, clearing away heat and toxic materials, removing dampness and alleviating edema, eliminating water by purgation, activating blood circulation and dissipating the stasis. Treatments to support healthy qi, such as invigorating the spleen, tonifying the kidneys, nourishing yin, warming yang, replenishing qi and nourishing blood are selectively used according to the condition of the deficiency of healthy qi.

1. Invasion by Wind and Overflow of Water

Chief Manifestations: Abrupt onset with rapid exacerbation of edema, fever, aversion to cold, soreness of limbs, cough, dyspnea, oliguria, sore throat, red tongue with thin and yellow coating, floating and rapid pulse.

Therapeutic Methods: To disperse wind, relieve superficies syndromes, release the lung and induce diuresis.

Prescription: Modified Yuebi Jia Zhu Tang (Yuebi Decoction with Atractylodis Macrocephalae) and Mahuang Lianyao Chixiaodou Tang (Decoction of Ephedrae, Forsythiae and Phaseoli), composed of Shigao (*Gypsum Fibrosum*, to be decocted first) 30 g, Mahuang (*Herba Ephedrae*) 5 g, Shengjiang (*Rhizoma Zingiberis Recens*) 3 pcs, Xingren (*Semen Armeniacae Amarum*) 10 g, Shengzibaipi (*Cortex Catalpae Ovatae Radicis*) 12 g, Lianyao (*Radix Forsythiae*) 12 g, Chixiaodou (*Semen Phaseoli*) 12 g and Shenggancao (*Radix Glycyrrhizae*) 5 g.

Modifications: In cases of sore throat, add Jinyinhua (*Flos Lonicerae*) 15 g, Niubangzi (*Fructus Arctii*) 6 g and Zaoxiu (*Rhizoma Paridis*) 20 g; in cases of pyrogenic and pruritic skin, add Mudanpi (*Cortex Moutan*

肿、攻下逐水、活血化瘀等法。扶正培本法多按正虚的不同情况选用健脾、补肾、滋阴、温阳、益气、养血等法。

1. 风水泛溢证

主要证候　水肿突然发作并加重,恶寒发热,肢体酸痛,咳嗽气粗,尿少,咽部发红或疼痛,舌苔薄黄,舌质偏红,脉浮数。

治　法　疏风解表,宣肺利水。

方　药　越婢加术汤合麻黄连轺赤小豆汤加减:石膏(先煎)30 g,麻黄5 g,生姜3片,杏仁10 g,生梓白皮10 g,连轺12 g,赤小豆12 g,生甘草5 g。

加　减　咽痛明显者,加金银花15 g,牛蒡子6 g,蚤休20 g;若皮肤痒疹红赤灼热,加牡丹皮10 g,赤芍药10 g;血尿

Radicis) 10 g and Chishaoyao (*Radix Paeoniae Rubra*) 10 g; in cases of pronounced hematuria, add Baimaogen (*Rhizoma Imperatae*) 20 g, Daji (*Herba seu Radix Cirsii Japonici*) 10 g and Xiaoji (*Herba Cirsii*) 15 g; in cases of headache and vertigo, add Gouteng (*Ramulus Uncariae cum Uncis*) 10 g and Shijueming (*Concha Haliotidis*, to be decocted first) 30 g.

2. Accumulation of Damp Heat

Chief Manifestations: Edema all over the body with strained skin, feeling of stuffiness and oppression in the chest and epigastrium, dyspnea, restless fever, thirst, scanty dark urine and dry stools, red tongue with yellow greasy coating, deep and rapid pulse.

Therapeutic Methods: To clear away heat, remove dampness and promote the flow of qi.

Prescription: Modified Shuzao Yinzi (Decoction for Diuresis), composed of Shanglu (*Radix Phytolaccae*) 10 g, Zexie (*Rhizoma Alismatis*) 10 g, Chixiaodou (*Semen Phaseoli*) 12 g, Jiaomu (*Semen Zanthoxyli*) 6 g, Mutong (*Caulis Akebiae*) 6 g, Fulingpi (*Cortex Sclerotii Poriae*) 12 g, Dafupi (*Pericarpium Arecae*) 10 g and Binglang (*Semen Arecae*) 10 g.

Modifications: If there is retained water in the middle and lower energizers, abdominal distention, difficulty and scantiness in micturition and defication, add Shengdahuang (*Radix et Rhizoma Rhei*, to be decocted later) 5 g or Heichoufen (*Semen Pharbitidis Nigrum*, *powdered* and to be infused separately) 3 g; if there is severe edema accompanied by feeling of stuffiness in the chest, dyspnea with difficulty in lying on back, add Tinglizi (*Semen Lepidii seu Descurainiae*, wrapped) 10 g and Sangbaipi (*Cortex mori*) 10 g; if damp heat turns into dryness and further damages yin, with manifestations of dry mouth and throat, red tongue and dry stools, do

明显者,加白茅根20 g,大蓟10 g,小蓟15 g;头痛、眩晕者,加钩藤10 g,石决明(先煎)30 g。

2. 湿热壅盛证

主要证候　全身水肿,皮肤绷急光亮,胸脘痞闷,呼吸气粗,烦热口干,小便短赤,大便干结,舌质红,苔黄腻,脉沉数。

治　法　清热利湿,疏理气机。

方　药　疏凿饮子加减:商陆10 g,泽泻10 g,赤小豆12 g,椒目6 g,木通6 g,茯苓皮12 g,大腹皮10 g,槟榔10 g。

加　减　若水邪壅阻中、下焦,腹胀,大、小便涩少者,可酌加生大黄(后下)5 g,或黑丑粉(另冲)3 g;若肿势严重,兼见气粗胸满,喘促不得平卧者,酌加葶苈子(包煎)10 g,桑白皮10 g;若湿热化燥伤阴,口咽干燥,舌质红,大便干结者,不宜过于利水,可用熟地黄12 g,山药12 g,茯苓10 g,牡丹皮10 g,泽泻10 g,山茱萸10 g,麦门冬10 g,阿胶(烊化冲服)

not over-induce diuresis, but add Shudihuang (*Radix Rehmanniae Preparata*) 12 g, Shanyao (*Rhizoma Dioscoreae*) 12 g, Fuling (*Poriae*) 10 g, Mudanpi (*Cortex
Moutan Radicis*) 10 g, Zexie (*Rhizoma Alismatis*)
10 g, Shanzhuyu (*Fructus Corni*) 10 g, Maimendong
(*Radix Ophiopogonis*) 10 g, Ejiao (*Colla Corri Asini*,
to be melted and taken separately) 10 g, Zhuling (*Polyporus*) 10 g and Huashi (*Talcum*, wrapped) 10 g; if
blood vessels are injured and hematuria occurs, add Daji
(*Herba seu Radix Cirsii Japonici*) 10 g, Xiaoji (*Herba
Cirsii*) 10 g and Baimaogen (*Rhizoma Imperatae*) 15 g.

3. Retention of Water and Dampness

Chief Manifestations: Pitted edema all over the
body or of the limbs, especially of the lower limbs, oliguria, fatigue and bodily heaviness, feeling of oppression in
the chest, impaired appetite, abdominal distention, nausea, white and thin tongue coating, slow and soft-superficial pulse.

Therapeutic Methods: To eliminate dampness,
strengthen the spleen, activate yang and induce diuresis.

Prescription: Modified Wupi San (Five Peels Powder) and Weiling Tang (Poriae Decoction for Regulating
Stomach), composed of Sangbaipi (*Cortex Mori*) 10 g,
Jupi (*Pericarpium Citri Reticulatae*) 6 g, Shengjiangpi
(*Cortex Zingiberis*) 3 g, Dafupi (*Pericarpium Arecae*)
10 g, Fulingpi (*Cortex Sclerotii Poriaee*) 12 g, Cangzhu
(*Rhizoma Atractylodis*) 10 g, Houpo (*Cortex Magnoliae Officinalis*) 10 g, Guizhi (*Ramulus Cinnamomi*)
5 g, Zexie (*Rhizoma Alismatis*) 10 g and Zhuling (*Polyporus*) 10 g.

Modifications: If there is retention of cold dampness and deficiency of middle energizer yang, with feeling
of stuffiness and fullness in the epigastrium and abdomen,
anorexia, add Ganjiang (*Rhizoma Zingiberis*) 3 g and

10 g,猪苓10 g,滑石（包煎）
10 g。若伤及血络而见尿血，
可加大蓟10 g,小蓟10 g,白茅
根15 g。

3. 水湿浸渍证

主要证候　四肢或全身
水肿，以下肢为明显，按之凹
陷，小便短少，身重困倦，胸
闷，纳谷减少，腹胀，泛恶，舌
苔薄白，脉濡缓。

治　法　化湿健脾，通阳
利水。

方　药　五皮散合胃苓
汤加减：桑白皮10 g,橘皮6 g,
生姜皮3 g,大腹皮10 g,茯苓
皮12 g,苍术10 g,厚朴10 g,桂
枝5 g,泽泻10 g,猪苓10 g。

加　减　若寒湿内蕴，中
阳不运，见脘痞、食少、腹部满
胀者，加干姜3 g,川椒目6 g;
兼感风邪，面肿喘咳气逆者，

Chuanjiaomu (*Semen Zanthoxyli*) 6 g; if the above symptoms are complicated with facial edema and dyspneic cough which are caused by pathogenic wind, add Mahuang (*Herba Ephedrae*) 5 g, Xingren (*Semen Armeniacae Amarum*) 10 g and Tinglizi (*Semen Lepidii seu Descurainiae*) 10 g; if there is exterior deficiency manifested as sweating, aversion to wind as well as prolonged edema, add Shenghuangqi (*Radix Astragali*) 12 g and Fangji (*Radix Stephaniae Tetrandrae*) 10 g.

4. Spleen Deficiency and Dampness Retention

Chief Manifestations: Persistent edema, heaviness of the body and limbs, fatigue and weakness, anorexia, abdominal distention, oliguria, sallow complexion, swollen and pale tongue with white, thin coating, soft-superficial pulse.

Therapeutic Methods: To tonify qi, invigorate the spleen and induce diuresis.

Prescription: Modified Wuling San (Powder of Five Drugs Containing Poriae) and Fangji Huangqi Tang (Stephaniae Tetrandrae and Astragali Decoction), composed of Guizhi (*Ramulus Cinnamomi*) 6 g, Baizhu (*Rhizoma Atractylodis Macrocephalae*) 10 g, Fuling (*Poriae*) 10 g, Zhuling (*Polyporus*) 10 g, Zexie (*Rhizoma Alismatis*) 10 g, Fangji (*Radix Stephaniae Tetrandrae*) 10 g and Dazao (*Fructus Jujubae*) 5 pcs.

Modifications: For retention of dampness and water in the body, edema of the limbs, enlargement of the abdomen, feeling of oppression in the chest, loss of appetite, sticky mouth and nausea, add Houpo (*Cortex Magnoliae Officinalis*) 10 g, Cangzhu (*Rhizoma Atractylodis*) 10 g and Jiangbanxia (*Rhizoma Pinelliae, ginger prepared*) 10 g; for prolonged edema or intermittent edema, loose stools, pale, swollen and teeth-printed tongue, weak pulse, add Dangshen (*Radix Codonopsis*) 10 g,

加麻黄5 g,杏仁10 g,葶苈子10 g;表虚汗出怕风,水肿不退者,加生黄芪12 g,防己10 g。

4. 脾虚湿阻证

主要证候　肌肤水肿持续较久,身重肢沉,倦怠乏力,纳呆,腹胀,尿少,面色萎黄,舌淡胖,苔薄白,脉濡。

治　法　益气健脾利水。

方　药　五苓散合防己黄芪汤加减:桂枝6 g,白术10 g,茯苓10 g,猪苓10 g,泽泻10 g,防己10 g,大枣 5 枚。

加　减　若湿困水停,肢肿腹大,胸闷纳呆,口腻泛恶,可加厚朴10 g,苍术10 g,姜半夏10 g;若屡经治疗,水肿消而不尽,或水肿时有时无,大便溏薄,舌质淡胖,边有齿痕,脉象虚弱者,可用党参10 g,茯苓10 g,白术10 g,山药10 g,白扁豆10 g,薏苡仁12 g,砂仁(后

Fuling (*Poriae*) 10 g, Baizhu (*Rhizoma Atractylodis Macrocephalae*) 10 g, Shanyao (*Rhizoma Dioscoreae*) 10 g, Baibiandou (*Semen Lablab Album*) 10 g, Yiyiren (*Semen Coicis*) 12 g and Sharen (*Fructus Amomi*, to be decocted later) 3 g; for spleen deficiency leading to collapse of gastrosplenic qi, and weakened kidney qi causing release of essence, manifested as protracted proteinuria, add Huangqi (*Radix Astragali*) 30 g; for predisposition to colds due to qi deficiency, resulting in frequent recurrence of the disease, employ Yupingfeng San (Jade Screen Powder) which includes Huangqi (*Radix Astragali*) 15 g, Baizhu (*Rhizoma Atractylodis Macrocephalae*) 10 g and Fangfeng (*Radix Saposhnikoviae*) 6 g.

5. Deficiency of Spleen Yang and Kidney Yang

Chief Manifestations: Pale, or sallow or dark complexion, aversion to cold, cold limbs, anorexia, loose stools, soreness of loins and limbs, scanty urine, generalized pitted edema which is more pronounced below the ankle, pale, swollen tongue with thin, white coating or white, greasy and smooth coating, deep and thready pulse.

Therapeutic Method: To warm and tonify the spleen and kidney.

Prescription: Modified Shipi Ying (Decoction for Invigorating Spleen) and Jingui Shenqi Wan (Jingui Pill for Invigorating Kidney Qi from *Golden Cabinet*), composed of Shufuzi (*Radix Aconiti Preparata*) 6 g, Rougui (*Cortex Cinnamomi*) 6 g, Ganjiang (*Rhizoma Zingiberis*) 3 g, Baizhu (*Rhizoma Atractylodis Macrocephalae*) 10 g, Houpo (*Cortex Magnoliae Officinalis*) 10 g, Muxiang (*Radix Aucklandiae*) 10 g, Caoguo (*Fructus Tsaoko*) 6 g, Binglang (*Semen Arecae*) 10 g, Mugua (*Fructus Chaenomelis*) 10 g, Fuling (*Poriae*) 10 g and Zexie (*Rhizoma Alismatis*) 12 g.

下）3 g。若脾虚气陷,肾气不固,致使精气外泄,症见持续蛋白尿者,可重用黄芪30 g;若气虚容易感冒而致病情常有反复者,可加用玉屏风散,药如黄芪15 g,白术10 g,防风6 g。

5. 脾肾阳虚证

主要证候 面色发白或萎黄或灰黯,怯寒肢冷,食欲不振,大便稀溏,腰膝酸软,小便量少,周身浮肿,尤以两足跗为甚,按之凹陷,久久不起,舌质淡胖,苔薄白或白腻而滑,脉沉细。

治 法 温补脾肾。

方 药 实脾饮合《金匮》肾气丸加减:熟附子6 g,肉桂6 g,干姜3 g,白术10 g,厚朴10 g,木香10 g,草果6 g,槟榔10 g,木瓜10 g,茯苓10 g,泽泻12 g。

Modifications: In cases of yang deficiency and fluid retention causing distinct edema all over the body or of the limbs, and scanty urine, add Huangqi (*Radix Astragali*) 15 g, Zhuling (*Polyporus*) 10 g, Niuxi (*Radix Achyranthis Bidentatae*) 10 g and Cheqianzi (*Semen Plantaginis*, wrapped) 10 g; in cases of upward overflow of fluid, manifested as cough, stuffiness in the chest, shortness of breath and inability to lie flat, add Tinglizi (*Semen Lepidii seu Descurainiae*) 10 g and Shiwei (*Folium Pyrrosiae*) 10 g; in cases of copious, clear urine, add Tusizi (*Semen Cuscutae*) 10 g and Buguzhi (*Fructus Psoraleae*) 10 g.

6. Deficiency of Kdney Yin

Chief Manifestations: Persistent moderate edema, weak and sore loins and knees, feverish sensation in the palms and soles, dry mouth and throat, vertigo and tinnitus, red tougue with little coating, deep, thready or wiry, thready pulse.

Therapeutic Methods: To nourish kidney yin.

Prescription: Modified Liuwei Dihuang Wan (Bolus of Six Drugs Containing Rehmanniae) and Da Buyin Wan (Bolus for Replenishing Yin), composed of Shudihuang (*Radix Rehmanniae Preparata*) 12 g, Shanyao (*Rhizoma Dioscoreae*) 12 g, Fuling (*Poriae*) 10 g, Mudanpi (*Cortex Moutan Radicis*) 10 g, Zexie (*Rhizoma Alismatis*) 10 g, Shanzhuyu (*Fructus Corni*) 10 g, Zhimu (*Rhizoma Anemarrhenae*) 10 g and Huangbai (*Cortex Phellodendri*) 10 g.

Modifications: For headache, vertigo, dry eyes, irritability, restlessness, and wiry pulse, add Huainiuxi (*Radix Achyranthis Bidentatae*) 10 g, Daizheshi (*Haematitum*, to be decocted first) 30 g, Shenglonggu (*Os Draconis*, to be decocted first) 30 g, Shengmuli (*Concha Ostreae*, to be decocted first) 15 g and

加　减　阳虚水泛,肢体或全身明显浮肿,尿少者,加黄芪15 g,猪苓10 g,牛膝10 g,车前子(包煎)10 g;若水湿上泛,兼见咳嗽,胸满气促不能平卧,可加葶苈子10 g,石韦10 g;若尿多色清,加菟丝子10 g,补骨脂10 g。

6. 肾阴亏虚证

主要证候　水肿日久,肿势不甚,腰膝酸软,手足心热,口咽干燥,头晕耳鸣,舌红少苔,脉象沉细或弦细。

治　法　滋养肾阴。

方　药　六味地黄丸合大补阴丸加减:熟地黄12 g,山药12 g,茯苓10 g,牡丹皮10 g,泽泻10 g,山茱萸10 g,知母10 g,黄柏10 g。

加　减　若见头晕头痛,目涩,心烦易怒,脉弦等,加怀牛膝10 g,代赭石(先煎)30 g,生龙骨(先煎)30 g,生牡蛎(先煎)15 g,白芍药12 g;若阴虚挟有湿热,见身体倦怠,烦热,

Baishaoyao (*Radix Paeoniae Alba*) 12 g; for deficiency of yin accompanied by damp heat, manifested as fatigue, feverish sensation with restlessness, yellowish urine, red tongue with yellowish greasy coating, add Shiwei (*Folium Pyrrosiae*) 10 g, Pugongying (*Herba Taraxaci*) 15 g, Yiyiren (*Semen Coicis*) 15 g and Cangzhu (*Rhizoma Atractylodis*) 10 g; for hematuria, add Xiaoji (*Herba Cirsii*) 10 g, Oujie (*Nodus Nelumbinis Rhizomatis*) 10 g, Baimaogen (*Rhizoma Imperatae*) 20 g, Puhuang (*Pollen Typhae*, wrapped) 10 g, Danshen (*Radix Salviae Miltiorrhizae*) 15 g and Qiancaogen (*Radix Rubiae*) 15 g.

7. Obstruction of Blood Stasis

Chief Manifestations: Protracted edema, localized lumbago, dark purple tongue or with petechia, and thready, unsmooth pulse.

Therapeutic Methods: To activate blood circulation and dissipate blood stasis.

Prescription: Modified Tao Hong Siwu Tang (Four-Ingredient Decoction with Persicae and Carthami), composed of Taoren (*Semen Persicae*) 10 g, Danggui (*Radix Angelicae Sinensis*) 10 g, Shudihuang (*Radix Rehmanniae Preparata*) 12 g, Baishaoyao (*Radix Paeoniae Alba*) 10 g, Honghua (*Flos Carthami*) 10 g and Chuanxiong (*Rhizoma Chuanxiong*) 6 g.

Modifications: For predominant excess, add Chishaoyao (*Radix Paeoniae Rubra*) 10 g, Yimucao (*Herba Leonuri*) 12 g and Dilong (*Pheretima*) 6 g; for predominant deficiency, add Jixueteng (*Caulis Spatholobi*) 10 g, Danshen (*Radix Salviae Miltiorrhizae*) 12 g, Shensanqifen (*Radix Notoginseng*, to be powdered and infused separately) 3 g, Puhuang (*Pollen Typhae*, wrapped) 10 g and Huainiuxi (*Radix Achyranthis Bidentatae*) 10 g; for the case with damp heat, add Huangbai

小便黄,舌质红,苔黄腻者,可酌加石韦10 g,蒲公英15 g,薏苡仁15 g,苍术10 g;若兼血尿者,可加用小蓟10 g,藕节10 g,白茅根20 g,蒲黄(包煎)10 g,丹参15 g,茜草根15 g。

7. 瘀血内阻证

主要证候 水肿日久不退,腰痛固定不移,舌质紫黯或有瘀点,脉细涩。

治 法 活血化瘀。

方 药 桃红四物汤加减:桃仁10 g,当归10 g,熟地黄12 g,白芍药10 g,红花10 g,川芎6 g。

加 减 若病证偏实者,加赤芍药10 g,益母草12 g,地龙6 g;若病证偏虚者,加鸡血藤10 g,丹参12 g,参三七粉(另冲)3 g,蒲黄(包煎)10 g,怀牛膝10 g;若挟有湿热者,加黄柏10 g,蒲公英15 g,石韦10 g,金银花15 g,板蓝根15 g;若兼气虚者,加党参10 g,山药

(*Cortex Phellodendri*) 10 g, Pugongying (*Herba Tarax-aci*) 15 g, Shiwei (*Folium Pyrrosiae*) 10 g, Jinyinhua (*Flos Lonicera*) 15 g and Banlangen (*Radix Isatidis*) 15 g; for the case accompanied by deficiency of qi, add Dangshen (*Radix Codonopsis*) 10 g, Shanyao (*Rhizoma Dioscoreae*) 12 g and Huangqi (*Radix Astragali*) 15 g.

Other Treatments

1. Chinese Patent Drugs

(1) Puhuang Wan (Pollen Typhae Pill): 6 g each time, twice daily; indicated for chronic nephritis characterized by obstruction of blood stasis with damp heat, manifested as edema, oliguria, persistent proteinuria, as well as microscopic hematuria, or accompanied by vertigo, fatigue, low fever, dark-red tongue with yellow coating, small, rapid or smooth, rapid pulse.

(2) Danggui Wan (Angelicae Sinensis Pill): 6 g each time, twice daily; indicated for chronic nephritis characterized by obstruction of blood stasis with damp heat, manifested as persistent proteinuria, microscopic hematuria, accompanied by vertigo, fatigue and dry stools.

(3) Shuilu Erxian Dan (Euryales and Rosae Laevigatae Pill): 6 g each time, twice daily; indicated for chronic nephritis characterized by disability of kidney qi.

(4) Zisheng Wan (Zisheng Pill): 6 g each time, twice daily; indicated for chronic nephritis characterized by deficiency of the spleen and kidneys.

(5) Tongxuan Lifei Wan (Pill for Regulating Lung Qi): 6 g each time, twice daily; indicated for sudden onset of chronic nephritis resulting from invasion of wind and retention of water, which lead to failure of the lung in regulating water passages, marked by fever, aversion to cold, sore limbs, dyspneic cough, edema starting from the face, then spreading to all over the body, scanty urine, thin and smooth tongue coating, superficial and

12 g,黄芪15 g。

【其他疗法】

1. 中成药

（1）蒲黄丸　每服6 g,每日2次。适用于慢性肾炎瘀血内阻,挟有湿热证,症见水肿,小便不利,长期蛋白尿、镜下血尿,或伴有头昏,身倦,低热,舌质暗红,苔黄,脉小数或滑数。

（2）当归丸　每服6 g,每日2次。适用于慢性肾炎瘀血内阻,挟有湿热,症见长期蛋白尿、镜下血尿,伴头昏、身倦、大便秘结。

（3）水陆二仙丹　每服6 g,每日2次。适用于慢性肾炎、肾气不固证。

（4）资生丸　每服6 g,每日2次。适用于慢性肾炎脾肾两虚证。

（5）通宣理肺丸　每服6 g,每日2次。适用于慢性肾炎急性发作,风遏水阻,肺失通调,症见恶寒发热,肢体酸痛,咳嗽气粗,水肿先从颜面开始,继而波及全身,尿少,舌苔薄而滑,脉浮紧。

tense pulse.

(6) Simiao Wan (Four Wonder-Drug Pill): 6 g each time, twice daily; indicated for chronic nephritis caused by damp heat.

2. Single-drug or Experiential Prescriptions

(1) Grind Xishuai (*Gryllus Chinensis*) 3 pcs and Lougu (*Gryllotalpa Africana*) 3 pcs to powder, decoct Chantui (*Periostracum Cicadae*) 10 g and Fuping (*Herba Spirodelae*) 9 g in water, infuse the powder with the decoction for oral use. This is indicated for chronic nephritis characterized by edema, scanty urine and anuresis.

(2) Decoct Chencandou (*Semen Viciae Fabae*, long-stocked) 120 g with 90g of brown sugar in 2,000 ml of clean water in a pottery pot on a slow fire to obtain 400 ml of the decoction, take the decoction as a daily drink. This is indicated for chronic nephritis with edema.

(3) Mix a cup of fresh celery juice with an appropriate amount of honey and take the juice twice daily. This is indicated for chronic nephritis marked by edema and high blood pressure.

(4) First decoct Zhiguiban (*Plastrum Testudinis*, roasted) 30 g for an hour, then add Huangqi (*Radix Astragali*) 30 g and Shanyao (*Rhizoma Dioscoreae*) 30 g to decoct for another 40 minutes, then take the decoction in 2 divided doses. This is indicated for chronic nephritis characterized by edema due to deficiency of the spleen and kidneys.

(5) Shudihuang (*Radix Rehmanniae Preparata*) 12 g, Shanzhuyu (*Fructus Corni*) 10 g, Fuling (*Poriae*) 10 g, Danggui (*Radix Angelicae Sinensis*) 10 g, Baishaoyao (*Radix Paeoniae Alba*) 10 g, Baizhu (*Rhizoma Atractylodis Macrocephalae*) 10 g, Yiyiren (*Semen Coicis*) 15 g, Suanzaoren (*Semen Ziziphi Spinosae*)

（6）四妙丸　每服6g,每日 2 次。适用于慢性肾炎湿热证。

2. 单验方

（1）蟋蟀、蝼蛄各 3 只,研末,用蝉蜕10 g,浮萍9 g,煎汤冲服。适用于慢性肾炎水肿、尿少、尿闭者。

（2）陈蚕豆(连壳)120 g,红糖90 g,同放沙锅内,加清水2 000 ml,文火熬至400 ml时,代茶饮服。适用于慢性肾炎水肿。

（3）鲜芹菜汁 1 小杯,加蜂蜜适量,口服,每日 2 次。适用于慢性肾炎水肿伴高血压者。

（4）黄芪30 g,山药30 g,炙龟版30 g,先煎龟版 1 小时后,加入黄芪、山药,再煎 40 分钟,每日 1 剂,分 2 次口服。适用于慢性肾炎脾肾两虚型水肿者。

（5）熟地黄12 g,山茱萸10 g,茯苓10 g,当归10 g,白芍药10 g,白术10 g,薏苡仁15 g,酸枣仁10 g,五味子6 g,白芥子5 g,肉桂3 g,黄连3 g。水煎服,每日 1 剂,分 2～3 次服。

10 g, Wuweizi (*Fructus Schisandrae*) 6 g, Baijiezi (*Semen Sinapis Albae*) 5 g, Rougui (*Cortex Cinnamomi*) 3 g and Huanglian (*Rhizoma Coptidis*) 3 g. Decoct the above drugs with water and take the decoction in 2 - 3 divided doses daily. This is indicated for chronic nephritis characterized by edema pertaining to deficiency of kidney yin.

(6) Decoct Yumixu (*Stylus Zeae Maydis*) 60 g in water, and take the decoction daily for six consecutive months. This is indicated for chronic nephritis marked by edema and preteinuria.

(7) Decoct Wubeizi (*Galla Chinensis*) 5 g and Qianshi (*Semen Euryales*) 10 g in water, and take the decoction daily. This is indicated for proteinuria due to kidney defficiency and emission of semen.

(8) Decoct Jicaihua (*Inflorescentia Capsellae Bursa-Pastoris*) 30 g and Mutouhui (*Radix Patriniae*) 30 g in water, and take the decoction daily. This is indicated for proteinuria due to retention of pathogenic heat.

(9) Decoct Baiji (*Rhizoma Bletillae*) 10 g and Oujie (*Nodus Nelumbinis Rhizomatis*) 10 g in water, and take the decoction daily. This is indicated for hematuria due to blood stasis and collateral injuries.

(10) Decoct Diyu (*Radix Sanguisorbae*) 15 g and Baimaogen (*Rhizoma Imperatae*) 30 g in water, and take the decoction daily. This is indicated for hematuria due to blood stasis and retention of damp heat.

3. External Therapy

(1) Decoct Fuzi (*Radix Aconiti Lateralis Preparata*) 10 - 30 g, Muli (*Concha Ostreae*) 30 g and Tufuling (*Rhizoma Smilacis Glabrae*) 30 g in water, concentrate the decoction to 200 ml, then add Shengdahuang (*Radix et Rhizoma Rhei*) 10 g to decoct for 1 - 3 minutes, collect the decoction in a bottle for later use. Apply the decoction for retention enema at 2 to 3 PM. Control the

适用于慢性肾炎水肿属肾阴不足者。

(6) 玉米须60 g,洗净,水煎服,连服 6 个月。适用于慢性肾炎之水肿、蛋白尿。

(7) 五倍子5 g,芡实10 g,水煎服。适用于蛋白尿明显属于肾虚精泄者。

(8) 荠菜花30 g,墓头回30 g,水煎服。适用于蛋白尿明显属于热毒内蕴者。

(9) 白及10 g,藕节10 g,水煎服。适用于血尿明显属于瘀阻络损者。

(10) 地榆15 g,白茅根30 g,水煎服。适用于血尿明显属于瘀阻湿热者。

3. 外治法

(1) 生大黄10 g,附子10~30 g,牡蛎30 g,土茯苓30 g。先煎后 3 味,取其汁,浓缩至 200 ml,再入煎生大黄1~3分钟,取汁装瓶备用。保留灌肠宜于下午 2~3 时进行,速度要慢,控制滴速在每

drop speed at about 100 drops per minute, complete the process in about 20 - 30 minutes, and retain for 2 - 4 hours. It is advisable to induce 2 or 3 motions daily. This can be adjusted by the amount of Sheng Dahuang (*Radix et Rhizoma Rhei*) as well as the time of decocting it. A course of treatment usually lasts two consecutive weeks, then the second course may be resumed after an interval of 5 to 7 days. Usually 2 to 4 courses of treatment are necessary for azotemia and uremia.

(2) Decoct Muli (*Concha Ostreae*) 30 g and Pugongying (*Herba Taraxaci*) 30 g in water, then add Dahuang (*Radix et Rhizoma Rhei*) 10 g to collect about 200 ml of the decoction for retention enema once daily. This is indicated for chronic nephritis with renal failure.

(3) Apply Shexiang (*Moschus*, artificial) 0.3 g on the umbilicus, crush a live crucian into a mash, spread the mashed crucian on Shexiang (*Moschus*, *artificial*) and cover it with oil paper, then with gauze and adhesive plaster, and immobilize the dressing with bandage. Remove the dressing after 24 hours. This is indicated for acute onset of chronic nephritis with generalized edema, scanty urine, dyspnea, etc.

(4) Crush Cheqianzi (*Semen Plantaginis*, wrapped and decocted) 10 g, Tianluorou (*Viviparus seu Cipangopaludina*, shell-moved) 4 pcs and Dasuan (*Bulbus Allii*) 5 cloves into a mash, shape the mixture into a pancake, then apply it on the umbilicus once daily to induce diuresis and alleviate edema. This is indicated for chronic nephritis with distinct edema.

(5) Crush Dasuan (*Bulbus Allii*) 120 g and Mangxiao (*Natrii Sulphas*) 60 g into a mash, wrap the mash with a piece of gauze, and put it on the renal regions for 4 hours. Apply the therapy for 3 consecutive days. This is indicated for chronic nephritis with severe edema.

分钟 100 滴左右,20～30 分钟滴完,保留 2～4 小时。灌肠时间大便以每日 2～3 次为宜,这可以通过增减生大黄量或煎煮时间来调节。连续 2 个星期为 1 个疗程,间隔 5～7 日,再行第 2 个疗程。一般治疗 2～4 个疗程。适用于慢性肾炎所致的氮质血症、尿毒症。

(2) 大黄(后下)10 g,牡蛎 30 g,蒲公英 30 g,水煎取汁 200 ml左右,保留灌肠,每日 1 次。适用于慢性肾炎肾功能衰竭。

(3) 麝香 0.3 g,置于脐当中,用活鲫鱼肉剁成泥酱,敷于麝香上面,外罩油纸,再覆纱布,胶布粘贴,绷带固定,经 24 小时后将药除去。适用于慢性肾炎急性发作而出现全身浮肿、尿少、气急等症。

(4) 田螺肉 4 个,大蒜(去皮)5 瓣,车前子(包煎)10 g,共捣如泥,作饼敷脐。每日 1 次。功效利水消肿,适用于慢性肾炎水肿明显者。

(5) 生大蒜 120 g,芒硝 60 g,拌和捣烂,用纱布包好,外敷双肾区,4 小时后取下,连用 3 日。适用于慢性肾炎水肿重者。

2.5.2 Chronic Renal Failure

General Description

Chronic renal failure refers to the syndromes resulting from decreased renal function at the late stage of various types of chronic kidney diseases. It is clinically manifested as a series of toxic symptoms caused by water-electrolyte imbalance, acid and alkali disturbance as well as retention of toxic substances. In the light of the impairment of renal functions, the disease can be classified into four stages: stage of decreasing renal reserve capacity, compensation stage of renal insufficiency, decompensation stage of renal insufficiency (the stage of azotemia) and stage of uremia.

By its clinical manifestations, in TCM the disease pertains to "long bi" (retention of urine), "guan ge" (dysuria and constipation with frequent vomiting), "shui zhong" (edema) and "xu lao" (consumptive diseases). It is believed that deficiency of the spleen and kidneys is the principal cause of the disease, with other causes like seven emotional upsets, attack of exogenous pathogenic factors, improper diet, alcohol and sex addiction and overstrain. The pathogenic factors vary, which may include wind, dampness, heat, turbid pathogenic factors, blood stasis. The impaired organs are the spleen and kidneys, often involving the lungs, liver and heart. The pathogenic feature of the disease is characterized by deficiency of healthy qi and excess of pathogenic factors. Deficiency of healthy qi is primarily manifested as deficiency of kidney yang and spleen yang, deficiency of liver yin and kidney yin, deficiency of both qi and yin, deficiency of both yin and yang. Excess of pathogenic factors exhibits attack of

第二节 慢性
肾功能衰竭

【概述】

慢性肾功能衰竭是由于各种慢性肾脏疾病晚期肾功能减退引起的综合征。临床表现为水、电解质和酸碱平衡失调,以及由毒素贮留引起的一系列全身中毒症状。本病按肾功能损害的程度分为肾储备功能减退期、肾功能不全代偿期、肾功能失代偿期(氮质血症期)和尿毒症期四期。

根据本病的临床表现,与中医学中的"癃闭"、"关格"、"水肿"、"虚劳"等病证相类似。中医学认为,脾肾虚衰是发病的根本,常因七情、外感、饮食、酒色、劳累等诱因而反复发作。病邪有风、湿、热、浊、瘀等不同。病位以脾、肾为主,常波及肺、肝、心。病理性质为正虚邪实,正虚多为脾肾阳虚、肝肾阴虚、气阴两虚、阴阳两虚,邪实可有外感、水停、湿热、湿浊、瘀血、痰湿、肝风等。

exogenous pathogenic factors, retention of water within the body, damp heat, blood stasis, dampness, phlegm dampness, liver wind, etc.

Essentials for Diagnosis

(1) The patient usually has a history of kidney diseases such as chronic nephritis.

(2) There must be symptoms reflecting the impaired function of multiple organs which are attributive to various metabolic disturbances and retention of toxic product of metabolism. These symptoms include poor appetite, nausea, vomiting, upper abdominal distention, anemia, marked decrease in packed cell volume, subdermal bleeding, epistaxis, profuse menstruation, various degrees of high blood pressure, fatigue, insomnia, cutaneous pruritus, hypothermia, hypometabolism, hyperlithuria, etc.

(3) Laboratory examinations may find increase in urea nitrogen, creatinine and endogenous creatinine clearance rate.

Syndrome Differentiation and Treatment

Chronic renal failure is most often caused by deficiency of healthy qi and excess of pathogenic factors, deficiency of the kidneys and spleen and retention of turbid pathogenic factors. So the treatment usually aims at supporting healthy qi to eliminate pathogenic factors. Supporting healthy qi means regulating the deficiency of yin, yang, qi and blood. Eliminating the pathogenic factors refers to activating blood circulation, clearing away heat, inducing diuresis, dispelling dampness, calming down endopathic wind, purging turbid pathogenic factors and removing toxic substances, which should be adopted in the light of the nature of pathogenic factors.

1. Deficiency of Spleen Yang and Kidney Yang

Chief Manifestations: Pale complexion, lassitude, anorexia, abdominal flatulence, aversion to cold, cold limbs, cold pain in the loins and knees, nocturia, impo-

【诊断要点】

（1）多有慢性肾炎等肾脏病史。

（2）各种代谢障碍及由毒性代谢产物潴留所产生的各系统症状。如食欲不振,上腹饱胀,恶心呕吐,贫血,红细胞压积明显下降,皮下出血,鼻衄,月经过多,不同程度高血压,疲乏,失眠,皮肤瘙痒,体温过低,基础代谢率下降,高尿酸等。

（3）实验室检查有尿素氮、肌酐、内生肌酐清除率等升高。

【辨证论治】

慢性肾功能衰竭总属正虚邪实,脾肾虚竭,浊邪壅塞,因而治疗上以扶正祛邪为原则。扶正即调整阴阳气血之虚;祛邪可根据邪之种类及性质而分别采用活血、清热、利水、化湿、熄风、泄浊、解毒等法。

1. 脾肾阳虚证

主要证候 面色㿠白,神疲乏力,纳少腹胀,畏寒肢冷,腰膝冷痛,夜尿清长,阳痿,下

tence, diarrhea with undigested food in stools or morning diarrhea, swollen, pale and teeth-printed tongue with thin coating, and thready, week or sunken, slow pulse.

Therapeutic Methods: To tonify qi, invigorate the spleen, warm the kidney and assist yang.

Prescription: Modified Sijunzi Tang (Four Mild-Drug Decoction) and Yougui Wan (Bolus for Replenishing Kidney Yang), composed of Zhihuangqi (*Radix Astragli*, roasted) 12 g, Dangshen (*Radix Codonopsis*) 10 g, Baizhu (*Rhizoma Atractylodis Macrocephalae*) 10 g, Fuling (*Poriae*) 10 g, Zhi Gancao (*Radix Glycyrrhizae*, roasted) 3 g, Yinyanghuo (*Herba Epimedii*) 10 g, Lujiao (*Cornu Cervi*) 10 g, Shudihuang (*Radix Rehmanniae Preparata*) 12 g, Gouqizi (*Fructus Lycii*) 10 g, Shanyao (*Rhizoma Dioscoreae*) 12 g, Shanzhuyu (*Fructus Corni*) 10 g and Paojiang (*Rhizoma Zingiberis Recens*, roasted in hot cinders) 3 g.

Modifications: For edema, add Shufuzi (*Radix Aconiti Lateralis Preparata*) 6 g, Rougui (*Cortex Cinnamomi*) 3 g, Niuxi (*Radix Achyranthis Bidentatae*) 10 g and Cheqianzi (*Semen Plantaginis*, wrapped) 12 g; for nausea and vomiting, add Shengjiang (*Rhizoma Zingiberis Recens*) 5 g, Zhibanxia (*Rhizoma Pinelliae Preparata*) 10 g and Chenpi (*Pericarpium Citri Reticulatae*) 6 g; for severe diarrhea, add Buguzhi (*Fructus Psoraleae*) 10 g and Roudoukou (*Semen Myristicae*) 10 g.

2. Deficiency of Liver Yin and Kidney Yin

Chief Manifestations: Flushed cheeks, feverish sensation in the palms, soles and chest, vertigo, headache, dry eyes, tinnitus, dry mouth and throat, weak and sore loins and knees, insomnia and dreamful sleep, red tongue with little coating, thready, wiry and rapid pulse.

Therapeutic Methods: To nourish yin, invigorate

利清谷或五更泄泻,舌胖质淡,边有齿痕,苔薄,脉细弱或沉迟。

治 法 补气健脾,温肾助阳。

方 药 四君子汤合右归丸加减:炙黄芪12 g,党参10 g,白术10 g,茯苓10 g,炙甘草3 g,淫羊藿10 g,鹿角10 g,熟地黄12 g,枸杞子10 g,山药12 g,山茱萸10 g,炮姜3 g。

加 减 伴水肿者,加熟附子6 g,肉桂3 g,牛膝10 g,车前子(包煎)12 g;恶心呕吐者,加生姜5 g,制半夏10 g,陈皮6 g;腹泻甚者,加补骨脂10 g,肉豆蔻10 g。

2. 肝肾阴虚证

主要证候 两颧红赤,五心烦热,头晕头痛,两目干涩,耳聋耳鸣,口干咽燥,腰膝酸软,失眠多梦,舌红少苔,脉细弦数。

治 法 滋阴补肾,养肝

the kidney, tonify the liver and suppress hyperactive yang.

Prescription: Modified Maiwei Dihuang Wan (Pill of Ophiopogonis, Schisandrae and Rehmanniae), composed of Shengdihuang (*Radix Rehmanniae*) 12 g, Gouqizi (*Fructus Lycii*) 10 g, Shanyao (*Rhizoma Dioscoreae*) 12 g, Shanzhuyu (*Fructus Corni*) 10 g, Maimendong (*Radix Ophiopogonis*) 10 g, Wuweizi (*Fructus Schisandrae*) 6 g, Baishaoyao (*Radix Paeoniae Alba*) 12 g, Quandanggui (*Radix Angelicae Sinensis*) 10 g, Danshen (*Radix Salviae Miltiorrhizae*) 12 g, Longgu (*Os Draconis*, to be decocted first) 15 g, Muli (*Concha Ostreae*, to be decocted first) 15 g.

Modification: For severe headache and vertigo, add Juhua (*Flos Chrysanthemi*) 6 g, Gouteng (*Ramulus Uncariae cum Uncis*, to be decocted later) 12 g and Duzhong (*Cortex Eucommiae*) 10 g.

3. Deficiency of Both Qi and Blood

Chief Manifestations: Sallow complexion, shortness of breath, reluctance to talk, lassitude, weakness, spontaneous perspiration, dizziness, vertigo, pale lips, numbness of hands and feet, palpitation, insomnia, pale and tender tongue, weak and thready pulse.

Therapeutic Methods: To strengthen middle energizer, replenish qi, nourish blood and tranquilize the mind.

Prescription: Modified Shiquan Dabu Tang (Decoction of Ten Powerful Tonics), composed of Zhihuangqi (*Radix Astragli*, roasted) 12 g, Dangshen (*Radix Codonopsis*) 10 g, Baizhu (*Rhizoma Atractylodis Macrocephalae*) 10 g, Fuling (*Poriae*) 12 g, Shenggancao (*Radix Glycyrrhizae*) 5 g, Quandanggui (*Radix Angelicae Sinensis*) 10 g, Chuanxiong (*Rhizoma Chuanxiong*) 10 g, Baishaoyao (*Radix Paeoniae Alba*) 10 g, Shudi-

潜阳。

方 药 麦味地黄丸加减:生地黄12 g,枸杞子10 g,山药12 g,山茱萸10 g,麦门冬10 g,五味子6 g,白芍药12 g,全当归10 g,丹参12 g,龙骨(先煎)15 g,牡蛎(先煎)15 g。

加 减 头晕头痛甚者,加菊花6 g,钩藤(后下)12 g,杜仲10 g。

3. 气血两虚证

主要证候 面色萎黄,少气懒言,神疲乏力,自汗,头晕目眩,唇色淡白,手足发麻,心悸失眠,舌淡而嫩,脉细弱。

治 法 补中益气,养血宁心。

方 药 十全大补汤加减:炙黄芪12 g,党参10 g,白术10 g,茯苓12 g,生甘草5 g,全当归10 g,川芎10 g,白芍药10 g,熟地黄12 g,五味子6 g,柏子仁10 g,酸枣仁10 g。

huang (*Radix Rehmanniae Preparata*) 12 g, Wuweizi (*Fructus Schisandrae*) 6 g, Baiziren (*Semen Platycladi*) 10 g and Suanzaoren (*Semen Ziziphi Spinosae*) 10 g.

Modifications: For aversion to cold, cold limbs and loose stools, add Rougui (*Cortex Cinnamomi*) 3 g; for low fever, dark red tongue with little coating, add Baiwei (*Radix Cynanchi Atrati*) 10 g and Digupi (*Cortex Lycii*) 10 g; for constipation, add Gualouren (*Semen Trichosanthis*) 10 g and Huomaren (*Semen Cannabis*) 10 g; for anorexia, add Shenqu (*Massa Medicata Fermentata*) 12 g and Shanzha (*Fructus Crataegi*) 10 g.

4. Deficiency of Both Yin and Yang

Chief Manifestations: Edema, aversion to cold, cold limbs, dark and dull complexion, loose or dry stools, nocturia, or scanty yellow urine, feverish sensation in the palms and soles, insomnia, spontaneous perspiration, pale, swollen and teeth-printed tongue with scanty saliva, thready or rapid pulse.

Therapeutic Methods: To warm and replenish kidney qi and regulate yin and yang.

Prescription: Modified Jisheng Shenqi Wan (Pill for Replenishing Kidney Qi from *Prescriptions for Saving Life*), composed of Rougui (*Cortex Cinnamomi*) 3 g, Shufuzi (*Radix Aconiti Lateralis Preparata*) 6 g, Yinyanghuo (*Herba Epimedii*) 10 g, Shudihuang (*Radix Rehmanniae Preparata*) 12 g, Shanyao (*Rhizoma Dioscoreae*) 12 g, Shanzhuyu (*Fructus Corni*) 10 g, Gouqizi (*Fructus Lycii*) 10 g and Heshouwu (*Radix Polygoni Multiflori*) 12 g.

Modifications: For edema, add Guizhi (*Ramulus Cinnamomi*) 6 g, Niuxi (*Radix Achyranthis Bidentatae*) 10 g and Cheqianzi (*Semen Plantaginis*, wrapped) 12 g; for loose stools or morning diarrhea, add Roudoukou

加　减　畏寒肢冷，便溏者,加肉桂3 g;低热,舌质暗红,苔少者,加白薇10 g,地骨皮10 g;便秘者,加瓜蒌仁10 g,火麻仁10 g;纳呆者,加神曲12 g,山楂10 g。

4. 阴阳两虚证

主要证候　浮肿,畏寒肢冷,面色晦滞黧黑,便溏或便秘,夜尿清长或尿少色黄,手足心热,失眠盗汗,舌淡胖而少津,有齿痕,脉细或数。

治　法　温补肾气,调摄阴阳。

方　药　《济生》肾气丸加减:肉桂3 g,熟附子6 g,淫羊藿10 g,熟地黄12 g,山药12 g,山茱萸10 g,枸杞子10 g,何首乌12 g。

加　减　有水肿者,加桂枝6 g,牛膝10 g,车前子(包煎)12 g;大便溏薄或五更泻者,加肉豆蔻6 g,补骨脂10 g;

(Semen Myristicae) 6 g and Buguzhi (Fructus Psoraleae) 10 g; for constipation, add Zhidahuang (Radix et Rhizoma Rhei Preparata) 6 g; for anorexia, add Jineijin (Endothelium Corneum Gigeriae Galli) 6 g and Shenqu (Massa Medicata Fermentata) 12 g; for hectic fever and spontaneous perspiration, add Digupi (Cortex Lycii) 10 g and Baiwei (Radix Cynanchi Atrati) 10 g.

5. Retention of Cold and Dampness in the Spleen

Chief Manifestations: Shortness of breath, weakness, lusterless complexion, nausea, vomiting, anorexia, abdominal flatulence, generalized edema, scanty urine, loose stools, swollen, pale tongue with thick, greasy coating, deep, thready or soft-superficial, thready pulse.

Therapeutic Methods: To warm and reinforce the middle energizer, remove dampness and stop vomiting.

Prescription: Modified Wuzhuyu Tang (Evodiae Decoction) and Ercheng Tan (Erchen Decoction), composed of Wuzhuyu (Fructus Evodiae) 3 g, Dangshen (Radix Codonopsis) 12 g, Fuling (Poriae) 12 g, Chenpi (Pericarpium Citri Reticulatae) 6 g, Shengjiang (Rhizoma Zingiberis Recens) 3 g, Zhibanxia (Rhizoma Pinelliae Preparata) 10 g, Houpo (Cortex Magnoliae Officinalis) 10 g, Muxiang (Radix Aucklandiae) 10 g and Shenggancao (Radix Glycyrrhizae) 3 g.

Modifications: For severe edema, add Cheqianzi (Semen Plantaginis, wrapped) 12 g and Niuxi (Radix Achyranthis Bidentatae) 10 g; for anorexia, add Shenqu (Massa Medicata Fermentata) 12 g and Shanzha (Fructus Crataegi) 10 g; for severe diarrhea, add Roudoukou (Semen Myristicae) 6 g and Wuweizi (Fructus Schisandrae) 6 g; for nausea and vomiting, increase the amount of Shengjiang (Rhizoma Zingiberis Recens) to 6 g, and add Zhishi (Fructus Aurantii Immaturus) 10 g.

大便秘结者,加制大黄6 g;纳差者,加鸡内金6 g,神曲12 g;潮热盗汗者,加地骨皮10 g,白薇10 g。

5. 寒湿困脾证

主要证候　少气乏力,面色无华,恶心呕吐,厌食腹胀,全身水肿,尿少便溏,舌体胖大,色淡,舌苔厚腻,脉沉细或濡细。

治　法　温中补虚,降浊止呕。

方　药　吴茱萸汤合二陈汤加减:吴茱萸3 g,党参12 g,茯苓12 g,陈皮6 g,生姜3 g,制半夏10 g,厚朴10 g,木香10 g,生甘草3 g。

加　减　水肿甚者,加车前子(包煎)12 g,牛膝10 g;纳食不香者,加神曲12 g,山楂10 g;腹泻甚者,加肉豆蔻6 g,五味子6 g;恶心呕吐者,重用生姜6 g,加枳实10 g。

6. Retention of Damp Heat in the Body

Chief Manifestations: Lassitude, weakness, nausea with retching, or frequent vomiting, anorexia, abdominal flatulence, constipation, red tongue with yellow, greasy or dry, coarse coating, thready, rapid or wiry, rapid pulse.

Therapeutic Methods: To support healthy qi, send stomach qi downward, relieve constipation and remove turbid pathogenic factors.

Prescription: Modified Wenpi Tang (Decoction for Warming Spleen Yang) and Wendan Tang (Decoction for Clearing away Gallbladder Heat), composed of Dangshen (*Radix Codonopsis*) 12 g, Fuling (*Poriae*) 12 g, Shenggancao (*Radix Glycyrrhizae*) 3 g, Shufuzi (*Radix Aconiti Lateralis Preparata*) 6 g, Shengjiang (*Rhizoma Zingiberis Recens*) 3 g, Zhibanxia (*Rhizoma Pinelliae Preparata*) 6 g, Chenpi (*Pericarpium Citri Reticulatae*) 6 g, Shengdahuang (*Radix et Rhizoma Rhei*, to be decocted later) 6 g, Huanglian (*Rhizoma Coptidis*) 3 g, Zhuru (*Caulis Bambusae in Taeniam*) 10 g, Zhishi (*Fructus Aurantii Immaturus*) 10 g.

Modifications: For severe vomiting, add Xuanfuhua (*Flos Inulae*, wrapped) 6 g and Wuzhuyu (*Fructus Evodiae*) 3 g; for anorexia, add Shengguya (*Fructus Oryzae Germinatus*) 12 g, Shengmaiya (*Fructus Hordei Germinatus*) 12 g and Jineijin (*Endothelium Corneum Gigeriae Galli*) 6 g; for dry stools, add Mangxiao (*Natrii Sulphas*, to be infused separately) 6 g.

7. Invasion of the Heart by Kidney Water

Chief Manifestations: Palpitation, feeling of oppression in the chest, dyspnea with disability to lie supine, cold body and limbs, profuse perspiration, coma, pale tongue with thin coating, faint and impalpable or hidden, deep pulse.

6. 湿热内蕴证

主要证候　神疲乏力,恶心干呕,或呕吐频作,纳呆腹胀,便结不通,舌质红,苔黄腻或干糙,脉细数或弦数。

治　法　扶正降逆,通腑泄浊。

方　药　温脾汤合温胆汤加减:党参12 g,茯苓12 g,生甘草3 g,熟附子6 g,生姜3 g,制半夏6 g,陈皮6 g,生大黄(后下)6 g,黄连3 g,竹茹10 g,枳实10 g。

加　减　呕吐甚者,加旋覆花(包煎)6 g,吴茱萸3 g;食欲不振者,加生谷芽12 g,生麦芽12 g,鸡内金6 g;大便燥结者,加芒硝(另冲)6 g。

7. 肾水凌心证

主要证候　心悸胸闷,气急不能平卧,形寒肢冷,大汗淋漓,神志昏迷,舌质淡,苔薄,脉微细欲绝或伏沉。

Therapeutic Methods: To warm yang, induce diuresis, replenish qi and arrest discharges.

Prescription: Modified Zhenwu Tang (Zhenwu Decoction for Strengthening Kidney Yang and Spleen Yang) and Shen Fu Tang (Decoction of Ginseng and Aconiti Lateralis), composed of Shufuzi (*Radix Aconiti Lateralis Preparata*) 6 g, Rougui (*Cortex Cinnamomi*) 3 g, Fuling (*Poria*) 10 g, Chaobaizhu (*Rhizoma Atractylodis Macrocephalae*, stir-baked) 10 g, Ganjiang (*Rhizoma Zingiberis*) 3 g, Dangshen (*Radix Codonopsis*) 12 g, Shenggancao (*Radix Glycyrrhizae*) 3 g, Baishaoyao (*Radix Paeoniae Alba*) 12 g, Longgu (*Os Draconis*, to be decocted first) 15 g and Muli (*Concha Ostreae*, to be decocted first) 15 g.

Modifications: In cases of coma, swollen tongue with white or greasy coating, add Shichangpu (*Rhizoma Acori Tatarinowii*) 6 g and Yujin (*Radix Curcumae*) 10 g; in cases of dyspneic cough, add Zhibanxia (*Rhizoma Pinelliae Preparata*) 10 g and Xixin (*Herba Asari*) 3 g; in cases of dyspnea with feeling of oppression in the chest, add Chenxiangfen (*Lignum Aquilariae Resinatum*, to be powdered and taken separately) 3 g; in cases of dark tongue with ecchymosis or petechiae, add Danshen (*Radix Salviae Miltiorrhizae*) 20 g.

8. Invasion of the Heart by Turbid Heat

Chief Manifestations: Coma, restlessness, epistaxis, gingival atrophy, hematuria, hemafecia, skin ecchymosis, stiff tongue resulting in disability to speak; in severe cases, anuresis, red tongue with brownish yellow coating, thready and rapid pulse.

Therapeutic Methods: To clear away heat, remove toxic substance, cool blood and dissipate stasis.

Prescription: Modified Xijiao Dihuang Tang (Cornu Rhinocerotis and Rehmanniae Decoction), composed of

治 法 温阳利水,益气固脱。

方 药 真武汤合参附汤加减:熟附子6 g,肉桂3 g,茯苓10 g,炒白术10 g,干姜3 g,党参12 g,生甘草3 g,白芍药12 g,龙骨(先煎)15 g,牡蛎(先煎)15 g。

加 减 神志昏迷,舌胖苔白或腻者,加石菖蒲6 g,郁金10 g;咳喘者,加制半夏10 g,细辛3 g;胸闷喘息者,加沉香粉(另吞)3 g;舌暗有瘀点、瘀斑者,加丹参20 g。

8. 热浊陷心证

主要证候 神志昏迷,烦躁不安,鼻衄牙宣,尿血便血,肌肤紫斑,舌强不语,甚则尿闭,舌质红,苔焦黄,脉细数。

治 法 清热解毒,凉血散瘀。

方 药 犀角地黄汤加减:水牛角(先煎)30 g,黄连

Shuiniujiao (*Cornu Rhinocerotis*, to be decocted first) 30 g, Huanglian (*Rhizoma Coptidis*) 3 g, Shengdihuang (*Radix Rehmanniae*) 12 g, Xuanshen (*Radix Scrophulariae*) 10 g, Maimendong (*Radix Ophiopogonis*) 10 g, Danshen (*Radix Salviae Miltiorrhizae*) 12 g, Chishaoyao (*Radix Paeoniae Rubra*) 10 g and Mudanpi (*Cortex Moutan Radicis*) 10 g.

Modifications: For hematemesis, hemoptysis and epistaxis, add Jinyinhuatan (*Flos Lonicerae*, charred) 15 g, Lianqiaotan (*Fructus Forsythiae*, charred) 12 g and Oujietan (*Nodus Nelumbinis Rhizomatis*, charred) 10 g; for hemafecia, add Diyutan (*Radix Sanguisorbae*, charred) 10 g and Huaihuatan (*Flos Sophorae*, charred) 10 g; for hematuria, add Nüzhenzitan (*Fructus Ligustri Lucidi*, charred) 10 g and Hanliancao (*Herba Ecliptae*) 10 g; for constipation, add Shengdahuang (*Radix et Rhizoma Rhei*, to be decocted later) 6 g; for accumulation of phlegm heat, add Zhulishui (*Succus Bambosae*) 20 ml and Tianzhuhuang (*Concretio Silicea Bambusae*) 10 g.

9. Invasion of the Liver by Turbid Heat

Chief Manifestations: Anuresis, tremor of fingers, trembling or curled tongue, headache and vertigo, gingival atrophy, aphthous stomatitis, cutaneous pruritus, restlessness, even coma and convulsion, dry, red tongue without coating, or dry, yellow tongue without much saliva, thready, wiry and rapid pulse.

Therapeutic Methods: To calm the liver to stop wind, and nourish yin to suppress hyperactive yang.

Prescription: Modified Zhengan Xifeng Tang (Decoction for Suppressing Liver Wind), composed of Longgu (*Os Draconis*, to be decocted first) 15 g, Muli (*Concha Ostreae*, to be decocted first) 15 g, Baishaoyao (*Radix Paeoniae Alba*) 10 g, Huainiuxi (*Radix Achy-*

3 g,生地黄12 g,玄参10 g,麦门冬10 g,丹参12 g,赤芍药10 g,牡丹皮10 g。

加 减 吐血、咳血、衄血者,加金银花炭15 g,连翘炭12 g,藕节炭10 g;便血者,加地榆炭10 g,槐花炭10 g;尿血者,加女贞子炭10 g,旱莲草10 g;腑实便秘者,加生大黄(后下)6 g;痰热壅盛者,加竹沥水 20 ml,天竺黄10 g。

9. 热浊犯肝证

主要证候 尿闭指颤,舌抖或卷缩,头痛头晕,牙宣口糜,皮肤瘙痒,烦躁不安,甚则神昏抽搐,舌干光红,或黄燥无津,脉细弦数。

治 法 平肝熄风,滋阴潜阳。

方 药 镇肝熄风汤加减:龙骨(先煎)15 g,牡蛎(先煎)15 g,白芍药10 g,怀牛膝10 g,玄参10 g,天门冬10 g,麦门冬10 g,生地黄10 g,生甘草

ranthis Bidentatae) 10 g, Xuanshen (*Radix Scrophulariae*) 10 g, Tianmendong (*Radix Asparagi*) 10 g, Maimendong (*Radix Ophiopogonis*) 10 g, Shengdihuang (*Radix Rehmanniae*) 10 g, Shenggancao (*Radix Glycyrrhizae*) 3 g and Shengguiban (*Plastrum Testudinis*, to be decocted first) 15 g.

Modification: For pronounced convulsion of limbs, add Quanxiefen (*Scorpio*, to be powdered and infused separately)0.5 g and Gouteng (*Ramulus Uncariae cum Uncis*) 12 g.

10. Stagnation of Phlegm in the Heart

Chief Manifestations: Dull and dirty complexion, dementia, incoherent or slurred speech, even deep coma, no fever in most cases, wheezing sound of sputum, nausea and vomiting, white greasy or grey greasy tongue coating, deep and smooth pulse.

Therapeutic Methods: To remove phlegm to restore resuscitation and regulate the stomach to eliminate turbid pathogenic factors.

Prescription: Modified Ditan Tang (Decoction for Eliminating Phlegm), composed of Zhibanxia (*Rhizoma Pinelliae Preparata*) 10 g, Juhong (*Exocarpium Citri Rubrum*) 6 g, Dangshen (*Radix Codonopsis*) 10 g, Fuling (*Poriae*) 12 g, Shenggancao (*Radix Glycyrrhizae*) 5 g, Huanglian (*Rhizoma Coptidis*) 3 g, Zhishi (*Fructus Aurantii Immaturus*) 10 g, Zhuru (*Caulis Bambusae in Taeniam*) 10 g, Shichangpu (*Rhizoma Acori Tatarinowii*) 6 g, Shengjiang (*Rhizoma Zingiberis Recens*) 3 g and Zhinanxing (*Arisaematis cum Bile*, processed) 10 g.

Modifications: For coma, immediately administer one bolus of Suhexiang Wan (Styrax Bolus) or Yushu Dan (Bolus for Relieving Swelling and Restoring Resusitation); for unceasing vomiting, add Banxia (*Rhizoma*

3 g,生龟版(先煎)15 g。

　　加　减　四肢抽搐明显者,加全蝎粉(另冲)0.5 g,钩藤12 g。

10. 痰浊蒙窍证

　　主要证候　面色垢滞,神志痴呆,语言错乱或不清,甚则深度昏迷,多不发热,静而不烦,痰声辘辘,恶心呕吐,舌苔白腻或灰腻,脉沉滑。

　　治　法　涤痰开窍,和胃降浊。

　　方　药　涤痰汤加减:制半夏10 g,橘红6 g,党参10 g,茯苓12 g,生甘草5 g,黄连3 g,枳实10 g,竹茹10 g,石菖蒲6 g,生姜3 g,制南星10 g。

　　加　减　神昏者,当急用苏合香丸或玉枢丹1粒;呕吐不止者,可加用半夏10 g。

Pinelliae) 10 g.

Other Treatments

1. Chinese Patent Drugs

(1) Shen Ling Baizhu Wan (Pill of Ginseng, Poriae and Atractylodis Macrocephalae): 6 g each time, twice a day; indicated for the case with diarrhea.

(2) Xiang Sha Liujun Wan (Pill of Aucklandiae, Amomi and Six Mild Drugs): 6 g each time, twice a day; indicated for deficiency of the spleen and stomach with loss of appetite.

(3) Liuwei Dihuang Wan (Bolus of Six Drugs containing Rehmanniae): 6 g each time, twice a day; indicated for deficiency of liver yin and kidney yin.

(4) Qi Ju Dihuang Koufuye (Oral Liquid of Lycii, Chrysanthemi and Rehmanniae): 1 vial each time, twice a day; indicated for deficiency of liver yin with vertigo and dizziness.

(5) Zhiling Jiaonang (Zhiling Capsule): 2 capsules each time, thrice a day; indicated for chronic renal failure.

(6) Fufang Danshen Pian (Compound Salviae Miltiorrhizae Tablet): 3 tablets each time, thrice a day; indicated for the cases with blood stasis.

2. Single-drug or Experiential Prescriptions

(1) Grind Shufuzi (*Radix Aconiti Lateralis Preparata*) 30 g and Renshen (*Radix Ginseng*) 90 g into powder, mix the powder with long-stocked rice gruel, shape the mixture to boluses as big as phoenix tree seeds, coat them with little Shexiang (*Moschus*, artificial) and take the boluses with rice gruel in 10 to 15 days. It is indicated for "guan ge" (dysuria and constipation with frequent vomiting), deep and thready pulse and extremely cold limbs.

(2) Jiangzhi Huanglian (*Rhizoma Coptidis*, pre-

【其他疗法】

1. 中成药

(1) 参苓白术丸　每服 6 g,每日 2 次。适用于以泄泻为主要症状者。

(2) 香砂六君丸　每服 6 g,每日 2 次。适用于以纳呆、食少为主的脾胃虚弱证。

(3) 六味地黄丸　每次 6 g,每日 2 次。适用于肝肾阴虚证。

(4) 杞菊地黄口服液　每服 1 支,每日 2 次。适用于肝阴不足,头晕目眩者。

(5) 至灵胶囊　每服 2 粒,每日 3 次。适用于慢性肾功能衰竭者。

(6) 复方丹参片　每服 3 片,每日 3 次。适用于以瘀血证为主者。

2. 单验方

(1) 熟附子 30 g,人参 90 g,研为细末,陈米饮糊丸,如梧桐子大,麝香少许为衣,分 10～15 日服完,米饮汤下服。治关格,脉沉细,手足厥冷者。

(2) 姜汁黄连 4.5 g,炮姜

pared with ginger juice) 4.5 g, Paojiang (*Rhizoma Zineris Recens*, roasted in hot cinders) 4.5 g, Renshen (*Radix Ginseng*) 4.5 g, Guizhi (*Ramulus Cinnamomi*) 3 g, Jiangbanxia (*Rhizoma Pinelliae*, ginger prepared) 4.5 g and Dazao (*Fructus Jujubae*) 5 pcs. Decoct the above drugs in water, 1 dose daily. It is indicated for renal failure with severe vomiting.

(3) Zisu (*Herba Perillae*) 10 g, Dangshen (*Radix Codonopsis*) 10 g, Baizhu (*Rhizoma Atractylodis Macrocephalae*) 10 g, Zhibanxia (*Rhizoma Pinelliae Preparata*) 10 g, Huanglian (*Rhizoma Coptidis*) 3 g, Liuyuexue (*Herba Serissae*) 30 g, Lüdou (*Semen Phaseoli Radiati*) 15 g, Danshen (*Radix Salviae iltiorrhizae*) 15 g, Shufuzi (*Radix Aconiti Preparata*) 6 g, Tudahuang (*Radix Rumicis Nepalensis*) 10 g, Sharen (*Fructus Amomi*, to be decocted later) 5 g and Shengjiang (*Rhizoma Zingiberis Recens*) 3 g. Decoct the above drugs in water, 1 dose daily. It is indicated for deficiency of spleen yang and kidney yang as well as retention of dampness in the body.

3. External Therapy

(1) Dahuang (*Radix et Rhizoma Rhei*) 30 g, Yimucao (*Herba Leonuri*) 30 g, Muli (*Concha Ostreae*) 30 g, Kunbu (*Thallus Laminariae et Eckloniae*) 30 g and Huaihua (*Flos Sophorae*) 30 g. Decoct the above drugs in water to collect 100 - 150 ml of the decoction, and use the decoction for high retention enema, once daily or every other day. This is indicated for renal failure at azotemic stage.

(2) Danshen (*Radix Salviae Miltiorrhizae*) 60 g, Yimucao (*Herba Leonuri*) 60 g, Huanglian (*Rhizoma Coptidis*) 30 g and Baizhi (*Radix Angelicae Dahuricae*) 30 g. Soak the above drugs in water, wrap the soaked drugs in a cloth bag, steam the bag for 20 - 30 minutes,

4.5 g,人参 4.5 g,桂枝 3 g,姜半夏 4.5 g,大枣 5 枚,水煎服,每日 1 剂。适用于肾功能衰竭呕吐明显者。

(3) 紫苏 10 g,党参 10 g,白术 10 g,制半夏 10 g,黄连 3 g,六月雪 30 g,绿豆 15 g,丹参 15 g,熟附子 6 g,土大黄 10 g,砂仁(后下) 5 g,生姜 3 g。水煎服,每日 1 剂。适用于脾肾阳虚、湿浊内停者。

3. 外治法

(1) 大黄 30 g,益母草 30 g,牡蛎 30 g,昆布 30 g,槐花 30 g。加水浓煎至 100 ～ 150 ml,高位保留灌肠。每日 1 次,或隔日 1 次。适用于慢性肾功能衰竭氮质血症期。

(2) 丹参 60 g,益母草 60 g,黄连 30 g,白芷 30 g。先将药用水浸潮,置于布袋中,用蒸锅蒸 20 ～ 30 分钟,然后将药袋直接热敷于双肾区,外

then foment the bag on renal regions, and keep the bag warm by employing a hot water bag. This can be used as the auxiliary treatment for renal failure.

2.5.3   Urinary Infection

General description

Urinary infection is one of the common infective diseases, referring to the inflammation caused by the reproduction of the pathogens in the urine involving the mucous membrane or tissue of the urinary tract. It is clinically categorized into upper urinary tract infection (ureteritis and pyelitis) and lower urinary tract infection (cystitis and urethritis). Lower urinary tract infection may be present alone, while the upper urinary tract infection is often complicated with the inflammatory symptoms of the lower urinary tract, which makes it difficult to differentiate between the two clinically. Urinary infection occurs more often in women, with the ratio of 1 man to 10 women. Pyelitis can be further classified into the chronic stage and the acute stage which are mostly attributive to the infection of lower urinary tract. Chronic pyelitisis is one of the major causes of chronic renal dysfunction.

In TCM, urinary infection pertains to the categories of "lin zheng"(stranguria), "long bi"(uroschesis), "yao tong"(lumbago). It is mainly caused by inversion of dirty pathogenic factors from the urethra leading to retention of heat in the bladder, which is then transmitted from zang to fu organs; improper diet with excessive intake of greasy, sweet or pungent food leading to dysfunction of the spleen and production of damp heat which moves downward to the lower energizer; weakness of the elderly people with deficiency of kidney qi leading to failure of the

加热水袋以保持温度。用于肾功能衰竭的辅助治疗。

第三节   泌尿系感染

【概述】

泌尿系感染是常见的感染性疾病,指病原体在尿中生长繁殖并侵犯泌尿道黏膜或组织而引起的炎症。临床分为上泌尿道感染(输尿管炎和肾盂肾炎)和下泌尿道感染(膀胱炎和尿道炎)。下泌尿道感染可单独存在,上泌尿道感染则多伴发下泌尿道炎性症状,临床上不易严格区分。临床发病以女性为多,男女之比为1:10。肾盂肾炎又分为急性和慢性两期,大都由下尿道感染引起。慢性肾盂肾炎是导致慢性肾功能不全的一个重要原因。

本病属于中医学"淋证"、"癃闭"、"腰痛"等病证范畴。主要因下阴不洁,秽浊之邪从下入侵,热蕴膀胱,由腑及脏;饮食不节,过食肥甘辛辣,脾失健运,酿湿生热,湿热下注;年老体衰,肾气亏虚,膀胱气化无权。病位在肾和膀胱,主要病机是湿热蕴结下焦,膀胱气化失调。病久不愈,湿热耗

urinary bladder to control urination. The diseased parts are the kidneys and bladder, while the pathogenesis is the accumulation of damp heat in the lower energizer and obstruction of qi activities in the urinary bladder. In prolonged cases, healthy qi is consumed by damp heat, resulting in deficiency of the kidneys and spleen.

Essentials for Diagnosis

(1) Urinary infection, at the acute stage, is primarily manifested as the general symptoms like frequent, urgent and painful urination, lumbago or abdominal pain radiating down to the urethra, often accompanied by chills, fever, headache, lassitude, loss of appetite, nausea, etc. At the chronic stage, there may appear the same symptoms as those at the acute stage, but at a sudden onset of chronic urinary infection, the symptoms can be just as severe at the acute stage.

(2) There may be tenderness on costovertebral point, and positive percussion pain in the renal regions.

(3) Pyuria can be found in routine urine test. Under the high power lens, white cell count is often more than 5 per field, and leukocyte cast can also be found. Midstream urine reveals culture colony count$>10^5$/ml.

Syndrome Differentiation and Treatment

Syndrome differentiation of this disease mainly concerns with whether the syndromes are excess or deficiency ones. Excess syndromes result from the accumulation of damp heat in the lower energizer as well as obstruction of qi activities in the urinary bladder. The disease does not persist very long, often with difficult and painful urination, red tongue with yellow tongue coating, and rapid, full pulse. Deficiency syndromes are caused by

伤正气,可致脾肾亏虚。

【诊断要点】

(1) 本病急性期主要表现为尿频、尿急、尿痛,腰痛或向阴部下传的腹痛,常伴寒战、发热、头痛、乏力、食欲不振、恶心等全身症状。慢性期患者平日也常有尿频、尿急、尿痛、腰痛等不适症状。慢性期急性发作时,全身症状可与急性期一样剧烈。

(2) 体征主要有脊肋点(腰大肌外缘与十二肋交叉点)压痛,肾区叩击痛阳性。

(3) 尿常规检查可见脓尿,高倍镜下每视野白细胞数常在 5 个以上,并常出现白细胞管型。尿细菌培养(清洁中段尿培养),菌落计数$>10^5$/ml。

【辨证论治】

本病临床辨证主要是辨虚实。实证系湿热蕴结下焦,膀胱气化不利所致,病程较短,小便涩痛不利,苔黄舌红脉实数;虚证系脾肾两虚,膀胱气化无权,病程长,小便频急,痛涩不甚,苔薄舌淡,脉细数。实证治予清热利湿,虚证

deficiency of both the spleen and kidneys, and obstruction of qi activities in the urinary bladder, usually with a long course, frequent and urgent, but not very difficult and painful urination, pale tongue with thin coating, and rapid, thready pulse. For excess syndromes, the therapeutic method of clearing away heat is employed; for deficiency syndromes, that of nourishing the kidney and spleen is applied.

1. Damp Heat in the Urinary Bladder

Chief Manifestations: Frequent, dripping, and urgent urination with burning pain around the umbilicus, distending pain in the lower abdomen, and discharge of dark yellow urine, or bitter taste in the mouth and dry throat, nausea, vomiting, constipation, thin, yellow tongue coating, and soft-superficial, rapid pulse.

Therapeutic Methods: To induce diuresis, treat stranguria, clear away heat and remove toxic substances.

Prescription: Modified Bazheng San (Eight Health Restoring Powder), composed of Cheqianzi (*Semen Plantaginis*, wrapped) 12 g, Qumai (*Herba Dianthi*) 12 g, Mutong (*Caulis Akebiae*) 6 g, Huashi (*Talcum*, wrapped) 15 g, Bianxu (*Herba Polygoni Avicularis*) 12 g, Shengdahuang (*Radix et Rhizoma Rhei*, to be decocted later) 6 g, Gancaoshao (*Apex Radicis Glycyrrhizae*) 5 g and Dengxincao (*Medulla Junci*) 6 g.

Modifications: In cases of urinary stones, add Shiwei (*Folium Pyrrosiae*) 15 g, Jineijin (*Endothelium Corneum Gigeriae Galli*) 10 g, Jinqiancao (*Herba Lysimachiae*) 30 g and Yujin (*Radix Curcumae*) 10 g; in cases of high fever, add Jinyinhua (*Flos Lonicera*) 15 g, Huangqin (*Radix Scutellariae*) 12 g and Huangbai (*Cortex Phellodendri*) 10 g; for thick, greasy tongue coating and retention of damp heat, add Yiyiren (*Semen Coicis*) 20 g and Zhizi (*Fructus Gardeniae*) 10 g.

治当培补脾肾。

1. 膀胱湿热证

主要证候 小便频数,淋漓不爽,尿色黄赤,灼热刺痛,急迫不舒,痛引脐中,少腹满痛,或口苦咽干,恶心呕吐,大便秘结,苔薄黄,脉濡数。

治 法 利湿通淋,清热解毒。

方 药 八正散加减:车前子(包煎)12 g,瞿麦12 g,木通6 g,滑石(包煎)15 g,萹蓄12 g,生大黄(后下)6 g,甘草梢5 g,灯心草6 g。

加 减 若伴有泌尿系结石者,加石韦15 g,鸡内金10 g,金钱草30 g,郁金10 g;若发热重,加金银花15 g,黄芩12 g,黄柏10 g;若舌苔厚腻,湿热困重者,加薏苡仁20 g,栀子10 g。

2. Impairment of Blood Vessels by Heat

Chief Manifestations: Frequent, urgent and difficult urination with stabbing pain, discharge of scanty, dark red urine, sometimes with blood clot or urethral spasm, or restlessness, lumbago with tenderness, high fever with aversion to cold, red tongue with thick, dry and yellow coating, smooth and rapid pulse.

Therapeutic Methods: To clear away heat, induce diuresis, cool blood to stop bleeding.

Prescription: Modified Xiaoji Yinzi (*Cirsii Decoction*), composed of Shengdihuang (*Radix Rehmanniae*) 15 g, Xiaoji (*Herba Cirsii*) 15 g, Huashi (*Talcum*, wrapped) 12 g, Mutong (*Caulis Akebiae*) 3 g, Puhuang (*Pollen Typhae*, wrapped) 10 g, Danzhuye (*Herba Lophatheri*) 6 g, Danggui (*Radix Angelicae Sinensis*) 10 g, Zhizi (*Fructus Gardeniae*) 10 g and Zhigancao (*Radix Glycyrrhizae*, roasted) 3 g.

Modification: For predominant heat, high fever and aversion to cold, add Jinyinhua (*Flos Lonicera*) 30 g and Lianqiao (*Fructus Forsythiae*) 15 g; for conspitation, add Shengdahuang (*Radix et Rhizoma Rhei*, to be decocted later) 6 g; for impaired yin by heat, hyperactivity of fire due to yin deficiency, restlessness and dreamful sleep, sore loins and seminal emission, add Zhimu (*Rhizoma Anemarrhenae*) 10 g, Huangbai (*Cortex Phellodendri*) 10 g, Nüzhenzi (*Fructus Ligustri Lucidi*) 12 g and Hanliancao (*Herba Ecliptae*) 12 g.

3. Deficiency of Both the Spleen and Kidneys

Chief Manifestations: Prolonged course with alternation in severity, aggravated by overwork and cold, difficult and painful urination lessened with discharge of dark yellow urine, persistent dripping urination, listlessness, dull pain in the lower abdomen, nocturia, pale tongue, and feeble and rapid pulse.

2. 热伤血络证

主要证候 小便热涩刺痛,尿色深红,甚则夹有血块,溲频短急,甚则尿道挛急疼痛,或见心烦,腰痛拒按,高热恶寒,舌质红,苔黄厚燥,脉滑数。

治　法 清热利湿,凉血止血。

方　药 小蓟饮子加减:生地黄15 g,小蓟15 g,滑石(包煎)12 g,木通3 g,蒲黄(包煎)10 g,淡竹叶6 g,当归10 g,栀子10 g,炙甘草3 g。

加　减 若热邪较重,高热恶寒,加金银花30 g,连翘15 g;大便秘结者,加生大黄(后下)6 g;热邪伤阴,阴虚火旺,心烦多梦,腰酸遗精者,加知母10 g,黄柏10 g,女贞子12 g,旱莲草12 g。

3. 脾肾两虚证

主要证候 发病日久,缠绵难愈,时轻时重,遇劳及遇寒加重,小便赤涩不甚,溺痛不著,淋沥不已,精神困惫,小腹隐隐作痛,夜尿次数增多,舌淡,脉虚数。

Therapeutic Methods: To strengthen the spleen and nourish the kidney.

Prescription: Modified Wubi Shanyao Wan (Powerful Dioscoreae Pill), composed of Shanyao (*Rhizoma Dioscoreae*) 20 g, Fuling (*Poriae*) 12 g, Zexie (*Rhizoma Alismatis*) 12 g, Shudihuang (*Radix Rehmanniae Preparata*) 15 g, Shanzhuyu (*Fructus Corni*) 12 g, Bajitian (*Radix Morindae Officinalis*) 12 g, Tusizi (*Semen Cuscutae*) 12 g, Duzhong (*Cortex Eucommiae*) 12 g, Niuxi (*Radix Achyranthis Bidentatae*) 12 g, Wuweizi (*Fructus Schisandrae*) 5 g and Roucongrong (*Herba Cistanchis*) 10 g.

Modifications: For yin deficiency and retention of damp heat, manifested as vertigo, tinnitus, sore and weak loins and knees, dry throat and lips, frequent and scanty urine and painful, difficult urination, add Zhimu (*Rhizoma Anemarrhenae*) 10 g and Huangbai (*Cortex Phellodendri*) 10 g; for the case deteriorated by overstrain with distending and bearing-down sensation in the lower abdomen, dripping urine, mental fatigue, shortness of breath and unwillingness to speak, add Dangshen (*Radix Codonopsis*) 10 g, Huangqi (*Radix Astragali*) 12 g, Baizhu (*Rhizoma Atractylodis Macrocephalae*) 10 g, Shengma (*Rhizoma Cimicifugae*) 6 g and Chaihu (*Radix Bupleuri*) 6 g; for deficiency of kidney yang, aversion to cold in lower limbs and edema of limbs, add Lujiaofen (*Cornu Cervi*, to be powdered and taken separately) 3 g; for retention of damp heat, add Bianxu (*Herba Polygoni Avicularis*) 15 g and Qumai (*Herba Dianthi*) 15 g.

Other Treatments

1. Chinese Patent Drugs

(1) Fenqing Zhilin Wan (Pill for Relieving Stranguria): 6 g each time, twice or thrice daily; indicated for

治　法　健脾益肾。

方　药　无比山药丸加减：山药20 g,茯苓12 g,泽泻12 g,熟地黄15 g,山茱萸12 g,巴戟天12 g,菟丝子12 g,杜仲12 g,牛膝12 g,五味子5 g,肉苁蓉10 g。

加　减　若肾阴不足,湿热留恋,头晕耳鸣,腰膝酸软,咽干唇燥,尿频而短,小便涩痛者,加知母10 g,黄柏10 g;若因劳倦病情加重,小腹坠胀,迫注肛门,便意不尽,小便点滴而出,精神疲惫,少气懒言者,加党参10 g,黄芪12 g,白术10 g,升麻6 g,柴胡6 g。若肾阳不足,下肢怕凉,肢体浮肿,可加用鹿角粉(吞服)3 g。若湿热未尽者,加萹蓄15 g,瞿麦15 g。

【其他疗法】

1. 中成药

(1) 分清止淋丸　每服6 g,每日 2～3 次。适用于膀

the case with damp heat in the bladder, frequent, urgent and painful urination.

(2) Liuwei Dihuang Wan (Pill of Six Drugs Containing Rehmanniae): 9 g each time, twice a day; indicated for prolonged cases with deficiency of both the spleen and kidney.

(3) Buzhong Yiqi Wan (Pill for Strengthening Middle Energizer and Benefiting Qi): 9 g each time, twice a day; indicated for the case with distending and bearing-down sensation in the lower abdomen and dripping urine due to deficiency of spleen qi.

(4) Zhi Bai Dihuang Wan (Pill of Anemarrhena, Phellodendron and Rehmannia): 9 g each time, twice a day; indicated for the case with hyperactivity of fire and deficiency of yin.

(5) Sanmiao Wan (Three Wonder-Drug Pill): 6 g each time, twice a day; indicated for the case with excessive damp heat.

2. Simple-drug or Experiential Prescriptions

(1) Daqingye (*Folium Isatidis*) 30 g, Pugongying (*Herba Taraxaci*) 15 g, Lianqiao (*Fructus Forsythiae*) 10 g, Hanliancao (*Herba Ecliptae*) 15 g, Chuanduan (*Radix Dipsaci*) 12 g, Niuxi (*Radix Achyranthis Bidentatae*) 12 g, Huangbai (*Cortex Phellodendri*) 10 g, Zhimu (*Rhizoma Anemarrhenae*) 10 g, Huashi (*Talcum*, wrapped) 10 g, Zhizi (*Radix Gardeniae*) 4.5 g, Gancao (*Radix Glycyrrhizae*) 3 g and Haijinsha (*Spora Lygodii*, wrapped) 10 g. Decoct the above drugs in water, 1 dose daily. It is indicated for fever, frequent, urgent and painful urination at the early stage of urinary infection.

(2) Pugongying (*Herba Taraxaci*) 30 g, Jinyinhua (*Flos Lonicera*) 20 g, Jinqiancao (*Herba Lysimachiae*) 30 g, Danshen (*Radix Salviae Miltiorrhizae*) 12 g,

胱湿热所致的尿频、尿急、尿痛者。

（2）六味地黄丸　每服9 g,每日 2 次。适用于本病病久脾肾两虚者。

（3）补中益气丸　每服9 g,每日 2 次。适用于脾气虚弱所致的小腹坠胀,下迫肛门,小便淋沥之症。

（4）知柏地黄丸　每服9 g,每日 2 次。适用于本病阴虚火旺者。

（5）三妙丸　每服6 g,每日 2 次。适用于本病湿热偏盛者。

2. 单验方

（1）大青叶30 g,蒲公英15 g,连翘10 g,旱莲草15 g,川断12 g,牛膝12 g,黄柏10 g,知母10 g,滑石(包煎)10 g,栀子4.5 g,甘草3 g,海金沙(包煎)10 g。水煎服,每日 1 剂。适用于泌尿系感染初起,发热、尿频、尿急、尿痛者。

（2）蒲公英30 g,金银花20 g,金钱草30 g,丹参12 g,香附6 g,大腹皮10 g,小蓟15 g,

Xiangfu (*Rhizoma Cyperi*) 6 g, Dafupi (*Pericarpium Arecae*) 10 g, Xiaoji (*Herba Cirsii*) 15 g, Fuping (*Herba Spirodelae*) 15 g and Baimaogen (*Rhizoma Imperatae*) 15 g. Decoct the above drugs in water, one dose a day. It is indicated for urinary infection with severe hematuria.

(3) Danggui (*Radix Angelicae Sinensis*) 15 g, Chuanbeimu (*Bulbus Fritillariae Cirrhosae*) 9 g, Kushen (*Radix Sophorae Flavescentis*) 15 g, Mutong (*Caulis Akebiae*) 9 g, Zhuye (*Herba Lophatheri*) 9 g, Shengdihuang (*Radix Rehmanniae*) 9 g and Gancaoshao (*Apex Radicis Glycyrrhizae*) 9 g. Decoct the above drugs in water, one dose a day. It is indicated for acute nephropyelitis and cystitis.

(4) Shengdihuang (*Radix Rehmanniae*) 12 g, Mutong (*Caulis Akebiae*) 10 g, Gancaoshao (*Apex Radicis Glycyrrhizae*) 9 g, Zhuye (*Herba Lophatheri*) 6 g, Bianxu (*Herba Polygoni Avicularis*) 15 g, Shiwei (*Folium Pyrrosiae*) 15 g, Daji (*Herba seu Radix Cirsii Japonici*) 12 g, Xiaoji (*Herba Cirsii*) 12 g, Haijinsha (*Spora Lygodii*, wrapped) 12 g and Baimaogen (*Rhizoma Imperatae*) 15 g. Decoct the above drugs in water, one dose a day. It is indicated for urinary infection with severe hematuria.

2.5.4 Urolithiasis

General Description

Urolithiasis refers to the formation of calculi in urinary system. In the light of locations of calculi, it can be classified into renal calculus, ureteral calculus, cystic calculus and urethral calculus. Clinically, it is characterized by dull pain in the loins and abdomen, hematuria, cloudy

浮萍15 g,白茅根15 g。水煎服,每日 1 剂。适用于泌尿系感染血尿严重者。

(3) 当归15 g,川贝母9 g,苦参15 g,木通9 g,竹叶9 g,生地黄9 g,甘草梢9 g。水煎服,每日 1 剂。适用于急性肾盂肾炎、膀胱炎。

(4) 生地黄12 g,木通10 g,甘草梢9 g,竹叶6 g,萹蓄15 g,石韦15 g,大蓟12 g,小蓟12 g,海金沙(包煎)12 g,白茅根15 g。水煎服,每日 1 剂。适用于泌尿系感染血尿明显者。

第四节　泌尿系结石

【概述】

泌尿系统结石是指在泌尿系统中出现晶体块而言。根据晶体块停留的不同部位,分别称为肾结石、输尿管结石、膀胱结石和尿道结石。临

urine, acute obstructive oliguria, anuresis, even renal colic and acute renal failure.

According to its clinical manifestations, the disease pertains to "sha lin" (sandy stranguria), "shi lin" (stony stranguria), "xue lin" (bloody stranguria), "yao tong" (lumbago) in TCM. It usually results from external invasion of damp heat, or addiction to pungent, greasy and sweet food, either of which results in the retention of damp heat in the bladder, causing the formation of stones. The impaired parts are the bladder and kidneys, often involving the spleen and liver. The pathogenesis of the disease is primarily the retention of damp heat in the lower energizer and obstruction of qi activities in the bladder. In prolonged cases, pathogenic damp blocks yang qi, pathogenic heat turns into fire and further injures yin, or yin injures qi, thus leading to deficiency of both the spleen and kidneys. The syndrome is then transformed from the excess one to the deficiency one, or a combination of both.

Essentials for Diagnosis

(1) There is sudden onset of typical colic of the kidney and ureter, accompanied by macroscopic or microscopic hematuria. Sometimes only dull pain occurs in the loins and abdomen, often accompanied by sore and distending sensation. A history of stone discharge can also be indicative of the disease. Cystic and urethral calculus often exhibits such symptoms as difficulty in urination, interruption of urine stream, retention of urine, terminal hematuria, etc.

(2) Percussion pain or tenderness may be felt at the renal and urerteral regions.

(3) Increase of RBC can be found in urine examina-

床特点是腰部或腹部钝痛、血尿、混浊尿、急性梗阻性少尿、无尿,甚至出现肾绞痛或导致急性肾功能衰竭。

根据本病的临床表现,与中医学中的"砂淋"、"石淋"、"血淋"、"腰痛"等病类似。本病的形成,常由于外感湿热,或恣食辛热肥甘,酿成湿热,湿热下注膀胱,煎熬尿液而成结石。病位以膀胱和肾为主,常涉及肝、脾。其病机主要是湿热蕴结下焦,膀胱气化不利。若病程迁延日久,湿邪阻遏阳气,热邪化火伤阴,或阴伤及气,导致脾肾两虚,则病证由实转虚,或虚实夹杂。

【诊断要点】

(1) 有典型突然发作的肾或输尿管绞痛伴肉眼或镜下血尿;或仅有腰腹部钝痛,酸胀不适,或有排石史。膀胱、尿道结石则有排尿困难,尿流中断,尿潴留及终末血尿等症状。

(2) 急性发作时肾区或输尿管部位有叩痛,或压痛。

(3) 尿液镜检红细胞常增

tion under microscopy, sometimes accompanied by saline crystals especially after the colic and increased white blood cells or pus cells in complicated infection.

(4) 95% of the cases show radio-opaque urinary stones in X-ray plain film with clear indication of stone size, location, shape and amount. If X-ray plain film shows a negative result, it can not rule out the possibility of urolithiasis. Excretion urography or retrograde urography should be conducted to confirm the existence of the stones and their locations. This can also provide further information on the anotomic morphology of renal pelvis, renal calyces, ureter, confirmation of hydronephrosis and its seriousness, thinness or thickness of renal parenchyma, condition of renal function or confirmation of the congenital abnormality in upper urinary tract and other organic diseases.

(5) Nuclein renagram examination can reveal the condition of renal function and obstruction of upper urinary tract. Supersonic examination can help detect the stone: its size, location as well as the seriousness of hydronephrosis.

Syndrome Differentiation and Treatment

The disease pertains to excess syndrome at its early stage or on acute onset of colic. It mainly results from retention of damp heat and accumulation of stones in the lower energizer as well as stagnation of qi. In treatment, clearing away heat to induce diuresis, treating stranguria to eliminate stones, promoting and regulating circulation of qi are often employed. If the disease persists, it usually turns into deficiency syndrome which is primarily manifested as deficiency of the spleen and kidneys. In this case, invigorating the spleen and nourishing the kidneys, treating stranguria and eliminating stones are often employed. For combination of both excess and deficiency syndromes,

多,尤其是绞痛发作后,有时可出现盐类晶体,并发感染时可见较多白细胞或脓细胞。

(4) X线检查约95%的尿路结石在平片上显影,可显示结石的大小、位置、形态、数目。平片阴性,尚不能完全排除尿路结石者,尚需作排泄性尿路造影或逆行性尿路造影,以了解结石之有无及位置,并能进一步了解肾盂、肾盏、输尿管解剖形态,有无肾积水及其程度,肾实质厚薄,肾功能好坏,上尿路有无先天性异常和其他器质性病。

(5) 核素肾图检查能反映肾功能情况和上尿路梗阻和存在及其程度。超声波检查辅助诊断结石的存在及其大小、位置、肾积水的程度。

【辨证论治】

本病初起或急性绞痛发作阶段属实证,多由下焦湿热蕴结,砂石结聚,气滞不利所致,治宜清热利湿,通淋排石,利气疏导;病程日久,多转变为虚证,以脾肾亏虚为主,治宜健脾益肾,通淋消石;虚实夹杂时,则要量虚实之多少,采取攻补兼施、标本同治的方法。

simultaneous application of purging and tonifying methods, or simultaneous treatment for the principal and the secondary symptoms should be used.

1. Damp Heat at the Lower Energizer

Chief Manifestations: Frequent urination with burning sensation and piercing pain, dark, yellow urine, interrupted urine stream with stones, or cramping pain in lumbar region which radiates to the lower abdomen and vulva, or accompanied by chills and fever, bitter taste in the mouth, nausea and vomiting, yellow and greasy tongue coating, and rapid, slippery pulse.

Therapeutic Methods: To clear away heat, induce diuresis, treat stranguria and eliminate stones.

Prescription: Modified Bazheng San (Eight Health Restoring Powder), composed of Cheqianzi (*Semen Plantaginis*, wrapped) 12 g, Qumai (*Herba Dianthi*) 12 g, Mutong (*Caulis Akebiae*) 6 g, Huashi (*Talcum*, wrapped) 15 g, Bianxu (*Herba Polygoni Avicularis*) 12 g, Sheng Dahuang (*Radix et Rhizoma Rhei*, to be decocted later) 6 g, Gancaoshao (*Apex Radicis Glycyrrhizae*) 5 g, Zhizi (*Radix Gardeniae*) 10 g and Dengxincao (*Medulla Junci*) 6 g.

Modifications: For hematuria, add Xiaoji (*Herba Cirsii*) 10 g, Oujie (*Nodus Nelumbinis Rhizomatis*) 10 g, Puhuang (*Pollen Typhae*, wrapped) 10 g and Shiwei (*Folium Pyrrosiae*) 10 g; for yellow, cloudy and smelly urine, accompanied by conjunctival congestion, bitter taste in the mouth, and irritability, add Longdancao (*Radix Gentianae*) 6 g and Huangqin (*Radix Scutellariae*) 10 g.

2. Qi Stagnation and Blood Stasis

Chief Manifestations: Difficult micturition with dribbling urine and blood clot, distending or piercing pain in the lower abdomen, colic in the loins and abdomen,

1. 下焦湿热证

主要证候 小便频数,灼热刺痛,尿色黄赤,小便涩滞不畅,时有中断,或夹有砂石,或腰痛如绞,牵引少腹,连及外阴,可伴寒热、口苦、恶心呕吐,舌苔黄腻,脉滑数。

治 法 清热利湿,通淋排石。

方 药 八正散加减:车前子(包煎)12 g,瞿麦12 g,木通6 g,滑石(包煎)15 g,萹蓄12 g,生大黄(后下)6 g,甘草梢5 g,栀子10 g,灯心草6 g。

加 减 以血尿为主时,加小蓟10 g,藕节10 g,蒲黄(包煎)10 g,石韦10 g;若见小便黄浊臭秽,伴目赤口苦,心烦易怒者,加龙胆草6 g,黄芩10 g。

2. 气滞血瘀证

主要证候 小便涩滞,淋漓不畅,尿中夹有血块,少腹胀痛或刺痛,甚至腰腹绞痛,

dark purplish tongue with ecchymosis or petechia, deep, wiry or unsmooth pulse.

Therapeutic Methods: To activate qi and blood circulation, treat stranguria and eliminate stones.

Prescription: Modified Chenxiang San (Aquilariae Resinatum Powder) and Xuefu Zhuyu Tang (Decoction for Removing Blood Stasis in Chest), composed of Chenxiang (*Lignum Aquilariae Resinatum*) 6 g, Qingpi (*Pericarpium Citri Reticulatae Viride*) 6 g, Chenpi (*Pericarpium Citri Reticulatae*) 6 g, Wuyao (*Radix Linderae*) 10 g, Taoren (*Semen Persicae*) 10 g, Honghua (*Flos Carthami*) 10 g, Zhike (*Fructus Aurantii*) 10 g, Niuxi (*Radix Achyranthis Bidentatae*) 10 g, Dang-gui (*Radix Angelicae Sinensis*) 10 g and Chishaoyao (*Radix Paeoniae Rubra*) 10 g.

Modifications: For fullness in the chest and hypochondrium, add Chaihu (*Radix Bupleuri*) 6 g and Xiangfu (*Rhizoma Cyperi*) 6 g; for severe blood stasis and colic pain, add Zhiruxiang (*Resina Olibani Preparata*) 6 g and Zhimoyao (*Myrrha*) 6 g.

3. Deficiency of Spleen Qi and Kidney Qi

Chief Manifestations: Less difficulty in micturition with light red, dribbling urine, which occurs when the patient is overworked, or tiny stones in urine, sore and weak loins and knees, lassitude, pale tongue, thready and weak pulse.

Therapeutic Methods: To strengthen the spleen, tonify the kidney, replenish qi and remove stones.

Prescription: Modified Wubi Shanyao Wan (Powerful Dioscoreae Pill), composed of Dangshen (*Radix Codonopsis*) 10 g, Huangqi (*Radix Astragali*) 12 g, Baizhu (*Rhizoma Atractylodis Macrocephalae*) 10 g, Shanyao (*Rhizoma Dioscoreae*) 12 g, Qianshi (*Semen Euryales*) 10 g, Lianzirou (*Semen Nelumbinis*) 10 g, Shanzhuyu

舌质紫黯,或有瘀点、瘀斑,脉沉弦或涩。

治　法　行气活血,通淋排石。

方　药　沉香散合血府逐瘀汤加减:沉香6g,青皮6g,陈皮6g,乌药10g,桃仁10g,红花10g,枳壳10g,牛膝10g,当归10g,赤芍药10g。

加　减　兼胸闷胁胀者,加柴胡6g,香附6g;瘀血明显,疼痛较甚时,可加制乳香6g,制没药6g。

3. 脾肾气虚证

主要证候　小便不甚赤涩,但淋漓不已,时作时止,遇劳即发,或尿中有细砂石排出,腰膝酸软,神疲乏力,舌质淡,脉细弱。

治　法　健脾益肾,补气消石。

方　药　无比山药丸加减:党参10g,黄芪12g,白术10g,山药12g,芡实10g,莲子肉10g,山茱萸10g,杜仲10g,菟丝子10g,金樱子10g,煅牡蛎(先煎)15g。

(*Fructus Corni*) 10 g, Duzhong (*Cortex Eucommiae*) 10 g, Tusizi (*Semen Cuscutae*) 10 g, Jinyingzi (*Fructus Rosae Laevigatae*) 10 g and Duanmuli (*Concha Ostreae Usta*, to be decocted first) 15 g.

Modification: In case of sinking qi of the middle energizer, distending and bearing-down sensation of the lower abdomen, and dribbling urine, add Shengma (*Rhizoma Cimicifugae*) 6 g and Chaihu (*Radix Bupleuri*) 6 g.

4. Deficiency of Liver Yin and Kidney Yin

Chief Manifestations: Sore loins, weak knees, vertigo, tinnitus, tidal fever, night sweating, flushed cheeks and red lips, dry mouth, sore throat, dribbling urine occasionally with stones, red tongue with thin coating or no coating, deep, thready and rapid pulse.

Therapeutic Methods: To nourish yin, clear away heat, reinforce the kidney and remove stones.

Prescription: Modified Liuwei Dihuang Wan (Bolus of Six Drugs Containing Rehmanniae), composed of Shudihuang (*Radix Rehmanniae Preparata*) 12 g, Shanyao (*Rhizoma Dioscoreae*) 12 g, Shanzhuyu (*Fructus Corni*) 10 g, Mudanpi (*Cortex Moutan Radicis*) 10 g, Fuling (*Poriae*) 12 g, Zexie (*Rhizoma Alismatis*) 12 g, Hutaorou (*Semen Juglandis*) 10 g, Niuxi (*Radix Achyranthis Bidentatae*) 10 g and Jinqiancao (*Herba Lysimachiae*) 15 g.

Modifications: For deficient yin and hyperactive fire, add Zhimu (*Rhizoma Anemarrhenae*) 10 g and Huangbai (*Cortex Phellodendri*) 10 g; for hyperactive liver yang with dizziness and blurred vision, add Gouqizi (*Fructus Lycii*) 10 g and Juhua (*Flos Chrysanthemi*) 6 g.

5. Deficiency of Kidney Yang

Chief Manifestations: Sore and weak loins and

加　减　若中气下陷,小腹坠胀,尿滴而下,加升麻6 g,柴胡6 g。

4. 肝肾阴虚证

主要证候　腰酸膝软,头晕耳鸣,潮热盗汗,颧红唇赤,口干咽痛,小便淋漓不爽,或有砂石排出,舌质红,少苔或无苔,脉沉细数。

治　法　滋阴清热,益肾消石。

方　药　六味地黄丸加减:熟地黄12 g,山药12 g,山茱萸10 g,牡丹皮10 g,茯苓12 g,泽泻12 g,胡桃肉10 g,牛膝10 g,金钱草15 g。

加　减　阴虚火旺者,加知母10 g,黄柏10 g;肝阳上亢,头晕目眩者,加枸杞子10 g,菊花6 g。

5. 肾阳亏损证

主要证候　腰膝酸软,倦

knees, lassitude, aversion to cold, cold limbs, pale complexion, frequent and difficult urination or dribbling urine, pale tongue, deep, and thready pulse.

Therapeutic Methods: To warm kidney yang, treat stranguria and remove stones.

Prescription: Modified Jingui Shenqi Wan (Pill for Invigorating Kidney Qi from *Golden Cabinet*), composed of Shufuzi (*Radix Aconiti Lateralis Preparata*) 6 g, Rougui (*Cortex Cinnamomi*) 5 g, Shudihuang (*Radix Rehmanniae Preparata*) 12 g, Shanyao (*Rhizoma Dioscoreae*) 12 g, Shanzhuyu (*Fructus Corni*) 10 g, Mudanpi (*Cortex Moutan Radicis*) 10 g, Fuling (*Poria*) 12 g, Zexie (*Rhizoma Alismatis*) 12 g, Hutaorou (*Semen Juglandis*) 10 g, Jineijin (*Endothelium Corneum Gigeriae Galli*) 10 g and Jinqiancao (*Herba Lysimachiae*) 15 g.

Modification: In case of edema in the lower limbs, add Fangji (*Radix Stephaniae Tetrandrae*) 10 g, Yiyiren (*Semen Coicis*) 15 g and Cheqianzi (*Semen Plantaginis*, wrapped) 12 g.

Other Treatments

1. Chinese Patent Drugs

(1) Paishi Chongji (Granule for Removing Stones): 1 sachet each time, three times daily; indicated for urolithrasis.

(2) Jinqiancao Chongji (Lysimachiae Granule): 1 sachet each time, three times daily; indicated for urolithrasis.

2. Single-drug or Experiential Prescriptions

(1) Decoct Hetaoren (*Semen Persicae*) 60 g and Zhihuangqi (*Radix Astragali*, roasted) 30 g in water, 1 dose daily. It is indicated for renal calculus.

(2) Decoct Maoxucao (*Herba Clerodendranthi Spicati*, dried whole plant) 60 g in water, 1 dose daily. It is

倦乏力,畏寒肢冷,面色苍白,小便频数而排出无力,或余沥不尽,舌质淡,脉沉细。

治　法　温补肾阳,通淋消石。

方　药　《金匮》肾气丸加减:熟附子6 g,肉桂5 g,熟地黄12 g,山药12 g,山茱萸10 g,牡丹皮10 g,茯苓12 g,泽泻12 g,胡桃肉10 g,鸡内金10 g,金钱草15 g。

加　减　下肢浮肿者,加防己10 g,薏苡仁15 g,车前子(包煎)12 g。

【其他疗法】

1. 中成药

(1) 排石冲剂　每服1包,每日3次。适用于泌尿系结石。

(2) 金钱草冲剂　每服1包,每日3次。适用于泌尿系结石。

2. 单验方

(1) 核桃仁60 g,炙黄芪30 g,水煎服,每日1剂。适用于肾结石。

(2) 猫须草全草(干燥品)60 g,水煎服,每日1剂。适用

indicated for urinary calculus.

(3) Grind the same amount of Jineijin (*Endotheli-um Corneum Gigeriae Galli*) and Mangxiao (*Natrii Sulphas*) into fine powder, decoct Jinqiancao (*Herba Ly-simachiae*) 60 g in water, and take 6 g of the powder with the decoction, once or twice daily. It is indicated for urolithrasis with difficulty in discharging stones.

(4) Crush Hulugua (*Fructus Lagenaria Sicerar-rae*, fresh) to collect juice, mix the juice with honey and take half a cup to one cup each time, twice daily, or boil Hulugua (*Fructus Lagenaria Sicerarrae*) in water and take the soup. It is indicated for urolithasis with difficulty in discharging stones.

(5) Dongkuizi (*Fructus Malvae Vertillatae*) 18 g, Shiwei (*Folium Pyrrosiae*) 12 g, Huashi (*Talcum*, wrapped) 12 g, Chuanduan (*Radix Dipsaci*) 12 g, Baizhu (*Rhizoma Atractylodis Macrocephalae*) 12 g, Biejia (*Carapax Trionycis*, to be decocted first) 15 g, Wang-buliuxing (*Semen Vaccariae*) 12 g, Niuxi (*Radix Achy-ranthis Bidentatae*) 10 g, Hutaorou (*Semen Juglandis*) 10 g, Hupomo (*Succinum*, powdered and to be infused separately) 1.5 g and Cheqiancao (*Herba Plantaginis*) 12 g. Decoct the above drugs in water, 1 dose daily. The recipe is effective for dissolving stones and can be used to treat urolithiasis.

(6) Biejia (*Carapax Trionycis*, to be decocted first) 15 g, Xiakucao (*Spica Prunellae*) 10 g, Shengyi-yiren (*Semen Coicis*) 15 g, Baizhi (*Radix Angelicae Dahuricae*) 10 g, Jinqiancao (*Herba Lysimachiae*) 30 g, Shensanqifen (*Radix Notoginseng*, powdered and to be infused separately) 3 g, Haijinsha (*Spora Lygodii*, wrapped) 30 g, Cangzhu (*Rhizoma Atractylodis*) 15 g, Huashi (*Talcum*, wrapped) 15 g. Decoct the above drugs in water, take the decoction in 2 divided doses a

于尿路结石。

(3) 鸡内金、芒硝等量,共研极细末,每次取药粉6g,用金钱草60g煎汤送服。每日1~2次。适用于泌尿系统结石难以排出者。

(4) 鲜葫芦瓜捣烂取汁,用蜂蜜调服,每次半杯至1杯,每日 2 次,或用葫芦瓜煮汤服食。适用于泌尿系结石难以排出者。

(5) 冬葵子18g,石韦12g,滑石(包煎)12g,川断12g,白术12g,鳖甲(先煎)15g,王不留行12g,牛膝10g,胡桃肉10g,琥珀末(另冲)1.5g,车前草12g,水煎服,每日 1 剂。本方有一定的溶石作用,可用于泌尿系结石。

(6) 鳖甲(先煎)15g,夏枯草10g,生薏苡仁15g,白芷10g,金钱草30g,参三七粉(另冲)3g,海金沙(包煎)30g,苍术15g,滑石(包煎)15g。水煎服,每日 1 剂,分 2次服。本方有一定的溶石作用,可用于泌尿系结石而结石较大者。

day. This recipe is effective for dissolving stones and can be employed to remove bigger stones of urinary system.

2.5.5   Impotence

General Description

Impotence refers to the inability to have an erection of the penis or the weak erection of the penis in males before climacteric.

The disease is usually attributive to excessive sexual activities and masturbation or frequent seminal emission that characterizes deficiency of essence. It may also be caused by anxiety and fright which impair the heart and spleen or the heart and kidneys. In some cases, it may result from the downward movement of damp heat. Its pathogenesis is flaccidity of penis which fails to achieve a satisfactory erection. Its pathological nature pertains to deficiency syndrome in most cases and in some cases, excess ones. The deficiency syndrome is caused by damage of essence, decline of fire of the life gate, deficiency of qi and blood, as well as lack of nourishment in the genita, with most of the cases characterized by decline of fire of the life gate. The downward movement of damp heat, however, is indicative of excess syndrome, but not as common as deficiency one. The pathogenesis of excess syndrome is the decline of fire of the life gate in most cases and the downflow of damp heat in less cases.

Impotence, in western medicine, can occur in male sexual disorder or some chronic diseases.

Essentials for Diagnosis

(1) The disease is characterized by inability to have an erection of penis during sexual intercourse in males before climacteric.

第五节　阳痿

【概述】

阳痿是指阴茎萎软不举，或临房举而不坚的病证。

本病的病因主要有纵欲过度、严重手淫，或遗精频作导致精气虚损；或因思虑、惊恐，损伤心脾、心肾；少数可因湿热下注所致。主要病机为宗筋弛纵，萎软不举，病理性质虚多实少。因精气虚损，命门火衰，气血不荣，宗筋失润者为虚证，尤以命门火衰者居多；湿热下注致痿者属实，但较少见。其病机以命门火衰较为多见，而湿热下注较为少见。

阳痿可见于西医学的男子性功能障碍和某些慢性疾病等。

【诊断要点】

（1）青壮年男子性交时，由于阴茎不能有效地勃起，无法进行正常的性生活，即可诊

(2) It can be attributive to excessive sexual activities, prolonged illness, weak constitution, frequent masturbation in youngsters, accompanied by lassitude, weak loins and knees, aversion to cold, cold limbs, or difficulty in urination with dribbling urine.

(3) Impotence due to hypoplasia of sex organ or the use of drugs should be excluded.

(4) Distinguish impotence from premature ejaculation. Premature ejaculation refers to early ejaculation of semen at the beginning of sexual intercourse and inability to carry on sexual intercourse because of flaccidity of the penis immediately after the ejaculation. However, impotence means the inability to achieve a satisfactory penile erection. They present marked differences. Nonetheless, if premature ejaculation persists, impotance may ensue.

Syndrome Differentiation and Treatment

Differentiation of the disease primarily concerns whether or not impotence pertains to deficiency syndrome or excess one, whether or not there exists the hyperactive fire. Impotence attributive to sex excess, anxiety, depression and fright is mainly indicative of deficiency of the spleen and kidneys, decline of fire of the life gate, thus pertaining to deficiency syndrome. Impotence due to the transformation of stagnant liver qi into fire, downward movement of damp heat and flaccidity of penis pertains to excess syndrome. Impotence with pale complexion, aversion to cold, cold limbs, pale tongue with white coating, deep and thready pulse is indicative of the nonexistence of fire; while the one with irritability, dark yellow urine, greasy and yellowish tongue coating, soft-superficial, rapid or wiry, rapid pulse is indicative of the hyperactive fire. To treat impotence, tonifying method should be employed for deficiency syndrome and purgative method for

断为本病。

（2）多有房事太过，久病体虚，或青少年频犯手淫史，常伴有神疲乏力，腰酸膝软，畏寒肢冷，或小便不畅，滴沥不尽等症。

（3）排除性器官发育不全，或药物引起的阳痿。

（4）要注意与早泄相区别。早泄是指在性交之初，阴茎虽能勃起，挺而不坚，旋即排精，不能完成正常性生活的现象。阳痿是指性交时阴茎不能勃起，两者有所不同，但早泄日久，可进一步导致阳痿的发生。

【辨证论治】

阳痿的辨证主要是辨其属虚属实和有火无火。由于恣情纵欲，思虑忧郁、惊恐所伤者，多为脾肾亏虚，命门火衰，属于虚证；由于肝郁化火，湿热下注，综筋弛纵者，属于实证。阳痿而兼见面色㿠白，畏寒肢冷，舌淡苔白，脉沉细者，是为无火；阳痿而兼见烦躁易怒，小便黄赤，苔黄腻，脉濡数或弦数者，是为有火。阳痿的治疗，属虚者宜补，属实者宜泻；有火者宜清，无火者宜温。

excess syndrome; heat clearing method for hyperactive fire and warming method for non-existence of fire.

1. Decline of Fire of the Life Gate

Chief Manifestations: Inability to have penis erection, thinness of seminal fluid, dizziness, tinnitus, pale complexion, listlessness, weak and sore loins and knees, aversion to cold, cold limbs, pale tongue with white coating, deep and thready pulse.

Therapeutic Method: To warm and nourish the kidney.

Prescription: Modified Zanyu Dan (Zanyu Pill), composed of Bajitian (*Radix Morindae Officinalis*) 10 g, Xianmao (*Rhizoma Curculiginis*) 10 g, Yinyanghuo (*Herba Epimedii*) 10 g, Jiucaizi (*Semen Allii Tuberosi*) 10 g, Tusizi (*Semen Cuscutae*) 10 g, Roucongrong (*Herba Cistanchis*) 10 g, Shudihuang (*Radix Rehmanniae Preparata*) 12 g, Shanyao (*Rhizoma Dioscoreae*) 12 g, Shanzhuyu (*Fructus Corni*) 10 g and Gouqizi (*Fructus Lycii*) 10 g.

Modification: For very weak and sore loins and knees, add Duzhong (*Cortex Eucommiae*) 10 g and Niuxi (*Radix Achyranthis Bidentatae*) 10 g.

2. Impairment of the Heart and Spleen

Chief Manifestations: Inability to have penis erection, listlessness, disturbed sleep, impaired appetite, lusterless complexion, pale tongue with thin, greasy coating, thready pulse.

Therapeutic Method: To tonify and nourish the heart and spleen.

Prescription: Modified Guipi Tang (Decoction for Invigorating Spleen and Nourishing Heart), composed of Dangshen (*Radix Codonopsis*) 10 g, Baizhu (*Rhizoma Atractylodis Macrocephalae*), Huangqi (*Radix Astragali*) 12 g, Danggui (*Radix Angelicae Sinensis*)

1. 命门火衰证

主要证候　阳事不举,精薄清冷,头晕耳鸣,面色㿠白,精神委靡,腰膝酸软,畏寒肢冷,舌质淡,苔白,脉沉细。

治　法　温补下元。

方　药　赞育丹加减:巴戟天10 g,仙茅10 g,淫羊藿10 g,韭菜子10 g,菟丝子10 g,肉苁蓉10 g,熟地黄12 g,山药12 g,山茱萸10 g,枸杞子10 g。

加　减　若腰膝酸软明显者,加杜仲10 g,牛膝10 g。

2. 心脾受损证

主要证候　阳事不举,精神不振,夜寐不安,胃纳不佳,面色不华,苔薄腻,舌质淡,脉细。

治　法　补益心脾。

方　药　归脾汤加减:党参10 g,白术10 g,黄芪12 g,当归10 g,白芍药10 g,桂圆肉10 g,远志6 g,茯神10 g,夜交藤10 g,陈皮6 g,大枣 5 枚,炙

10 g, Baishaoyao (*Radix Paeoniae Alba*) 10 g, Guiyuanrou (*Arillus Longan*) 10 g, Yuanzhi (*Radix Polygalae*) 6 g, Fushen (*Sclerotium Poriae Circum Radicem Pini*) 10 g, Yiejiaoteng (*Caulis et Folium Polygoni Multiflori*) 10 g, Chenpi (*Pericarpium Citri Reticulatae*) 6 g, Dazao (*Fructus Jujubae*) 5 pcs and Zhigancao (*Radix Glycyrrhizae, roasted*) 3 g.

Modification: For palpitation and insomnia, add Baihe (*Bulbus Lilli*) 10 g and Hehuanpi (*Cortex Albiziae*) 6 g.

3. Impairment of the Kidney due to Fright

Chief Manifestations: Inability to have penis erection or weak erection of the penis, timidity, oversentiveness, palpitation, insomnia, thin and greasy tongue coating, wiry and thready pulse.

Therapeutic Methods: To nourish the kidney and tranquilize the mind.

Prescription: Modified Da Buyuan Jian (Potent Decoction for Replenishing Primordial Qi), composed of Shudihuang (*Radix Rehmanniae Preparata*) 12 g, Shanzhuyu (*Fructus Corni*) 10 g, Shanyao (*Rhizoma Dioscoreae*) 10 g, Gouqizi (*Fructus Lycii*) 10 g, Dangshen (*Radix Codonopsis*) 10 g, Danggui (*Radix Angelicaer Sinensis*) 10 g and Duzhong (*Cortex Eucommiae*) 10 g.

Modifications: For restlessness, add Suanzaoren (*Semen Ziziphi Spinosae*) 10 g and Yuanzhi (*Radix Polygalae*) 6 g; for descent of qi due to fright, add Shengma (*Rhizoma Cimicifugae*) 6 g and Chaihu (*Radix Bupleuri*) 6 g.

4. Stagnation of Liver Qi

Chief Manifestations: Inability to have penis erection, depression or irritability, feeling of discomfort in the chest, distention and fullness in hypochondrum, poor

甘草3 g。

加 减 心悸失眠者,加百合10 g,合欢皮6 g。

3. 恐惧伤肾证

主要证候 阳痿不举,举而不刚,胆怯多疑,心悸易惊,寐不安宁,苔薄腻,脉弦细。

治 法 益肾宁神。

方 药 大补元煎加减:熟地黄12 g,山茱萸10 g,山药10 g,枸杞子10 g,党参10 g,当归10 g,杜仲10 g。

加 减 若心神不宁,可加酸枣仁10 g,远志6 g;因恐则气下,加升麻6 g,柴胡6 g。

4. 肝郁不舒证

主要证候 阳痿不举,情绪抑郁或烦躁易怒,胸脘不适,胁肋胀闷,食少便溏,苔

appetite, loose stools, thin tongue coating, wiry pulse.

Therapeutic Methods: To soothe liver qi and relieve depression.

Prescription: Modified Xiaoyao San (Xiaoyao Powder), composed of Chaihu (*Radix Bupleuri*, stir-baked with vinegar) 6 g, Danggui (*Radix Angelicae Sinensis*) 10 g, Baishaoyao (*Radix Paeoniae Alba*) 10 g, Fuling (*Poria*) 10 g, Guangyujin (*Radix Curcumae*) 10 g, Chaobaizhu (*Rhizoma Atractylodis Macrocephalae*, stir-baked) 10 g, Chaoyiyiren (*Semen Coicis*, stir-baked) 15 g, Chaoguya (*Fructus Oryzae Germinatus*, stir-baked) 15 g and Chaomaiya (*Fructus Hordei Germinatus*, stir-baked) 15 g.

Modifications: For transformation of stagnant liver qi into fire, add Mudanpi (*Cortex Moutan Radicis*) 10 g and Zhizi (*Fructus Gardeniae*) 10 g; for yin impairment due to fire, add Heshouwu (*Radix Polygoni Multiflori*) 10 g, Gouqizi (*Fructus Lycii*) 10 g and Shudihuang (*Radix Rehmanniae Preparata*) 10 g.

5. Downward Movement of Damp Heat

Chief Manifestations: Inability to have penis erection, damp and smelly scrotum, soreness of lower limbs, dark yellow urine, yellow and greasy tongue coating, and soft-superficial, rapid pulse.

Therapeutic Method: To remove damp heat.

Prescription: Longdan Xiegan Tang (Gentianae Decoction for Purging Liver Fire), composed of Longdancao (*Radix Gentianae*) 6 g, Zhizi (*Fructus Gardeniae*) 10 g, Huangqin (*Radix Scutellariae*) 10 g, Chaihu (*Radix Bupleuri*) 6 g, Gancao (*Radix Glycyrrhizae*) 3 g, Mutong (*Caulis Akebiae*) 3 g, Zexie (*Rhizoma Alismatis*) 10 g, Cheqianzi (*Semen Plantaginis*, wrapped) 10 g, Shengdihuang (*Radix Rehmanniae*) 12 g and Danggui (*Radix Angelicae Sinensis*) 10 g.

薄,脉弦。

治 法 疏肝解郁。

方 药 逍遥散加减:
醋炒柴胡6 g,当归10 g,白芍药10 g,茯苓10 g,广郁金10 g,炒白术10 g,炒薏苡仁15 g,炒谷芽15 g,炒麦芽15 g。

加 减 气郁化火者,加牡丹皮10 g,栀子10 g;郁火伤阴者,加何首乌10 g,枸杞子10 g,熟地黄10 g。

5. 湿热下注证

主要证候 阴茎萎软,阴囊潮湿、臊臭,下肢酸困,小便黄赤,苔黄腻,脉濡数。

治 法 清化湿热。

方 药 龙胆泻肝汤:
龙胆草6 g,栀子10 g,黄芩10 g,柴胡6 g,甘草3 g,木通3 g,泽泻10 g,车前子(包煎)10 g,生地黄12 g,当归10 g。

Modifications：For impaired liver yin and kidney yin and disturbance of deficient fire, marked by penis erection and seminal emission in the dream, spontaneous perspiration during sleep, restlesness with feverish sensation in the chest, palms and soles, soreness of the loins and knees, red tongue with reduced saliva, and wiry, thready, rapid pulse, use the following to nourish yin and purge fire：Zhimu (*Rhizoma Anemarrhenae*) 10 g, Huangbai (*Cortex Phellodendri*) 10 g, Shudihuang (*Radix Rehmanniae Preparata*) 10 g, Shanyao (*Rhizoma Dioscoreae*) 10 g, Shanzhuyu (*Fructus Corni*) 10 g, Gouqizi (*Fructus Lycii*) 12 g, Fuling (*Poria*) 10 g, Mudanpi (*Cortex Moutan Radicis*) 10 g and Zexie (*Rhizoma Alismatis*) 10 g.

Other Treatments
1. Chinese Patent Drugs
(1) Jingui Shenqi Wan (Pill for Invigorating Kidney Qi from *Golden Cabinet*)：6 g each time, twice a day; indicated for impotence attributive to deficiency of kidney yang.

(2) Quan Lu Wan (Quan Lu Pill)：6 g each time, twice a day; indicated for impotence attributive to deficiency of kidney yang.

2. Single-drug or Experiential Prescriptions
(1) Niubian (*Testis et Pennis Bovis*) 1 piece, Jiucaizi (*Semen Allii Tuberosi*) 25 g, Yinyanghuo (*Herba Epimedii*) 15 g and Tusizi (*Semen Cuscutae*) 15 g. Put Niubian (*Testis et Pennis Bovis*) on a tile, bake it dry on a slow fire, then grind it into powder; stir-bake Yinyanghuo (*Herba Epimedii*) with a small amount of sheep oil in an iron pot on a slow fire until it turns yellow, and grind it with Tusizi (*Semen Cuscutae*) and Jiucaizi (*Semen Allii Tuberosi*) into powder. Mix up the above ingredients, infuse one spoon of the mixed powder with yellow rice

加　减　若症见梦中阳举,举则遗精,寐则盗汗,五心烦热,腰酸膝软,舌红少津,脉弦细数,为肝肾阴伤,虚火妄动,治宜滋阴降火,用知母10 g,黄柏10 g,熟地黄10 g,山药10 g,山茱萸10 g,枸杞子12 g,茯苓10 g,牡丹皮10 g,泽泻10 g。

【其他疗法】
1. 中成药
(1)《金匮》肾气丸　每服6 g,每日2次。用于肾阳亏虚之阳痿。

(2) 全鹿丸　每服6 g,每日2次。用于肾阳亏虚之阳痿。

2. 单验方
(1) 牛鞭1根,韭菜子25 g,淫羊藿15 g,菟丝子15 g。将牛鞭置于瓦上用文火焙干,磨细;淫羊藿放入铁锅,加少许羊油,文火炒黄,再和菟丝子、韭菜子磨成细面;将上药混匀。每晚用黄酒冲服1匙,或将1匙药粉用蜂蜜和成丸,用黄酒送服。适用于肾阳虚之阳痿。

wine and take it every night, or prepare one spoon of the mixed powder with honey, shape it to pills and take it with yellow rice wine. It is indicated for impotence attributive to deficiency of kidney yang.

(2) Yanggaowan (*Testis Caprinus*) 2 pcs and a small amount of old wine. Steam Yanggaowan (*Testis Caprinus*) with old wine, and take it every morning for a month as a course of treatment. It is indicated for impotence due to decline of fire of the life gate.

3. External Therapy

(1) Grind Xiaohuixiang (*Fructus Foenicuii*) 5 g and Paojiang (*Rhizoma Zingiberis Recens*, roasted in hot cinders) 5 g into powder, mix the powder with a small amount of salt and a proper amount of breast milk(or honey or chicken blood). Apply the paste on the umbilicus and change the dressing every 5 - 7 days, ten times being a course of treatment. It is indicated for impotence due to deficiency of kidney yang.

(2) Grind the same amount of Shechuangzi (*Fructus Cnidii*), Yuanzhi (*Radix Polygalae*), Fengfang (*Nidus Vespae*), Xixin (*Herba Asari*) and Dilong (*Pheretima*) together into powder, and apply a little to the penis each time. It is indicated for impotence due to decline of fire of the life gate.

2.5.6 Spermatorrhea

General Description

Spermatorrhea refers to involuntary discharge of seminal fluid without sexual intercourse. It is usually caused by kidney deficiency and weakness of the seminal gate or hyperactive monarch fire and minister fire, downward movement of damp heat, which disturb the seminal vesicle. Seminal emission during dreamful sleep is referred to

（2）羊睾丸 2 只，加陈酒少许，每晨蒸服，连服 1 个月为 1 个疗程。适用于命火衰微之阳痿。

3. 外治法

（1）小茴香5 g，炮姜5 g，研末，加食盐少许，用适量人乳调和（也可用蜂蜜或鸡血），敷于肚脐，5～7 日更换 1 次，10 次为 1 个疗程。适用于阳痿肾阳虚型。

（2）蛇床子、远志、蜂房、细辛、地龙各等分，共为细末，每用少许涂阴茎上。适用于阳痿命门火衰型。

第六节　遗精

【概述】

遗精是指不因性生活而精液频繁遗泄的病证。多因肾虚精关不固，或君相火旺、湿热下注等，扰动精室所致。有梦而遗精，称为梦遗；无梦而遗精，甚至清醒时精液流

as nocturnal emission; while that during dreamless sleep or when being awake is termed as spontaneous emission.

The major causes of the disease may be indulgence in sexual activities, weak congenital constitution, mental strain, anxiety for seeking sexual pleasure and improper diet. Etiologically, its occurrence is usually closely relevant to the impaired heart, liver and kidneys. Apart from deficiency of the kidneys and inability to arrest semen, hyperactivity of heart fire and liver fire can also impair the renal ability to store essence.

Spermatorrhea, in western medicine, may be present in neurasthenia and prostatitis.

Essentials for Diagnosis

(1) If emission of semen occurs in married males more than once a week, and often during sleep without sexual activities, or if the unmarried have seminal emission more than twice a week, accompanied by tinnitus, vertigo, lassitude, soreness of loins and knees which persist for over a month, these can be indicative of the disease.

(2) Rectum digital examination, ultrasonography B over the prostate and seminal fluid examination can help determine the diagnosis.

(3) Spermatorrhea should be distinguished from overflow of seminal fluid and premature ejaculation. Overflow of seminal fluid is a physiological phenomenon where the unmarried or the healthy man who has not had sexual intercourse for a long time has seminal emission once or twice a month without any indisposition or other symptoms the following day. Premature ejaculation refers to the early ejaculation of sperm during sexual activity and inability to carry on sexual intercourse.

出,称滑精。

本病的病因主要有恣情纵欲、禀赋不足、劳心过度、思欲不遂、饮食不节等。遗精的发病机理,主要责之于心、肝、肾三脏。本病除肾脏自虚,精关不固外,心肝之火内动,也能影响肾的封藏。

遗精可见于西医学的神经衰弱、前列腺炎等。

【诊断要点】

(1) 已婚男子不因性生活而排泄精液,多在睡眠中发生,每星期超过 1 次以上;或未婚男子频繁发生精液遗泄,每星期超过 2 次以上者,伴有耳鸣、头昏、神倦乏力、腰酸膝软等症,持续 1 个月以上,即可诊断为本病证。

(2) 直肠指诊、前列腺 B 超及精液常规等检查,可协助病因诊断。

(3) 本病要与溢精和早泄相区别。溢精是指成年未婚男子,或婚后夫妻分居者,1 个月遗精 1～2 次,次日并无不适感觉或其他症状,属于精满自溢的生理现象,并非病态。早泄是指性交时精液过早泄出而不能完成正常的性生活。

Syndrome Differentiation and Treatment

At the early stage, spermatorrhea is mainly attributive to hyperactivity of monarch fire and minister fire and downward movement of damp heat which disturbs seminal vesicle, thus pertaining to excess syndrome. If the disease persists and is caused by deficiency of yin, hyperactivity of fire, inability to store essence due to kidney deficiency, it pertains to deficiency syndrome. To treat excess syndrome, heat-clearing methods such as removing heart fire and clearing away damp heat should be employed. To treat deficiency syndrome, kidney-reinforcing methods such as nourishing yin, purging fire, tonifying the kidneys and consolidating essence should be used. However, both should be used simultaneously in case of excess syndrome combined with deficiency one.

1. Hyperactivity of Monarch Fire and Minister Fire

Chief Manifestations: Insomnia with dreamful sleep, nocturnal emission during sleep, accompanied by feverish sensation in the heart, dizziness, blurred vision, listlessness, lassitude, palpitation, fright and forgetfulness, dry mouth, scanty and deep-colored urine, red tongue, and thready, rapid pulse.

Therapeutic Methods: To clear away heart fire, tranquilize the mind, nourish yin and remove heat.

Prescription: Modified Huanglian Qingxin Yin (Coptidis Decoction for Clearing Heart Fire), composed of Huanglian (*Rhizoma Coptidis*) 3 g, Zhizi (*Fructus Gardeniae*) 10 g, Zhimu (*Rhizoma Anemarrhenae*) 10 g, Huangbai (*Cortex Phellodendri*) 10 g, Shengdihuang (*Radix Rehmanniae*) 10 g, Yuanzhi (*Radix Polygalae*) 6 g, Suanzaoren (*Semen Ziziphi Spinosae*) 10 g and Lianzi (*Semen Nelumbinis*) 10 g.

Modifications: In cases of hyperactive liver fire

【辨证论治】

遗精初起者,多因君相火旺、湿热下注,拢动精室而遗,属实;久病,以阴虚火旺、肾虚不固、封藏失职致遗,属虚。在治疗方法上,实证宜清,分别治予清心泻火、清利湿热法;虚证宜固,治以滋阴降火、补肾固精等法。虚实夹杂者酌情兼顾。

1. 君相火旺证

主要证候 少寐多梦,梦则遗精,伴有心中烦热,头晕目眩,精神不振,倦怠乏力,心悸不宁,善恐健忘,口干,小溲短赤,舌质红,脉细数。

治 法 清心安神,滋阴清热。

方 药 黄连清心饮加减:黄连3g,栀子10g,知母10g,黄柏10g,生地黄10g,远志6g,酸枣仁10g,莲子10g。

加 减 肝火偏旺,面红

with flushed face, conjunctival congestion, restlessness, irritability, wiry and rapid pulse, add Xiakucao (*Spica Prunellae*) 10 g and Longdancao (*Radix Gentianae*) 5 g; in cases of deficient yin with vertigo, tinnitus and red tongue, add Tianmendong (*Radix Asparagi*) 10 g and Xuanshen (*Radix Scrophulariae*) 10 g.

2. Downward Movement of Damp Heat

Chief Manifestations: Frequent seminal emission, or discharge of small amount of seminal fluid during urination, difficult micturition with a burning sensation and deep-colored or dribbling urine, bitter taste in the mouth or thirst, restlessness, insomnia, orolingual ulceration, loose and foul stools, or feeling of oppression and fullness in the chest and abdomen, nausea, yellow, greasy tongue coating, and soft-superficial, rapid pulse.

Therapeutic Methods: To remove heat and induce diuresis.

Prescription: Modified Chengshi Bixie Fenqing Yin (Cheng's Decoction of Dioscoreae Septemlobae for Clearing Turbid Urine), composed of Bixie (*Rhizoma Dioscoreae Septemlobae*) 10 g, Huangbai (*Cortex Phellodendri*) 10 g, Fuling (*Poria*) 10 g, Shengyiyiren (*Semen Coicis*) 12 g, Cheqianzi (*Semen Plantaginis*, wrapped) 10 g, Lianzi (*Semen Nelumbinis*) 10 g, Shichangpu (*Rhizoma Acori Tatarinowii*) 6 g and Baizhu (*Rhizoma Atractylodis Macrocephalae*) 10 g.

Modifications: For retention of damp heat in the liver meridian, dark-yellow urine, itching and pain of penis, add Longdancao (*Radix Gentianae*) 5 g, Kushen (*Radix Sophorae Flavescentis*) 10 g and Mutong (*Caulis Akebiae*) 6 g; for prolonged illness with stagnant heat, manifested as dribbling urine, fullness in the lower abdomen and pudendum, add Baijiangcao (*Herba Patriniae cum Radice*) 10 g and Chishaoyao (*Radix Paeoniae*

目赤,烦躁易怒,脉弦数,加夏枯草10 g,龙胆草5 g;兼有阴虚,眩晕耳鸣,舌红,加天门冬10 g,玄参10 g。

2. 湿热下注证

主要证候　遗精频作,或尿时少量精液外流,小溲热赤浑浊,或尿涩不爽,口苦或渴,心烦少寐,口舌生疮,大便溏臭,或见脘腹痞闷,恶心,苔黄腻,脉濡数。

治　法　清热利湿。

方　药　程氏萆薢分清饮加减:萆薢10 g,黄柏10 g,茯苓10 g,生薏苡仁12 g,车前子(包煎)10 g,莲子10 g,石菖蒲6 g,白术10 g。

加　减　若湿热流注肝脉,尿黄赤,茎中痒痛者,加龙胆草5 g,苦参10 g,木通6 g;若患者尿时不爽,少腹及阴部作胀,为病久挟有瘀热之征,可加败酱草10 g,赤芍药10 g。

Rubra) 10 g.

3. Inability of Qi to Arrest Semen

Chief Manifestations: Seminal emission due to overwork, palpitation, insomnia, forgetfulness, sallow complexion, weakness and fatigue of the limbs, poor appetite, loose stools, pale tongue with thin coating, thready and weak pulse.

Therapeutic Methods: To regulate and strengthen the heart and spleen, nourish qi and arrest semen.

Prescription: Modified Miaoxiang San (Miaoxiang Powder), composed of Dangshen (*Radix Codonopsis*) 10 g, Huangqi (*Radix Astragali*) 10 g, Shanyao (*Rhizoma Dioscoreae*) 10 g, Fuling (*Poria*) 10 g, Yuanzhi (*Radix Polygalae*) 6 g, Muxiang (*Radix Aucklandiae*) 8 g and Jiegeng (*Radix Platycodi*) 6 g.

Modification: For failure of middle energizer qi to ascend, add Shengma (*Rhizoma Cimicifugae*) 6 g and Chaihu (*Radix Bupleuri*) 6 g.

4. Inability to Store Essence due to Kidney Deficiency

Chief Manifestations: Frequent nocturnal emission, even spontaneous emission, soreness and weakness of loins and knees, dry throat, restlessness, vertigo, tinnitus, forgetfulness, insomnia, low fever, flushed cheeks, emaciation, night perspiration, loss of hair, odontoseisis, red tongue with little coating, thready and rapid pulse; in some cases with persistent spermatorrhoea, often accompanied by aversion to cold, cold limbs, impotence, premature ejaculation, cold sperm, scanty urine or frequent urination at night, edema, clean or dribbling urine, pale or lusterless complexion, pale, tender teeth-printed tongue with white and smooth coating, deep and thready pulse.

Therapeutic Methods: To nourish kidney essence,

3. 气不摄精证

主要证候　劳则遗精,心悸不宁,失眠健忘,面色萎黄,四肢困倦,食少便溏,舌质淡,苔薄,脉细弱。

治　法　调补心脾,益气摄精。

方　药　妙香散加减:党参10 g,黄芪10 g,山药10 g,茯苓10 g,远志6 g,木香8 g,桔梗6 g。

加　减　若中气不升,加升麻6 g,柴胡6 g。

4. 肾虚不固证

主要证候　梦遗频作,甚至滑精,腰膝酸软,咽干,心烦,眩晕,耳鸣,健忘,失眠,低热,颧赤,形瘦盗汗,发落齿摇,舌红少苔,脉细数。部分患者久遗滑精,可兼见形寒肢冷,阳痿早泄,精冷,夜尿多或尿少,浮肿,溲色清白,或余沥不尽,面色㿠白或枯槁无华,舌淡嫩有齿痕,苔白滑,脉沉细。

治　法　补益肾精,固涩

induce astringency and stop nocturnal emission.

Prescription: Modified Zuogui Yin (Decoction for Invigorating Kidney Yin), Jinsuo Gujing Wan (Golden Lock Pill for Keeping Kidney Essence) and Shuilu Erxian Dan (Euryales and Rosae Laevigatae Pill), composed of Shudihuang (*Radix Rehmanniae Preparata*) 12 g, Shanyao (*Rhizoma Dioscoreae*) 10 g, Shanzhuyu (*Fructus Corni*) 10 g, Gouqizi (*Fructus Lycii*) 10 g, Tongjili (*Fructus Tribuli*) 10 g, Sangjisheng (*Herba Taxilli*) 10 g, Duanlonggu (*Os Draconis Usta*, to be decocted first) 30 g, Duanmuli (*Concha Ostreae Usta*, to be decocted first) 30 g, Lianzirou (*Semen Nelumbinis*) 10 g, Qianshi (*Semen Euryales*) 10 g and Jinyingzi (*Fructus Rosae Laevigatae*) 10 g.

Modification: If yin deficiency involves yang, leading to deficiency of both yin and yang, add Buguzhi (*Fructus Psoraleae*) 10 g, Suoyang (*Herba Cynormorii*) 10 g, Jiucaizi (*Semen Allii Tuberosi*) 10 g and Lujiaoshuang (*Cornu Cervi Degelatinatum*) 10 g.

Other Treatments

1. Chinese Patent Drugs

(1) Longdan Xiegan Wan (Gentianae Pill for Purging Liver Fire): 6 g each time, twice a day; indicated for seminal emission due to downward movement of damp heat in the liver meridian.

(2) Zhi Bai Dihuang Wan (Pill of Anemarrhenae, Phellodendron and Rehmanniae): 6 g each time, twice a day; indicated for seminal emission due to deficiency of yin and hyperactivity of fire.

(3) Jinsuo Gujing Wan (Golden Lock Bolus for Keeping Kidney Essence): 6 g each time, twice a day; indicated for seminal emission due to kidney deficiency.

(4) Shuilu Erxian Dan (Euryales and Rosae Laevigatae Pill): 6 g each time, twice a day; indicated for per-

止遗。

方　药　左归饮合金锁固精丸、水陆二仙丹加减：熟地黄12 g，山药10 g，山茱萸10 g，枸杞子10 g，潼蒺藜10 g，桑寄生10 g，煅龙骨（先煎）30 g，煅牡蛎（先煎）30 g，莲子肉10 g，芡实10 g，金樱子10 g。

加　减　若阴虚及阳，阴阳俱虚者，加补骨脂10 g，锁阳10 g，韭菜子10 g，鹿角霜10 g。

【其他疗法】

1. 中成药

（1）龙胆泻肝丸　每服6 g，每日2次。适用于肝经湿热下注之遗精。

（2）知柏地黄丸　每服6 g，每日2次。适用于阴虚火旺之遗精。

（3）金锁固精丸　每服6 g，每日2次。适用于肾虚遗精。

（4）水陆二仙丹　每服6 g，每日2次。适用于遗精日

sistent seminal emission or spontaneous emission.

2. Simple-drug or Experiential Prescriptions

(1) Take Jiucaizi (*Semen Allii Tuberosi*) 20 - 30 pcs every night with dilute salt water. It is indicated for spontaneous emission and impotence attributive to unconsolidation of kidney qi.

(2) Chew Lianzi (*Semen Nelumbinis*) 10 g each time, twice daily. It is indicated for nocturnal emission due to a desire for sexual pleasure.

(3) Bake Ciweipi (*Corium Erinacei*) until it becomes dry and grind it into powder, take 1.5 - 3 g every night. It is indicated for seminal emission due to kidney deficiency.

3. External Therapy

(1) Mix the same amount of Wubeizifen (*Galla Chinensis, powdered*) and Shengmulifen (*Concha Ostreae*, powdered) with warm water to make pills, apply it on the umbilicus before sleep, immobilize it with adhesive tape, change the dressing every 2 - 3 days. It is indicated for seminal emission due to kidney deficiency.

(2) Equal amounts of Shengdihuang (*Radix Rehmanniae*), Baishaoyao (*Radix Paeoniae Alba*), Chuanxiong (*Rhizoma Chuanxiong*), Maimendong (*Radix Ophiopogonis*), Huangbai (*Cortex Phellodendri*), Zhimu (*Rhizoma Anemarrhenae*), Huanglian (*Rhizoma Coptidis*), Zhizi (*Fructus Gardeniae*), Paojiang (*Rhizoma Zingiberis Recens*, roasted in hot cinders), Shanzhuyu (*Fructus Corni*) and Duanmuli (*Concha Ostreae Usta*). Simmer the above drugs in sesame oil, add red lead to collect extract, apply it on Shenshu (BL 23). It is indicated for seminal emission due to hyperactivity of fire due to yin deficiency.

(3) Grind Duanlonggu (*Os Draconis Usta*) 50 g and Wubeizi (*Galla Chinensis*) 40 g into powder, add water

2. 单验方

(1) 韭菜子20~30粒,每晚淡盐汤送下。治肾气不固的滑精、阳痿。

(2) 莲子,每服10 g,每日2次,嚼服。治心动梦遗。

(3) 刺猬皮,焙干研细末,每晚服1.5 ~ 3 g。治肾虚遗精。

3. 外治法

(1) 五倍子、生牡蛎粉等分,临卧时用温开水少许,搓成弹子大小,置脐中,用胶布固定,每2~3日更换1次。适用于肾虚遗精。

(2) 生地黄、白芍药、川芎、麦门冬、黄柏、知母、黄连、栀子、炮姜、山茱萸、煅牡蛎各等分。用麻油熬,铅丹收,贴肾俞穴。适用于阴虚火旺之遗精。

(3) 煅龙骨50 g,五倍子40 g。将两药研成细末,用水调

to make a paste, fill the umbilicus with the paste and fix it with adhesive tape before sleep. Apply the method for 1 - 2 consecutive weeks. It is indicated for seminal emission due to kidney deficiency.

（4）Jinyingzi（*Fructus Rosae Laevigatae*）10 g, Shengmuli（*Concha Ostreae*）15 g, Qianshi（*Semen Euryales*）20 g, Lianzirou（*Semen Nelumbinis*）10 g, Yizhiren（*Fructus Alpiniae Oxyphyllae*）10 g and Baijili（*Fructus Tribuli*）15 g. Grind the above drugs into powder, fill a belt-like cloth bag with the powder, place the bag around the loins and lower abdomen, refill the bag with the powder every 3 - 5 days, employ the method 5 - 7 times for a course. It is indicated for seminal emission due to unconsolidation of kidney qi.

成糊状，每晚睡前填药于脐中，然后用胶布贴紧，连用 1～2 个星期。适用于肾虚遗精。

（4）金樱子 10 g，生牡蛎 15 g，芡实 20 g，莲子肉 10 g，益智仁 10 g，白蒺藜 15 g。将诸药共研末，装入细长如带的布袋中，用制成的药带缚于腰间及下腹部。每 3～5 日换药 1 次，5～7 次为 1 个疗程。适用于肾气不固之遗精。

2.6 General Disease and Acropathy

第六章 全身与肢体病证

2.6.1 Fever due to Internal Disorders

第一节 内伤发热

General Description

Fever due to internal disorders is marked by fever, with the dysfunction of the zang-fu organs and deficiency of qi, blood, yin and yang as its pathogenesis. It usually has a gradual onset and a long duration. Clinically it is manifested as a low fever in most cases, but as a high fever in some cases.

This kind of fever is mainly caused by internal disorders like emotional stress, improper diet and overstrain. In occasional cases, it is first caused by exogenous factors but afterwards prolonged fever may lead to the impairment of zang-fu organs and fever due to internal disorders occurs. The pathogenesis of fever due to internal disorders mainly includes stagnation of heat in liver meridians, stagnation of blood, retention of dampness, insufficiency of middle energizer qi, deficiency of blood, depletion of yin essence and deficiency of yang qi.

Fever that is not caused by exogenous factors is considered to be of the category of fever due to internal disorders. It may be present in some cases of functional low fever, tumor, hemotopathy, desmosis, endocrinopathy, chronic infective diseases and fever of unknown causes in western medicine.

【概述】

内伤发热是指因内伤所致,以脏腑功能失调、气血阴阳亏虚为基本病机,以发热为主要表现的病证。本病一般起病较缓,病程较长。临床上多表现为低热,但有时也可以是高热。

本病主要因情志、饮食、劳倦等内因所致,但也有少数始为外感,日久导致脏腑亏虚而引起。发生内伤发热的共同病机是气血阴精亏虚,脏腑功能失调。主要有肝经郁热、瘀血阻滞、内湿停聚、中气不足、血虚失养、阴精亏耗、阳气虚衰等。

凡是不因感受外邪所导致的发热,均属内伤发热的范畴。本病证可见于西医学所称的功能性低热,肿瘤、血液病、结缔组织疾病、内分泌疾病、部分慢性感染性疾病所引

Essentials for Diagnosis

(1) Fever due to internal disorders develops slowly and has a long duration, mostly characterized by low fever or subjective fever and high fever in rare cases, no chilliness, or aversion to cold which can be relieved by wearing more clothes. Accompanying symptoms are dizziness, listlessness, spontaneous sweating, night sweating and weak pulse.

(2) In general, the patient has a background of stagnation of qi, blood, and fluids, or deficiency of qi, blood, yin and yang, or a recurrent fever.

(3) Examinations of blood, urine, blood biochemistry, immunology, serology and endocrine function should be done, which help make accurate diagnosis.

(4) Fever due to internal disorders should be differentiated from fever caused by exogenous factors, which has an acute onset, a shorter course, and a higher temperature (>38℃). The fevers vary with different diseases. In most cases, fever comes with chilliness at the initial stage and can not be relieved by wearing more clothes. Accompanying symptoms include headache, bodily pain, nasal stuffiness with discharge, cough, and superficial pulse. If the case is attacked by exogenous pathogenic factors resulting in the conflict between healthy qi and pathogenic factors, it is attributed to an excess syndrome.

Syndrome Differentiation and Treatment

The differentiation of fever due to internal disorders is to determine whether the case is of the deficiency or of the excess syndromes. It is a deficiency syndrome if it is caused by deficiency of qi, blood, yin and yang, and an

起的发热,以及某些原因不明的发热。

【诊断要点】

(1) 内伤发热起病缓慢,病程较长,多为低热,或自觉发热,表现为高热者较少,不恶寒,或虽有怯冷,但得衣被则暖,常兼见头晕、神疲、自汗、盗汗、脉弱等症。

(2) 一般有气、血、水壅遏或气血阴阳亏虚的病史,或有反复发热的病史。

(3) 血、尿常规,以及血液生化、免疫学、血清学、激素类等检查,有助于明确病因诊断。

(4) 内伤发热主要应与外感发热相鉴别。外感发热表现的特点是起病较急,病程较短,体温一般超过 38℃,发热类型随病种的不同而有所差异,发热初期大多伴有恶寒,其恶寒得衣被而不减,常兼有头身疼痛、鼻塞、流涕、咳嗽、脉浮等症;由感受外邪,正邪相争所致,属实证者较多。

【辨证论治】

对内伤发热的辨证主要是辨证候的虚实。如属气血阴阳亏虚所致者属虚,因气郁、瘀血所致者属实。实证治

excess syndrome if it is caused by stagnation of qi and blood. Treatment for the excess syndrome centers on dispersing the stagnant liver qi, relieving blood stagnation and clearing away heat; while treatment for deficiency syndrome should be replenishing yin, yang, qi and blood to clear deficient heat.

1. Fever Caused by Stagnation of Qi

Chief Manifestations: Low fever or hectic fever which fluctuates with emotions, emotional depression, a feeling of fullness and oppression over the chest and hypochondrium, restlessness, irritability, dry mouth with bitter taste, impaired appetite, red tongue with yellow coating, wiry and rapid pulse.

Therapeutic Methods: To soothe the liver, regulate qi, alleviate depression and purge heat.

Prescription: Modified Dan Zhi Xiaoyao San (Xiaoyao Powder with Moutan and Gardeniae), composed of Chaihu (*Radix Bupleuri*) 6 g, Bohe (*Herba Menthae*) 6 g, Mudanpi (*Cortex Moutan Radicis*) 10 g, Zhizi (*Fructus Gardeniae*) 10 g, Baizhu (*Rhizoma Atractylodis Macrocephalae*) 10 g, Fuling (*Poria*) 10 g, Danggui (*Radix Angelicae Sinensis*) 10 g and Baishaoyao (*Radix Paeoniae Alba*) 10 g.

Modifications: For pronounced stagnation of qi, add Yujin (*Radix Curcumae*) 10 g, Xiangfu (*Rhizoma Cyperi*) 10 g and Qingpi (*Pericarpium Citri Reticulatae Viride*) 6 g; for pronounced heat-syndrome manifested with red tongue, dry mouth and constipation, remove Baizhu, add Longdancao (*Radix Gentianae*) 6 g and Huangqin (*Radix Scutellariae*) 10 g; for female cases with irregular menstruation, add Zelan (*Herba Lycopi*) 10 g and Yimucao (*Herba Leonuri*) 10 g.

2. Fever Caused by Blood Stagnation

Chief Manifestations: Fever in the afternoon or at

疗以疏肝解郁、化瘀清热为主,虚证当补益阴阳气血,以退虚热。

1. 气郁发热证

主要证候　发热多为低热或潮热,热势常随情绪波动而起伏,精神抑郁,胸胁胀满,烦躁易怒,口干而苦,纳食减少,舌红,苔黄,脉弦数。

治　法　疏肝理气,解郁泄热。

方　药　丹栀逍遥散加减:柴胡6 g,薄荷6 g,牡丹皮10 g,栀子10 g,白术10 g,茯苓10 g,当归10 g,白芍药10 g。

加　减　气郁较甚,可加郁金10 g,香附10 g,青皮6 g;热象较甚,舌红、口干、便秘者,可去白术,加龙胆草6 g,黄芩10 g;妇女若兼月经不调,可加泽兰10 g,益母草10 g。

2. 血瘀发热证

主要证候　午后或夜晚

night, subjective fever in some parts of the body, dry
mouth and throat, but with a desire to drink a little, localized pain or masses in the body or limbs, sallow or lusterless complexion, bluish-purple tongue with occasional
macules or ecchymosis, wiry or unsmooth pulse.

Therapeutic Methods: To activate blood circulation
and remove blood stasis.

Prescription: Modified Xuefu Zhuyu Tang (Decoction for Removing Blood Stasis in Chest), composed of
Taoren (*Semen Persicae*) 10 g, Honghua (*Flos Carthami*) 10 g, Chishaoyao (*Radix Paeoniae Rubra*) 10 g,
Mudanpi (*Cortex Moutan Radicis*) 10 g, Niuxi (*Radix
Achyranthis Bidentatae*) 10 g, Zhidahuang (*Radix et
Rhizoma Rhei Preparata*) 10 g, Danggui (*Radix Angelicae Sinensis*) 10 g, Chuanxiong (*Rhizoma Chuanxiong*) 10 g, Shengdihuang (*Radix Rehmanniae*) 10 g,
Chaihu (*Radix Bupleuri*) 6 g, Zhike (*Fructus Aurantii*) 6 g and Jiegeng (*Radix Platycodi*) 6 g.

Modifications: For high fever, add Qinjiao (*Radix
Gentianae Macrophyllae*) 10 g, Baiwei (*Radix Cynan-
chi Atrati*) 10 g and Mudanpi (*Cortex Moutan Radicis*)
10 g; for edema of limbs, add Danshen (*Radix Salviae
Miltiorrhizae*) 10 g, Yujin (*Radix Curcumae*) 10 g and
Yanhusuo (*Rhizoma Corydalis*) 10 g.

3. Fever Due to Retension of Dampness

Chief Manifestations: Low fever which is prominent in the afternoon, fullness and oppression in the
chest, bodily heaviness, poor appetite, thirst but with no
desire to drink, nausea, vomiting, loose or sticky stools,
yellow greasy or white greasy tongue coating, soft-superficial and rapid pulse.

Therapeutic Methods: To promote diuresis and
clear away heat.

Prescription: Modified Sanren Tang (Three-Seed

发热,或自觉身体某些部位发
热,口燥咽干,但不多饮,肢体
或躯干有固定痛处或肿块,面
色萎黄或晦暗,舌质青紫或有
瘀点、瘀斑,脉弦或涩。

治 法 活血化瘀。

方 药 血府逐瘀汤加
减:桃仁10 g,红花10 g,赤芍
药10 g,牡丹皮10 g,牛膝10 g,
制大黄10 g,当归10 g,川芎
10 g,生地黄10 g,柴胡6 g,枳
壳6 g,桔梗6 g。

加 减 发热较甚者,可
加秦艽10 g,白薇10 g,牡丹皮
10 g;肢体肿痛者,可加丹参
10 g,郁金10 g,延胡索10 g。

3. 湿郁发热证

主要证候 低热,午后热
甚,胸闷脘痞,全身重着,不思
饮食,渴不欲饮,呕恶,大便稀
薄或黏滞不爽,舌苔白腻或黄
腻,脉濡数。

治 法 利湿清热。

方 药 三仁汤加减:杏

Decoction）, composed of Xingren （*Semen Armeniacae*）10 g, Yiyiren （*Semen Coicis*）12 g, Baikouren （*Semen Amomi Rotundus*）3 g, Chuanhoupo （*Cortex Magnoliae Officinalis*）6 g, Tongcao （*Medulla Tetrapanacis*）6 g, Huashi （*Talcum*, wrapped）10 g, Zhibanxia （*Rhizoma Pinelliae Preparata*）10 g and Zhuye （*Herba Lophatheri*）10 g.

Modifications：For pronounced vomiting, add Zhuru （*Caulis Bambusae in Taeniam*）10 g, Huoxiang （*Herba Agastachis*）10 g and Chenpi （*Pericarpium Citri Reticulatae*）6 g; for fullness in the chest and greasy tongue coating, add Yujin （*Radix Curcumae*）10 g and Peilan （*Herba Eupatorii*）10 g; for retention of damp heat in shaoyang meridian manifested as pronounced fever like malaria, bitter taste in the mouth and vomiting, add Qinghao （*Herba Artemisiae*）10 g and Huangqin （*Radix Scutellariae*）10 g.

4. Fever Due to Deficiency of Qi

Chief Manifestations：Low fever or high fever which is induced or aggravated by overwork, lassitude, shortness of breath, hypologia, spontaneous sweating, susceptibility to the colds, poor appetite, loose stools, pale tongue with thin white coating, thready and weak pulse.

Therapeutic Methods：To replenish qi, invigorate the spleen and clear away heat with sweet warm herbs.

Prescription：Modified Buzhong Yiqi Tang （Decoction for Strengthening Middle Energizer and Benefiting Qi）, composed of Huangqi （*Radix Astragali*）12 g, Dangshen （*Radix Codonopsis*）10 g, Baizhu （*Rhizoma Atractylodis Macrocephalae*）10 g, Zhigancao （*Radix Glycyrrhizae*, roasted）3 g, Danggui （*Radix Angelicae Sinensis*）10 g, Chenpi （*Pericarpium Citri Reticulatae*）6 g, Shengma （*Rhizoma Cimicifugae*）6 g and

仁10 g, 薏苡仁12 g, 白蔻仁3 g, 川厚朴6 g, 通草6 g, 滑石（包煎）10 g, 制半夏10 g, 竹叶10 g。

加 减 呕恶明显者, 加竹茹10 g, 藿香10 g, 陈皮6 g; 胸闷、苔腻明显者, 加郁金10 g, 佩兰10 g; 湿热阻滞少阳枢机, 症见寒热如疟, 寒轻热重, 口苦呕逆者, 加青蒿10 g, 黄芩10 g。

4. 气虚发热证

主要证候 发热, 热势或低或高, 常在劳累后发作或加剧, 倦怠乏力, 气短懒言, 自汗, 易于感冒, 食少便溏, 舌质淡, 苔薄白, 脉细弱。

治 法 益气健脾, 甘温除热。

方 药 补中益气汤加减: 黄芪12 g, 党参10 g, 白术10 g, 炙甘草3 g, 当归10 g, 陈皮6 g, 升麻6 g, 柴胡6 g。

Chaihu (*Radix Bupleuri*) 6 g.

Modifications: For pronounced spontaneous sweating, add Muli (*Concha Ostreae*, to be decocted first) 20 g, Fuxiaomai (*Fructus Tritici Levis*) 12 g and Nuodaogen (*Rhizoma et Radix Oryzae Glutinosae*) 20 g; for alteration of chills and fever, accompanied with sweating and aversion to wind, add Guizhi (*Ramulus Cinnamomi*) 6 g and Baishaoyao (*Radix Paeoniae Alba*) 10 g; for spleen deficiency complicated by dampness retention, manifested as fullness and oppression in the chest, white and greasy tongue coating, add Cangzhu (*Rhizoma Atractylodis*) 10 g, Fuling (*Poria*) 10 g and Houpo (*Cortex Magnoliae Officinalis*) 10 g.

5. Fever Due to Deficiency of Blood

Chief Manifestations: Fever and mostly low fever, dizziness, lassitude, palpitation, pale complexion, pale lips and nails, pale tongue, thready and weak pulse.

Therapeutic Methods: To replenish qi and nourish blood.

Prescription: Modified Guipi Tang (Decoction for Invigorating Spleen and Nourishing Heart), composed of Dangshen (*Radix Codonopsis*) 10 g, Baizhu (*Rhizoma Atractylodis Macrocephalae*) 10 g, Huangqi (*Radix Astragali*) 12 g, Danggui (*Radix Angelicae Sinensis*) 10 g, Baishaoyao (*Radix Paeoniae Alba*) 10 g, Guiyuanrou (*Arillus Longan*) 10 g, Yuanzhi (*Radix Polygalae*) 6 g, Fushen (*Sclerotium Poriae circum Radicem Pini*) 10 g, Yejiaoteng (*Caulis et Folium Polygoni Multiflori*) 10 g, Chenpi (*Pericarpium Citri Reticulatae*) 6 g, Dazao (*Fructus Jujubae*) 5 pcs and Zhigancao (*Radix Glycyrrhizae*, roasted) 3 g.

Modifications: For pronounced blood deficiency, add Shudihuang (*Radix Rehmanniae Preparata*) 12 g,

加 减 自汗较多者,加牡蛎(先煎)20 g,浮小麦12 g,糯稻根20 g;时冷时热,汗出恶风者,加桂枝6 g,白芍药10 g;脾虚挟湿,而见胸闷脘痞,舌苔白腻者,加苍术10 g,茯苓10 g,厚朴10 g。

5. 血虚发热证

主要证候 发热,热势多为低热,头晕眼花,身倦乏力,心悸不宁,面白少华,唇甲色淡,舌质淡,脉细弱。

治 法 益气养血。

方 药 归脾汤加减:党参10 g,白术10 g,黄芪12 g,当归10 g,白芍药10 g,桂圆肉10 g,远志6 g,茯神10 g,夜交藤10 g,陈皮6 g,大枣 5 枚,炙甘草3 g。

加 减 血虚较甚者,加熟地黄12 g,枸杞子12 g,制何

Gouqizi (*Fructus Lycii*) 12 g and Zhiheshuwu (*Radix Polygoni Multiflori Preparata*) 12 g; for high fever, add Yinchaihu (*Radix Stellariae*) 10 g and Baiwei (*Radix Cynanchi Atrati*) 10 g; for blood deficiency due to chronic hemorrhage with little bleeding, add Shensanqifen (*Radix Notoginseng*, powdered and to be taken separately) 3 g, Xianhecao (*Herba Agrimoniae*) 10 g and Qiancao (*Radix Rubiae*) 10 g.

6. Fever Due to Deficiency of Yin

Chief Manifestations: Afternoon or night fever, no desire for clothes, hot feeling of the palms and soles, restlessness, dreamful sleep, night sweating, dry throat and mouth, red tongue with fissures, or with little coating, even no coating, thready and rapid pulse.

Therapeutic Methods: To nourish yin and clear away heat.

Prescription: Modified Qinggu San (Powder for Clearing away Heat in Bones), composed of Yinchaihu (*Radix Stellariae*) 10 g, Digupi (*Cortex Lycii*) 10 g, Huhuanglian (*Rhizoma Picrorhizae*) 10 g, Zhimu (*Rhizoma Anemarrhenae*) 10 g, Qinjiao (*Radix Gentianae Macrophyllae*) 10 g, Biejia (*Carapax Trionycis*, to be decocted first) 15 g, Xuanshen (*Radix Scrophulariae*) 12 g and Shengdihuang (*Radix Rehmanniae*) 12 g.

Modifications: For night sweating, add Duanmuli (*Concha Ostreae Usta*, to be decocted first) 20 g, Fuxiaomai (*Fructus Tritici Levis*) 12 g and Nuodaogen (*Radix Oryzae Glutinosae*) 20 g; for predominant yin deficiency, add Xuanshen (*Radix Scrophulariae*) 10 g, Shengdihuang (*Radix Rhemanniae*) 10 g and Zhiheshuwu (*Radix Polygoni Multiflori Preparata*) 10 g; for pronounced insomnia, add Suanzaoren (*Semen Ziziphi Spinosae*) 10 g, Baiziren (*Semen Platycladi*) 10 g and Yejiaoteng (*Caulis et Folium Polygoni Multiflori*)

首乌12 g;发热较甚者,可加银柴胡10 g,白薇10 g;由慢性失血所致的血虚,若仍有少许出血者,可酌加参三七粉(另吞)3 g,仙鹤草10 g,茜草10 g。

6. 阴虚发热证

主要证候 午后潮热,或夜间发热,不欲近衣,手足心热,烦躁,少寐多梦,盗汗,口干咽燥,舌质红,或有裂纹,苔少甚至无苔,脉细数。

治 法 滋阴清热。

方 药 清骨散加减:银柴胡10 g,地骨皮10 g,胡黄连10 g,知母10 g,秦艽10 g,鳖甲(先煎)15 g,玄参12 g,生地黄12 g。

加 减 盗汗较甚者,加煅牡蛎(先煎)20 g,浮小麦12 g,糯稻根20 g;阴虚较甚者,加玄参10 g,生地黄10 g,制何首乌10 g;失眠明显者,加酸枣仁10 g,柏子仁10 g,夜交藤10 g。

10 g.

7. Fever Due to Deficiency of Yang

Chief Manifestations: Fever with a desire for being covered up, aversion to cold, cold limbs, hypologia, dizziness, somnolence, soreness and weakness of loins and knees, poor appetite, loose stools, pale complexion, swollen pale tongue with white and moist coating, or teeth marks on its margin, and deep, thready and forceless pulse.

Therapeutic Methods: To warm and replenish yang qi and direct the fire back to its origin.

Prescription: Modified Jingui Shenqi Wan (Pill for Invigorating Kidney Qi from *Golden* Cabinet), composed of Zhifuzi (*Radix Aconiti Lateralis Preparata*) 6 g, Rougui (*Cortex Cinnamomi*) 3 g, Shudihuang (*Radix Rehmanniae Preparata*) 12 g, Shanzhuyu (*Fructus Corni*) 12 g, Shanyao (*Rhizoma Dioscoreae*) 12 g, Zexie (*Rhizoma Alismatis*) 10 g, Mudanpi (*Cortex Moutan Radicis*) 10 g and Fuling (*Poria*) 10 g.

Modifications: For shortness of breath, add Hongshen (*Radix Ginseng Rubra*, to be decocted separately) 10 g; for loose stools and diarrhea, add Baizhu (*Rhizoma Atractylodis Macrocephalae*) 10 g and Paoganjiang (*Rhizoma Zingiberis*, roasted in hot cinders) 3 g.

Other Treatments

1. Chinese Patent Drugs

(1) Liuwei Dihuang Wan (Pill of Six Drugs Containing Rehmanniae): 6 g each time, twice daily; indicated for fever due to yin dificiency.

(2) Dan Zhi Xiaoyao Wan (Xiaoyao Pill with Moutan and Gardeniae): 6 g each time, twice daily; indicated for fever due to stagnation of liver qi.

(3) Buzhong Yiqi Wan (Pill for Strengthening Middle Energizer and Benefiting Qi): 6 g each time, twice

7. 阳虚发热证

主要证候 发热而欲近衣,形寒怯冷,四肢不温,少气懒言,头晕嗜卧,腰膝酸软,纳少便溏,面色㿠白,舌质淡胖,或有齿痕,苔白润,脉沉细无力。

治 法 温补阳气,引火归元。

方 药 《金匮》肾气丸加减:制附子6 g,肉桂3 g,熟地黄12 g,山茱萸12 g,山药12 g,泽泻10 g,牡丹皮10 g,茯苓10 g。

加 减 短气甚者,加红参(另煎)10 g;便溏腹泻者,加白术10 g,炮干姜3 g。

【其他疗法】

1. 中成药

(1) 六味地黄丸 每服6 g,每日 2 次。适用于阴虚发热。

(2) 丹栀逍遥丸 每服6 g,每日 2 次。适用于肝郁化火之发热。

(3) 补中益气丸 每服6 g,每日 2 次。适用于气虚

daily; indicated for fever due to qi deficiency.

2. Single-drug or Experiential Prescriptions

(1) Take one tortoise and one carapax trionycis, remove their heads and viscera, then stew them in water and take the soup, once per week. It is indicated for fever due to yin deficiency.

(2) Soak 10 g of tremella in boiled water and cook it over a slow fire until it is soft enough, and then put some crystal sugar and take the soup, once or twice a week. It is indicated for fever due to yin deficiency.

2.6.2 Consumptive Disease

General Description

Consumptive disease is a general term for various chronic deficiency syndromes due to impaired function of the zang-fu organs, and deficiency of qi, blood, yin and yang.

Consumptive disease is either caused by weak resistance or by various diseases, both of which result in exhaustion of primordial qi of the body. Pathogenically, it is related to the consumption of qi, blood, yin and yang. The involved parts are the five zang-fu organs, especially the spleen and kidneys. Since the five zang-fu organs are related to one another, qi and blood are of the same origin and yin and yang interdepend on each other, the consumption of qi, blood, yin and yang in one of the zang-fu organs may involve the other ones and deficient qi fails to generate blood and in turn deficient blood fails to generate qi. In the case of prolonged deficiency of qi, yang insufficiency occurs and in the case of prolonged deficiency of blood, yin insufficiency occurs. Then persistent depletion of yang will involve yin and persistent depletion of yin will involve yang, leading to deterioration of the disease.

发热。

2. 单验方

（1）乌龟、鳖甲各 1 只，去头及内脏，炖服。每星期 1 次。适用于阴虚发热。

（2）银耳10 g，用开水泡开，细火煮烂，并放冰糖少许，每星期服 1～2 次。适用于阴虚发热。

第二节 虚 劳

【概述】

虚劳又称虚损，是以脏腑功能衰退，气血阴阳不足为主要病机的多种慢性虚弱证候的总称。

虚劳或是因虚致病，因病成劳；或是因病致虚，久虚不复成劳。而其病性，主要为气、血、阴、阳的亏耗。病损部位主要在五脏，尤以脾肾两脏更为重要。引起虚损的病因，往往首先导致某一脏气、血、阴、阳的亏损，而由于五脏相关，气血同源，阴阳互根，所以在虚劳的病变过程中常互相影响。一脏受病，累及他脏；气虚不能生血，血虚无以生气；气虚者，日久阳也渐衰；血虚者，日久阴也不足；阳损日久，累及于阴；阴虚日久，累及于阳，以致病势日渐发展，而

Consumptive diseases in traditional Chinese medicine include chronic and consumptive diseases of various systems in western medicine.

Essentials for Diagnosis

(1) Common manifestations are lassitude, fatigue, shortness of breath, palpitation, sallow complexion, spontaneous sweating, night sweating, feverish sensation in the palms, soles and chest, aversion to cold, cold limbs, and feeble, forceless pulse. If the disease lasts long and deficiency is persistent, the symptoms will gradually deteriorate.

(2) There are pathogenic factors that lead to consumptive diseases and the patient has contracted an illness for quite a long time.

(3) Similar syndromes, especially pulmonary tuberculosis and other diseases of deficiency type, should be differentiated from consumptive diseases.

Syndrome Differentiation and Treatment

The key to the differentiation of consumptive diseases lies in the differentiation of the state of yin, yang, qi and blood of the five zang-fu organs. Its treatment should focus on reinforcement and different treatments like replenishing qi, nourishing yin and blood, and warming yang should be adopted according to different cases. Meanwhile selection of herbs and prescriptions should be based on different condition of the impaired organs, so as to enhance the therapeutic effect. Besides, much attention should be paid to invigorate the kidneys as well as the spleen and stomach.

1. Deficiency of Qi

(1) Deficiency of Lung Qi

Chief Manifestations: Shortness of breath, spontaneous sweating, low voice, alteration of chills and fever,

病情趋于复杂。

虚劳可见于西医学中多个系统的各种慢性、消耗性疾病。

【诊断要点】

(1) 本病多见神疲体倦，心悸气短，面容憔悴，自汗盗汗，或五心烦热，或畏寒肢冷，脉虚无力等症。若病程较长，久虚不复，症状可逐渐加重。

(2) 具有引起虚劳的致病因素及较长的病史。

(3) 排除类似病证。应着重排除肺痨及其他病证中的虚证类型。

【辨证论治】

虚劳的辨证当以气血阴阳为纲，五脏虚候为目。治疗当以补益为原则。应根据其病理属性的不同，分别采取益气、养血、滋阴、温阳的治疗方法。同时要密切结合五脏病位的不同而选方用药，以增强治疗的针对性，尤其要重视补益先天之肾和后天脾胃。

1. 气虚证

(1) 肺气虚证

主要证候　短气自汗，声音低怯，时寒时热，经常感冒，

susceptibility to colds, pale complexion, pale tongue and weak pulse.

Therapeutic Method: To replenish and restore lung qi.

Prescription: Modified Bufei Tang (Decoction for Replenishing Lung Qi), composed of Dangshen (*Radix Codonopsis*) 10 g, Huangqi (*Radix Astragali*) 12 g, Shudihuang (*Radix Rehmanniae Preparata*) 12 g, Wu-weizi (*Fructus Schisandrae*) 6 g, Sangbaipi (*Cortex Mori*) 10 g and Ziwan (*Radix Asteris*) 10 g.

Modifications: For absense of no cough, remove Sangbaipi and Ziwan; for profuse spontaneous sweating, add Duanmuli (*Concha Ostreae Usta*, to be decocted first) 20 g and Mahuanggen (*Radix Ephedrae*) 12 g; for deficiency of qi and yin complicated with hectic fever and night sweating, add Biejia (*Carapax Trionycis*, to be decocted first) 15 g, Digupi (*Cortex Lycii*) 10 g and Qin-jiao (*Radix Gentianae Macrophyllae*) 10 g.

(2) Deficiency of Heart Qi

Chief Manifestations: Palpitation, shortness of breath which is aggravated on exertion, lassitude, sponta-neous sweating, pale tongue and weak pulse.

Therapeutic Method: To replenish qi and nourish the heart.

Prescription: Modified Qifu Yin (Seven-Happiness Decoction), composed of Dangshen (*Radix Codonopsis*) 10 g, Baizhu (*Rhizoma Atractylodis Macrocephalae*) 10 g, Zhigancao (*Radix Glycyrrhizae*, roasted) 3 g, Shudihuang (*Radix Rehmanniae Preparata*) 10 g, Dang-gui (*Radix Angelicae Sinensis*) 10 g, Suanzaoren (*Semen Ziziphi Spinosae*) 10 g and Yuanzhi (*Radix Polyga-lae*) 6 g.

Modifications: For profuse spontaneous sweating, add Huangqi (*Radix Astragali*) 12 g and Wuweizi

面白,舌质淡,脉弱。

治　法　补益肺气。

方　药　补肺汤加减:党参10 g,黄芪12 g,熟地黄12 g,五味子6 g,桑白皮10 g,紫菀10 g。

加　减　无咳嗽者,可去桑白皮、紫菀。自汗较多者,加煅牡蛎(先煎)20 g,麻黄根12 g;若气阴两虚而兼见潮热、盗汗者,加鳖甲(先煎)15 g,地骨皮10 g,秦艽10 g。

(2) 心气虚证

主要证候　心悸,气短,劳则尤甚,神疲体倦,自汗,舌质淡,脉弱。

治　法　益气养心。

方　药　七福饮加减:党参10 g,白术10 g,炙甘草3 g,熟地黄10 g,当归10 g,酸枣仁10 g,远志6 g。

加　减　自汗多者,可加黄芪12 g,五味子6 g;饮食少

(*Fructus Schisandrae*) 6 g; for poor appetite, add Sharen (*Fructus Amomi*, to be decocted later) 3 g and Fuling (*Poria*) 10 g.

(3) Deficiency of Spleen Qi

Chief Manifestations: Impaired appetite, abdominal flatulence after eating, lassitude, loose stools, sallow complexion, pale tongue with thin white coating, and weak pulse.

Therapeutic Methods: To invigorate the spleen and benefit qi.

Prescription: Modified Jiawei Sijunzi Tang (Four Mild-Drug Decoction with Additions), composed of Dangshen (*Radix Codonopsis*) 10 g, Baizhu (*Rhizoma Atractylodis Macrocephalae*) 10 g, Huangqi (*Radix Astragali*) 10 g, Zhigancao (*Radix Glycyrrhizae*, roasted) 3 g, Fuling (*Poria*) 12 g and Biandou (*Semen Dolichoris*) 12 g.

Modifications: If stomach qi fails to descend and there is abdominal flatulence, belching and vomiting, add Chenpi (*Pericarpium Citri Reticulatae*) 6 g and Zhibanxia (*Rhizoma Pinelliae Preparata*) 10 g; if there is dyspepsia and abdominal flatulence, belching with fetid odor and greasy tongue, add Shenqu (*Massa Medicata Fermentata*) 10 g, Maiya (*Fructus Hordei Germinatus*) 10 g, Shanzha (*Fructus Crataegi*) 10 g and Jineijin (*Endothelium Corneum Gigeriae Galli*) 6 g; if deficient qi involves yang and deficient spleen yang follows, manifested as abdominal pain with immediate diarrhea and cold limbs, add Rougui (*Cortex Cinnamomi*) 3 g and Paojiang (*Rhzioma Zingiberis*, roasted in hot cinders) 3 g.

(4) Deficiency of Kidney Qi

Chief Manifestations: Lassitude, soreness and weakness of the loins and knees, frequent urination with clear urine, thin leucorrhea, pale tongue and weak pulse.

思,加砂仁(后下)3 g,茯苓10 g。

（3）脾气虚证

主要证候 饮食减少,食后胃脘不舒,倦怠乏力,大便溏薄,面色萎黄,舌质淡,苔薄白,脉弱。

治 法 健脾益气。

方 药 加味四君子汤加减:党参10 g,黄芪10 g,白术10 g,炙甘草3 g,茯苓12 g,扁豆12 g。

加 减 胃失和降而兼见胃脘胀满,嗳气呕吐者,加陈皮6 g,制半夏10 g;食积停滞而兼见脘闷腹胀,嗳气酸腐,苔腻者,加神曲10 g,麦芽10 g,山楂10 g,鸡内金6 g;气虚及阳,脾阳渐虚而兼见腹痛即泻,手足欠温者,加肉桂3 g,炮姜3 g。

（4）肾气虚证

主要证候 神疲乏力,腰膝酸软,小便频数而清,白带清稀,舌质淡,脉弱。

Therapeutic Methods: To benefit qi and nourish the kidney.

Prescription: Da Buyuan Jian (Potent Decoction for Replenishing Primordial Qi), composed of Shudihuang (*Radix Rehmanniae Preparata*) 12 g, Shanzhuyu (*Fructus Corni*) 10 g, Shanyao (*Rhizoma Dioscoreae*) 10 g, Gouqizi (*Fructus Lycii*) 10 g, Dangshen (*Radix Codonopsis*) 10 g, Danggui (*Radix Angelicae Sinensis*) 10 g and Duzhong (*Cortex Eucommiae*) 10 g.

Modifications: For pronounced lassitude, add Huangqi (*Radix Astragali*) 12 g; for frequent urination and incontinence of urine, add Tusizi (*Semen Cusutae*) 10 g, Wuweizi (*Fructus Schisandrae*) 6 g and Yizhiren (*Semen Alpiniae Oxyphyllae*) 10 g; for failure of the spleen to transport and convert, accompanied by loose stools, remove Shudihuang and Danggui, add Roudoukou (*Semen Myristicae*) 10 g and Buguzhi (*Fructus Psoraleae*) 10 g.

2. Deficiency of Blood

(1) Deficiency of Heart Blood

Chief Manifestations: Palpitation, amnesia, insomnia, dreamfulness, lusterless complexion, pale tongue, thready pulse or slow-irregular and intermittent pulse.

Therapeutic Methods: To nourish blood and tranquilize the mind.

Prescription: Modified Yangxin Tang (Decoction for Nourishing Heart), composed of Dangshen (*Radix Codonopsis*) 10 g, Huangqi (*Radix Astragali*) 12 g, Fuling (*Poria*) 10 g, Zhigancao (*Radix Glycyrrhizae*, roasted) 3 g, Danggui (*Radix Angelicae Sinensis*) 10 g, Chuanxiong (*Rhizoma Chuanxiong*) 10 g, Wuweizi (*Fructus Schisandrae*) 6 g, Baiziren (*Semen Platycladi*) 10 g, Suanzaoren (*Semen Ziziphi Spinosae*)

治　法　益气补肾。

方　药　大补元煎：熟地黄12 g,山茱萸10 g,山药10 g,枸杞子10 g,党参10 g,当归10 g,杜仲10 g。

加　减　神疲乏力甚者,加黄芪12 g;尿频较甚及小便失禁者,加菟丝子10 g,五味子6 g,益智仁10 g;脾失健运而兼见大便溏薄者,去熟地黄、当归,加肉豆蔻10 g,补骨脂10 g。

2. 血虚

(1) 心血虚证

主要证候　心悸怔忡,健忘,失眠,多梦,面色不华,舌质淡,脉细或结代。

治　法　养血宁心。

方　药　养心汤加减：党参10 g,黄芪12 g,茯苓10 g,炙甘草3 g,当归10 g,川芎10 g,五味子6 g,柏子仁10 g,酸枣仁10 g,远志6 g,肉桂3 g。

10 g, Yuanzhi (*Radix Polygalae*) 6 g and Rougui (*Cortex Cinnamomi*) 3 g.

Modification: For insomnia and dreamfulness, add Hehuanhua (*Flos Albiziae*) 6 g and Yejiaoteng (*Caulis et Folium Polygoni Multiflori*) 10 g.

(2) Deficiency of Spleen Blood

Chief Manifestations: Lassitude, poor appetite, palpitation, shortness of breath, amnesia, insomnia, sallow complexion, pale tongue with thin and white coating, thready and slow pulse.

Therapeutic Methods: To invigorate the spleen and nourish blood.

Prescrioption: Modified Guipi Tang (Decoction for Invigorating Spleen and Nourishing Heart), composed of Dangshen (*Radix Codonopsis*) 12 g, Baizhu (*Rhizoma Atractylodis Macrocephalae*) 10 g, Huangqi (*Radix Astragali*) 12 g, Danggui (*Radix Angelicae Sinensis*) 10 g, Baishaoyao (*Radix Paeoniae Alba*) 10 g, Guiyuanrou (*Arillus Longan*) 10 g, Yuanzhi (*Radix Polygalae*) 6 g, Fushen (*Sclerotium Poriae circum Radicem Pini*) 10 g, Yejiaoteng (*Cualis et Folium Polygoni Multiflori*) 10 g, Chenpi (*Pericarpium Citri Reticulatae*) 6 g, Dazao (*Fructus Jujubae*) 5 pcs and Zhigancao (*Radix Glycyrrhizae*, roasted) 3 g.

Modification: For insomnia, add Suanzaoren (*Semen Ziziphi Spinosae*) 10 g and Hehuanpi (*Cortex Albiziae*) 6 g.

(3) Deficiency of Liver Blood

Chief Manifestations: Dizziness, blurred vision, hypochondriac pain, numbness of limbs, muscular spasm or muscular twitching and cramps, irregular menstruation or even amenorrhea, lusterless complexion, pale tongue, wiry and thready pulse or thready and unsmooth pulse.

Therapeutic Methods: To replenish blood and

加 减 失眠、多梦,可加合欢花6 g,夜交藤10 g。

(2) 脾血虚证

主要证候 体倦乏力,纳差食少,心悸气短,健忘,失眠,面色萎黄,舌质淡,苔薄白,脉细缓。

治 法 补脾养血。

方 药 归脾汤加减:党参12 g,白术10 g,黄芪12 g,当归10 g,白芍药10 g,桂圆肉10 g,远志6 g,茯神10 g,夜交藤10 g,陈皮6 g,大枣 5 枚,炙甘草3 g。

加 减 失眠,加酸枣仁10 g,合欢皮6 g。

(3) 肝血虚证

主要证候 头晕,目眩,胁痛,肢体麻木,筋脉拘急,或惊惕肉𥆧,妇女月经不调甚则闭经,面色不华,舌质淡,脉弦细或细涩。

治 法 补血养肝。

nourish the liver.

Prescription: Modified Siwu Tang (Four-Ingredient Decoction), composed of Danggui (*Radix Angelicae Sinensis*) 10 g, Baishaoyao (*Radix Paeoniae Alba*) 10 g, Chuanxiong (*Rhizoma Chuanxiong*) 10 g, Shudi-huang (*Radix Rehmanniae Preparata*) 12 g and Ejiao (*Colla Corii Asini*, to be melted in the finished decoc-tion) 10 g.

Modifications: For severe deficiency of blood, add Zhiheshouwu (*Radix Polygoni Multiflori Preparata*) 10 g, Gouqizi (*Fructus Lycii*) 10 g and Jixueteng (*Caulis Spatholobi*) 10 g; for hypochondriac pain, add Sigualuo (*Retinervus Luffae Fructus*) 6 g, Yujin (*Radix Curcumae*) 8 g and Xiangfu (*Rhizoma Cyperi*) 8 g; for blurred vision due to failure of liver blood to nourish the eyes, add Zhushizi (*Fructus Broussonetiae*) 10 g, Gouqizi (*Fructus Lycii*) 10 g and Juemingzi (*Semen Cassiae*) 15 g.

3. Yin Deficiency

(1) Deficiency of Lung Yin

Chief Manifestations: Dry cough, dry throat and even loss of voice, hemoptysis, hectic fever, night swea-ting, flushed face, red tongue with little saliva, thready and rapid pulse.

Therapeutic Methods: To nourish yin and moistur-ize the lung.

Prescription: Modified Shashen Maidong Tang (Gle-hniae and Ophiopogonis Decoction), composed of Shashen (*Radix Glehniae*) 10 g, Maimendong (*Radix Ophiopog-onis*) 10 g, Yuzhu (*Rhizoma Polygonati Odorati*) 10 g, Tianhuafen (*Radix Trichosanthis*) 10 g, Sangye (*Folium Mori*) 10 g and Zhigancao (*Radix Glycyrrhizae*, roasted) 3 g.

Modifications: For severe cough, add Baibu (*Ra-

方 药 四物汤加减：当归10 g,白芍药10 g,川芎10 g,熟地黄12 g,阿胶（烊化冲服）10 g。

加 减 血虚甚者,加制何首乌10 g,枸杞子10 g,鸡血藤10 g；胁痛,加丝瓜络6 g,郁金8 g,香附8 g；目失所养,视物模糊,加楮实子10 g,枸杞子10 g,决明子15 g。

3. 阴虚

(1) 肺阴虚证

主要证候 干咳,咽燥,甚或失音,咯血,潮热,盗汗,面色潮红,舌红少津,脉细数。

治 法 养阴润肺。

方 药 沙参麦冬汤加减：沙参10 g,麦门冬10 g,玉竹10 g,天花粉10 g,桑叶10 g,炙甘草3 g。

加 减 咳嗽甚者,加百

dix Stemonae）10 g and Kuandonghua（*Flos Farfarae*）10 g; for hemoptysis, add Baiji（*Rhizoma Bletillae*）10 g, Xianhecao（*Herba Agrimoniae*）10 g and Xiaoji（*Herba Cirsii*）10 g; for pronounced hectic fever, add Digupi（*Cortex lycii*）10 g, Yinchaihu（*Radix Stellariae*）10 g, Qinjiao（*Radix Gentianae Macrophyllae*）10 g and Biejia（*Carapax Trionycis*, to be decocted first）15 g; for night sweating, add Duanmuli（*Concha Ostreae Usta*, to be decocted first）20 g and Fuxiaomai（*Fructus Tritici Levis*）12 g.

(2) Deficiency of Heart Yin

Chief Manifestations: Palpitation, insomnia, restlessness, hectic fever, night sweating or ulcers on the tongue, flushed face, red tongue with little saliva, thready and rapid pulse.

Therapeutic Method: To nourish yin and the heart.

Prescription: Modified Tianwang Buxin Dan（Tianwang Pill for Tonifying Heart）, composed of Shengdihuang（*Radix Rehmanniae*）10 g, Xuanshen（*Radix Scrophulariae*）10 g, Maimendong（*Radix Ophiopogonis*）10 g, Tianmendong（*Radix Asparagi*）10 g, Dangshen（*Radix Codonopsis*）10 g, Fuling（*Poria*）10 g, Wuweizi（*Fructus Schisandrae*）6 g, Danggui（*Radix Angelicae Sinensis*）10 g, Danshen（*Radix Salviae Miltiorrhizae*）12 g, Baiziren（*Semen Platycladi*）10 g, Suanzaoren（*Semen Ziziphi Spinosae*）10 g, Yuanzhi（*Radix Polygalae*）6 g and Jiegeng（*Radix Platycodi*）6 g.

Modifications: For predominant heat with manifestations as restlessness and ulcers on the tongue, remove Danggui and Yuanzhi which are acrid-tasted and warmnatured, add Huanglian（*Rhizoma Coptidis*）3 g, Mutong（*Caulis Akebiae*）6 g and Danzhuye（*Herba Lophatheri*）10 g; for hectic fever, add Digupi（*Cortex Lycii*）10 g,

部10 g,款冬花10 g;咯血,加白及10 g,仙鹤草10 g,小蓟10 g;潮热明显者,加地骨皮10 g,银柴胡10 g,秦艽10 g,鳖甲(先煎)15 g;盗汗,加煅牡蛎(先煎)20 g,浮小麦12 g。

(2) 心阴虚证
主要证候 心悸,失眠,烦躁,潮热,盗汗,或口舌生疮,面色潮红,舌红少津,脉细数。

治 法 滋阴养心。

方 药 天王补心丹加减:生地黄10 g,玄参10 g,麦门冬10 g,天门冬10 g,党参10 g,茯苓10 g,五味子6 g,当归10 g,丹参12 g,柏子仁10 g,酸枣仁10 g,远志6 g,桔梗6 g。

加 减 火热偏盛而见烦躁不安,口舌生疮者,去当归、远志之辛温,加黄连3 g,木通6 g,淡竹叶10 g;潮热明显者,加地骨皮10 g,银柴胡10 g,秦艽10 g;盗汗者,加煅

Yinchaihu (*Radix Stellariae*) 10 g and Qinjiao (*Radix Gentianae Macrophyllae*) 10 g; for night sweating, add Duanmuli (*Concha Ostreae Usta*, to be decocted first) 15 g and Fuxiaomai (*Fructus Tritici Levis*) 12 g.

(3) Deficiency of Spleen Yin and Stomach Yin

Chief Manifestations: Dry mouth and lips, poor appetite, dry stools, even retch, hiccup, flushed face, dry tongue with little coating or no coating, thready and rapid pulse.

Therapeutic Methods: To nourish yin and regulate stomach qi.

Prescription: Modified Yiwei Tang (Decoction for Nourishing Stomach), composed of Shashen (*Radix Adenophorae*) 12 g, Maimendong (*Radix Ophiopogonis*) 12 g, Shengdihuang (*Radix Rehmanniae*) 12 g, Yuzhu (*Rhizoma Polygonati Odorati*) 10 g, Shanyao (*Rhiaoma Dioscoreae*) 12 g and Biandou (*Semen Dolichoris*) 12 g.

Modifications: For consumption of body fluids manifested as dry mouth and lips, add Shihu (*Herba Dendrobii*) 10 g and Tianhuafen (*Radix Trichosanthis*) 10 g; for poor appetite, add Maiya (*Fructus Hordei Germinatus*) 12 g and Guya (*Fructus Oryzae Germinatus*) 12 g; for hiccup, add Daodou (*Semen Canavaliae*) 6 g, Shidi (*Calyx Kaki*) 6 g and Zhuru (*Caulis Bambusae in Taeniam*) 6 g.

(4) Deficiency of Liver Yin

Chief Manifestations: Headache, dizziness, tinnitus, dry eyes, photophobia, impaired vision, irritability, or numbness of limbs, muscular twitching and cramps, flushed cheeks, dry red tongue, wiry, thready and rapid pulse.

Therapeutic Method: To nourish liver yin.

Prescription: Modified Bugan Tang (Decoction for

牡蛎(先煎)15 g,浮小麦12 g。

（3）脾胃阴虚证

主要证候　口干唇燥,不思饮食,大便燥结,甚则干呕,呃逆,面色潮红,舌干,苔少或无苔,脉细数。

治　法　养阴和胃。

方　药　益胃汤加减:沙参12 g,麦门冬12 g,生地黄12 g,玉竹10 g,山药12 g,扁豆12 g。

加　减　口干唇燥,为津亏较甚,加石斛10 g,天花粉10 g;不思饮食,加麦芽12 g,谷芽12 g;呃逆较甚者,加刀豆6 g,柿蒂6 g,竹茹6 g。

（4）肝阴虚证

主要证候　头痛,眩晕,耳鸣,目干畏光,视物不明,急躁易怒,或肢体麻木,筋惕肉瞤,面色潮红,舌干红,脉弦细数。

治　法　滋养肝阴。

方　药　补肝汤加减:当

Nourishing Liver), composed of Danggui (*Radix Angelicae Sinensis*) 10 g, Baishaoyao (*Radix Paeoniae Alba*) 10 g, Chuanxiong (*Rhizoma Chuanxiong*) 10 g, Shudihuang (*Radix Rehmanniae Preparata*) 12 g, Mugua (*Fructus Chaenomelis*) 10 g, Zhigancao (*Radix Glycyrrhizae, roasted*) 3 g, Maimendong (*Radix Ophiopogonis*) 10 g and Suanzaoren (*Semen Ziziphi Spinosae*) 10 g.

Modifications: For disturbance of liver wind inside the body, manifested as pronounced headache, dizziness, tinnitus, or muscular twitching and cramps, add Shijueming (*Concha Haliotidis*, to be decocted first) 15 g, Juhua (*Flos Chrysanthemi*) 6 g, Gouteng (*Ramulus Uncariae cum Uncis*) 12 g and Cijili (*Fructus Tribuli*) 12 g; for dryness of eyes and photophobia, or impaired vision, add Gouqizi (*Fructus Lycii*) 10 g, Nüzhenzi (*Fructus Ligustri Lucidi*) 10 g and Caojueming (*Cemen Cassiae*) 15 g; for hyperactive liver fire manifested as irritability, deep-coloured urine, constipation, red tongue and rapid pulse, add Longdancao (*Radix Gentianae*) 5 g, Huangqin (*Radix Scutellariae*) 10 g and Zhizi (*Fructus Gardeniae*) 10 g.

(5) Deficiency of Kidney Yin

Chief Manifestations: Soreness of loins, nocturnal emission, weakness of legs, dizziness, tinnitus, even deaf, dryness of mouth, sore throat, flushed cheeks, red tongue with little moisture , deep and thready pulse.

Therapeutic Method: To nourish kidney yin.

Prescription: Modified Zuogui Wan (Pill for Replenishing Kidney Yin), composed of Shudihuang (*Radix Rehmanniae Preparata*) 10 g, Gouqizi (*Fructus Lycii*) 10 g, Shanyao (*Rhizoma Dioscoreae*) 10 g, Guiban (*Plastrum Testudinis*, to be decocted first) 15 g, Niuxi (*Radix Achyranthis Bidentatae*) 10 g, Shanzhuyu

归10 g,白芍药10 g,川芎10 g,熟地黄12 g,木瓜10 g,炙甘草3 g,麦门冬10 g,酸枣仁10 g。

加　减　头痛、眩晕、耳鸣,或筋惕肉瞤者,为风阳内扰,加石决明(先煎)15 g,菊花6 g,钩藤12 g,刺蒺藜12 g;目干涩畏光,或视物不明者,加枸杞子10 g,女贞子10 g,草决明15 g;急躁易怒,尿赤便秘,舌红脉数者,为肝火亢盛,加龙胆草5 g,黄芩10 g,栀子10 g。

(5) 肾阴虚证

主要证候　腰酸,遗精,两足萎弱,眩晕,耳鸣,甚则耳聋,口干,咽痛,颧红,舌红,少津,脉沉细。

治　法　滋补肾阴。

方　药　左归丸加减。熟地黄10 g,枸杞子10 g,山药10 g,龟版(先煎)15 g,牛膝10 g,山茱萸10 g,菟丝子10 g,鹿角胶(烊化冲)10 g。

(*Fructus Corni*) 10 g, Tusizi (*Semen Cuscutae*) 10 g
and Lujiaojiao (*Colla Cornus Cervi*, to be melted in the
finished decoction) 10 g.

Modifications: For frequent nocturnal emission,
add Duanmuli (*Concha Ostreae Usta*, to be decocted
first) 20 g, Jinyingzi (*Fructus Rosae Laevigatae*) 10 g,
Qianshi (*Semen Euryales*) 10 g and Lianxu (*Stamen
Nelumbinis*) 10 g; for deficiency of yin and hyperactivity
of fire, manifested as hectic fever, dryness of mouth,
sore throat and rapid pulse, remove Lujiaojiao, add Zhimu
(*Rhizoma Anemarrhenae*) 10 g, Huangbai (*Cortex
Phellodendri*) 10 g and Digupi (*Cortex Lycii*) 10 g.

4. Yang Deficiency

(1) Deficiency of Heart Yang

Chief Manifestations: Palpitation, spontaneous
sweating, lassitude, sleepiness, stuffiness and pain in the
heart and chest, chills, cold limbs, pale complexion, pale
or dark purple tongue, thready and weak pulse or deep
and slow pulse.

Therapeutic Methods: To benefit qi and warm
yang.

Prescription: Modified Baoyuan Tang (Decoction
for Preserving Primordial Qi), composed of Hongshen
(*Radix Ginseng*, to be decocted separately) 10 g, Huangqi (*Radix Astragali*) 10 g, Zhigancao (*Radix Glycyr-
rhizai*, roasted) 3 g, Rougui (*Cortex Cinnamomi*) 6 g
and Shengjiang (*Rhizoma Zingiberis Recens*) 3 g.

Modifications: For pain in the heart and chest, add
Yujin (*Radix Curcumae*) 10 g, Chuanxiong (*Rhizoma
Chuanxiong*) 10 g and Danshen (*Radix Salviae Miltiorrhizae*) 10 g; for predominance of deficient yang, manifested as chills, cold limbs and slow pulse, add Zhifuzi
(*Radix Aconiti Lateralis Preparata*) 8 g, Bajitian (*Radix Morindae Officinalis*) 10 g, Xianmao (*Rhizoma

加　减　遗精较频者,加
煅牡蛎(先煎)20 g,金樱子
10 g,芡实10 g,莲须10 g;潮
热、口干、咽痛、脉数,为阴虚
火旺,去鹿角胶,加知母10 g,
黄柏10 g,地骨皮10 g。

4. 阳虚

(1) 心阳虚证

主要证候　心悸,自汗,
神倦嗜卧,心胸憋闷疼痛,形
寒肢冷,面色苍白,舌质淡或
紫暗,脉细弱或沉迟。

治　法　益气温阳。

方　药　保元汤加减:
红参(另煎)10 g,黄芪10 g,炙
甘草3 g,肉桂6 g,生姜3 g。

加　减　心胸疼痛者,加
郁金10 g,川芎10 g,丹参10 g;
形寒肢冷,脉迟,为阳虚较甚,
酌加制附子8 g,巴戟天10 g,
仙茅10 g,淫羊藿10 g。

Curculiginis) 10 g and Yinyanghuo (*Herba Epimedii*)
10 g.

(2) Deficiency of Spleen Yang

Chief Manifestations: Sallow complexion, poor appetite, chills, lassitude, shortness of breath, hypologia, loose
stools, borborymus, abdominal pain which is aggravated by
exposure to cold and improper diet, pale tongue with
white coating, weak pulse.

Therapeutic Methods: To warm the middle energizer and invigorate the spleen.

Prescription: Modified Fuzi Lizhong Tang (Aconiti
Lateralis Decoction for Regulating Middle Energizer),
composed of Dangshen (*Radix Codonopsis*) 10 g, Baizhu
(*Rhizoma Atractylodis Macrocephalae*) 10 g, Zhigancao
(*Radix Glycyrrhizae, roasted*) 3 g, Ganjiang (*Rhizo-
ma Zingiberis*) 6 g and Zhifuzi (*Radix Aconiti Lateralis
Preparata*) 6 g.

Modifications: For stagnation of qi due to pathogenic cold manifested as severe cold pain in the abdomen,
add Gaoliangjiang (*Rhizoma Alpiniae Officinarum*)
6 g, Xiangfu (*Rhizoma Cyperi*) 10 g and Wuzhuyu
(*Frutus Evodiae*) 3 g; for adverse flow of qi due to
stomach cold, manifested as abdominal flatulence and
vomiting after eating, add Sharen (*Fructus Amomi*, to
be decocted later) 3 g, Zhibanxia (*Rhizoma Pinelliae
Preparata*) 10 g and Chenpi (*Pericarpium Citri Reticulatae*) 6 g; for retention of dampness due to yang deficiency manifested as severe diarrhea, add Roudoukou
(*Semen Myristicae*) 10 g, Buguzhi (*Fructus Psoraleae*) 10 g and Yiyiren (*Semen Coicis*) 12 g.

(3) Deficiency of Kidney Yang

Chief Manifestations: Soreness and pain of back
and loins, nocturnal emission, impotence, polyuria or incontinence, pale complexion, chills and cold limbs, dys-

（2）脾阳虚证

主要证候　面色萎黄,食
少,形寒,神倦乏力,少气懒
言,大便溏泻,肠鸣腹痛,每因
受寒或饮食不慎而加剧,舌质
淡,苔白,脉弱。

治　法　温中健脾。

方　药　附子理中汤加
减:党参10 g,白术10 g,炙甘
草3 g,干姜6 g,制附子6 g。

加　减　腹中冷痛较甚,
为寒凝气滞,可加高良姜6 g,
香附10 g,吴茱萸3 g;食后腹
胀及呕逆者,为胃寒气逆,加
砂仁(后下)3 g,制半夏10 g,
陈皮6 g;腹泻,为阳虚湿甚,加
肉豆蔻10 g,补骨脂10 g,薏苡
仁12 g。

（3）肾阳虚证

主要证候　腰背酸痛,遗
精,阳痿,多尿或失禁,面色苍
白,畏寒肢冷,下利清谷或五

peptic diarrhea or morning diarrhea, swollen pale tongue with white coating and teeth marks on its margin, deep and slow pulse.

Therapeutic Method: To warm and nourish kidney yang.

Prescription: Modified Yougui Wan (Bolus for Replenishing Kidney Yang), composed of Zhifuzi (*Radix Aconiti Preparata*) 6 g, Rougui (*Cortex Cinnamomi*) 3 g, Duzhong (*Cortex Eucommiae*) 10 g, Shanzhuyu (*Fructus Corni*) 10 g, Tusizi (*Semen Cuscutae*) 10 g, Lujiaojiao (*Colla Cornus Cervi*, to be melted in the finished decoction) 10 g, Shudihuang (*Radix Rehmanniae Preparata*) 12 g, Shanyao (*Rhizoma Dioscoreae*) 12 g, Gouqizi (*Fructus Lycii*) 10 g and Danggui (*Radix Angelicae Sinensis*) 10 g.

Modifications: For frequent nocturnal emission, add Jinyingzi (*Fructus Rosae Laevigatae*) 10 g, Sangpiaoxiao (*Oötheca Mantidis*) 10 g and Lianxu (*Stamen Nelumbinis*) 10 g; for predominant dampness due to deficiency of the spleen manifested as dyspeptic diarrhea, remove those lubricious and sticky drugs such as Shudihuang and Danggui, add Chaodangshen (*Radix Codonopsis*, stir-baked) 10 g, Baizhu (*Rhizoma Atractylodis Macrocephalae*) 10 g and Yiyiren (*Semen Coicis*) 10 g; for morning diarrhea resulting from deficiency of kidney yang, add Buguzhi (*Fructus Psoraleae*) 10 g, Yinyanghuo (*Herba Epimedii*) 10 g and Roudoukou (*Semen Myristicae*) 10 g; for water retention caused by yang deficiency, manifested as edema and oliguria, add Fuling (*Poria*) 12 g, Zexie (*Rhizoma Alismatis*) 12 g and Cheqianzi (*Semen Plantaginis*, wrapped) 10 g; for failure of the kidney to promote inspiration manifested as dyspnea, shortness of breath which is aggravated on exertion, add Buguzhi (*Fructus Psoraleae*) 10 g and Wuweizi (*Fructus*

更泄泻，舌质淡胖，有齿痕，苔白，脉沉迟。

治　法　温补肾阳。

方　药　右归丸加减：制附子6 g，肉桂3 g，杜仲10 g，山茱萸10 g，菟丝子10 g，鹿角胶（烊化冲服）10 g，熟地黄12 g，山药12 g，枸杞子10 g，当归10 g。

加　减　遗精较频者，加金樱子10 g，桑螵蛸10 g，莲须10 g；脾虚湿盛以致下利清谷者，减去熟地黄、当归等滋润滑腻之品，加炒党参10 g，白术10 g，薏苡仁10 g；命门火衰以致五更泄泻者，加补骨脂10 g，淫羊藿10 g，肉豆蔻10 g；阳虚水泛以致浮肿、尿少者，加茯苓12 g，泽泻12 g，车前子（包煎）10 g；肾不纳气而见喘促、短气，动则更甚者，加补骨脂10 g，五味子6 g。

Schisandrae) 6 g.

Other Treatments

1. Chinese Patent Drugs

(1) Renshen Jing (Ginseng Essence): 2 - 3 ml each time, thrice daily, taken before meals; indicated for poor appetite due to spleen deficiency and cough due to lung deficiency.

(2) Huangqijing Koufuye (Oral Liquid of Astragali Essence): 10 ml each time, twice daily; indicated for deficiency of qi and blood, spontaneous sweating due to exterior deficiency and weakness of limbs.

(3) Jingui Shenqi Wan (Pill for Invigorating Kidney Qi from *Golden Cabinet*): 6 g each time, twice daily; indicated for deficiency of kidney yang manifested as dizziness, soreness and weakness of loins and knees.

(4) Shiquan Dabu Jiu (Powerful Medicated Wine of Ten Tonics): 15 - 30 ml each time, twice daily; indicated for deficiency of both qi and blood manifested as pallor, shortness of breath, palpitation, dizziness, spontaneous sweating and fatigue.

(5) Shengmai Yin (Oral Liquid for Reinforcing Qi and Nourishing Yin): 10 ml each time, 3 times daily; indicated for deficiency of both qi and yin.

(6) Shouwu Pian (Tablet of Polygoni Multiflori): 5 tablets each time, taken with warm water, 3 times daily; indicated for deficiency of blood manifested as dizziness, tinnitus, soreness and weakness of the loins and knees.

(7) Danggui Yangxue Gao (Angelicae Sinensis Extract for Nourishing Blood): 15 ml each time, 3 times daily; indicated for deficiency of both qi and blood manifested as sallow complexion, dizziness and emaciaton.

(8) Liuwei Dihuang Wan (Pill of Six Drugs Containing Rehmanniae): 6 g each time, twice daily; indicated for deficiency of kidney yin manifested as dizziness, tinni-

【其他疗法】

1. 中成药

(1) 人参精　每服 2～3 ml,每日 3 次,饭前服。适用于脾虚食少,肺虚喘咳者。

(2) 黄芪精口服液　每服 10 ml,每日 2 次。适用于气虚血少,表虚自汗,四肢乏力者。

(3)《金匮》肾气丸　每服 6 g,每日 2 次。适用于肾阳不足,头晕目眩,腰膝酸软者。

(4) 十全大补酒　每服 15～30 ml,每日 2 次。适用于气血两亏,面色苍白,气短心悸,头晕自汗,体倦乏力者。

(5) 生脉饮　每服 10 ml,每日 3 次。适用于气阴不足之证。

(6) 首乌片　每服 5 片,每日 3 次,温开水送服。适用于血虚体弱,头晕耳鸣,腰膝酸软。

(7) 当归养血膏　每服 15 ml,每日 3 次。适用于气虚血亏,面色萎黄,眩晕乏力,肌肉消瘦者。

(8) 六味地黄丸　每服 6 g,每日 2 次。适用于肾阴亏虚,头晕耳鸣,腰膝酸软,骨蒸

tus, soreness and weakness of loins and knees, hectic fever, night sweating and nocturnal emission.

(9) Zhuangyao Jianshen Wan (Pill for Strengthening Loins and Invigorating Kidney): 6 g each time, twice daily; indicated for kidney deficiency manifested as soreness and pain of the loins, frequent micturition, impotence and nocturnal emission.

2. Single-drug or Experiential Prescriptions

(1) Soak 10 g of American ginseng with 300 ml of hot water for two hours and take the warm ginseng tea at any time, and eat the ginseng, one dose daily. It is indicated for consumptive diseases due to deficiency of both qi and yin.

(2) Take Taipanfen (*Placenta Hominis*, powdered) 30 g, capsulize the powder, 0.5 g for each capsule. Take 6 capsules each time, 4 times daily. It is indicated for consumptive diseases due to deficiency of qi and blood and deficiency of the kidney.

(3) Take one tortoise, wash it and remove the viscera, then bake it on an iron plate over a gentle fire until the shell and flesh turn scorched-yellow. Grind them into powder and take 3 – 5 g each time, 3 times daily. It is indicated for consumptive diseases due to deficiency of blood and yin.

2.6.3　Systemic Lupus Erythematosus (SLE)

General Description

SLE is a kind of autoimmune disease that affects many systems of the body. It is found more often in young females. Clinically it has a variety of symptoms which occur repeatedly and tissues and organs like joints, muscles, skin and the kidneys are mostly involved. The cause of

潮热,盗汗遗精者。

（9）壮腰健肾丸　每服6 g,每日 2 次。适用于肾亏腰痛,腰软无力,小便频数,阳痿遗精者。

2.　单验方

（1）西洋参 10 g,以水300 ml,浸泡 2 小时后,温服,不拘时,最后将渣全部食用,每日 1 剂。适用于气阴两虚之虚劳。

（2）胎盘粉 30 g,装胶囊,每粒 0.5 g,每次 6 粒,每日 4 次。适用于气血双亏及肾虚之虚劳。

（3）乌龟 1 只,洗净,去肠杂,放在低温的铁板上烘烤,待壳、肉呈焦黄时研末备用。每次服 3～5 g,每日 3 次。适用于血虚阴亏之虚劳。

第三节　系统性红斑狼疮

【概述】

系统性红斑狼疮是一种可侵犯全身多系统的自身免疫性疾病。本病多发于青年女性,临床症状多种多样,反复发作,以关节、肌肉、皮肤、

SLE is unknown, but generally it is believed to be related to heredity, virus infection, intake of some medicines, exposure to ultraviolet ray and disturbance of endocrine function.

SLE is considered to be of the category of "bi zheng" (arthralgia-syndrome), "yin yang du" (lupus erythematosus discoides), "gui lian chuang" (facial erythema). Insufficiency of congenital disposition , lack of nourishment after birth, or seven emotional upsets complicated by exposure to sunlight and attack of six exogenous factors are the causes of the disease; imbalance of yin and yang, stagnation of qi and blood and blockage of meridians are its pathogenesis. When toxic heat flares up the face, facial erythema occurs; when it deeply attacks yingfen and xuefen, the zang-fu organs are injured and complicated syndromes of the body ensue.

Essentials for Diagnosis

(1) Early symptoms include fever and lesion of the skin and joints. Typical skin lesion shows the symmetrical butterfly erthema on both cheeks and nose. In severe cases, skin lesion spreads all over the body, mucous membranes of the mouth and vulva erode and ulcerate, and the hair falls out. In most cases, there appears irregular low fever and high fever in occasional cases. Arthralgia mostly involves the joint of the limbs and Raynaud phenomenon may occur in those cases who are exposed to cold. At the later stage, injury and even failure of multiple organs appear.

(2) Different symptoms are seen when various organs are involved at the later stage. The kidneys are first involved and injured severely. So nephritis and nephrotic syndrome occur and ultimately uremia may appear. In addition, the cardiovascular system, the respiratory sys-

肾脏等为主要累及的组织或器官。本病病因尚未清楚，一般认为与遗传、病毒感染、服用某些药物、紫外线照射、内分泌失调等原因有关。

根据本病的症状特点，可归属于中医学"痹证"、"阴阳毒"、"鬼脸疮"等范畴。先天禀赋不足，后天失于调养，或七情内伤，加之日光阳毒，六淫侵袭为本病之因；机体阴阳失衡，气血瘀滞，经络阻滞是本病主要病机。热毒上炎面肤，则发红斑；入里灼伤营血，薰蒸脏腑，故致脏腑全身错综复杂之证候出现。

【诊断要点】

(1) 本病早期多为发热，皮肤和关节损害。典型皮损为鼻和两颊部对称性蝶形红斑，严重时皮损可泛发全身，口腔外阴黏膜糜烂、破溃，头发脱落。发热多为不规则低热，也可出现高热。关节痛以四肢关节为主，部分患者遇寒冷出现雷诺现象。晚期则可见多脏器损伤甚至衰竭。

(2) 晚期侵犯各脏器而出现不同的症状。肾脏是发生最早和损害最严重的脏器，主要表现为肾炎和肾病综合征，后期可形成尿毒症。此外，心

tem, the digestive system and the nervous system may get involved and corresponding symptoms are seen.

(3) Laboratory examination: anemia, decreased numbers of white blood cells, lymphocytic cells and platelets, and increased ESR; elevated serum gamma globulin, IgG, IgM, IgA and circulatory immunocomplex; decreased complement; positive ANA and anti-ds-DNA-antibody; proteinuria seen in the patients with the kidneys involved.

(4) Skin LBT is positive or specific change is found in renal tissue biopsy.

Syndrome Differentiation and Treatment

Clinically the disease is characterized by principal deficiency and secondary excess and the differentiation should focus on whether principal deficiency or secondary excess is dominant. If it is a case of secondary excess, a further differentiation is needed as to identify the location of the disease as whether it is at qifen, yingfen or xuefen, the severity and urgency of the case and the involved organ; if it is a case of principal deficiency, a further differentiation should be made to identify the location of the disease and the dominant aspect as whether it is qi deficiency, yang deficiency or yin deficiency. Then corresponding principles should be established according to whether principal deficiency or secondary excess is dominant. As most of the cases are caused by deficiency of liver yin and kidney yin and the attack of pathogenic heat, nourishing yin, subduing fire, clearing away heat and toxic substance are the common therapeutic principles.

1. Yin Deficiency Generating Internal Heat

Chief Manifestations: Facial erythema which is

血管系统、呼吸系统、消化系统、神经系统也可受累而出现相应症状。

（3）实验室检查可见贫血、白细胞、淋巴细胞、血小板减少，血沉增快。血清丙种球蛋白升高，免疫球蛋白 IgG、IgM、IgA 升高，循环免疫复合物升高，补体降低。抗核抗体阳性，抗 ds－DNA 抗体阳性。肾脏受累者可见蛋白尿。

（4）皮肤狼疮带试验阳性，或肾组织活检有特异性改变。

【辨证论治】

本病临床多属本虚标实之证，故必须辨明本虚和标实的主次。标实为主者，须进一步辨明在气、在营、在血，何脏受累，病之轻重缓急；本虚为主者，还须进一步辨其气虚、阳虚、阴虚何者为主以及病位所在。治疗当根据标本虚实的主次，确立相应的治法。由于本病多见肝肾阴虚，热毒侵袭，故滋阴降火、清热解毒实为本病临床常用之治疗大法。

1. 阴虚内热证

主要证候 面部红斑，边

well-demarcated and mildly swollen, bright red or deep red, covered with scales and aggravated by exposure to sunlight or overstrain, associated with flushed cheeks, low fever, weakness, feverish sensation of five centers, insomnia and night sweating, red tongue with little coating, thready and rapid pulse.

Therapeutic Methods: To nourish yin, tonify the kidney, clear away heat and cool blood.

Prescription: Modified Zhi Bai Dihuang Wan (Pill of Anemarrhenae, Phellodendri and Rehmanniae), composed of Zhimu (*Rhizoma Anemarrhenae*) 10 g, Huangbai (*Cortex Phellodendri*) 10 g, Shengdihuang (*Radix Rehmanniae*) 12 g, Mudanpi (*Cortex Moutan Radicis*) 10 g, Zexie (*Rhizoma Alismatis*) 10 g, Digupi (*Cortex Lycii*) 12 g, Xuanshen (*Radix Scrophulariae*) 10 g, Shihu (*Herba Dendrobii*) 10 g, Qinghao (*Herba Artemisiae Annuae*) 12 g and Maimendong (*Radix Ophiopogonis*) 10 g.

Modifications: For persistent low fever, add Yinchaihu (*Radix Stellariae*) 6 g and Baiwei (*Radix Cynanchi Atrati*) 10 g; for pronounced night sweating, add Wuweizi (*Fructus Schisandrae*) 6 g and Fuxiaomai (*Fructus Tritici Levis*) 12 g; for baldness, add Heshouwu (*Radix Polygoni Multiflori*) 12 g and Nüzhenzi (*Fructus Ligustri Lucidi*) 10 g; for pronounced arthralgia, add Qinjiao (*Radix Gentianae Macrophyllae*) 10 g and Jixueteng (*Caulis Spatholobi*) 12 g; for more facial erythema, add Chishaoyao (*Radix Paeoniae Rubra*) 10 g and Qiancao (*Radix Rubiae*) 10 g.

2. Qi Stagnation and Blood Stasis

Chief Manifestations: Symmetrical butterfly facial erythema, which is red and covered with adhesive greyish-white scales, associated with hypochondriac distension and pain, headache, eye pain, abdominal distension, poor

缘清楚隆起微肿,鲜红或黯红,上覆鳞屑,日晒或劳累加重。伴两颊潮红,低热乏力,五心烦热,失眠盗汗,舌质红,少苔,脉细数。

治　法　滋阴补肾,清热凉血。

方　药　知柏地黄丸加减:知母10 g,黄柏10 g,生地黄12 g,牡丹皮10 g,泽泻10 g,地骨皮12 g,玄参10 g,石斛10 g,青蒿12 g,麦门冬10 g。

加　减　低热不退者,加银柴胡6 g,白薇10 g;盗汗明显者,加五味子6 g,浮小麦12 g;脱发者,加何首乌12 g,女贞子10 g;关节疼痛明显,加秦艽10 g,鸡血藤12 g;面颊红斑较多者,加赤芍药10 g,茜草10 g。

2. 气滞血瘀证

主要证候　面部红斑呈蝶型对称,颜色红,鳞屑灰白,粘着难剥,伴胸胁胀痛,头目晕痛,腹胀纳呆,月经不调或

appetite, irregular menstruation or dysmenorrhea, deep red tongue or with petechia, yellow and thin coating, wiry and unsmooth pulse or wiry and rapid pulse.

Therapeutic Methods: To soothe the liver, regulate qi, promote blood circulation and remove blood stasis.

Prescription: Modified Xiaoyao San (Xiaoyao Powder), composed of Chaihu (*Radix Bupleuri*) 6 g, Danggui (*Radix Angelicae Sinensis*) 10 g, Baishaoyao (*Radix Paeoniae Alba*) 10 g, Yujin (*Radix Curcumae*) 10 g, Baizhu (*Rhizoma Atractylodis macrocephalae*) 10 g, Fuling (*Poria*) 12 g, Taoren (*Semen Persicae*) 10 g, Honghua (*Flos Carthami*) 10 g, Zhike (*Fructus Aurantii*) 6 g, Chuanlianzi (*Fructus Meliae Toosendan*) 10 g, Bohe (*Herba Menthae*) 6 g, Shenggancao (*Radix Glycyrrhizae*) 5 g and Weijiang (*Rhizoma Zingiberis Recens*, roasted in fresh cinders) 3 g.

Modifications: For more severe hypochondriac pain, add Danshen (*Radix Salviae Miltiorrhizae*) 12 g and Gouqizi (*Fructus Lycii*) 10 g; for irregular menstruation, add Yimucao (*Herba Leonuri*) 12 g and Zelan (*Herba Lycopi*) 10 g.

3. Excessive Toxic Heat

Chief Manifestations: Acute onset, persistent high fever, erythema or ecchymosis on the skin, associated with hematemesis, epistaxis, hemafecia, purpura, soreness and pain of muscles, arthralgia, irritability and sleeplessness, even coma, delirium and convulsion in severe cases, deep red tongue with yellow or exfoliated coating, bounding and rapid pulse.

Therapeutic Methods: To clear away heat, cool blood, remove toxic substance and dissipate erythema.

Prescription: Modified Xijiao Dihuang Tang (Cornu Rhinocerotis and Rehmanniae Decoction), composed of Shuiniujiao (*Cornu Bubali*, to be decocted first) 30 g,

痛经,舌质黯红或有瘀点,苔薄黄,脉弦涩或弦数。

治　法　疏肝理气,活血化瘀。

方　药　逍遥散加减:柴胡6 g,当归10 g,白芍药10 g,郁金10 g,白术10 g,茯苓12 g,桃仁10 g,红花10 g,枳壳6 g,川楝子10 g,薄荷6 g,生甘草5 g,煨姜3 g。

加　减　胁肋疼痛较甚者,加丹参12 g,枸杞子10 g;月经不调,加益母草12 g,泽兰10 g。

3. 热毒炽盛证

主要证候　发病急促,持续高热,皮肤出现红斑或瘀斑,可有吐血、衄血、便血、紫斑、肌肉酸痛、关节疼痛、烦躁不眠,严重时神昏、谵语、抽搐,舌质红绛,苔黄或光剥,脉洪数。

治　法　清热凉血,解毒化斑。

方　药　犀角地黄汤加减:水牛角(先煎)30 g,生地黄12 g,牡丹皮10 g,赤芍药10 g,

Shengdihuang （ *Radix Rehmanniae* ） 12 g, Mudanpi （*Cortex Moutan Radicis*） 10 g, Chishaoyao （*Radix Paeoniae Rubra*） 10 g, Jingyinhua （*Flos Lonicerae*） 15 g, Xuanshen （*Radix Scrophulariae*） 12 g, Zicao （*Radix Arnebiae seu Lithospermi*） 10 g, Shengshigao （*Gypsum Fibrosum*, to be decocted first） 30 g, Zhimu （*Rhizoma Anemarrhenae*） 10 g and Shenggancao （*Radix Glycyrrhizae*） 5 g.

Modifications: For pronounced hemorrhage, add Jinyinhuatan （*Flos Lonicerae*, charred） 10 g, Shengdihuangtan （*Radix Rehmanniae*, charred） 10 g and Cebaiye （*Cacumen Platycladi*） 10 g; for persistent high fever, add Huanglian （*Rhizoma Coptidis*） 3 g, Huangbai （*Cortex Phellodendri*） 10 g and Shengdahuang （*Radix et Rhizoma Rhei*, to be decocted later） 5 g; for convulsion, add Lingyangjiaofen （*Cornu Saigae Tataricae*, powdered and to be infused separately） 1 g and Gouteng （*Ramulus Uncariae cum Uncis*） 12 g.

4. Deficiency of Both Qi and Yin

Chief Manifestations: Sustained bright-red erythema, persistent high fever followed by low fever, feverish sensation in the palms and soles, dry throat and thirst, irritability, insomnia, shortness of breath, hypologia, lusterless complexion, soreness of joints, baldness, red tongue with thin or no coating, thready, rapid pulse or soft-superficial, rapid pulse.

Therapeutic Methods: To replenish qi, nourish yin and activate the collaterals.

Prescription: Modified Shengmai Yin (Decoction for Reinforcing Qi and Nourishing Yin), composed of Taizishen （*Radix Pseudostellariae*） 12 g, Maimendong （ *Radix Ophiopogonis* ） 10 g, Wuweizi （ *Fructus Schisandrae*） 6 g, Shengdihuang （*Radix Rehmanniae*） 12 g, Xuanshen （*Radix Scrophulariae*） 10 g, Huangqi

金银花15 g, 玄参12 g, 紫草10 g, 生石膏(先煎)30 g, 知母10 g, 生甘草5 g。

加　减　衄血明显者, 加金银花炭10 g, 生地黄炭10 g, 侧柏叶10 g; 壮热不退者, 加黄连3 g, 黄柏10 g, 生大黄(后下)5 g; 抽搐者, 加羚羊角粉(另冲)1 g, 钩藤12 g。

4. 气阴两虚证

主要证候　皮损红斑不退, 色鲜红, 高热后持续低热, 手足心热, 口渴咽干, 心烦不眠, 少气懒言, 面色不华, 关节酸痛, 毛发脱失, 舌红苔薄或无, 脉细数或濡数。

治　法　益气养阴, 通经活络。

方　药　生脉饮加减: 太子参12 g, 麦门冬10 g, 五味子6 g, 生地黄12 g, 玄参10 g, 黄芪12 g, 沙参10 g, 石斛10 g, 当归10 g, 丹参12 g, 鸡血藤12 g。

(*Radix Astragali*) 12 g, Shashen (*Radix Adenophorae*) 10 g, Shihu (*Herba Dendrobii*) 10 g, Danggui (*Radix Angelicae Sinensis*) 10 g, Danshen (*Radix Salviae Miltiorrhizae*) 12 g and Jixueteng (*Caulis Spatholobi*) 12 g.

Modifications: For persistent low fever, add Digupi (*Cortex Lycii*) 10 g and Yinchaihu (*Radix Stellariae*) 6 g; for more severe arthralgia, add Sangjisheng (*Herba Taxilli*) 10 g and Qinjiao (*Radix Gentianae Macrophyllae*) 10 g; for erythema on the cheeks, add Jingyinhua (*Flos Lonicerae*) 15 g and Lingxiaohua (*Flos Campsis*) 10 g; for weakness of limbs, add Chaoduzhong (*Cortex Eucommiae*, stir-baked) 10 g and Xuduan (*Radix Dipsaci*) 10 g; for insomnia, add Hehuanhua (*Flos Albiziae*) 6 g and Yejiaoteng (*Caulis et Folium Polygoni Multiflori*) 12 g.

5. Deficiency of Heart Yang and Kidney Yang

Chief Manifestations: Indistinct or no erythema, chills, cold limbs, painful loins and knees, lassitude, puffy face, edema of limbs, palpitation, shortness of breath, cold abdomen and loose stools, swollen, tender and pale tongue with white coating and teeth marks on its margin, deep, thready and weak pulse.

Therapeutic Methods: To warm yang, invigorate the kidney, promote blood circulation and activate collaterals.

Prescription: Modified Jisheng Shenqi Wan (Pill for Replenishing Kidney Qi from *Prescriptions for Saving Life*) and Sijunzi Tang (Four Mild-Drug Decoction), composed of Shufuzi (*Radix Aconiti Lateralis Preparata*) 6 g, Rougui (*Cortex Cinnamomi*) 3 g, Shudihuang (*Radix Rehmanniae Preparata*) 12 g, Shanzhuyu (*Fructus Corni*) 10 g, Shanyao (*Rhizoma Dioscoreae*) 12 g, Mudanpi (*Cortex Moutan Radicis*) 10 g, Fuling

加　减　低热不退者,加地骨皮10 g,银柴胡6 g;关节疼痛明显,加桑寄生10 g,秦艽10 g;面颊红斑,加金银花15 g,凌霄花10 g;肢软乏力加炒杜仲10 g,续断10 g;失眠,加合欢花6 g,夜交藤12 g。

5. 心肾阳虚证

主要证候　皮损红斑不显或无红斑,形寒肢冷,腰膝疼痛,神疲乏力,面浮肢肿,心悸气短,腹冷便溏,舌体胖嫩,舌质淡有齿痕,苔白,脉沉细弱。

治　法　温阳补肾,活血通络。

方　药　《济生》肾气丸合四君子汤加减:熟附子6 g,肉桂3 g,熟地黄12 g,山茱萸10 g,山药12 g,牡丹皮10 g,茯苓10 g,泽泻12 g,党参10 g,黄芪12 g,白术10 g,丹参12 g,车前子(包煎)12 g。

(*Poria*) 10 g, Zexie (*Rhizoma Alismatis*) 12 g, Dang-shen (*Radix Codonopsis*) 10 g, Huangqi (*Radix Astra-gali*) 12 g, Baizhu (*Rhizoma Atractylodis Macrocepha-lae*) 10 g, Danshen (*Radix Salviae Miltiorrhizae*) 12 g and Cheqianzi (*Semen Plantaginis*, wrapped) 12 g.

Modifications: For pronounced edema, add Zhuling (*Polyporus*) 10 g and Dafupi (*Pericarpium Arecae*) 10 g; for scanty urine, add Guizhi (*Ramulus Cinnamo-mi*) 6 g and Shengyiyiren (*Semen Coicis*) 12 g; for se-vere palpitation, add Fushen (*Sclerotium Poriae circum Radicem Pini*) 12 g; for cold and painful limbs, add Qianghuo (*Rhizoma et Radix Notopterygii*) 10 g and Du-huo (*Radix Angelicae Pubescentis*) 10 g.

Other Treatments
1. Chinese Patent Drugs

（1）Hongteng Zhusheye (Sargentodoxae Injection)：4 ampules (2 ml/ampule, containing 4 g of crude drug) are added to 500 ml of 5%–10% glucose solution for in-travenous drip, once daily; or 1 – 2 ampules, once or twice daily for muscle injection; indicated for SLE with pronounced blood stasis.

（2）Leigongteng Pian (Tripterygii Wilfordii Tablet)：2 tablets each time, 3 times daily; indicated for SLE with-out any damage of liver function.

（3）Kunming Shanhaitang Pian (Tripterygium Hypo-glaucum Tablet)：2 to 4 tablets each time, 3 times daily; indicated for milder SLE.

2. Single-drug or Experiential Prescriptions

（1）Huangqi (*Radix Astragali*) 30 – 60 g. Decoct the herb with water, and take the decoction daily. It is indicated for SLE manifested as qi deficiency.

（2）Dangshen (*Radix Codonopsis*) 30 g, Huangqi (*Radix Astragali*) 30 g, Shashen (*Radix Glehniae*)

加 减 水肿明显,加猪苓10 g,大腹皮10 g;小便量少,加桂枝6 g,生薏苡仁12 g;心悸较著,加茯神12 g;肢冷疼痛者,加羌活10 g,独活10 g。

【其他疗法】
1. 中成药

（1）红藤注射液 每次4支(每支2毫升,含生药4克),加入5%～10%葡萄糖溶液500 ml 中,静脉滴注,每日1次。或肌肉注射,每次1～2支,每日1～2次。适用于系统性红斑狼疮血瘀较甚者。

（2）雷公藤片 每服2片,每日3次。适用于系统性红斑狼疮无肝功能损害者。

（3）昆明山海棠片 每服2～4片,每日3次。适用于系统性红斑狼疮病情较轻者。

2. 单验方

（1）黄芪 30～60 g,水煎服,每日1剂。适用于系统性红斑狼疮表现为气虚者。

（2）党参30 g,黄芪30 g,沙参30 g,玄参30 g,生地黄

30 g, Xuanshen (*Radix Scrophulariae*) 30 g, Shengdi-huang (*Radix Rehmanniae*) 30 g, Mudanpi (*Cortex Moutan Radicis*) 30 g, Chishaoyao (*Radix Paeoniae Rubra*) 12 g, Danggui (*Radix Angelicae Sinensis*) 12 g, Taoren (*Semen Persicae*) 6 g, Honghua (*Flos Cartha-mi*) 15 g, Yujin (*Radix Curcumae*) 6 g, Chuanhuanglian (*Rhizoma Coptidis*) 6 g, Lianzixin (*Plumula Nelumbi-nis*) 6 g, Xuejie (*Resina Draconis*) 3 g and Gancao (*Ra-dix Glycyrrhizae*) 6 g. Decoct the above herbs with wa-ter, and take the decoction daily. It is indicated for SLE with deficiency of both qi and yin associated with blood stasis.

3. External Therapy

(1) Shengdahuang (*Radix et Rhizoma Rhei*) 12 g, Shufuzi (*Radix Aconiti Lateralis Preparata*) 10 g and Muli (*Concha Ostreae*) 10 g. Decoct the above herbs with 500 - 800 ml of water to 200 ml of the decoction. Then use the decoction for retention enema one time daily and discharge it 30 minutes later. It is indicated for SLE with renal lesion.

(2) Baifan (*Alumen*) 0.5 g, Kufan (*Alumen Us-ta*) 0.5 g and Wubeizi (*Galla Chinensis*) 2 g. Grind the drugs into fine powder and apply the powder onto the ero-sive and ulcerated area of the skin. It is indicated for SLE with pronounced skin lesion.

2.6.4 Hypertension

General Description

Hypertension, also known as essential hypertension, is a clinical syndrome marked by elevated arterial pressure in the systematic circulation. It is an independent disease manifested mainly as the elevation of the blood pressure with unidentified cause.

30 g,牡丹皮30 g,赤芍药12 g,当归12 g,桃仁6 g,红花15 g,郁金6 g,川黄连6 g,莲子心6 g,血竭3 g,甘草6 g。水煎服,每日1剂。适用于系统性红斑狼疮辨证属气阴两虚兼有血瘀证者。

3. 外治法

(1) 生大黄12 g,熟附子10 g,牡蛎10 g,加水 500 ～ 800 ml,煎至200 ml,保留灌肠,每日1次,保留30分钟后排出。适用于系统性红斑狼疮肾脏损害者。

(2) 白矾 0.5 g,枯矾0.5 g,五倍子2 g,混合研细末,在皮肤糜烂或溃疡处外敷。适用于皮损较著者。

第四节　高血压病

【概述】

高血压病是以体循环动脉压增高为主要表现的临床综合征,是一种以血压升高为主要临床表现而病因尚未明确的独立性疾病,又称原发性

Hypertension is the most common cardiovascular disease with approximately 100 million of hypertensive patients in China. It may lead to severe complication of the heart, brain and kidneys and it is one of the risk factors for stroke, coronary heart disease and renal insufficiency. Hypertension can be classified into benign hypertension and accelerated hypertension according to the urgency and the duration and the latter is also known as malignant hypertension with unfavorable prognosis.

According to its clinical manifestations, this disease falls into the categories of "xuan yun" (vertigo), "tou tong" (headache), "gan yang" (liver yang) and "gan feng" (liver wind) in TCM. The causes of hypertension are mainly emotional disorders, improper diet, prolonged illness and overstrain. Its pathogenesis includes deficiency of liver yin and kidney yin or deficiency of yin and yang, hyperactivity of liver yang, accumulation of turbid phlegm and obstruction of collaterals by blood stasis. I female patients it is related to disorders of conception and thoroughfare vessels. The location of the disease is at the liver, kidney and heart, with incoordination between yin and yang as the principal aspect and wind, fire, phlegm or stasis as the secondary aspect. Pathogenically, it is mainly a case of principal deficiency and secondary excess, deficiency with concomitant excess. For the young, the middle-aged and new patients, their cases are mostly attributed to excess syndrome; and for the old and prolonged patients, their cases chiefly attributed to principal deficiency and secondary excess.

Essentials for Diagnosis

(1) Hypertension has a gradual onset often with no symptom at the early stage, manifested as dizziness,

高血压。

高血压病是最常见的心血管疾病,中国高血压病患者约有1亿之多。本病可引起严重的心、脑、肾并发症,是脑卒中、冠心病、肾功能不全的主要危险因素之一。根据起病的缓急及病程的长短可分为缓进型和急进型两型,急进型又称恶性高血压,预后多不良。

根据高血压病的临床表现,本病属于中医学"眩晕"、"头痛"、"肝阳"、"肝风"等病证。本病的主要病因是情志失调、饮食不节和久病过劳。主要病机是肝肾阴虚或阴阳两虚,肝阳上亢,痰浊内阻,瘀血阻络,女性与冲任失调有关。病位在肝、肾、心,病之本为阴阳失调,病之标为风、火、痰、瘀,病理性质多为本虚标实,虚实相兼。中青年人和新病者多为实证,老年人和久病者多为本虚标实。

【诊断要点】

(1) 高血压病起病缓慢,早期多无症状,有的患者可有

headache, blurred vision, tinnitus, insomnia and lassitude in some cases.

(2) Upon physical examination, the aortic second sound is accentuated and in elderly cases, metallic sound may be heard. Besides, there may be the fourth heart sound and aortic early systolic ejection sound. In a case with prolonged hypertension, there appears left ventricular hypertrophy.

(3) According to the 1999 World Health Organization (WHO)/International Society of Hypertention (ISH) Guidelines, hypertension is defined with the systolic pressure (SP) $\geqslant$ 18.7 kPa (140 mmHg) and/or diastolic pressure (DP) $\geqslant$ 12.0 kPa (90 mmHg) and without taking antihypertensive medication.

(4) Accelerated (malignant) hypertension progresses rapidly with a persistent DP greater than 17.3 kPa (130 mmHg), usually manifested as fundus bleeding or exudation, or edema of the optic disc. There may appear severe damage to the heart, brain and kidneys in a short time and even death.

(5) Routine urine examination: usually normal at the early stage, but when renal function is impaired, protein, erythrocyte, and cast, in occassional cases, may be found in the urine and the concentration of creatinine may increase.

(6) Chest X-ray may reflect the appearance and size of the heart, the change of the width and density (calcification) of the aorta. Echocardiogram is a reliable means to evaluate hypertrophy of the left ventricular. Besides electrocardiogram discloses the involvement of the heart (left ventricular hypertrophy, strain, ischemia and infarction) and arrhythmia, which are caused by high blood

头晕、头痛、眼花、耳鸣、失眠、乏力等症状。

（2）体检时，可听到主动脉瓣第二音亢进，年龄大者可呈金属音，可有第四心音，主动脉收缩早期喷射音。高血压持续时间长时，有左心室肥厚征象。

（3）高血压的诊断，依据1999年世界卫生组织（WHO）/国际高血压联盟高血压治疗的标准，是指在未服用抗高血压药物的情况下，收缩压≥18.7 kPa(140 mmHg)和（或）舒张压≥12.0 kPa（90 mmHg）。

（4）急进性（恶性）高血压，病情多急骤发展，舒张压常持续在 17.3 kPa（130 mm-Hg)以上，可有眼底出血、渗出或视乳头水肿，短时间内可出现心、脑、肾的严重损害，甚至危及生命。

（5）实验室检查尿常规，早期患者多正常，肾功能受损时，尿中可出现蛋白、红细胞，偶见管型。当肾功能受损时血肌酐浓度可增高。

（6）胸部 X 线摄片可显示心脏外形和大小、主动脉宽度和密度（钙化）的变化。超声心动图为评价左心室肥厚的一个可靠的方法。心电图检查可发现由于高血压所致的心脏受累（左心室肥厚和劳

pressure.

Syndrome Differentiation and Treatment

　　Wind, fire, phlegm and blood stasis are the secondary aspect while deficiency of the liver and kidneys is the principal aspect. In clinical practice, cases of the deficiency type are more than those of the excess type; yin deficiency is more often seen than yang deficiency. Generally, hyperactivity of yang is the secondary aspect and deficiency of yin is the principal aspect. However, in the course of the disease, hyperactivity of yang is concurrent with deficiency of yin, with predominance of hyperactivity of yang or with predominance of deficiency of yin and associated with liver wind, turbid phlegm and blood stasis. Therefore, the theraputic principle should primarily aim at nourishing yin and calming the liver and different methods like calming wind, clearing away fire, resolving phlegm and removing blood stasis, should be used accordingly.

1. Hyperactivity of Liver Yang

　　Chief Manifestations: Distending pain of head and eyes, dizziness, flushed face, red eyes, restlessness, irritability, tinnitus, deafness, bitter taste, deep yellow urine, constipation, dry red tongue with thick, yellow coating or greasy, yellow coating, wiry, rapid and forceful pulse.

　　Therapeutic Methods: To calm the liver, suppress yang, clear away heat and reduce fire.

　　Prescription: Modified Longdan Xiegan Tang (Gentianae Decoction for Purging Liver Fire), composed of Longdancao (*Herba Radix Gentianae*) 6 g, Juhua (*Flos Chrysanthemi*) 10 g, Huangqin (*Radix Scutellariae*) 10 g, Zhizi (*Fructus Gardeniae*) 10 g, Zexie (*Rhizoma Alismatis*) 10 g, Caojueming (*Semen Cassiae*) 15 g, Shengdihuang (*Radix Rehemanniae*) 12 g, Sheng-

损、缺血和梗死)和心律失常。

【辨证论治】

　　本病是以风、火、痰、瘀为标,肝肾亏虚为本。从临床实践看来,本病虚证多于实证,阴虚多于阳虚。一般而言,阳亢为标,阴虚是本,就其病程的演变却往往是阳亢与阴虚同时互见,或偏于阳亢,或偏于阴虚,其间并有挟风、挟痰、挟瘀之兼证相伴随。治疗上当以养阴平肝为主要大法,并根据风、火、痰、瘀等病理因素的不同,分别施以熄风、清火、化痰、祛瘀的方法。

1. 肝阳上亢证

　　主要证候　头目胀痛,眩晕,面红目赤,烦躁易怒,耳鸣耳聋,口苦舌干,尿赤便结,舌质红,苔黄厚或黄腻,脉弦数有力。

　　治　法　平肝潜阳,清热降火。

　　方　药　龙胆泻肝汤加减:龙胆草6 g,菊花10 g,黄芩10 g,栀子10 g,泽泻10 g,草决明15 g,生地黄12 g,生大黄(后下)3～10 g,牡丹皮10 g,钩藤(后下)15 g。

dahuang (*Radix et Rhizoma Rhei*, to be decocted later)
3 - 10 g, Mudanpi (*Cortex Moutan Radicis*) 10 g and
Gouteng (*Ramulus Uncariae cum Uncis*, to be decocted
later) 15 g.

Modifications: For severe headache and dizziness,
add Zhenzhumu (*Concha Margaritifera Usta*, to be decocted first) 30 g and Shengshijueming (*Concha Haliotidis*, to be decocted first) 30 g; for pronounced numbness
of limbs, add Dilong (*Pheretima*) 10 g; for stiffness and
pain of the head and neck, add Gegen (*Radix Puerariae*)
10 g.

2. Yin Deficiency Causing Hyperactivity of Yang

Chief Manifestations: Headache, dizziness, tinnitus, blurred vision, heaviness of the head, palpitation, insomnia, restlessness, dreamfulness, soreness and weakness of loins and knees, dry throat and mouth, red tongue
with little coating or yellow, thin coating, wiry, thready
and rapid pulse.

Therapeutic Methods: To nourish yin and calm the
liver.

Prescription: Modified Tianma Gouteng Yin (Gastrodiae and Uncariae Decoction) and Qiju Dihuang Wan
(Rehmanniae Bolus with Lycii and Chrysanthemi), composed of Tianma (*Rhizoma Gastrodiae*) 10 g, Gouteng
(*Ramulus Uncariae cum Uncis*, to be decocted later)
15 g, Shengshijueming (*Concha Haliotidis*, to be decocted first) 30 g, Chuanniuxi (*Radix Cyathulae*) 10 g,
Sangjisheng (*Herba Taxilli*) 15 g, Fushen (*Sclerotium
Poriae circum Radicem Pini*) 15 g, Shengdihuang (*Radix Rehmanniae*) 15 g, Juhua (*Flos Chrysanthemi*)
12 g, Gegen (*Radix Puerariae*) 15 g and Shanzhuyu
(*Fructus Corni*) 12 g.

Modifications: For severe pain in the loins, add
Duzhong (*Cortex Eucommiae*) 10 g; for pronounced dry

加 减 头痛眩晕甚者，
加珍珠母(先煎)30 g,生石决
明(先煎)30 g;肢麻明显者,加
地龙10 g;头项强痛者,加葛根
10 g。

2. 阴虚阳亢证

主要证候 头痛眩晕,耳
鸣眼花,头重脚轻,心悸失眠,
心烦多梦,腰膝酸软,咽干口
燥,舌红苔少或薄黄,脉弦
细数。

治 法 滋阴平肝。

方 药 天麻钩藤饮合
杞菊地黄丸加减:天麻10 g,
钩藤(后下)15 g,生石决明(先
煎)30 g,川牛膝10 g,桑寄生
15 g,茯神15 g,生地黄15 g,菊
花12 g,葛根15 g,山茱萸12 g。

加 减 腰痛甚者,加杜
仲10 g;口干明显者,加石斛

mouth, add Shihu (*Herba Dendrobii*) 10 g; for constipation, add Huomaren (*Semen Cannabis*) 10 g; for numbness of limbs, add Xixiancao (*Herba Siegesbeckiae*) 15 g and Luoshiteng (*Caulis Trachelospermi*) 15 g.

3. Retention of Phlegm Damp in the Body

Chief Manifestations: Dizziness, headache, heaviness of the head with a feeling that the head is tightly wrapped, abdominal distention, poor appetite, nausea, palpitation, edema, weak limbs, white and greasy or yellow and greasy tongue coating, thready and smooth pulse.

Therapeutic Methods: To resolve phlegm and calm wind.

Prescription: Banxia Baizhu Tianma Tang Jiawei (Decoction of Pinelliae, Atractylodis Macrocephalae and Gastrodiae with Additions), composed of Fabanxia (*Rhizoma Pinelliae Preparata*) 10 g, Baizhu (*Rhizoma Atractylodis Macrocephalae*) 12 g, Tianma (*Rhizoma Gastrodiae*) 6 g, Fuling (*Poria*) 15 g, Chenpi (*Pericarpium Citri Reticulatae*) 10 g, Gouteng (*Ramulus Uncariae cum Uncis*, to be decocted later) 15 g, Shichangpu (*Rhizoma Acori Tatarinowii*) 10 g, Zhike (*Fructus Aurantii*) 10 g and Gancao (*Radix Glycyrrhizae*) 6 g.

Modifications: For dizziness, feeling of oppression over the chest, profuse sputum and numbness of limbs, add Beimu (*Bulbus Fritillariae*) 10 g, Tianzhuhuang (*Concretio Silicea Bambusae*) 6 g and Huangqin (*Radix Scutellariae*) 10 g; for scanty urine and pronounced swollen limbs, add Cheqiancao (*Herba Plantaginis*) 15 g; for predominant heat in the liver and gallbladder, add Yinchen (*Herba Artemisiae Scopariae*) 12 g and Huangqin (*Radix Scutellariae*) 10 g.

10 g;大便干结较甚者,加火麻仁10 g;肢体麻木者,加豨莶草15 g,络石藤15 g。

3. 痰湿内盛证

主要证候 头晕头痛,头重如裹,胸闷脘胀,食少欲吐,心悸浮肿,四肢无力,舌苔白腻或黄腻,脉细滑。

治 法 化痰熄风。

方 药 半夏白术天麻汤加味:法半夏10 g,白术12 g,天麻6 g,茯苓15 g,陈皮10 g,钩藤(后下)15 g,石菖蒲10 g,枳壳10 g,甘草6 g。

加 减 头晕、胸闷、痰多、肢体麻木者,加贝母10 g,天竺黄6 g,黄芩10 g;尿少肢肿明显者,加车前草15 g;肝胆湿热明显者,加茵陈12 g,黄芩10 g。

4. Deficiency of Both Yin and Yang

Chief Manifestations: Dizziness, soreness and weakness of the loins and legs, deafness, tinnitus, palpitation, insomnia, short breath on exertion, cold and numb limbs, nocturia , cold feeling of external genitals, impotence, pale tongue with no coating, thready and weak pulse or slow-irregular and intermittent pulse.

Therapeutic Methods: To replenish yin and assist yang.

Prescription: Modified Erxian Tang (Curculiginis and Epimedii Decoction) and Jingui Shenqi Wan (Pill for Invigorating Kidney Qi from *Golden Cabinet*), composed of Xianmao (*Rhizoma Curculiginis*) 12 g, Yinyanghuo (*Herba Epimedii*) 12 g, Bajirou (*Radix Morindae Officinalis, lignin removed*) 12 g, Gouqizi (*Fructus Lycii*) 12 g, Shanzhuyu (*Fructus Corni*) 12 g, Shengdihuang (*Radix Rehmanniae*) 15 g, Shudihuang (*Radix Rehmanniae Preparata*) 15 g, Mudanpi (*Cortex Moutan Radicis*) 10 g, Zhimu (*Rhizoma Anemarrhenae*) 10 g, Danggui (*Radix Angelicae Sinensis*) 10 g, Wuweizi (*Fructus Schisandrae*) 6 g and Shengmuli (*Concha Ostreae*, to be decocted first) 30 g.

Modifications: For deficiency of kidney yang, add Paofuzi (*Radix Aconiti Lateralis*, roasted in hot cinders) 6 g and Rougui (*Cortex Cinnamomi*) 3 g; for deficiency of the spleen, add Fuling (*Poria*) 15 g and Baizhu (*Rhizoma Atractylodis Macrocephalae*) 10 g; for predominant qi deficiency, add Huangqi (*Radix Astragali*) 30 g; for frequent micturition, add Yizhiren (*Semen Alpiniae Oxyphyllae*) 10 g and Buguzhi (*Fructus Psoraleae*) 10 g.

5. Incoordination of Thoroughfare and Conception Vessels

Chief Manifestations: Dizziness, headache, rest-

4. 阴阳两虚证

主要证候 头目眩晕,腰酸腿软,耳聋耳鸣,心悸健忘,动则气促,肢凉麻木,夜尿频数,或见阴冷阳痿,舌淡苔净,脉细弱或结代。

治 法 益阴助阳。

方 药 二仙汤合《金匮》肾气丸加减:仙茅12 g,淫羊藿12 g,巴戟肉12 g,枸杞子12 g,山茱萸12 g,生地黄15 g,熟地黄15 g,牡丹皮10 g,知母10 g,当归10 g,五味子6 g,生牡蛎(先煎)30 g。

加 减 肾阳虚者,加炮附子6 g,肉桂3 g;脾虚者,加茯苓15 g,白术10 g;气虚明显,加黄芪30 g;尿频数者,加益智仁10 g,补骨脂10 g。

5. 冲任失调证

主要证候 头晕头痛,心

lessness, insomnia, tinnitus, irritability, feverish sensation in the palms and soles, amnesia, shortness of breath, irregular menstruation, red tongue with thin coating, wiry and thready pulse.

Therapeutic Methods: To regulate and nourish the thoroughfare and conception vessels.

Prescription: Erxian Tang Jiawei (Curculiginis and Epimedii Decoction with Additions), composed of Xianmao (*Rhizoma Curculiginis*) 10 g, Yinyanghuo (*Herba Epimedii*) 12 g, Bajitian (*Radix Morindae Officinalis*) 12 g, Danggui (*Radix Angelicae Sinensis*) 15 g, Zhimu (*Rhizoma Anemarrhenae*) 10 g and Huangbai (*Cortex Phellodendri*) 10 g.

Modifications: For severe dizziness, add Gouteng (*Ramulus Uncariae cum Uncis*, to be decocted later) 12 g; for restlessness and insomnia, add Suanzaoren (*Semen Ziziphi Spinosae*) 15 g, Yejiaoteng (*Caulis et Folium Polygoni Multiflori*) 12 g and Baiziren (*Semen Platycladi*) 10 g; for irritability, add Chaihu (*Radix Bupleuri*) 6 g and Zisugeng (*Caulis Perillae*) 10 g; for dizziness and distending pain in the head, add Xiakucao (*Spica Prunellae*) 12 g.

Other Treatments

1. Chinese Patent Drugs

(1) Niuhuang Qingxin Wan (Calculus Bovis Bolus for Clearing Heart Fire): 1 bolus each time, taken with boiled water, twice daily; indicated for dizziness and headache due to hyperactivity of liver yang and accumulation of phlegm fire.

(2) Niuhuang Jiangya Wan (Calculus Bovis Bolus for Lowering Blood Pressure): 1 bolus each time, twice daily; indicated for hypertension due to hyperactivity of liver yang.

(3) Naoliqing (Pill for Lowering Blood Pressure): 10

烦失眠,耳鸣易怒,手足心热,记忆力减退,心慌气短,月经失调,舌质红,苔薄,脉弦细。

治　法　调补冲任。

方　药　二仙汤加味:仙茅10 g,淫羊藿12 g,巴戟天12 g,当归15 g,知母10 g,黄柏10 g。

加　减　头晕甚者,加钩藤(后下)12 g;心烦不寐者,加酸枣仁15 g,夜交藤12 g,柏子仁10 g;烦躁易怒者,加柴胡6 g,紫苏梗10 g;头晕胀痛者,加夏枯草12 g。

【其他疗法】

1. 中成药

(1) 牛黄清心丸　每服1丸,每日 2 次,白开水送服。适用于肝阳上亢及痰火壅盛致眩晕头痛。

(2) 牛黄降压丸　每服1丸,每日 2 次。适用于肝阳上亢型高血压病。

(3) 脑立清　每服 10 粒,

pills each time, twice daily; indicated for hypertension due to hyperactivity of liver yang, contraindicated in pregnancy and not suitable for weak constitution with deficient cold.

(4) Quan Tianma Jiaonang (Gastrodiae Capsule): 4 capsules each time, 3 times daily; indicated for hypertension due to hyperactivity of liver yang and upward disturbance of liver wind.

(5) Shanlücha Jiangya Pian (Ilicis Hainanensis Tablet for Lowering Blood Pressure): 3 tablets each time, 3 times daily; indicated for hypertension due to hyperactivity of liver yang.

(6) Qi Ju Dihuang Ye (Oral Liquid of Lycii, Chysanthemi and Rehmanniae): 1 ampule each time, 3 times daily; indicated for hypertension due to deficiency of liver yin and kidney yi.

(7) Tianma Shouwu Pian (Tablet of Gastrodiae and Polygoni Multiflori): 6 tablets each time, 3 times daily; indicated for hypertension due to deficiency of liver yin and kidney yin.

(8) Jiangya Jiaonang (Capsule for Lowering Blood Pressure): 2 - 4 capsules each time, 3 times daily, 30 days as a course of treatment; indicated for hypertension due to deficiency of yin leading to hyperactivity of fire.

(9) Xiakucao Tangjiang (Prunellae Syrup): 30 ml each time, 3 times daily, 30 days as a course of treatment; indicated for hypertension complicated with hyperlipemia.

2. Single-drug or Experiential Prescriptions

(1) Cebaiye (*Cacumen Platycladi*) 30 g, Chouwutong (*Clerodendri Trichotomi*) 30 g and Sangshugen (*Radix Mori*) 30 g. Decoct the above herbs with water and take the decoction daily. It is indicated for mild hypertension.

每日 2 次。适用于肝阳上亢之高血压病。孕妇忌服,体弱虚寒者不宜使用。

(4) 全天麻胶囊　每服 4 粒,每日 3 次。适用于高血压病属于肝阳上亢,肝风上扰者。

(5) 山绿茶降压片　每服 3 片,每日 3 次。适用于肝阳上亢之高血压病患者。

(6) 杞菊地黄液　每服 1 支,每日 3 次。适用于肝肾阴虚型高血压病。

(7) 天麻首乌片 每服 6 片,每日 3 次。适用于高血压病属于肝肾阴虚者。

(8) 降压胶囊　每服2～4 粒,每日 3 次,30 日为 1 个疗程。适用于阴虚火旺之高血压病患者。

(9) 夏枯草糖浆　每服 30 ml,每日 3 次,30 日为 1 个疗程。适用于高血压病伴有高血脂者。

2. 单验方

(1) 侧柏叶30 g,臭梧桐 30 g,桑树根30 g,水煎服,每日 1 剂。适用于轻度高血压患者。

(2) Xiaojicao (*Herba Cirsii*) 30 g, Cheqiancao (*Herba Plantaginis*) 30 g and Xixiancao (*Herba Siegesbeckiae*) 15 g. Decoct the above herbs with water and take the decoction daily. It is indicated for hypertension complicated by edema.

(3) Jicai (*Herba Capsellae Bursa-Pastoris cum Radice*) 100 g and fresh Shuqucao (*Herba Gnaphalii Affinis*) 30 g. Decoct the above herbs with water and take the decoction. It is indicated for mild hypertension.

(4) Hanqincai (*Herba Apii Graveolentis*, tassels removed) 2 - 3 kg. Remove the old leaves and fibrous roots, chop it up and decoct it with water. Pour the decoction into an earthen pot and seal it. Then add 60 - 120 g of sugar when the decoction turns sour. Take one bowl of the decoction daily. It is indicated for mild hypertension.

(5) Luobumaye (*Folium Apocyni Veneti*) 6 - 9 g, Gouteng (*Ramulus Uncariae cum Uncis*) 3 - 6 g, and Dazao (*Fructus Jujubae*) 4 pcs. Decoct the herbs with water and take the decoction, 2 - 3 times daily. It is indicated for hypertension associated with headache and insomnia.

(6) Juhua (*Flos Chrysanthemi*) 9 g. Decoct it with water and take the decoction as a subsititute of daily drink, one dose daily. This is indicated for hypertension due to hyperactivity of liver yang.

(7) Yama (*Herba Lini*) 10 - 20 g. Decoct it with water and take the decoction twice daily. This is indicated for hypertension with increased cholesterol.

(8) Pingjiang Tang (Decoction for Relieving Hypertension): composed of Zexie (*Rhizoma Alismatis*) 60 g, Yimucao (*Herba Leonuri*) 30 g, Huainiuxi (*Radix Achyranthis Bidentatae*) 15 g, Gouteng (*Ramulus Uncariae cum Uncis*, to be decocted later) 15 g, Xiakucao (*Spica*

(2) 小蓟草30 g, 车前草30 g, 豨莶草15 g, 水煎服, 每日 1 剂。适用于高血压病并有水肿者。

(3) 荠菜100 g, 鲜鼠曲草30 g, 水煎服。适用于轻度高血压患者。

(4) 旱芹菜(去根须)2～3 kg, 切碎加水煎, 入罐密封, 变酸后加糖 60～120 g。每日 1 次, 每服 1 碗。适用于轻度高血压患者。

(5) 罗布麻叶6～9 g, 钩藤3～6 g, 大枣 4 枚, 加水煎服, 每日 2～3 次。适用于高血压病伴头痛、失眠者。

(6) 菊花9 g, 水煎代茶, 每日 1 剂。适用于高血压病属于肝阳偏亢者。

(7) 亚麻10～20 g, 水煎去渣, 日服 2 次。适用于高血压病伴有血胆固醇增高者。

(8) 平降汤 泽泻60 g, 益母草30 g, 怀牛膝15 g, 钩藤(后下)15 g, 夏枯草15 g, 桑寄生15 g, 生石决明(先煎)30 g, 天麻10 g, 青木香10 g。水煎

Prunellae) 15 g, Sangjisheng (*Herba Taxilli*) 15 g, Shengshijueming (*Concha Haliotidis*, to be decocted first) 30 g, Tianma (*Rhizoma Gastrodiae*) 10 g and Qingmuxiang (*Radix Aristolochiae*) 10 g. Decoct Shengshijueming alone for over 30 minutes, add the other herbs except Gouteng, simmer for about 40 minutes, then add Gouteng, and simmer for another 5 - 10 minutes, each dose being decocted twice to collect 500 ml of the decoction. Take 250 ml of the decoction after breakfast and dinner, 20 doses making up a course of treatment. This is indicated for hypertension with deficienct yin and hyperactive yang.

(9) Fufang Huaihua Jiangya Tang (Compound Decoction of Sophorae for Lowering Blood Pressure): composed of Huaihua (*Flos Sophorae*) 25 g, Sangjisheng (*Herba Taxilli*) 25 g, Chuanxiong (*Rhizoma Chuanxiong*) 15 g and Dilong (*Pheretima*) 15 g. Decoct the herbs with water and take the decoction daily. It is indicated for hypertension with stagnation of liver qi, blood stasis, deficiency of liver yin and kidney yin and hyperactivity of yang.

(10) Jiangya Fang (Prescription for Lowering Blood Pressure): composed of Shengshijueming (*Concha Haliotidis*) 30 g, Luobumaye (*Folium Apocyni Veneti*) 30 g, Xixiancao (*Herba Siegesbeckiae*) 30 g, Baishaoyao (*Radix Paeoniae Alba*) 10 g, Yimucao (*Herba Leonuri*) 10 g, Hanfangji (*Radix Stephaniae Tetrandrae*) 10 g, Sangjisheng (*Herba Taxilli*) 15 g and Danshen (*Radix Salviae Miltiorrhizae*) 15 g. Decoct the herbs with water and take the decoction daily. It is indicated for various types of hypertension.

3. External Therapy

(1) Wuzhuyu (*Fructus Evodiae*, *prepared with bile*) 500 g, Longdancao (*Herba Radix Gentianae*, *extracted with alcohol*) 6 g, Liuhuang (*Sulfur*) 50 g, Bai-

服,煎时将先煎的药物先煎 30 分钟以上,再入群药,用文火煎 40 分钟左右,再加后入之品,再煎 5～10 分钟,即可。每日 1 剂,每剂煎 2 次,共取汁 500 ml。每次 250 ml,早、晚饭后服,20 剂为 1 个疗程。适用于阴虚阳亢之高血压患者。

(9)复方槐花降压汤 槐花25 g,桑寄生25 g,川芎15 g,地龙15 g。水煎服,每日 1 剂。适用于肝郁血瘀,肝肾阴虚阳亢之高血压病患者。

(10) 降压方 生石决明 30 g,罗布麻叶 30 g,豨莶草 30 g,白芍药10 g,益母草10 g,汉防己10 g,桑寄生15 g,丹参 15 g。水煎服,每日 1 剂。适用于各型高血压病患者。

3. 外治法

(1)胆汁制吴茱萸500 g,龙胆草醇提取物 6 g,硫黄 50 g,醋制白矾 100 g,朱砂

fan (*Alumen，prepared with vinegar*) 100 g, Zhusha
(*Cinnabaris*) 50 g and Ultraminzil 175 mg. Mix the
above ingredients and grind them into fine powder for later use. Apply 200 mg of the powder at the navel, then
cover it with soft paper and fix it with adhesive tape.
Change the powder once a week and continue the treatment for about 3 weeks. It is indicated for mild and moderate hypertension.

　(2) Baihuasheshecao (*Herba Hedyotis Diffusae*)
15 g, Wugong (*Scolopendra*) 3 g, Chantui (*Periostracum Cicadae*) 6 g, Dilong (*Pheretima*) 10 g, Zhechong
(*Eupolyphaga seu Steleophaga*) 5 g, Huanglian (*Rhizoma Coptidis*) 3 g, Baijiezi (*Semen Sinapis Albae*) 6 g,
Yanhusuo (*Rhizoma Corydalis*) 10 g, Gegen (*Radix
Puerariae*) 10 g, Gansui (*Radix Kansui*) 3 g, Xixin
(*Herba Asari*) 3 g and Shensanqi (*Radix Notoginseng*)
6 g. Grind all the herbs into fine powder, then mix it with
a proper amount of ginger juice to make medicated cakes
and put a little Shexiang (*Moschus Powder*) on the center
of each cake. Apply the cakes on bilateral acupoints of
Xinshu (BL 15), Ganshu (BL 18), Shenshu (BL 23) and
Guanyuan (CV 4), for 8 - 12 hours. It is indicated for
mild and moderate hypertension.

　(3) Wuzhuyu (*Fructus Evodiae*). Grind the herb
into powder and mix it with vinegar, then apply it to the
center of both soles. It is effective for lowering blood
pressure and indicated for mild hypertension.

　(4) Chongweizi (*Fructus Leonuri*) 50 g, Gouteng
(*Ramulus Uncariae cum Uncis*) 50 g and Sangshupi
(*Radix Mori*) 50 g. Decoct the herbs in water and soak
the feet in the decoction for 30 minutes. It is indicated for
mild hypertension.

　(5) Gouteng (*Ramulus Uncariae cum Uncis*) 20 g
and a little amount of Bingpian (*Borneolum Synthetic-*

50 g,环戊甲噻嗪175 mg。将
上方按量混合研成细面,备
用。每次取200 mg,置于脐
中,外用软纸敷盖加胶布固
定,每星期更换1次,用药3个
星期左右。适用于轻、中度高
血压患者。

　(2) 白花蛇舌草15 g,蜈
蚣3 g,蝉蜕6 g,地龙10 g,䗪虫
5 g,黄连3 g,白芥子6 g,延胡
索10 g,葛根10 g,甘遂3 g,细
辛3 g,参三七6 g,共研细末,
拌以姜汁适量,做成药饼。中
心放少许麝香末。将上药饼
贴于两侧心俞、肝俞、肾俞及
关元穴,8～12 小时取下。适
用于轻、中度高血压患者。

　(3) 吴茱萸研末,醋调贴
于两脚心,有降压作用。适用
于轻度高血压患者。

　(4) 茺蔚子50 g,钩藤
50 g,桑树皮50 g,水煎备用。
用温热药水浸泡双足 30 分
钟。适用于轻度高血压患者。

　(5) 钩藤20 g,冰片少许。
取钩藤20 g剪碎,布包冰片少

um). Cut Gouteng into small pieces and wrap Bingpian in a piece of cloth, put them together in a basin and add in warm water to soak the feet for 30 - 45 minutes after rising in the morning and at bed time every day, 10 days making up a treatment course. It is indicated for mild and moderate hypertension.

(6) Bohe (*Herba Menthae*), Yejuhua (*Flos Chrysanthemi Indici*), Qingmuxiang (*Radix Aristolochiae*), Danzhuye (*Herba Lophatheri*), Shengshigao (*Gypsum Fibrosum*), Baishaoyao (*Radix Paeoniae Alba*), Chuanxiong (*Rhizoma Chuanxiong*), Dongsangye (*Folium Mori*), Manjingzi (*Fructus Viticis*), Cishi (*Magnetitum*) and Wanchansha (*Feculae Bombycis*). Crush equal amounts of each of the above herbs into small pieces, fill a cloth bag with the crushed herbs to make a medicated pillow and use it for at least 6 hours each day. It is indicated for hypertension with hyperactivity of liver yang.

(7) Juhua (*Flos Chrysanthemi*), Chuanxiong (*Rhizoma Chuanxiong*), Mudanpi (*Cortex Moutan Radicis*) and Baizhi (*Radix Angelicae Dahuricae*). Crush equal amounts of each of the above herbs, fill a cloth bag with the crushed herbs to make a medicated pillow. It is indicated for mild and moderate hypertension.

2.6.5 Apoplexy

General Description

Apoplexy is mainly characterized by sudden syncope, loss of conciousness, hemiplegia and deviation of the eyes and mouth. In a mild case, only hemiplegia together with contortion of the facial muscles can be seen, without occurrence of syncope.

The disease is caused by long-term internal disorders, overstrain, improper diet and emotional disorders

许,于每日晨起和晚睡前放入盆内,并加温水浴脚,每次30~45分钟,早晚各1次,10日为1个疗程。适用于轻、中度高血压患者。

(6) 薄荷、野菊花、青木香、淡竹叶、生石膏、白芍药、川芎、冬桑叶、蔓荆子、磁石、晚蚕沙,等量研碎后装入布袋制成药枕,每昼夜使用时间不少于6小时。适用于高血压肝阳上亢型。

(7) 菊花、川芎、牡丹皮、白芷,等量研碎后装入布袋内制成药枕。适用于轻、中度高血压患者。

第五节   中风

【概述】

中风以猝然昏仆,不省人事,半身不遂,口眼歪斜为主症;病轻者可无昏仆而仅见口眼歪斜及半身不遂等症状。

本病的病因有长期劳倦内伤、饮食不节、情志失调等。

and is usually induced by sudden change of weather, over-strain, emotional upsets and trauma. In general, the pathogenesis includes deficiency, fire, wind, phlegm, qi and blood. Although the brain is the involved organ, the disease is closely related to the heart, kidneys, liver and spleen. In terms of the nature, it is mainly a case of principal deficiency and secondary excess, upper excess and lower deficiency. Deficiency of liver yin and kidney yin and deficiency of qi and blood are the principal; while fire and wind stirring up each other, accumulation of phlegm dampness, obstruction of blood stasis and disorders of qi and blood are the secondary. But above all, the basic pathogenesis of the disease is disorder of qi and blood involving the brain.

Clinically, manifestations of apoplexy are similar to those of acute cerebrovascular disease in western medicine, including ischemic and hemorrhagic cerebrovascular diseases.

Essentials for Diagnosis

(1) Chief manifestations are trance even coma or mental confusion, hemiplegia, distortion of the mouth and tongue, stiff tongue and dysphasia, numbness in one side of the body.

(2) Abrupt onset.

(3) The disease is often caused by some precipitating factors and such aural symptoms as dizziness, headache, numbness of limbs and weakness are commonly seen.

(4) It is mostly seen in people aged 40 and older.

(5) Cerebrospinal fluid examination, brain CT scanning and MRI are helpful in making a diagnosis.

Syndrome Differentiation and Treatment

It is essential to clarify whether the meridians or zang-fu organs have been involved. If zang and fu organs

常见的诱因为气候骤变、烦劳过度、情志相激及跌仆努力等。其病机概而论之有虚、火、风、痰、气、血六端。病位在脑，与心、肾、肝、脾密切相关。病性多为本虚标实，上盛下虚。病本为肝肾阴虚，气血衰少；其标为风火相煽，痰湿壅盛，瘀血阻滞，气血逆乱。基本病机为气血逆乱，上犯于脑。

中风的临床表现与西医的急性脑血管病相似，包括缺血性脑血管病和出血性脑血管病两大类型。

【诊断要点】

（1）以神志恍惚、迷蒙，甚或昏迷，不省人事，半身不遂，口舌歪斜，舌强言謇或不语，偏身麻木为主症。

（2）多急性起病。

（3）病发多有诱因，病前常有头晕、头痛、肢体麻木、无力等先兆症状。

（4）好发于 40 岁以上中老年人。

（5）脑脊液检查，颅脑CT、MRI 等有助于明确诊断。

【辨证论治】

本病辨证上应分清中经络与中脏腑；中脏腑者又当分

have been involved, there can be two different categories: excess syndrome of apoplexy and collapse syndrome
of apoplexy, and the former may be further divided into
yin type and yang type. At the acute stage, the treatment
should focus on the secondary symptoms. The principle
should be eliminating pathogenic factors and the common
methods are calming the liver to suppress pathogenic
wind, clearing away heat and phlegm, dissipating phlegm
to remove obstructions from the fu organs, promoting
blood circulation to activate meridians and waking up the
patient from unconciousness. In the case of excess syndrome of apoplexy, it should be treated by eliminating
pathogenic factors and waking up the patient from unconciousness, while in the case of collapse syndrome of apoplexy, supporting healthy qi to relieve collapse and restoring yin to revive yang should be adopted. At the stage of
restoration and sequela, more often seen is deficiency
complicated with excess. In this case, the treatment
should focus on supporting healthy qi and emilinating pathogenic factors, for instance, the methods of nourishing
yin and calming wind, replenishing qi and activating blood
circulation are usually recommended.

1. Apoplexy Involving the Meridians

(1) Wind Phelgm Blocking the Meridians

Chief Manifestation: Abrupt onset of hemiplegia,
distortion of the face, stiff tongue, dysphasia, numbness
in one side of the body, dizziness, blurred vision, dull
pale tongue with thin and white coating, or white and
greasy coating, wiry and smooth pluse.

Therapeutic Methods: To dispell wind, resolve
blood stasis and activate blood to remove obstruction from
the collaterals.

Prescription: Modified Qianzheng San (Powder for
Treating Wry-Mouth) and Daotan Tang (Decoction for

辨闭证与脱证；闭证者又当辨
阴闭与阳闭。治疗原则，急性
期标实症状突出，急则治其
标，治疗当以祛邪为主，常用
平肝熄风、清化痰热、化痰通
腑、活血通络、醒神开窍等治
疗方法。闭、脱二证当分别治
以祛邪开窍醒神和扶正固脱、
救阴固阳。恢复期及后遗症
期，多为虚实夹杂，治宜扶正
祛邪，常用育阴熄风、益气活
血等法。

1. 中经络

（1）风痰阻络证

主要证候　突然半身不
遂，口舌歪斜，舌强言謇或不
语，偏身麻木，头晕目眩，舌质
暗淡，苔薄白或白腻，脉弦滑。

治　法　祛风化痰，活血
通络。

方　药　牵正散合导痰
汤加减：天麻10 g，钩藤10 g，

Expelling Phlegm), composed of Tianma (*Rhizoma Gastrodiae*) 10 g, Gouteng (*Ramulus Uncariae cum Uncis*) 10 g, Baijili (*Fructus Tribuli*) 10 g, Juhua (*Flos Chrysanthemi*) 6 g, Zhibanxia (*Rhizoma Pinelliae Preparata*) 10 g, Chenpi (*Pericarpium Citri Reticulatae*) 6 g, Chendanxing (*Arisaema cum Bile*) 6 g, Dilong (*Pheretima*) 10 g, Baijiangcan (*Bombyx Batryticatus*) 6 g and Quanxie (*Scorpio*) 3 g.

Modifications: For pronounced stasis of blood, dark purplish tongue or with petechia on it, add Taoren (*Semen Persicae*) 10 g, Honghua (*Flos Carthami*) 6 g and Chishaoyao (*Radix Paeoniae Rubra*) 10 g; for yellow greasy tongue coating and restlessness, add Huangqin (*Radix Scutellariae*) 10 g and Zhizi (*Fructus Gardeniae*) 10 g; for slurred speech, add Shichangpu (*Acori Tatarinowii*) 6 g and Yuanzhi (*Radix Polygalae*) 10 g.

(2) Hyperactivity of Liver Yang

Chief Manifestations: Hemiplegia, numbness in one side of the body, stiff tongue, dysphasia, distortion of the mouth and tongue, dizziness, headache, flushed face, red eyes, bitter taste in the mouth, dry throat, restlessness, irritability, dark urine and dry stools, red or crimsom tongue with thin yellow, coating, and wiry, forceful pulse.

Therapeutic Methods: To calm the liver, purge the fire and remove obstructions from the collaterals.

Prescription: Modified Tianma Gouteng Yin (Gastrodiae and Uncariae Decoction), composed of Tianma (*Rhizoma Gastrodiae*) 10 g, Gouteng (*Ramulus Uncariae cum Uncis*) 10 g, Shijueming (*Concha Haliotidis*, to be decocted first) 30 g, Chuanniuxi (*Radix Cyathulae*) 10 g, Huangqin (*Radix Scutellariae*) 10 g, Zhizi (*Fructus Gardeniae*) 10 g and Xiakucao (*Spica Prunellae*) 10 g.

白蒺藜10 g,菊花6 g,制半夏10 g,陈皮6 g,陈胆星6 g,地龙10 g,白僵蚕6 g,全蝎3 g。

加 减 瘀血重,舌质紫暗或有瘀斑,加桃仁10 g,红花6 g,赤芍药10 g;舌苔黄腻,烦躁不安者,加黄芩10 g,栀子10 g;语言不清者,加石菖蒲6 g,远志10 g。

(2) 肝阳上亢证

主要证候 半身不遂,偏身麻木,舌强言謇或不语,或舌口歪斜,眩晕头痛,面红目赤,口苦咽干,心烦易怒,尿赤便干,舌质红或红绛,舌苔薄黄,脉弦有力。

治 法 平肝泻火通络。

方 药 天麻钩藤饮加减:天麻10 g,钩藤10 g,石决明(先煎)30 g,川牛膝10 g,黄芩10 g,栀子10 g,夏枯草10 g。

Modifications: For pronounced dizziness and headache, add Juhua (*Flos Chrysanthemi*) 6 g and Sangye (*Folium Mori*) 10 g; for restlessness and irritability, add Mudanpi (*Cortex Moutan Radicis*) 10 g and Baishaoyao (*Radix Paeoniae Alba*) 10 g; for dry stools, add Shengdahuang (*Radix et Rhizoma Rhei*, to be decocted later) 6 g.

(3) Excess Syndrome of Fu Organs due to Phlegm Heat

Chief Manifestations: Hemiplegia, distortion of the mouth and tongue, dysphasia, numbness in one side of the body, abdominal distention, constipation, dizziness, blurred vision, productive cough, dark red or dull pale tongue with yellow or yellow, greasy coating, and wiry and smooth pulse or wiry, smooth and large pulse.

Therapeutic Methods: To resolve phlegm and remove obstructions from fu organs.

Prescription: Modified Xing Lou Chengqi Tang (Arisaema and Trichosanthis Decoction for Purgation), composed of Shengdahuang (*Radix et Rhizoma Rhei*, to be decocted later) 6 g, Mangxiao (*Natrii Sulfas*, to be infused separately) 6 g, Quangualou (*Fructus Trichosanthis*) 10 g, Danxing (*Arisaema cum Bile*) 10 g and Danshen (*Radix Salviae Miltiorrhizae*) 12 g.

Modifications: For pronounced heat manifestation, add Zhizi (*Fructus Gardeniae*) 10 g and Huangqin (*Radix Scutellariae*) 10 g; for old patient with weak constitution and consumption of body fluid, add Shengdihuang (*Radix Rehmanniae*) 12 g, Maimendong (*Radix Ophiopogonis*) 10 g and Xuanshen (*Radix Scrophulariae*) 10 g.

(4) Stagnation of Blood due to Deficiency of Qi

Chief Manifestations: Hemiplegia, distortion of

加　减　头晕头痛明显，加菊花6 g，桑叶10 g；心烦易怒，加牡丹皮10 g，白芍药10 g；大便干，加生大黄（后下）6 g。

（3）痰热腑实证

主要证候　半身不遂，口舌歪斜，言语謇涩或不语，偏身麻木，腹胀便秘，头晕目眩，咯痰量多，舌质暗红或暗淡，苔黄或黄腻，脉弦滑或脉弦滑大。

治　法　化痰通腑。

方　药　星蒌承气汤加减：生大黄（后下）6 g，芒硝（另冲）6 g，全瓜蒌10 g，胆星10 g，丹参12 g。

加　减　热象明显者，加栀子10 g，黄芩10 g；年老体弱津亏者，加生地黄12 g，麦门冬10 g，玄参10 g。

（4）气虚血瘀证

主要证候　半身不遂，口

the mouth and tongue, dysphasia, numbness in one side of the body, pale complexion, shortness of breath, lassitude, angular salivation, spontaneous perspiration, palpitation, loose stools, swollen hands and feet, dull pale tongue with thin and white coating or white and greasy coating, deep and thready pulse, thready and even-soft or thready and wiry pulse.

Therapeutic Methods: To replenish qi, activate blood circulation and support healthy qi to eliminate pathogenic factors.

Prescription: Modified Buyang Huanwu Tang (Decoction for Invigorating Yang and Recuperation), composed of Huangqi (*Radix Astragali*) 15 g, Danggui (*Radix Angelicae Sinensis*) 10 g, Chishaoyao (*Radix Paeoniae Rubra*) 10 g, Chuanxiong (*Rhizoma Chuanxiong*) 10 g, Taoren (*Semen Persicae*) 10 g, Honghua (*Flos Carthami*) 10 g and Dilong (*Pheretima*) 10 g.

Modifications: For pronounced deficiency of qi, add Dangshen (*Radix Codonopsis*) 10 g and Taizishen (*Radix Pseudostellariae*) 12 g; for dysphasia, add Yuanzhi (*Radix Polygalae*) 6 g, Shichangpu (*Rhizoma Acori Tatarinowii*) 6 g and Yujin (*Radix Curcumae*) 10 g; for palpitation and dyspnea, add Guizhi (*Ramulus Cinnamomi*) 6 g and Zhigancao (*Radix Glycyrrhizae, roasted*) 3 g; for numbness in the limbs, add Mugua (*Fructus Chaenomelis*) 10 g, Shenjincao (*Herba Lycopodii*) 12 g and Hanfangji (*Radix Stephaniae Tetrandrae*) 10 g; for paralysis of upper limbs, add Guizhi (*Ramulus Cinnamomi*) 6 g; for flaccid paralysis of lower limbs, add Chuanxuduan (*Radix Dipsaci*) 10 g, Sangjisheng (*Herba Taxilli*) 10 g, Duzhong (*Cortex Eucommiae*) 10 g and Niuxi (*Radix Achyranthis Bidentatae*) 10 g; for incontinence of urine, add Sangpiaoxiao (*Oötheca Mantidis*) 10 g and Yizhiren (*Fructus Alpiniae Oxyphyllae*) 10 g; for se-

舌歪斜,言语謇涩或不语,偏身麻木,面色㿠白,气短乏力,口角流涎,自汗出,心悸便溏,手足肿胀,舌质暗淡,舌苔薄白或白腻,脉沉细、细缓或细弦。

治 法 益气活血,扶正祛邪。

方 药 补阳还五汤加减:黄芪15 g,当归10 g,赤芍药10 g,川芎10 g,桃仁10 g,红花10 g,地龙10 g。

加 减 气虚明显者,加党参10 g,太子参12 g;言语不利,加远志6 g,石菖蒲6 g,郁金10 g;心悸、喘息,加桂枝6 g,炙甘草3 g;肢体麻木,加木瓜10 g,伸筋草12 g,汉防己10 g;上肢偏废者,加桂枝6 g;下肢瘫软无力者,加川续断10 g,桑寄生10 g,杜仲10 g,牛膝10 g;小便失禁者,加桑螵蛸10 g,益智仁10 g;血瘀重者,加莪术10 g,水蛭5 g,鬼箭羽10 g,鸡血藤12 g。

vere stagnation of blood, add Ezhu (*Rhizoma Curcum-ae*) 10 g, Shuizhi (*Hirudo*) 5 g, Guijianyu (*Ramulus Euonymi Alati*) 10 g and Jixueteng (*Caulis Spatholobi*) 12 g.

(5) Stirring up of Endogenous Wind due to Deficiency of Yin

Chief Manifestations: Hemiplegia, distortion of the mouth and tongue, dysphasia, numbness in one side of the body, irritability, insomnia, dizziness, tinnitus, feverish sensation over the palms and soles, crimson or dark red tongue with little coating or no coating, thready and wiry pulse or thready, wiry and rapid pulse.

Therapeutic Methods: To nourish the liver and kidneys, suppress yang and calm wind.

Prescription: Modified Zhengan Xifeng Tang (Decoction for Suppressing Liver Wind), composed of Shenglonggu (*Os Dracomis*, to be decocted first) 20 g, Shengmuli (*Concha Ostreae*, to be decocted first) 20 g, Daizheshi (*Haematitum*, to be decocted first) 20 g, Guiban (*Plastrum Testudinis*, to be decocted first) 15 g, Baishaoyao (*Radix Paeoniae Alba*) 10 g, Xuanshen (*Radix Scrophulariae*) 10 g, Tianmendong (*Radix Asparagi*) 10 g, Niuxi (*Radix Achyranthis Bidentatae*) 10 g, Gouteng (*Ramulus Uncariae cum Uncis*) 10 g and Juhua (*Flos Chrysanthemi*) 6 g.

Modifications: For the case accompanied by phlegm heat, add Tianzhuhuang (*Conretio Silicea Bambusae*) 5 g, Zhulishui (*Succus Phyllostachydis Henonis*, to be taken separately) 30 g and Chuanbeimu (*Bulbus Fritillariae Cirrhosae*) 10 g; for restlessness and insomnia, add Huangqin (*Radix Scutellariae*) 10 g, Zhizi (*Fructus Gardeniae*) 10 g, Yejiaoteng (*Caulis et Folium Polygoni Multiflori*) 10 g and Zhenzhumu (*Concha Margaritifera Usta*, to be decocted first) 15 g; for severe

（5）阴虚风动证

主要证候 半身不遂，口舌歪斜，舌强言謇或不语，偏身麻木，烦躁失眠，眩晕耳鸣，手足心热，舌质红绛或暗红，少苔或无苔，脉细弦或细弦数。

治 法 滋养肝肾，潜阳熄风。

方 药 镇肝熄风汤加减：生龙骨（先煎）20 g，生牡蛎（先煎）20 g，代赭石（先煎）20 g，龟版（先煎）15 g，白芍药10 g，玄参10 g，天门冬10 g，牛膝10 g，钩藤10 g，菊花6 g。

加 减 挟有痰热者，加天竺黄5 g，竹沥水（另冲）30 g，川贝母10 g；心烦失眠者，加黄芩10 g，栀子10 g，夜交藤10 g，珍珠母（先煎）15 g；头痛重者，加生石决明（先煎）20 g，夏枯草10 g。

headache, add Shengshijueming (*Concha Haliotidis*, to be decocted first) 20 g and Xiakucao (*Spica Prunellae*) 10 g.

2. Apoplexy Involving Zang-fu Organs

(1) Phlegm Heat Blocking the Heart Orifice

Chief Manifestations: Abrrupt onset, coma or mental confusion, hemiplegia, coarse breathing, wheezing sound in the throat, spasms of limbs, feverish sensation in the neck and back, restlessness, even cold hands and feet, frequent convulsion, hematemesis in rare cases, crimson tongue with yellow, greasy or dry, greasy coating, wiry, smooth and rapid pulse.

Therapeutic Methods: To clear away heat, resolve phlegm and wake up the patient from unconsciousness.

Prescription: Modified Lingyangjiao Tang (*Cornu Saigae Tataricae Decoction*), composed of Lingyangjiaofen (*Cornu Saigae Tataricae*, powdered and to be infused separately) 0.5 g, Zhenzhumu (*Concha Margaritifera Usta*, to be decocted first) 30 g, Zhuru (*Caulis Bambusae in Taeniam*) 10 g, Tianzhuhuang (*Concretio Silicea Bambusae*) 5 g, Shichangpu (*Rhizoma Acori Tatarinowii*) 6 g, Yuanzhi (*Radix Polygalae*) 6 g, Xiakucao (*Spica Prunellae*) 10 g and Mudanpi (*Cortex Moutan Radicis*) 10 g.

Modifications: For profuse sputum, add Zhulishui (*Succus Phyllostachydis Henonis*, to be taken separately) 30 g and Danxing (*Arisaema cum Bile*) 10 g; for high fever, add Huangqin (*Radix Scutellariae*) 10 g and Zhizi (*Fructus Gardeniae*) 10 g; for coma, add Yujin (*Radix Curcumae*) 10 g.

(2) Phlegm Dampness Blocking the Heart Orifice

Chief Manifestations: Coma, hemiplegia with the involved side not warm enough, relaxed limbs and even

2. 中脏腑

(1) 痰热闭窍证

主要证候　起病骤急,神昏或昏愦,半身不遂,鼻鼾痰鸣,肢体强痉拘急,项背身热,躁扰不宁,甚则手足厥冷,频繁抽搐,偶见呕血,舌质红绛,舌苔黄腻或干腻,脉弦滑数。

治　法　清热化痰,醒神开窍。

方　药　羚羊角汤加减:羚羊角粉(另冲)0.5 g,珍珠母(先煎)30 g,竹茹10 g,天竺黄5 g,石菖蒲6 g,远志6 g,夏枯草10 g,牡丹皮10 g。

加　减　痰多者,加竹沥水(另饮)30 g,胆星10 g;热甚者,加黄芩10 g,栀子10 g;神昏重,加郁金10 g。

(2) 痰湿蒙窍证

主要证候　神昏,半身不遂,肢体松懈,瘫痪不温,甚则

cold hands and feet, pale complexion, dark lips, excessive sputum, dull pale tongue with white and greasy coating, deep and smooth pulse or deep and even-soft pulse.

Therapeutic Methods: To warm yang, resolve sputum and wake up the patient from unconsciousness.

Prescription: Modified Ditan Tang (Decoction for Eliminating Phlegm), composed of Zhibanxia (*Rhizoma Pinelliae Preparata*) 10 g, Chenpi (*Pericarpium Citri Reticulatae*) 6 g, Fuling (*Poria*) 10 g, Danxing (*Arisaema cum Bile*) 10 g, Zhuru (*Caulis Bambusae in Taeniam*) 10 g and Shichangpu (*Rhizoma Acori Tatarinowii*) 6 g.

Modification: For pronounced cold manifestations, add Guizhi (*Ramulus Cinnamomi*) 6 g.

(3) Exhaustion of Primordial Qi

Chief Manifestations: Sudden onset of coma or mental confusion, flaccid paralysis of limbs, cold limbs with hands stretching out, profuse sweating, even wet and cold body, incontinence of urine and stools, atrophy of dark purple tongue with white and greasy coating, deep and even-soft pulse or deep and indistinct pulse.

Therapeutic Methods: To replenish qi, revive yang and relieve collapse.

Prescription: Shen Fu Tang Jiawei (Decoction of Ginseng and Aconiti Laterali with Additions), composed of Hongshen (*Radix Ginseng Rubra*, to be decocted separately) 10 g, Zhifuzi (*Radix Aconiti Lateralis Preparata*) 10 g, Ganjiang (*Rhizoma Zingiberis*) 6 g and Zhigancao (*Radix Glycyrrhizae*, roasted) 6 g.

Modification: For profuse perspiration, add Shanzhuyu (*Fructus Corni*) 10 g, Huangqi (*Radix Astragali*) 12 g, Longgu (*Os Draconis*, to be decocted first) 15 g and Muli (*Concha Ostreae*, to be decocted first) 15 g.

四肢逆冷，面白唇暗，痰涎壅盛，舌质暗淡，舌苔白腻，脉沉滑或沉缓。

治　法　温阳化痰，醒神开窍。

方　药　涤痰汤加减：制半夏10 g，陈皮6 g，茯苓10 g，胆星10 g，竹茹10 g，石菖蒲6 g。

加　减　寒象明显者，加桂枝6 g。

（3）元气败脱证

主要证候　突然神昏或昏愦，肢体瘫软，手撒肢冷汗多，重则周身湿冷，二便失禁，舌萎，舌质紫暗，苔白腻，脉沉缓或沉微。

治　法　益气回阳固脱。

方　药　参附汤加味。红参（另煎）10 g，制附子10 g，干姜6 g，炙甘草6 g。

加　减　汗出不止，加山茱萸10 g，黄芪12 g，龙骨（先煎）15 g，牡蛎（先煎）15 g。

Other Treatments

1. Chinese Patent Drugs

（1）Angong Niuhuang Wan (Calculus Bovis Bolus for Resuscitation): 1 bolus by nasal feeding, once daily; indicated for yang type excess syndrome of apoplexy involving zang and fu organs.

（2）Niuhuang Qingxin Wan (Calculus Bovis Bolus for Clearing Heart Fire): 1 bolus by nasal feeding, once daily; indicated for yang type excess syndrome of apoplexy involving zang and fu organs.

（3）Suhexiang Wan (Styrax Bolus): 1 bolus by nasal feeding, once daily; indicated for yin type excess syndrome of apoplexy involving zang and fu organs.

（4）Xiaoshuan Zaizao Wan (Bolus for Eliminating Blood Stasis): 1 bolus, taken orally, twice daily; indicated for ischemic cerebrovascular disease.

（5）Xueshuan Xinmaining Jiaonang (Capsule for Eliminating Blood Stasis and Calming Heart): 4 capsules, taken orally, 3 times daily; indicated for ischemic cerebrovascular disease.

（6）Zhulishui (*Succus Phyllostachydis Henonis*): 10 - 20 ml, taken orally, twice or thrice daily; indicated for cases with profuse sputum.

（7）Qingkailing Zhusheye (Injection for Clearing away Heat and Inducing Resuscitation): 40 - 80 ml intravenous drip with 10% of 250 - 500 ml glucose solution, once or twice daily; indicated for yang-type excess syndrome of apoplexy involving zang and fu organs.

（8）Mailuoning Zhusheye (Injection for Promoting Blood Circulation): 10 - 20 ml, intravenous drip with 250 - 500 ml glucose solution, once daily; indicated for yang-type excess syndrome of apoplexy involving zang and fu organs.

【其他疗法】

1. 中成药

（1）安宫牛黄丸　每服1丸,每日1次,鼻饲。适用于中脏腑阳闭证。

（2）牛黄清心丸　每服1丸,每日1次,鼻饲。适用于中脏腑阳闭证。

（3）苏合香丸　每服1丸,每日1次,鼻饲。适用于中脏腑阴闭证。

（4）消栓再造丸　每服1丸,每日2次,口服。适用于缺血性脑血管病。

（5）血栓心脉宁胶囊　每服4粒,每日3次,口服。适用于缺血性脑血管病。

（6）竹沥水　每服10～20 ml,每日2～3次,口服。适用于本病痰多者。

（7）清开灵注射液 40～80 ml加入10%葡萄糖溶液250～500 ml,静脉滴注,每日1～2次。适用于中脏腑阳闭证。

（8）脉络宁注射液 10～20 ml加入10%葡萄糖溶液250～500 ml,静脉滴注,每日1次。适用于中脏腑阳闭证。

2. Single-drug or Experiential Prescriptions

（1）Taoren（*Semen Persicae*）10 g, Honghua（*Flos Carthami*）10 g, Danggui（*Radix Angelicae Sinensis*）10 g, Chishaoyao（*Radix Paeoniae Rubra*）10 g, Chuanxiong（*Rhizoma Chuanxiong*）10 g, Chuanshanjia（*Squama Manitis*）15 g and Jixueteng（*Caulis Spatholobi*）12 g. Decoct the above herbs in water for oral administration, 1 dose daily. It is indicated for cerebral thrombosis.

（2）Gualou（*Fructus Trichosanthis*）10 g, Danxing（*Arisaema cum Bile*）10 g, Shengdahuang（*Radix et Rhizoma Rhei*, to be decocted later）10 g and Mangxiao（*Natrii Sulfas*, to be infused separately）10 g. Decoct the above herbs in water for oral administration, 1 dose daily. It is indicated for acute ischemic apoplexy manifested as excess syndrome of fu organs due to phlegm heat.

（3）Shengruxiang（*Olibanum*）12 g, Shengmoyao（*Myrrhae*）12 g, Danggui（*Radix Angelicae Sinensis*）12 g and Danshen（*Radix Salviae Miltiorrhizae*）12 g. Decoct the above herbs in water for oral administration, 1 dose daily. It is indicated for ischemic apoplexy.

（4）Taoren（*Semen Persicae*）5 g, Honghua（*Flos Carthami*）15 g, Danggui（*Radix Angelicae Sinensis*）10 g, Chuanxiong（*Rhizoma Chuanxiong*）5 g, Chuanshanjia（*Squama Manitis*）5 g, Guizhi（*Ramulus Cinnamomi*）5 g, Shenghuangqi（*Radix Astragali*）15 g, Chishaoyao（*Radix Paeoniae Rubra*）10 g, Baishaoyao（*Radix Paeoniae Alba*）10 g, Dilong（*Pheretima*）10 g, Yujin（*Radix Curcumae*）10 g and Shichangpu（*Rhizoma Acori Tatarinowii*）5 g. Decoct the above herbs in water for oral administration, 1 dose daily. It is indicated for cerebral thrombosis.

（5）Xixiancao（*Herba Siegesbeckiae*）15 g, Lao-

2. 单验方

（1）桃仁10 g, 红花10 g, 当归10 g, 赤芍药10 g, 川芎10 g, 穿山甲15 g, 鸡血藤12 g。水煎服, 每日1剂。适用于脑血栓形成。

（2）瓜蒌10 g, 胆星10 g, 生大黄（后下）10 g, 芒硝（另冲）10 g。水煎服, 每日1剂。适用于急性缺血性中风痰热腑实者。

（3）生乳香12 g, 生没药12 g, 当归12 g, 丹参12 g。水煎服, 每日1剂。适用于缺血性中风。

（4）桃仁5 g, 红花15 g, 当归10 g, 川芎5 g, 穿山甲5 g, 桂枝5 g, 生黄芪15 g, 赤芍药10 g, 白芍药10 g, 地龙10 g, 郁金10 g, 石菖蒲5 g。水煎服, 每日1剂。适用于脑血栓形成。

（5）豨莶草15 g, 老鹳草

guancao（*Herba Erodii seu Ceranii*）12 g，Sangzhi（*Ramulus Mori*）20 g，Niuxi（*Radix Achyranthis Bidentatae*）12 g，Qinjiao（*Radix Gentianae Macrophyllae*）12 g，Mugua（*Fructus Chaenomelis*）10 g，Dilong（*Pheretima*）10 g，Haifengteng（*Caulis Piperis Kadsurae*）10 g，Danshen（*Radix Salviae Miltiorrhizae*）12 g，Chishaoyao（*Radix Paeoniae Rubra*）10 g，Zhechong（*Eupolyphaga seu Steleophaga*）10 g，Quanxie（*Scorpio*）6 g and Baijiangcan（*Bombyx Batryticatus*）10 g. Decoct the above herbs in water for oral administration，1 dose daily. It is indicated for the sequelae of cerebral thrombosis.

3. External Therapy

（1）Jixueteng（*Caulis Spatholobi*）15 g，Luoshiteng（*Caulis Trachelospermi*）10 g，Haifengteng（*Caulis Piperis Kadsurae*）10 g，Shinanteng（*Caulis Photiniae Serrulatae*）10 g，Sanleng（*Rhizoma Sparganii*）6 g，Ezhu（*Rhizoma Curcumae*）6 g，Hanfangji（*Radix Stephaniae Tetrandrae*）10 g，Tougucao（*Herba Speranskiae Tuberculatae*）15 g，Sangzhi（*Ramulus Mori*）30 g and Honghua（*Semen Carthami*）10 g. Decoct the above herbs in water and use the decoction for bathing the affected limbs，once or twice daily.

（2）Chuanwu（*Radix Aconiti*）10 g，Danggui（*Radix Angelicae Sinensis*）10 g，Chuanxiong（*Rhizoma Chuanxiong*）6 g and Sangzhi（*Ramulus Mori*）30 g. Soak the herbs in water for 30 minutes, then decoct the herbs for 40 minutes and use the decoction for bathing the affected limbs，once or twice daily.

12 g，桑枝20 g，牛膝12 g，秦艽12 g，木瓜10 g，地龙10 g，海风藤10 g，丹参12 g，赤芍药10 g，䗪虫10 g，全蝎6 g，白僵蚕10 g。水煎服，每日1剂。适用于脑血栓形成后遗症。

3. 外治法

（1）鸡血藤15 g，络石藤10 g，海风藤10 g，石南藤10 g，三棱6 g，莪术6 g，汉防己10 g，透骨草15 g，桑枝30 g，红花10 g。煎汤外洗患肢，每日1～2次。

（2）川乌10 g，当归10 g，川芎6 g，桑枝30 g，用水浸30分钟，煎煮40分钟，将患肢浸泡药液中外洗，每日1～2次。

2.6.6 Rheumatoid Arthritis

General Description

Rheumatoid arthritis is a chronic systemic autoimmune disease characterized by pathologic changes of the joints. It is clinically manifested as symmetric polyarthritis mostly with the joints of hands, wrists and feet involved. At the initial stage, there may be redness, swelling, a hot sensation, pain and limited motion in the affected joints, while at the advanced stage, rigidity and deformity of joints may be seen. In fact, the morbidity of rheumatoid arthritis is rather high, the incidence being 1% overseas and 0.1%-0.3% in China respectively; and most of the patients are the young and middle-aged (80% of the cases aged from 20 - 45). Moreover, the prognosis of the disease is unfavorable, and 60%- 70% of the patients are said to become disabled, 10% of whom lose their ability to labor within only a few years.

The etiology and pathogenesis of rheumatoid arthritis have not been fully known so far, but generally it is recognized as a kind of autoimmune disease with abnormity of humoral immunity and cellular immunity.

According to its clinical manifestations, rheumatoid arthritis is attributive to bi-syndrome. The external cause is the invasion of the muscles, joints and meridians by exogenous pathologic factors such as wind, cold, dampness and heat, while the endogenous factors are considered to be deficiency of qi and blood, and deficiency of the liver and kidneys. In terms of pathogenesis, it is the blockage of meridians by pathogenic factors and stagnation of qi and blood. In a prolonged case, phlegm stagnation and blood

第六节　类风湿
关节炎

【概述】

类风湿关节炎是一种以关节病变为主的慢性全身性自身免疫性疾病。临床主要表现为对称的多发性关节炎，以手、腕、足等关节最常受累，早期以红、肿、热、痛和运动障碍为主，至晚期可见关节僵硬和畸形。本病发病率一般为1.0%～0.3%，发病以青壮年为多，80%患者的发病年龄在20～45岁左右。本病预后欠佳，据报道其致残废率高达60%～70%，其中10%的患者在数年内丧失劳动力。

本病的病因和发病机理至今尚未完全明确，一般认为本病是一种既有体液免疫也有细胞免疫异常的自身免疫性疾病。

根据本病的临床表现，属于中医学"痹证"范畴。其外因为风、寒、湿、热等外邪的侵入，内因为素体气血不足、肝肾亏虚。主要病机为邪气痹阻经络，气血运行滞涩。病久可致痰浊瘀血痹阻，气血肝肾受损，表现为虚实夹杂。

stasis may occur, which results in deficiency of qi and blood and deficiency of the liver and kidneys, and the case is manifested as deficiency complicated by excess.

Essentials for Diagnosis

(1) Pain, swelling , rigidity which is aggravated in the morning and alleviated by exertion. The affected parts are usually the small joints of the hands (especially the interphalangeal joints and metacarpophalangeal joints), wrist joints and foot joints; sometimes, elbows, shoulders, ankles, knees and hips may also be affected.

(2) At the advanced stage, rigidity and deformity of joints can be seen. The affected joints are less flexible and the muscles around the joints are atrophic. In some cases, there may be subcutaneous nodules in the prominence of joints.

(3) Laboratory examination: blood sedimentation increased; serum albumin decreased and globulin increased; IgG, IgA and IgM increased in electrophoregram ; in most cases, blood RF positive.

(4) X-ray examination: swelling of periarticular tissue at the initial stage, followed by osteoporosis of joints and narrowing of joint space; at the advanced stage, dislocation of joints, disappearance of articular cartilage, erosion of subchondral bone substance and ultimately rigidity of joints.

Syndrome Differentiation and Treatment

Clinically there are five types of bi-syndromes, i.e., bi-syndrome caused by wind, cold and dampness; bi-syndrome caused by wind, dampness and heat; bi-syndrome with concurrence of cold and heat; bi-syndrome with phlegm stagnation and blood stasis; and bi-syndrome with deficient healthy qi and retained pathogenic factors. As far

【诊断要点】

(1) 关节疼痛、肿胀、僵硬（晨间显著，活动后可减轻）。受累关节以两手小关节（尤其是近端指间关节和掌指小关节）、腕、足关节为常见，肘、肩、踝、膝、髋等关节也常受累。

(2) 病变晚期，关节僵硬、畸形，功能受限，关节附近的肌肉萎缩。部分患者可在关节的隆突部位出现皮下小结。

(3) 实验室检查可见血沉加快；血清白蛋白降低、球蛋白增高；免疫蛋白电泳显示 IgG、IgA 及 IgM 增高；多数患者类风湿因子乳胶试验阳性。

(4) X 线检查早期仅见关节周围组织胀肿，进而关节部位骨质疏松，关节间隙狭窄。晚期关节脱位，关节软骨消失，软骨下骨质受侵蚀，最后导致关节强直。

【辨证论治】

本病临床主要分为风寒湿证、风湿热证、寒热夹杂证、痰瘀痹阻证及正虚邪恋证。治疗以祛邪通络为原则，根据病邪的偏胜，分别采用祛风、散寒、除湿、清热、化痰、祛瘀

as the treatment is concerned, it should primarily aim at eliminating pathogenic factors and activating meridians. Different methods, for example, dispelling wind, eliminating cold, removing dampness, clearing away heat, resolving phlegm and removing blood stasis, should be used according to different cases; for prolonged cases with healthy qi deficiency, herbs for replenishing qi and blood, nourishing the liver and kidneys should be used accordingly.

1. Bi-syndrome Caused by Wind, Cold and Dampness

Chief Manifestations: Wandering pain of joints with localized swelling and numbness, or with localized cold pain which is aggravated by cold, in cloudy and rainy days and alleviated by warmth, stiff joints in the morning, limited flexibility, aversion to wind and cold, pale tongue with thin and white, or white and greasy coating, superficial and tense, or deep and tense, or soft-superficial and even-soft pulse.

Therapeutic Methods: To dispel wind, eliminate cold, remove dampness and activate collaterals.

Prescription: Modified Yiyiren Tang (Coicis Decoction) and Wutou Tang (Aconiti Decoction), composed of Yiyiren (*Semen Coicis*) 12 g, Qianghuo (*Rhizoma et Radix Notopterygii*) 10 g, Duhuo (*Radix Angelicae Pubescentis*) 10 g, Mahuang (*Herba Ephedrae*) 6 g, Zhichuanwu (*Radix Aconiti Preparata*) 8 g, Cangzhu (*Rhizoma Atractylodis*) 10 g, Weilingxian (*Radix Clematidis*) 10 g, Chuanxiong (*Rhzioma Chuanxiong*) 10 g and Laoguancao (*Herba Erodii seu Geranii*) 15 g.

Modifications: For severe wandering pain, add Fangfeng (*Radix Saposhnikoviae*) 6 g, Baizhi (*Radix Angelicae Dahuricae*) 6 g and Xungufeng (*Rhizoma seu Herba Aristolochiae Mollissimae*) 10 g; for severe swol-

法;病久正虚者,则应配伍益气血、补肝肾之品。

1. 风寒湿证

主要证候 肢体关节疼痛,局部肿胀,麻木重着,痛处游走不定,或局部畏寒冷痛,遇寒痛增,得热痛减,阴雨天疼痛加剧,晨起关节僵硬,活动不利,恶风畏寒,舌质黯淡,苔薄白或白腻,脉浮紧或沉紧或濡缓。

治 法 祛风散寒,除湿通络。

方 药 薏苡仁汤合乌头汤加减:薏苡仁12 g,羌活10 g,独活10 g,麻黄6 g,制川乌8 g,苍术10 g,威灵仙 10 g,川芎10 g,老鹳草15 g。

加 减 疼痛游走不定明显者,加防风6 g,白芷6 g,寻骨风10 g;关节肿甚者,加防己10 g,晚蚕沙(包煎)10 g,萆

len joints, add Fangji (*Radix Stephaniae Tetrandrae*) 10 g, Wancansha (*Feculae Bombycis*, wrapped) 10 g and Bixie (*Rhizoma Dioscoreae Hypoglaucae*) 10 g; for severe pain, add Shufu Pian (*Radix Aconiti Lateralis Preparata*, sliced) 6 g, Guizhi (*Ramulus Cinnamomi*) 10 g and Xixin (*Herba Asari*) 3 g.

2. Bi-syndrome Caused by Wind, Dampness and Heat

Chief Manifestations: Red, feverish, swollen and painful joints which are aggravated by touching, rigidity, or subcutaneous nodules, feverish body with flushed face, excessive thirst, sore throat, scanty deep yellow urine, red tongue with thin and yellow, or yellow and greasy coating, smooth and rapid, or wiry and rapid pulse.

Therapeutic Methods: To clear away heat, activate collaterals, dispel wind and remove dampness.

Prescription: Modified Baihu Guizhi Tang (White Tiger Decoction with Cinnamomi) and Simiao Wan (Four Wonder-Drug Pill), composed of Shengshigao (*Gypsum Fibrosum*, to be decocted first) 30 g, Zhimu (*Rhizoma Anemarrhenae*) 10 g, Guizhi (*Ramulus Cinnamomi*) 6 g, Cangzhu (*Rhizoma Atractylodis*) 10 g, Huangbai (*Cortex Phellodendri*) 10 g, Rendongteng (*Caulis Lonicerae*) 12 g, Qinjiao (*Radix Gentianae Macrophyllae*) 10 g, Sangzhi (*Ramulus Mori*) 20 g, Shengyiyiren (*Semen Coicis*) 15 g and Luoshiteng (*Caulis Trachelospermi*) 15 g.

Modifications: For persistent high fever and excessive thirst with a desire to drink, add Lianqiao (*Fructus Forsythiae*) 12 g, Zhizi (*Fructus Gardeniae*) 10 g and Baihuasheshecao (*Herba Hedyotis Diffusae*) 20 g; for hot pain of the lower limb joints and difficult urination with deep yellow urine, add Niuxi (*Radix Achyranthis Bidentatae*) 10 g and Haitongpi (*Cortex Erythinae Ori-*

薜10 g;痛剧者,加熟附片6 g,桂枝10 g,细辛3 g。

2. 风湿热证

主要证候　肢体关节红肿疼痛,扪之觉热,痛不可近,屈伸不利,或见皮下结节,身热面赤,烦渴欲饮,咽喉疼痛,小溲短赤,舌质红,苔薄黄或黄腻,脉滑数或弦数。

治　法　清热通络,祛风除湿。

方　药　白虎桂枝汤合四妙丸加减:生石膏(先煎)30 g,知母10 g,桂枝6 g,苍术10 g,黄柏10 g,忍冬藤12 g,秦艽10 g,桑枝20 g,生薏苡仁15 g,络石藤15 g。

加　减　壮热不退,烦渴欲饮者,加连翘12 g,栀子10 g,白花蛇舌草20 g;下肢关节热痛,小溲赤涩者,加牛膝10 g,海桐皮10 g;若低热不退或午后潮热,舌质红,少苔,脉细数者,加龟版(先煎)15 g,熟

entalis) 10 g; for persistent slight fever or afternoon fever, red tongue with little coating, and thready, rapid pulse, add Guiban (*Plastrum Testudinis*, to be decocted first) 15 g, Shudihuang (*Radix Rehmanniae Preparata*) 12 g, Danggui (*Radix Angelicae Sinensis*) 10 g, Baishaoyao (*Radix Paeoniae Alba*) 10 g, Qinjiao (*Radix Gentianae Macrophyllae*) 10 g and Qinghao (*Herba Artemisiae Annuae*) 10 g; for subcutaneous nodules, add Huzhang (*Rhizoma Polygoni Cuspidati*) 15 g, Baijiezi (*Semen Sinapis Albae*) 6 g and Kunbu (*Thallus Laminariae et Eckloniae*) 10 g.

3. Bi-syndrome with Concurrence of Cold and Heat

Chief Manifestations: Redness, swelling and pain of joints, general fever but preference to warmth, rigidity of joints, thirst with desire for hot drink, red tongue with white coating or pale tongue with yellow coating, wiry and rapid or wiry and tense pulse.

Therapeutic Methods: To warm the meridians, eliminate cold, clear away heat and remove dampness.

Prescription: Modified Guizhi Shaoyao Zhimu Tang (Decoction of Cinnamomi, Paeoniae and Anemarrhenae), composed of Guizhi (*Ramulus Cinnamomi*) 6 g, Baishaoyao (*Radix Paeoniae Alba*) 10 g, Zhimu (*Rhizoma Anemarrhenae*) 10 g, Cangzhu (*Rhizoma Atractylodis*) 10 g, Shufuzi (*Radix Aconiti Lateralis Preparata*) 6 g, Huangbai (*Cortex Phellodendri*) 10 g, Qianghuo (*Rhizoma et Radix Notopterygii*) 10 g, Chuanxiong (*Rhizoma Chuanxiong*) 10 g, Haifengteng (*Caulis Piperis Kadsurae*) 10 g, Fangji (*Radix Stephaniae Tetrandrae*) 10 g and Qinjiao (*Radix Gentianae Macrophyllae*) 12 g.

Modifications: For the case with cold predominating over heat, add Zhichuanwu (*Radix Aconiti Preparata*)

地黄12 g,当归10 g,白芍药10 g,秦艽10 g,青蒿10 g;皮下结节者,加虎杖15 g,白芥子6 g,昆布10 g。

3. 寒热夹杂证

主要证候 肢体关节红肿热痛,但局部畏寒,虽有身热,却欲盖衣被,关节屈伸不利,口渴而欲热饮,舌红苔白或舌淡苔黄,脉弦数或弦紧。

治 法 温经散寒,清热除湿。

方 药 桂枝芍药知母汤加减:桂枝6 g,白芍药10 g,知母10 g,苍术10 g,熟附子6 g,黄柏10 g,羌活10 g,川芎10 g,海风藤10 g,防己10 g,秦艽12 g。

加 减 寒甚于热,加制川乌6 g,制草乌6 g,细辛3 g;

6 g, Zhicaowu (*Radix Aconiti Kusnezoffii Preparata*) 6 g and Xixin (*Herba Asari*) 3 g; for that with heat predominating over cold, add Shengshigao (*Gypsum Fibrosum*, to be decocted first) 30 g.

4. Bi-syndrome with Phlegm Stagnation and Blood Stasis

Chief Manifestations: Long-term intermittent arthralgia with swelling, rigidity and deformity of joints, numbness of limbs, darkish purple skin, purplish dim tongue with ecchymosis, white or greasy coating, thready and unsmooth pulse.

Therapeutic Methods: To resolve phlegm, remove blood stasis, expel wind and activate meridians.

Prescription: Modified Tao Hong Yin (Persicae and Carthami Decoction), composed of Danggui (*Radix Angelicae Sinensis*) 10 g, Taoren (*Semen Persicae*) 10 g, Honghua (*Flos Carthami*) 10 g, Shudihuang (*Radix Rehmanniae Preparata*) 12 g, Chuanxiong (*Rhizoma Chuanxiong*) 8 g, Chishaoyao (*Radix Paeoniae Rubra*) 10 g, Zhinanxing (*Arisaema cum Bile*) 6 g, Baijiezi (*Semen Sinapis Albae*) 6 g, Zhibaijiangcan (*Bombyx Batryticatus*, roasted) 10 g, Dilong (*Pheretima*) 10 g, Lufengfang (*Nidus Polistis Mandarini*) 10 g, Weilingxian (*Radix Clematidis*) 10 g and Lulutong (*Fructus Liquidambaris*) 10 g.

Modifications: For severe pain, add Quanxie (*Scorpio*) 3 g and Wugong (*Scolopendra*) 3 g; for the prolonged case with healthy qi deficiency, add Huangqi (*Radix Astragali*) 15 g and Danggui (*Radix Angelicae Sinensis*) 10 g.

5. Bi-syndrome with Deficient Healthy Qi and Retained Pathogenic Factors

Chief Manifestations: Prolonged arthralgia with

热甚于寒，加生石膏（先煎）30 g。

4. 痰瘀痹阻证

主要证候　病变日久不愈，疼痛时轻时重，关节肿大，僵硬畸形，屈伸不利，肢体麻木、肤色、舌质紫黯，或有瘀斑、瘀点，苔白或腻，脉象细涩。

治　法　化痰祛瘀、搜风通络。

方　药　桃红饮加减：当归10 g，桃仁10 g，红花10 g，熟地黄12 g，川芎8 g，赤芍药10 g，制南星6 g，白芥子6 g，炙白僵蚕10 g，地龙10 g，露蜂房10 g，威灵仙10 g，路路通10 g。

加　减　疼痛明显者，加全蝎3 g，蜈蚣3 g；病久正虚者，加黄芪15 g，当归10 g。

5. 正虚邪恋证

主要证候　病变日久，肢

intermittent pain of joints, lassitude, lusterless complexion, cold pain of lumber vertebrae, inflexibility of the joints, weakness of the knees, atrophy of muscles, pale tongue with white coating, thready and weak pulse.

Therapeutic Methods: To tonify qi and blood, nourish the liver and kidney, remove obstruction from the collaterals.

Prescription: Modified Duhuo Jisheng Tang (Angelicae Pubescentis and Taxilli Decoction) and Huangqi Guizhi Wuwu Tang (Five-Ingredient Decoction Containing Astragali and Cinnamomi), composed of Huangqi (*Radix Astragali*) 15 g, Dangshen (*Radix Codonopsis*) 10 g, Baizhu (*Rhizoma Atractylodis Macrocephalae*) 10 g, Danggui (*Radix Angelicae Sinensis*) 10 g, Baishaoyao (*Radix Paeoniae Alba*) 12 g, Duzhong (*Cortex Eucommiae*) 10 g, Sangjisheng (*Herba Taxilli*) 12 g, Niuxi (*Radix Achyranthis Bidentatae*) 10 g, Duhuo (*Radix Angelicae Pubescentis*) 6 g, Fangfeng (*Radix Saposhnikoviae*) 10 g, Jixueteng (*Caulis Spatholobi*) 12 g, Qiannianjian (*Rhizoma Homalomenae*) 15 g and Jingangci (*Rhizoma Smilacis*) 12 g.

Modifications: For weakness of the limbs, sallow complexion, pale tongue and thready pulse, add Heshouwu (*Radix Polygoni Multiflori*) 12 g and Shudihuang (*Radix Rehmanniae Preparata*) 12 g; for dizziness and tinnitus, add Gouqizi (*Fructus Lycii*) 10 g and Tusizi (*Semen Cuscutae*) 10 g; for cold limbs, cold pain of the joints and aversion to cold, add Shufuzi (*Radix Aconiti Lateralis Preparata*) 6 g, Lujiaopian (*Cornu Cervi*, sliced) 10 g and Bajitian (*Radix Morindae Officinalis*) 10 g.

Other Treatments

1. Chinese Patent Drugs

(1) Fengshi Hantong Pian (Tablet for Rheumatoid

体关节疼痛时轻时重,倦怠乏力,面色少华,腰脊冷痛,肢体屈伸不利,胫酸膝软,肌肉萎缩,舌质淡,苔白,脉细弱。

治　法　补气血,养肝肾,蠲痹通络。

方　药　独活寄生汤合黄芪桂枝五物汤加减:黄芪15 g,党参10 g,白术10 g,当归10 g,白芍药12 g,杜仲10 g,桑寄生12 g,牛膝10 g,独活6 g,防风10 g,鸡血藤12 g,千年健15 g,金刚刺12 g。

加　减　如肢倦乏力,面色萎黄,舌淡,脉细者,加何首乌12 g,熟地黄12 g;头晕耳鸣者,加枸杞子10 g,菟丝子10 g;畏寒肢冷,关节冷痛,加熟附子6 g,鹿角片10 g ,巴戟天10 g。

【其他疗法】

1. 中成药

(1) 风湿寒痛片　每服

Arthritis with Cold Pain): 6 - 8 tablets (a double dosage for the severe case) each time, twice or thrice daily; applicable to rheumatoid arthritis at the initial stage.

(2) Biku Naiting Pian (Tablet for Relieving Arthralgia): 5 - 7 tablets each time, 4 times daily; applicable to rheumatoid arthritis with predominance of cold and dampness.

(3) Shexiang Wan (Moschus (artificial) Pill): 7 pills (10 pills for the severe case) each time, 3 times daily; applicable to rheumatoid arthritis with wandering pain at the initial stage.

(4) Fangfeng Wan (Saposhnikovia Pill): 30 pills (gradually increased to 40 pills) each time, 3 times daily, taken with warm wine on empty stomach; applicable to rheumatoid arthritis with painful , red and feverish joints.

(5) Yishen Juanbi Wan (Pill for Nourishing Kidney and Relieving Arthralgia): 6 g (12 g for the severe case) each time, 3 times daily, taken after meals; applicable to the prolonged case of rheumatoid arthritis with deficiency of the kidney.

2. Single-drug or Experiential Prescriptions

(1) Huzhanggen (*Rhizoma Polygoni Cuspidati*, sliced) 250 g and 750 ml of white spirit. Soak the herb in white spirit and add a small amount of brown sugar to make the medicated wine. Take 15 g of the wine, twice daily. It is applicable to rheumatoid arthritis caused by wind, dampness and heat.

(2) Shengdihuang (*Radix Rehmanniae*) 90 - 100 g. Crush and boil the herb in 600 - 800 ml of water for one hour, filter and collect 300 ml of decoction. Take the decoction in one or two doses each day. It is applicable to rheumatoid arthritis with predominance of heat or with consumption of yin fluid.

(3) Qingfengteng (*Caulis Sinomenii*) 15 g and

6～8 片(病重者可加倍服用)，每日 2～3 次。适用于早期类风湿关节炎。

（2）痹苦乃停片　每服5～7 片，每日 4 次。适用于类风湿关节炎之寒湿偏重型。

（3）麝香丸　每服 7 丸(甚者 10 丸)，每日 3 次。适用于类风湿关节炎早期疼痛游走不定者。

（4）防风丸　每服 30 丸，渐加至 40 丸，每日 3 次，空腹温酒送服。适用于类风湿关节炎关节疼痛、红肿、微热者。

（5）益肾蠲痹丸　每服6 g(重症者可加至12 g)，每日 3 次，食后服用。适用于类风湿关节炎病久肾虚较甚者。

2. 单验方

（1）虎杖根切片泡白酒，250 g 生药泡 750 ml 白酒，加少量赤砂糖，每次15 ml，日服2 次。适用于类风湿关节炎风湿热证。

（2）生地黄90～100 g，切碎，加水 600～800 ml，煮沸 1 小时，滤出药液 300 ml，为 1 日量，分 1～2 次服完。适用于类风湿关节炎偏热证或有阴津耗伤者。

（3）青风藤15 g,麻黄(后

Mahuang (*Herba Ephedrae*, to be decocted later) 6 g. Decoct the herbs in water and take the decoction after meals. It is applicable to mild cases of rheumatoid arthritis.

(4) Shujin Huoxue San (Powder for Relaxing Tendons and Activating Blood Circulation), composed of Ruxiang (*Olibanum*) 15 g, Moyao (*Myrrha*) 15 g, Niuxi (*Radix Achyranthis Bidentatae*) 15 g, Duzhong (*Cortex Eucommiae*) 15 g, Qianghuo (*Rhizoma et Radix Notopterygii*) 15 g, Dilong (*Pheretima*) 15 g, Mugua (*Fructus Chaenomelis*) 15 g, Dangshen (*Radix Codonopsis*) 15 g, Guizhi (*Ramulus Cinnamomi*) 15 g and Danggui (*Radix Angelicae Sinensis*) 25 g. Dry and grind the above herbs into fine powder, take 3 g of the powder, 3 times daily. It is applicable to the prolonged case with pronounced rigidity of joints.

(5) Jiajian Tongfeng Fang (Modified Formula for Rigidity of Joints), composed of Mahuang (*Herba Ephedrae*) 6 g, Guizhi (*Ramulus Cinnamomi*) 10 g, Fangfeng (*Radix Saposhnikoviae*) 10 g, Fangji (*Radix Stephaniae Tetrandrae*) 10 g, Weilingxian (*Radix Clematidis*) 10 g, Cangzhu (*Rhizoma Atractylodis*) 10 g, Jixueteng (*Caulis Spatholobi*) 10 g, Quanxie (*Scorpio*) 3 g, Zhinanxing (*Arisaema cum Bile*) 6 g, Taoren (*Semen Persicae*) 10 g and Honghua (*Flos Carthami*). Decoct the above herbs in water and take the decoction. It is applicable to pronounced rigidity and deformity of joints.

3. External Therapy

(1) Shengjiang (*Rhizoma Zingiberis Recens*, liquidized) 250 g, Ruxiang (*Olibanum*, powdered) 15 g, Moyao (*Myrrha*, powdered) 15 g, Shexiang (*Moschus*, artificial) 3 g and Niupiguangjiao (*Colla Corium Bovis*) 60 g. Melt Niupiguangjiao with ginger juice and mix it

下)6 g,水煎,早晚饭后服。适用于类风湿关节炎轻症。

(4) 舒筋活血散   乳香15 g,没药15 g,牛膝15 g,杜仲15 g,羌活15 g,地龙15 g,木瓜15 g,党参15 g,桂枝15 g,当归25 g,干燥后研末。每次3 g,每日3次。适用于病程较长、关节僵硬明显者。

(5) 加减痛风方   麻黄6 g,桂枝10 g,防风10 g,防己10 g,威灵仙10 g,苍术10 g,鸡血藤10 g,全蝎3 g,制南星6 g,桃仁10 g,红花10 g,水煎服。适用于关节僵硬畸形明显者。

3. 外治法

(1) 生姜250 g(取汁),乳香(研末)15 g,没药(研末)15 g,麝香3 g,真牛皮广胶60 g。先将姜汁并广胶溶化,后下乳香、没药调匀,待少温,

evenly with Ruxiang and Moyao. When it is not so hot, add Shexiang to make paste. Apply the paste to the affected part. It is applicable to the case caused by wind, cold and dampness.

(2) Wutou (*Radix Aconiti*, raw) 30 g, Mubiezi (*Semen Momordicae*, shelled) 30 g, Baijiezi (*Semen Sinapis Albae*) 30 g, Biejia (*Carapax Trionycis*) 30 g and Xingren (*Semen Armeniacae Amarum*, raw) 40 g. Grind the above herbs into coarse powder, boil it in 3,000 ml of water for a while, remove the dregs, drip-wash the affected part while the decoction is still hot, warm the decoction again if it becomes cool and drip-wash the affected part again. This is applicable to pain and spasm of the muscles and tendons.

(3) Xionghuang (*Realgar*) 30 g, Banmao (*Mylabris*) 30 g and Shexiang (*Moschus*, artificial) 10 g. Grind the first two ingredients into fine powder, mix the powder with honey into paste, add Shexiang to the paste and mix them thoroughly, then bottle and seal the paste for future use. Decide and mark the acupoints in the affected part or the painful spots. Prepare some 3 cm x 3 cm adhesive plasters, each of which has the paste of a rice-grain size in the center. Apply the plasters to 4 - 8 acupoints or pain spots, at most 20 spots for all the joints each time. A hot sensation and stabbing pain will appear after the application for 2 - 4 hours and for another 6 - 10 hours, blisters appear. Do not break the blisters. To avoid infection, do not wash the affected part 1 - 7 days after the application. If the blister is more than 3 cm in diameter and the patient suffers severe pain, break the blister, let the fluid out and apply gentian violet to it. This method is applicable to localized swelling and pain.

下麝香成膏。摊贴患处。适用于风寒湿证。

（2）乌头（生用不去皮）30 g，木鳖子（去壳）30 g，白芥子30 g，鳖甲30 g，杏仁（生用）40 g。将上药研为粗末，加水3 000 ml，煎数沸去渣，趁热淋洗患处，冷后再加热，复淋洗。适用于筋骨疼痛挛急者。

（3）雄黄30 g，斑蝥30 g，麝香10 g。先将雄黄、斑蝥研成细末，用蜂蜜适量拌成糊状，再加入麝香拌均匀，装瓶盖紧备用。找好患部穴位或痛点作记号。将胶布剪成3 cm见方，正中放米粒大小药糊，对准穴位或痛点将胶布贴好。每次贴 4～8 个点，全身关节最多可贴 20 个点。贴后2～4 小时有热感和刺痛感。8～12小时起水泡，不要碰破。贴后 1～7 日不可洗患处，防止感染。若水泡直径超过3 cm，疼痛剧烈时，可挑破放液，涂龙胆紫即可。适用于局部肿痛明显者。

2.6.7 Gout

General Description

Gout is a kind of disease caused by prolonged purine metabolic disturbance, clinically characterized by hyperuricemia, repeated attack of acute arthritis, gouty tophus sedimentation, chronic arthritis with deformity of joints, pathogenic change of renal parenchyma and formation of tophus. The disease is grouped into two categories by different causes of increased uric acid in blood, i.e., primary and secondary. Primary gout is caused by congenital purine metabolic disturbance and secondary gout is caused by hyperuricemia due to the increase of uricopoiesis or hypoeccrisia of uric acid, which is induced by other diseases or drugs. The disease may occur in people at any age, mostly at the age between 30 - 40. Among the patients, 95% are male and usually they have a family history of gout.

Because gout is clinically manifested as recurrence of redness, swelling, a burning sensation, pain, and limited flexibility of joints, it is included in the category of bi-syndrome in TCM. As for the pathogenesis, this disease is externally caused by blockage of the meridians following invasion of the body by exogenous pathogenic wind, cold and damp heat; and internally caused by deficient healthy qi, overstrain, or exposure to wind while sweating and the weakened weiqi failing to protect the body from the exogenous pathogenic factors, giving rise to blockage of the meridians and stagnation of qi and blood. In a prolonged case, there may appear blood stasis and phlegm stagnation with the involvement from the meridians to the viscera, then visceral bi-syndrome occurs.

第七节　痛风

【概述】

痛风是由于长期嘌呤代谢紊乱所致的疾病,临床以高尿酸血症、急性关节炎反复发作、痛风石沉积、慢性关节炎和关节畸形、肾实质性病变和尿酸石形成为特点。根据血液中尿酸增高的原因,可分为原发性和继发性两大类。原发性痛风是由于先天性嘌呤代谢紊乱所致;继发性痛风是由于其他疾病、药物等引起尿酸生成增多或排出减少,形成高尿酸血症而致。本病以男性为多,约占95%。各种年龄均可发病,但发病高峰多在30~40岁之间。有家族遗传史。

根据本病临床以关节红、肿、热、痛反复发作,关节活动不灵活为主要表现,属于中医学"痹证"等病的范畴。中医认为本病的发生,外因多为风寒湿热之邪侵袭人体,痹阻经络。内因则为正气不足或劳倦过度或汗出当风,卫气不固,外邪乘虚而入,以致经络阻滞,气血运行不畅而成痹证。痹证日久不愈,血脉瘀阻,津聚痰凝,由经络及脏腑,可导致脏腑痹。

Essentials for Diagnosis

(1) At the initial stage, it is symptomless with only the increase of uric acid in blood. At the acute stage, its typical manifestation is sudden onset of arthralgia and most of the cases would suddenly be woken up by sharp arthralgia when sleeping. The affected parts are mostly the first metatarsophalangeal joint or other metatarsophalangeal joints with localized redness, swelling, a burning sensation, pain and limited flexibility. When the greater joint is involved, there may be some exudate. In addition, such symptoms as chills, fatigue, poor appetite and headache may appear. However, the above-mentioned symptoms would be relieved in 1-2 weeks.

(2) At the chronic stage, there may be gouty tophus, deformity and rigidity of joints, and renal lesions.

(3) Laboratory examination shows uric acid in blood increasing to over 420 μmol/L. In roentgenogram, a round or irregular transparent defective area can be found in the bone substance of the joint adjacent to osteochondral edge, which is characteristic of gout in X-ray examination.

Syndrome Differentiation and Treatment

The pathological factors of this disease are chiefly dampness, phlegm and blood stasis, and therefore removing dampness, resolving phlegm and eliminating blood stasis are the basic treatment principles. However, dampness is classified into cold dampness and damp heat and different treatments should be adopted according to syndrome differentiation. At the later stage, spleen yang and kidney yang are usually impaired. Thus it is advisable to eliminate pathogenic factors and support healthy qi as well.

【诊断要点】

(1) 本病初期可仅有血尿酸增高而无临床症状。急性关节炎期典型的表现是关节突发疼痛,多数患者在半夜因突感关节剧痛而惊醒,以第一跖趾关节及跖趾关节为多见,局部红、肿、热、痛及活动受限,大关节受累时常有渗液。可伴有发热,有时出现寒战、倦怠、厌食、头痛等症状。一般历时 1～2 个星期症状缓解。

(2) 慢性关节炎期主要可见痛风石形成、关节畸形僵硬和肾脏病变。

(3) 实验室检查可见血尿酸增高,超过 420 μmol/L。X 线摄片检查在受累关节可发现骨软骨缘邻近关节的骨质有圆形或不整齐的穿凿样透亮缺损区,为痛风的 X 线特征。

【辨证论治】

本病的病理因素以湿、痰、瘀为主,故祛湿、化痰、消瘀为本病的基本治疗大法。但湿有寒、热之分,因此应根据辨证选择不同的治法。本病后期多伤及脾肾阳气,治疗当以扶正祛邪兼施为要。

1. Obstruction of Damp Heat in the Meridians

Chief Manifestations: Redness, swelling, a burning sensation and pain of the joints which is alleviated by cold, tenderness, or fever, constipation, dark yellow urine, yellow and greasy tongue coating, and wiry and rapid or smooth and rapid pulse.

Therapeutic Methods: To clear away heat, eliminate dampness, and remove obstruction in the collaterals.

Prescription: Modified Simiao Wan (Four Wonder-Drug Pill), composed of Cangzhu (*Rhizoma Atractylodis*) 10 g, Huangbai (*Cortex Phellodendri*) 10 g, Yiyiren (*Semen Coicis*) 15 g, Chuanniuxi (*Radix Cyathulae*) 10 g, Rendongteng (*Caulis Lonicerae*) 15 g, Sangzhi (*Ramulus Mori*) 20 g, Wancansha (*Feculae Bombycis*, wrapped) 10 g and Xuanmugua (*Fructus Chaenomelis*) 10 g.

Modifications: For fever with thirst, add Zhimu (*Rhizoma Anemarrhenae*) 10 g, Shengshigao (*Gypsum Fibrosum*, to be decocted first) 30 g and Zhizi (*Fructus Gardeniae*) 10 g; for swollen joints, add Jianghuang (*Rhizoma Curcumae Longae*) 10 g and Weilingxian (*Radix Clematidis*) 10 g; for erythema around the joints, add Mudanpi (*Cortex Moutan Radicis*) 10 g, Shengdihuang (*Radix Rehmanniae*) 12 g and Chishaoyao (*Radix Paeoniae Rubra*) 10 g; for slight fever due to yin impairment by heat, dry mouth, feverish sensation over the palms, soles and chest, add Qinghao (*Herba Artemisiae Annuae*) 12 g, Qinjiao (*Radix Gentianae Macrophyllae*) 10 g and Shidagonglaoye (*Folium Mahoniae*) 15 g according to individual cases; for predominance of dampness, add Cheqiancao (*Herba Plantaginis*) 15 g and Fangji (*Radix Stephaniae Tetrandrae*) 10 g; for severe arthralgia, add Yanhusuo (*Rhizoma Corydalis*) 10 g and Dilong (*Pheretima*) 10 g.

1. 湿热痹阻证

主要证候 关节红肿热痛,得冷则舒,痛不可触,或有发热,大便秘结,小便黄赤,舌苔黄腻,脉弦数或滑数。

治 法 清热祛湿,宣痹通络。

方 药 四妙丸加减:苍术10 g,黄柏10 g,薏苡仁15 g,川牛膝10 g,忍冬藤15 g,嫩桑枝20 g,晚蚕沙(包煎)10 g,宣木瓜10 g。

加 减 发热口渴者,加知母10 g,生石膏(先煎)30 g,栀子10 g;关节肿大者,加姜黄10 g,威灵仙10 g;关节周围出现红斑者,加牡丹皮10 g,生地黄12 g,赤芍药10 g;邪热伤阴出现低热,口干,五心烦热者,酌加青蒿12 g,秦艽10 g,十大功劳叶15 g;湿重者,加车前草15 g,防己10 g;关节痛甚者,加延胡索10 g,地龙10 g。

2. Invasion of the Collaterals by Cold and Dampness

Chief Manifestations: Rigidity and deformity of the joints, limited flexibility, darkish red skin, aversion to cold and cold limbs, darkish tongue with ecchymosis, thin and white coating, deep and thready pulse.

Therapeutic Methods: To warm the meridians, eliminate cold, remove dampness and activate the collaterals.

Prescription: Modified Yiyiren Tang (Coicis Decoction), composed of Qianghuo (*Rhizoma et Radix Notopterygii*) 10 g, Duhuo (*Radix Angelicae Pubescentis*) 10 g, Fangfeng (*Radix Saposhnikoviae*) 10 g, Zhichuanwu (*Radix Aconiti Preparata*) 6 g, Mahuang (*Herba Ephedrae*) 5 g, Guizhi (*Ramulus Cinnamomi*) 10 g, Yiyiren (*Semen Coicis*) 15 g, Cangzhu (*Rhizoma Atractylodis*) 10 g, Danggui (*Radix Angelicae Sinensis*) 10 g, Chuanxiong (*Rhizoma Chuanxiong*) 10 g, Shengjiang (*Rhizoma Zingiberis Recens*) 3 pcs and Zhigancao (*Radix Glycyrrhizae*, roasted) 3 g.

Modifications: For the case with predominance of wind and marked by wandering pain of upper limbs, increase the amount of Qianghuo to 30 g and add Sangzhi (*Ramulus Mori*) 30 g and Pianjianghuang (*Rhizoma Curcumae Longae*, sliced) 10 g; for the case with predominance of cold and characterized by localized pain which is alleviated by warmth, add Xixin (*Herba Asari*) 3 g and Zhicaowu (*Radix Aconiti Kusnezoffii Preparata*) 6 g; for the case with predominance of dampness and characterized by swollen joints and heaviness of lower limbs, add Fangji (*Radix Stephaniae Tetrandrae*) 15 g, Tufuling (*Rhizoma Smilacis Glabrae*) 15 g, Mugua (*Fructus Chaenomelis*) 10 g and Bixie (*Rhizoma Dioscoreae Hypoglaucae*) 15 g.

2. 寒湿入络证

主要证候　关节僵硬畸形,屈伸不利,皮色暗红,畏寒肢凉,舌质暗或有瘀斑,苔薄白,脉沉细。

治　法　温经散寒,祛湿通络。

方　药　薏苡仁汤加减:羌活10 g,独活10 g,防风10 g,制川乌6 g,麻黄5 g,桂枝10 g,薏苡仁15 g,苍术10 g,当归10 g,川芎10 g,生姜3片,炙甘草3 g。

加　减　若风邪偏盛,以上肢游走痛为主者,重用羌活至30 g,并加桑枝30 g,片姜黄10 g;寒邪偏盛,痛处不移,得温则减者,可加细辛3 g,制草乌6 g;湿邪偏盛,关节肿胀,重着不利,以下肢为主者,加防己15 g,土茯苓15 g,木瓜10 g,萆薢15 g。

3. Phlegm Stagnation Blending with Blood Stasis

Chief Manifestations: Subcutaneous nodules which are normal-colored, tenderless or ruptured, darkish tongue with occasional ecchymosis, thin and white coating, and deep and smooth pulse.

Therapeutic Methods: To resolve phlegm, eliminate stagnation, activate blood circulation to dissipate stasis.

Prescription: Modified Xiaotan Tang (Phlegm-Resolving Decoction), composed of Kunbu (*Thallus Laminariae et Eckloniae*) 10 g, Haizao (*Sargassum*) 10 g, Baijiezi (*Semen Sinapis Albae*) 6 g, Zhebeimu (*Bulbus Fritillariae Thunbergii*) 10 g, Tiannanxing (*Rhizoma Arisaematis*) 10 g, Fuling (*Poria*) 12 g, Fabanxia (*Rhizoma Pinelliae*) 10 g, Shancigu (*Pseudobulbus Cremastrae seu Pleiones*) 15 g, Dangshen (*Radix Codonopsis*) 12 g and Taoren (*Semen Persicae*) 10 g.

Modifications: For blood stasis, add Danshen (*Radix Salviae Miltiorrhizae*) 15 g and Honghua (*Flos Carthami*) 10 g; for ulceration of subcutaneous nodules, add Huangqi (*Radix Astragali*) 15 g.

4. Retained Damp Heat in the Urinary Bladder

Chief Manifestations: Sandy stones in the urine; difficult, frequent and urgent urination; urethral pain and colicky pain of the loins and abdomen; even hematuria, red tongue with yellow coating, and rapid pulse.

Therapeutic Methods: To clear away heat, promote diuresis, relieve stranguria and expel stones.

Prescription: Modified Shiwei San (Pyrrosiae Powder), composed of Shiwei (*Folium Pyrrosiae*) 10 g, Qumai (*Herba Dianthi*) 10 g, Huashi (*Talcum*, wrapped) 10 g, Cheqianzi (*Semen Plantaginis*, wrapped) 15 g, Bianxu (*Herba Polygoni Avicularis*) 10 g, Huangbai

3. 痰瘀互结证

主要证候 皮下硬结,触之不痛,皮色不变,或溃破,舌质暗或有瘀斑,苔薄白,脉沉滑。

治 法 消痰散结,活血化瘀。

方 药 消痰汤加减:昆布10 g,海藻10 g,白芥子6 g,浙贝母10 g,天南星10 g,茯苓12 g,法半夏10 g,山慈姑15 g,党参12 g,桃仁10 g。

加 减 血瘀明显者,加丹参15 g,红花10 g;痰核破溃者,加黄芪15 g。

4. 膀胱湿热证

主要证候 尿中时夹砂石,小便难,尿频,尿急,尿道涩痛,腰腹绞痛,甚则尿血,舌红,苔黄,脉数。

治 法 清利湿热,通淋排石。

方 药 石韦散加减:石韦10 g,瞿麦10 g,滑石(包煎)10 g,车前子(包煎)15 g,萹蓄10 g,黄柏10 g,冬葵子10 g,海金沙(包煎)12 g,台乌

(*Cortex Phellodendri*) 10 g, Dongkuizi (*Semen Malvae*) 10 g, Haijinsha (*Spora Lygodii*, wrapped) 12 g and Taiwuyao (*Radix Linderae*) 6 g.

Modifications: For hematuria, add Baimaogen (*Rhizoma Imperatae*) 20 g and Xiaoji (*Herba Cirsii*) 15 g; for colicky pain of the loins and abdomen, add Yanhusuo (*Rhizoma Corydalis*) 10 g and Baishaoyao (*Radix Paeoniae Alba*) 15 g.

5. Deficiency of Spleen Yang and Kidney Yang

Chief Manifestations: Short breath, lassitude, loss of appetite, nausea, vomiting, abdominal flatulence, loose stools, sore and weak loins and knees, aversion to cold, cold limbs, edema of the face and lower limbs, pale complexion, pale swollen tongue with white and thin coating, and deep, thready and forceless pulse.

Therapeutic Methods: To invigorate the spleen, replenish qi, nourish the kidney and warm kidney yang.

Prescription: Modified Fuzi Tang (Aconiti Lateralis Decoction), composed of Zhifupian (*Radix Aconiti Lateralis Preparata*, sliced) 10 g, Dangshen (*Radix Codonopsis*) 10 g, Baizhu (*Rhizoma Atractylodis Macrocephalae*) 10 g, Fuling (*Poria*) 12 g, Baishaoyao (*Radix Paeoniae Alba*) 12 g, Huangqi (*Radix Astragali*) 15 g, Rougui (*Cortex Cinnamomi*) 5 g, Tusizi (*Semen Cuscutae*) 10 g and Zexie (*Rhizoma Alismatis*) 12 g.

Modifications: For severe vomiting, add Banxia (*Rhizoma Pinelliae*) 10 g and Shengjiang (*Rhizoma Zingiberis Recens*) 3 pcs; for pronounced edema, add Cheqianzi (*Semen Plantaginis*, wrapped) 10 g and Fangji (*Radix Stephaniae Tetrandrae*) 10 g.

Other Treatments

1. Chinese Patent Drugs

(1) Wangbi Chongji (Granule for Relieving Gout): 1 sachet each time, twice or thrice daily; applicable to gout

药6 g。

加　减　尿血者,加白茅根20 g,小蓟15 g;腰腹绞痛者,加延胡索10 g,白芍药15 g。

5. 脾肾阳虚证

主要证候　气短乏力,纳呆呕恶,腹胀便溏,腰膝酸软,畏寒肢冷,面部、下肢浮肿,面色㿠白,舌淡胖,苔薄白,脉沉细无力。

治　法　健脾益气,补肾温阳。

方　药　附子汤加减:制附片10 g,党参10 g,白术10 g,茯苓12 g,白芍药12 g,黄芪15 g,肉桂5 g,菟丝子10 g,泽泻12 g。

加　减　呕恶甚者,加半夏10 g,生姜 3 片;水肿明显者,加车前子(包煎)10 g,防己10 g。

【其他疗法】

1. 中成药

(1) 尪痹冲剂　每服 1 袋,每日 2～3 次。适用于痛

due to cold dampness.

(2) Yishen Juanbi Chongji (Granule for Nourishing Kidney and Relieving Arthralgia): 1 sachet each time, twice or thrice daily; applicable to prolonged case of gout.

(3) Shujin Huoxue Pian (Tablet for Relaxing Tendon and Activating Blood Circulation): 5 tablets each time, 3 times daily; applicable to gout with blood stasis.

2. Single-drug or Experiential Prescriptions

(1) Leigongtenggen (*Radix Tripterygii Wilfordii*, barked) 15 g and Shenggancao (*Radix Glycyrrhizae*) 5 g. Decoct the herbs in water for oral administration, 1 dose daily, 14 days being a course of treatment. It is applicable to gout due to cold dampness.

(2) Xixiancao (*Herba Siegesbeckiae*) 15 g and Chouwutong (*Folium Clerodendri Trichotomi*) 15 g. Decoct the herbs in water for oral administration, 1 dose daily, 14 days being a course of treatment. It is applicable to gout due to cold dampness.

风寒湿证。

(2) 益肾蠲痹冲剂　每服1袋，每日2～3次。适用于痛风病久者。

(3) 舒筋活血片　每次5片，每日3次。适用于痛风瘀血之证明显者。

2. 单验方

(1) 雷公藤根去皮15 g，生甘草5 g，煎水服用，每日1剂，14日为1个疗程。适用于痛风寒湿证。

(2) 豨莶草15 g，臭梧桐15 g，煎水服用，每日1剂，14日为1个疗程。适用于痛风寒湿证。

2.7 Syndrome Patterns of Qi, Blood and Body Fluid

第七章 气血津液病证

2.7.1 Depressive syndrome

第一节 郁证

General Description

Depressive syndrome is due to emotional upsets and stagnation of qi, clinically manifested as mental depression, restlessness, feeling of fullness and oppression over the chest, distending pain over hypochondrium or irritability and susceptibility to cry, or feeling of a foreign body in the throat.

The cause of depressive syndrome is emotional upsets. Pathogenically, if the liver fails to control the dispersion, the stagnant liver qi attacks the spleen, which impairs the spleen's function of transportation and transformation and the heart is deprived of nourishment. Thus, disorders of the viscera, yin, yang, qi and blood appear. At the initial stage, depressive syndrome is attributed to the excess type. It is usually caused by stagnation of qi, complicated by blood stagnation, fire transformation, phlegm accumulation and food retention. But prolonged cases will change from the excess type into the deficiency type, and there may appear different pathological changes of the heart, spleen, liver or kidneys, as a result of different conditions of the involved zang-fu organs and of the consumption of qi, blood, yin or yang.

According to the clinical manifestations and its pathogensis, depressive syndrome is mainly seen in neurasthe-

【概述】

郁证是由于情志不舒、气机郁滞所致的以心情抑郁、情绪不宁、胸部满闷、胁肋胀痛，或易怒易哭，或咽中如有异物梗塞等为主要临床表现的一类病证。

本病的病因是情志内伤。其病机主要为肝失疏泄，脾失健运，心失所养及脏腑阴阳气血失调。郁病初起病变以气滞为主，常兼血瘀、化火、痰结、食滞等，多属实证。病久则易由实转虚，随其影响的脏腑及损耗气血阴阳的不同，而形成心、脾、肝、肾亏虚的不同病变。

根据郁证的临床表现及其以情志内伤为致病原因的

nia, hysteria and anxiety in western medicine, and also in perimenopausal syndrome and reactive psychosis.

Essentials for Diagnosis

(1) The major symptoms are mental depression, restlessness, distending pain over chest and hypochondrium or irritability and susceptibility to cry, or feeling of a foreign body in the throat, mostly seen in young and middle-aged women.

(2) The patient usually has a history of emotional upsets, such as melancholy, anxiety, sorrow, terror and resentment. Its recurrence is closely related with the emotional factors.

(3) Examinations of various systems and laboratory examinations are normal. Organic diseases should be excluded.

Syndrome Differentiation and Treatment

At the initial stage, depressive syndrome is mostly of the excess type, and then the prolonged case changes from the excess to the deficiency type or the deficiency-excess type. The principle of the treatment is to regulate qi circulation. The case of the excess type should be treated by soothing liver qi and alleviating mental depression, and assisted by promoting blood circulation, resolving phlegm, promoting diuresis, clearing away heat and promoting digestion; the case of the deficiency type should be treated by nourishing the heart, tranquilizing the mind and nourishing the heart and kidneys.

1. Stagnation of Liver Qi

Chief Manifestations: Mental depression, restlessness, feeling of fullness and oppression over the chest, distending and wandering pain in the hypochondrium, abdominal flatulence, eructation, loss of appetite, irregular

特点,主要见于西医学中的神经衰弱、癔病及焦虑症等。另外,也可见于围绝经期综合征、反应性精神病等。

【诊断要点】

(1) 以忧郁不畅,情绪不宁,胸胁胀痛,或易怒易哭,或咽中如有异物梗塞为主症。多发于青中年女性。

(2) 患者大多数有忧愁、焦虑、悲哀、恐惧、愤懑等情志内伤的病史。并且其病情的反复常与情志因素密切相关。

(3) 各系统检查和实验室检查正常,除外器质性疾病。

【辨证论治】

郁证初起多实,病久转虚或虚实夹杂。治疗以疏通气机为原则。属实者除疏肝理气解郁外,还应配合行血、化痰、利湿、清热、消食等法;虚证者应佐以养心安神、滋养心肾等治法。

1. 肝气郁结证

主要证候 精神抑郁,情绪不宁,胸部满闷,胁肋胀痛,痛无定处,脘闷嗳气,不思饮食,大便不调,苔薄腻,脉弦。

bowel movements, thin and greasy tongue coating, and wiry pulse.

Therapeutic Methods: To soothe liver qi, alleviate mental depression and regulate middle energizer qi.

Prescription: Modified Chaihu Shugan San (Bupleuri Powder for Soothing Liver Qi), composed of Chaihu (*Radix Bupleuri*) 6 g, Zhike (*Fructus Aurantii*) 10 g, Xiangfu (*Rhizoma Cyperi*) 10 g, Qingpi (*Pericarpium Citri Reticulatae Viride*) 6 g, Zisugeng (*Caulis Perillae*) 10 g, Hehuanpi (*Cortex Albiziae*) 6 g, Lü'emei (*Flos Mume*) 3 g, Chuanxiong (*Rhizoma Chuanxiong*) 8 g, Baishaoyao (*Radix Paeoniae Alba*) 10 g and Zhigancao (*Radix Glycyrrhizae*, roasted) 3 g.

Modifications: For pronounced distending pain over the hypochondrium, add Yujin (*Radix Curcumae*) 10 g and Foshou (*Fructus Citri Sarcodactylis*) 6 g; for invasion of the stomach by liver qi, resulting in failure of the stomach qi to descend, manifested as frequent eructation and flatulence, add Xuanfuhua (*Flos Inulae*, wrapped) 6 g, Daizheshi (*Haematitum*, to be decocted first) 30 g, Zisugeng (*Caulis Perillae*) 10 g and Fabanxia (*Rhizoma Pinelliae Preparata*) 10 g; for the case accompanied by dyspepsia and flatulence, add Shenqu (*Massa Medicata Fermentata*) 12 g, Maiya (*Fructus Hordei Germinatus*) 12 g, Shanzha (*Fructus Crataegi*) 10 g and Jineijin (*Endothelium Corneum Gigeriae Galli*) 6 g; for hyperactive liver qi attacking the spleen manifested as abdominal flatulence and pain, and diarrhea, add Cangzhu (*Rhizoma Atractylodis*) 10 g, Fuling (*Poria*) 10 g, Wuyao (*Radix Linderae*) 6 g and Baidoukou (*Fructus Amomi Rotundus*) 3 g; for the case accompanied by blood stasis manifested as stabbing pain over the chest and hypochondria, petechia and ecchymosis on the tongue, add Danggui (*Radix Angelicae Sinensis*) 10 g, Danshen (*Radix*

治 法 疏肝解郁,理气畅中。

方 药 柴胡疏肝散加减:柴胡6 g,枳壳10 g,香附10 g,青皮6 g,紫苏梗10 g,合欢皮6 g,绿萼梅3 g,川芎8 g,白芍药10 g,炙甘草3 g。

加 减 胁肋胀满疼痛较甚者,可加郁金10 g,佛手6 g;肝气犯胃,胃失和降,而见嗳气频作,脘闷不舒者,可加旋覆花(包煎)6 g,代赭石(先煎)30 g,紫苏梗10 g,法半夏10 g;兼有食滞腹胀者,可加神曲12 g,麦芽12 g,山楂10 g,鸡内金6 g;肝气乘脾而见腹胀、腹痛、腹泻者,可加苍术10 g,茯苓10 g,乌药6 g,白豆蔻3 g;兼有血瘀而见胸胁刺痛,舌质有瘀点、瘀斑,可加当归10 g,丹参12 g,郁金10 g,红花10 g。

Salviae Miltiorrhizae) 12 g, Yujin (*Radix Curcumae*) 10 g and Honghua (*Flos Carthami*) 10 g.

2. Stagnant Qi Transforming into Fire

Chief Manifestations: Irritability, distention and fullness over the chest and hypochondrium, dry mouth and bitter taste, or headache, red eyes, tinnitus, or gastric upset and acid regurgitation, constipation, red tongue with yellow coating, wiry and rapid pulse.

Therapeutic Methods: To soothe liver qi, alleviate mental depression and clear away liver fire.

Prescription: Modified Dan Zhi Xiaoyao San (Xiaoyao Powder with Moutan and Gardeniae), composed of Chaihu (*Radix Bupleuri*) 6 g, Bohe (*Herba Menthae*) 6 g, Mudanpi (*Cortex Moutan Radicis*) 10 g, Zhizi (*Fructus Gardeniae*) 10 g, Baizhu (*Rhizoma Atractylodis Macrocephalae*) 10 g, Fuling (*Poria*) 12 g, Danggui (*Radix Angelicae Sinensis*) 10 g and Baishaoyao (*Radix Paeoniae Alba*) 10 g.

Modifications: For high fever, bitter taste in the mouth and constipation, add Longdancao (*Radix Gentianae*) 5 g, Zhidahung (*Radix et Rhizoma Rhei Preparata*) 6 g; for liver fire attacking the stomach manifested as pain over hypochondrium, bitter taste in the mouth, gastric upset, acid regurgitation, eructation and vomiting, add Huanglian (*Rhizoma Coptidis*) 3 g and Wuzhuyu (*Fructus Euodiae*) 1.5 g; for flaming-up of liver fire manifested as headache, red eyes and tinnitus, add Juhua (*Flos Chrysanthemi*) 6 g, Gouteng (*Ramulus Uncariae cum Uncis*) 10 g and Cijili (*Fructus Tribuli*) 10 g; for impairment of yin by excessive heat manifested as red tongue with little coating, thready and rapid pulse, add Shengdihuang (*Radix Rehmanniae*) 10 g, Maimendong (*Radix Ophiopogonis*) 10 g and Shanyao (*Rhizoma Dioscoreae*) 10 g.

2. 气郁化火证

主要证候　性情急躁易怒,胸胁胀满,口苦而干,或头痛、目赤、耳鸣,或嘈杂吞酸,大便秘结,舌质红,苔黄,脉弦数。

治　法　疏肝解郁,清肝泻火。

方　药　丹栀逍遥散加减:柴胡6 g,薄荷6 g,牡丹皮10 g,栀子10 g,白术10 g,茯苓12 g,当归10 g,白芍药10 g。

加　减　热势较甚,口苦、大便秘结者,可加龙胆草5 g,制大黄6 g;肝火犯胃而见胁肋疼痛、口苦、嘈杂吞酸、嗳气、呕吐者,可加黄连3 g,吴茱萸1.5 g;肝火上炎而见头痛、目赤、耳鸣者,加菊花6 g,钩藤10 g,刺蒺藜10 g;热盛伤阴,而见舌红少苔、脉细数者,加生地黄10 g,麦门冬10 g,山药10 g。

3. Stagnation of Blood

Chief Manifestations: Mental depression, irritability, headache, insomnia, amnesia, or pain over the chest and hypochondium, or chills or fever of some part of the body, dark purple tongue, with petechia and ecchymosis, wiry or unsmooth pulse.

Therapeutic Methods: To activate blood circulation, dissipate blood stasis, regulate qi and alleviate mental depression.

Prescription: Modified Xuefu Zhuyu Tang (Decoction for Removing Blood Stasis in Chest), composed of Taoren (*Semen Persicae*) 10 g, Honghua (*Flos Carthami*) 10 g, Chishaoyao (*Radix Paeoniae Rubra*) 10 g, Mudanpi (*Cortex Moutan Radicis*) 10 g, Niuxi (*Radix Achyranthis Bidentatae*) 10 g, Zhidahuang (*Radix et Rhizoma Rhei Preparata*) 10 g, Danggui (*Radix Angelicae Sinensis*) 10 g, Chuanxiong (*Rhizoma Chuanxiong*) 10 g, Shengdihuang (*Radix Rehmanniae*) 10 g, Chaihu (*Radix Bupleuri*) 6 g, Zhike (*Fructus Aurantii*) 10 g and Jiegeng (*Radix Platycodi*) 6 g.

Modification: For the case accompanied by deficiency of qi, add Dangshen (*Radix Codonopsis*) 10 g, Huangqi (*Radix Astragali*) 12 g and Baizhu (*Rhizoma Atractylodis Macrocephalae*) 10 g.

4. Stagnation of Qi and Retention of Phlegm

Chief Manifestations: Mental depression, feeling of oppression over the chest, distension and fullness over the hypochondrium, feeling of a foreign body in the throat with difficulty to swallow or spit out, white and greasy tongue coating, wiry and smooth pulse. This syndrome, in TCM, is also known as "mei he qi" (globus hystericus).

Therapeutic Methods: To promote circulation of qi, alleviate mental depression, resolve phlegm and re-

3. 血行郁滞证

主要证候 精神抑郁,性情急躁,头痛,失眠,健忘,或胸胁疼痛,或身体某部有发冷或发热感,舌质紫暗,或有瘀点、瘀斑,脉弦或涩。

治　法 活血化瘀,理气解郁。

方　药 血府逐瘀汤加减:桃仁10 g,红花10 g,赤芍药10 g,牡丹皮10 g,牛膝10 g,制大黄10 g,当归10 g,川芎10 g,生地黄10 g,柴胡6 g,枳壳10 g,桔梗6 g。

加　减 兼气虚者,加党参10 g,黄芪12 g,白术10 g。

4. 痰气郁结证

主要证候 精神抑郁,胸部闷塞,胁肋胀满,咽中如有物梗塞,吞之不下,咯之不出,苔白腻,脉弦滑。本证即"梅核气"。

治　法 行气开郁,化痰散结。

lieve stagnation.

Prescription: Modified Banxia Houpo Tang (Decoction of Pinelliae and Magnoliae Officinalis), composed of Fabanxia (*Rhizoma Pinelliae Preparata*) 10 g, Houpo (*Cortex Magnoliae Officinalis*) 10 g, Fuling (*Poria*) 10 g, Chenpi (*Pericarpium Citri Reticulatae*) 6 g, Foshou (*Fructus Citri Sarcodactylis*) 6 g, Xiangfu (*Rhizoma Cyperi*) 10 g, Zhike (*Fructus Aurantii*) 10 g and Zisugeng (*Caulis Perillae*) 10 g.

Modifications: For retention of dampness, stagnation of qi, accompanied by sensation of fullness and oppression over the chest and stomach, eructation and greasy tongue coating, add Cangzhu (*Rhizoma Atractylodis*) 10 g; for retention of phlegm transforming into heat, manifested as restlessness, red tongue with yellow coating, add Zhuru (*Caulis Bambusae in Taeniam*) 10 g, Gualou (*Fructus Trichosanthis*) 10 g, Huangqin (*Radix Scutellariae*) 10 g and Huanglian (*Rhizoma Coptidis*) 3 g; for the prolonged case manifested as blood stasis, stabbing pain over the chest and hypochondria, dark purple tongue or with petechia and ecchymosis, and unsmooth pulse, add Yujin (*Radix Curcumae*) 10 g, Danshen (*Radix Salviae Miltiorrhizae*) 10 g, Jiangxiang (*Lignum Dalbergiae Odoriferae*, to be decocted cater) 6 g and Jianghuang (*Rhizoma Curcumae Longae*) 6 g.

5. Mental Confusion

Chief Manifestations: Restlessness, trance, suspiciousness, timidness, sentimentality, liability to cry, changeable moods, or frequent stretching and yawning, or unrestrained flourishing and shouting, pale tongue, and wiry pulse.

Therapeutic Methods: To relieve the acute case with herbs of sweet taste and lubricant nature, and tranquilize the mind by nourishing the heart.

方　药　半夏厚朴汤加减：法半夏10 g，厚朴10 g，茯苓10 g，陈皮6 g，佛手6 g，香附10 g，枳壳10 g，紫苏梗10 g。

加　减　湿郁气滞而兼胸脘痞闷、嗳气、苔腻者，加苍术10 g；痰郁化热而见烦躁、舌红、苔黄者，加竹茹10 g，瓜蒌10 g，黄芩10 g，黄连3 g；病久入络而有瘀血征象，胸胁刺痛，舌质紫暗或有瘀点、瘀斑，脉涩者，加郁金10 g，丹参10 g，降香(后下)6 g，姜黄6 g。

5. 心神惑乱证

主要证候　精神恍惚，心神不宁，多疑易惊，悲忧善哭，喜怒无常，或时时欠伸，或手舞足蹈，骂詈喊叫，舌质淡，脉弦。

治　法　甘润缓急，养心安神。

Prescription: Modified Gan Mai Dazao Tang (Decoction of Glycyrrhizae, Tritici Levis and Jujubae), composed of Gancao (*Radix Glycyrrhizae*) 10 g, Xiaomai (*Fructus Tritici Aestivi*) 12 g, Dazao (*Fructus Jujubae*) 5 pcs, Baiziren (*Semen Biotae*) 10 g, Fushen (*Sclerotium Poriae Circum Radicem Pini*) 10 g, Yujin (*Radix Curcumae*) 10 g and Hehuanhua (*Flos Albiziae*) 6 g.

Modifications: For deficiency of blood causing wind, manifested as tremor of hands and feet or convulsion, add Danggui (*Radix Angelicae Sinensis*) 10 g, Shengdihuang (*Radix Rehmanniae*) 10 g, Zhenzhumu (*Concha Margaritifera Usta*, to be decocted first) 30 g and Gouteng (*Ramulus Uncariae cum Uncis*) 12 g; for restlessness and insomnia, add Suanzaoren (*Semen Ziziphi Spinosae*) 10 g, Baiziren (*Semen Biotae*) 10 g, Fushen (*Sclerotium Poriae Circum Radicem Pini*) 10 g and Zhiheshouwu (*Radix Polygoni Multiflori Preparata*) 12 g.

6. Deficiency of the Heart and Spleen

Chief Manifestations: Suspiciousness, dizziness, listlessness, palpitation, timidness, insomnia, amnesia, poor appetite, lusterless complexion, pale tongue with thin and white coating, and thready pulse.

Therapeutic Methods: To invigorate the spleen, nourish the heart and replenish qi and blood.

Prescription: Modified Guipi Tang (Decoction for Invigorating Spleen and Nourishing Heart), composed of Dangshen (*Radix Codonopsis*) 10 g, Baizhu (*Rhizoma Atractylodis Macrocephalae*) 10 g, Huangqi (*Radix Astragali*) 12 g, Danggui (*Radix Angelicae Sinensis*) 10 g, Baishaoyao (*Radix Paeoniae Alba*) 10 g, Guiyuanrou (*Arillus Longan*) 10 g, Yuanzhi (*Radix Polygalae*) 6 g, Fushen (*Sclerotium Poriae Circum Radi-*

方　药　甘麦大枣汤加减：甘草10 g,小麦12 g,大枣5枚,柏子仁10 g,茯神10 g,郁金10 g,合欢花6 g。

加　减　血虚生风而见手足蠕动或抽搐者,加当归10 g,生地黄10 g,珍珠母(先煎)30 g,钩藤12 g;见躁扰、失眠者,加酸枣仁10 g,柏子仁10 g,茯神10 g,制何首乌12 g。

6. 心脾两虚证

主要证候　多思善疑,头晕神疲,心悸胆怯,失眠,健忘,纳差,面色不华,舌质淡,苔薄白,脉细。

治　法　健脾养心,补益气血。

方　药　归脾汤加减：党参10 g,白术10 g,黄芪12 g,当归10 g,白芍药10 g,桂圆肉10 g,远志6 g,茯神10 g,夜交藤10 g,陈皮6 g,大枣5枚,炙甘草3 g。

cem Pini) 10 g, Yejiaoteng (Caulis et Folium Polygoni Multiflori) 10 g, Chenpi (Pericarpium Citri Reticulatae) 6 g, Dazao (Fructus Jujubae) 5 pcs and Zhigancao (Radix Glycyrrhizae, roasted) 3 g.

Modifications: For feeling of depression over the heart and chest and emotional upsets, add Yujin (Radix Curcumae) 10 g and Foshou (Fructus Citri Sarcodactylis) 6 g; for headache, add Chuanxiong (Rhizoma Chuanxiong) 6 g and Baizhi (Radix Angelicae Dahuricae) 6 g.

7. Consumption of Heart Yin

Chief Manifestations: Restlessness, palpitation, amnesia, insomnia, dreamfulness, burning sensation of the palms, soles and chest, night sweating, dryness of the mouth and throat, red and dry tongue, thready and rapid pulse.

Therapeutic Methods: To nourish yin and blood, tonify the heart and tranquilize the mind.

Prescription: Modified Tianwang Buxin Dan (Tianwang Pill for Tonifying Heart), composed of Shengdihuang (Radix Rehmanniae) 12 g, Xuanshen (Radix Scrophulariae) 12 g, Tianmendong (Radix Asparagi) 10 g, Maimendong (Radix Ophiopogonis) 10 g, Shanzhuyu (Fructus Corni) 10 g, Gouqizi (Fructus Lycii) 10 g, Suanzaoren (Semen Ziziphi Spinosae) 10 g, Yuanzhi (Radix Polygalae) 6 g, Fushen (Sclerotium Poriae Circum Radicem Pini) 10 g and Wuweizi (Fructus Schisandrae) 6 g.

Modifications: For incoordination between the heart and kidney, manifested as restlessness, insomnia, dreamfulness and nocturnal emission, add Huanglian (Rhizoma Coptidis) 3 g and Rougui (Cortex Cinnamomi) 1.5 g; for frequent nocturnal emission, add Qianshi (Semen Euryales) 10 g, Lianxu (Stamen Nelumbi-

加 减 见心胸郁闷,情志不舒者,加郁金10 g,佛手6 g;见头痛者,加川芎6 g,白芷6 g。

7. 心阴亏虚证

主要证候 情绪不宁,心悸,健忘,失眠,多梦,五心烦热,盗汗,口咽干燥,舌红少津,脉细数。

治 法 滋阴养血,补心安神。

方 药 天王补心丹加减:生地黄12 g,玄参12 g,天门冬10 g,麦门冬10 g,山茱萸10 g,枸杞子10 g,酸枣仁10 g,远志6 g,茯神10 g,五味子6 g。

加 减 心肾不交而见心烦失眠,多梦遗精者,可加黄连3 g,肉桂1.5 g;遗精较频者,可加芡实10 g,莲须10 g,金樱子10 g。

nis) 10 g and Jinyingzi (*Fructus Rosae Laevigatae*) 10 g.

8. Consumption of Liver Yin

Chief Manifestations: Restlessness, irritability, dizziness, tinnitus, dryness of the eyes, photophobia, blurred vision, or headache and feeling of distention in the head, flushed face, red eyes, dry and red tongue, wiry and thready or rapid pulse.

Therapeutic Methods: To nourish yin essence and invigorate the liver and kidney.

Prescription: Modified Zishui Qinggan Yin (Decoction for Nourishing Kidney and Clearing Liver Fire), composed of Shengdihuang (*Radix Rehmanniae*) 12 g, Shanzhuyu (*Fructus Corni*) 10 g, Fuling (*Poria*) 10 g, Danggui (*Radix Angelicae Sinensis*) 10 g, Shanyao (*Rhizoma Dioscoreae*) 12 g, Mudanpi (*Cortex Moutan Radicis*) 10 g, Zexie (*Rhizoma Alismatis*) 12 g, Baishaoyao (*Radix Paeoniae Alba*) 12 g, Chaihu (*Radix Bupleuri*) 6 g, Zhizi (*Fructus Gardeniae*) 10 g and Suanzaoren (*Semen Ziziphi Spinosae*) 10 g.

Modifications: For deficiency of liver yin resulting in hyperactivity of liver yang and upward disturbance of liver wind, manifested as headache, dizziness, flushed cheeks, or muscular twitching and cramp, add Cijili (*Fructus Tribuli*) 15 g, Caojueming (*Semen Cassiae*) 15 g, Gouteng (*Ramulus Uncariae cum Uncis*) 15 g, Shijueming (*Concha Haliotidis*, to be decocted first) 30 g; for predominant deficient fire, manifested as low fever, feverish sensation over the palms and soles, add Yinchaihu (*Radix Stellariae*) 6 g, Baiwei (*Radix Cynanchi Atrati*) 6 g and Maimendong (*Radix Ophiopogonis*) 10 g; for irregular menstruation, add Xiangfu (*Rhizoma Cyperi*) 10 g, Zelan (*Herba Lycopi*) 12 g and Yimucao (*Herba Leonuri*) 10 g.

8. 肝阴亏虚证

主要证候　情绪不宁,急躁易怒,眩晕,耳鸣,目干畏光,视物不明,或头痛且胀,面红目赤,舌干红,脉弦细或数。

治　法　滋养阴精,补益肝肾。

方　药　滋水清肝饮加减:生地黄12 g,山茱萸10 g,茯苓10 g,当归身10 g,山药12 g,牡丹皮10 g,泽泻12 g,白芍药12 g,柴胡6 g,栀子10 g,酸枣仁10 g。

加　减　肝阴不足而肝阳偏亢,肝风上扰,以致头痛、眩晕、面时潮红,或筋惕肉瞤者,加刺蒺藜15 g,草决明15 g,钩藤15 g,石决明(先煎)30 g。虚火较甚,表现低热,手足心热者,可加银柴胡6 g,白薇6 g,麦门冬10 g;月经不调者,可加香附10 g,泽兰12 g,益母草10 g。

Other Treatments

1. Chinese Patent Drugs

(1) Yueju Wan (Pill for Relieving Stagnancy): 6 g, twice daily; indicated for depressive syndrome caused by stagnation of liver qi.

(2) Xiaoyao Wan (Xiaoyao Pill): 6 g, twice daily; indicated for depressive syndrome caused by stagnation of liver qi and deficiency of the spleen.

(3) Chaihu Shugan Wan (Bupleuri Pill for Soothing Liver Qi): 6 g, twice daily; indicated for stagnation of liver qi and disharmony of the liver and stomach, manifested as fullness sensation in the hypochondrium, abdominal flatulence, eructation or distending pain over the hypochondrium and abdomen.

2. Single-drug or Experiential Prescriptions

(1) Xiaomai (*Fructus Tritici Aestivi*, macerated and crushed) 60 g, Dazao (*Fructus Jujubae*) 14 pcs and Gancao (*Radix Glycyrrhizae*) 20 g. Mix and boil the herbs for 1 hour, and take the decoction and Dazao. It is indicated for depressive syndrome caused by deficiency of both the heart and spleen.

(2) Baihe (*Bulbus Lilii*, fresh) 50 g. Mix it with 1-2 spoons of honey, steam it until it is well done and take it at times. It is indicated for prolonged case with restlessness due to insufficiency of blood.

2.7.2 Hemorrhagic Syndrome

General Description

Hemorrhagic syndrome refers to discharge of blood from nine orifices or extravasated blood diffusing in the skin, resulting from failure of blood to circulate in the vessels. It includes epistaxis, gingival hemorrhage, hemoptysis, hematemesis, hematuria, hemafecia and he-

【其他疗法】

1. 中成药

（1）越鞠丸　每服6 g,每日 2 次。适用于肝气郁结之郁证。

（2）逍遥丸　每服6 g,每日 2 次。适用于郁证属肝郁脾虚者。

（3）柴胡疏肝丸　每服 6 g,每日 2 次。适用于肝气郁结、肝胃不和之胁胀、脘闷嗳气或胁腹胀痛者。

2. 单验方

（1）小麦（浸软,研碎） 60 g,大枣 14 枚,甘草20 g,共煮 1 小时,喝汤食枣。适用于心脾不足之郁证。

（2）鲜百合50 g,加蜂蜜 1~2 匙拌合,蒸熟,不拘时服之。适用于郁证日久阴血不足,心神不宁者。

第二节　血证

【概述】

血证是指血不循经,自九窍排出体外,或渗溢于肌肤的一类出血性病证。在内科范围内常见鼻衄、齿衄、咳血、吐血、尿血、便血及紫斑等。

mokelidosis in internal medicine.

Hemorrhagic syndrome results from attack by exogenous pathogenic factors, emotional stress, improper diet, overwork, prolonged illness or febrile disease. Their common pathogenesis includes two types: reckless movement of blood caused by excessive pathogenic fire and extravasation of blood from the vessels due to deficiency of qi. As for the pathogenic fire, it is classified into excess-fire and deficiency-fire. The former includes fire caused by wind heat, retention of damp heat, and fire caused by stagnation of liver qi; while the latter is hyperactive fire caused by deficiency of yin. As for deficiency of qi, there is either deficiency of qi or deficiency of qi damaging yang.

Hemorrhagic syndrome covers a wide range. Clinically, those syndromes chiefly manifested as bleeding belong to this category. For instance, hemorrhage in various acute and chronic diseases in western medicine, including diseases in respiratory, digestive, or urinary systems as well as hemorrhagic diseases caused by the disorder of hematopoietic system.

Essentials for Diagnosis

(1) The patient has a history of suffering from some diseases in which bleeding is frequently seen. For instance, hemoptysis is indicative of a history of diseases of the pulmonary system, such as chronic cough, dyspnea due to retention of sputum, and tuberculosis; hematemesis and hemafecia are indicative of a history of stomachache, hypochondric pain, jaundice and abdominal mass.

(2) There may be different symptoms with bleeding from different areas of the body. For instance, epistaxis is manifested as bleeding from nasal cavity; gingival hemorrhage is manifested as bleeding from the dental diastema

血证的病因主要有感受外邪、情志过极、饮食不节、劳倦过度、久病或热病等。其共同的病机可以归结为火热熏灼、迫血妄行及气虚不摄、血溢脉外两类。在火热之中，又有实火及虚火之分。外感风热燥火，湿热内蕴，肝郁化火等，均属实火；而阴虚火旺之火，则属虚火。气虚之中，又有仅见气虚，以及气损及阳之别。

血证的范围相当广泛，凡以出血为主要临床表现的病证，均属本证的范围。如西医学中多种急、慢性疾病所引起的出血，包括呼吸、消化、泌尿等系统疾病有出血症状者，以及造血系统病变所引起的出血性疾病等。

【诊断要点】

（1）有易引起出血的疾病史，如咳血多有慢性咳嗽、痰喘、肺痨等肺系病证史；吐血、便血多有胃痛、胁痛、黄疸、癥积等疾病史等。

（2）有各个部位出血所出现的症状，如鼻衄可见鼻腔流血；齿衄可见齿龈或齿缝溢出；咳血者血经咳嗽而出，或

and gum; hemoptysis is manifested as spitting of blood by coughing, or itching of the throat and feeling of oppression over the chest, followed by coughing up bright red blood with foam, or blood-stained sputum; hematemesis is manifested as spitting of brown or dark purple blood by vomiting often with food residue from the stomach, and accompanied by pitch-black stools; hemafecia is manifested as discharge of bloody stools in bright red or dark red color, even as black as tar; hematuria is manifested as blood or blood streak in the urine; hemokelidosis is manifested as bluish purple spots which are as small as pinholes or become confluent to form a patch on the skin and do not fade on pressure.

(3) The following examinations are recommended to help ascertain the causes of hemorrhagic syndrome. They are blood and urine routine examinations, fecal occult blood test, platelet count, bleeding and coagulation times, vasoconstrictive time, prothrombin time, capillary fragility test, bone marrow smear, gastrofiberscopy, barium meal radiography of the upper digestive tract, ultrasonography (B mode), X-ray examination of chest, bronchoscopy or bronchography, and computerized tomography of chest and abdomen.

(4) Hemorrhagic syndrome should be differentiated from physiological hemorrhage. Retrograde menstruation may cause epistaxis, which is closely related with menstrual cycle and often occurs ahead of or during menstrual cycle.

Syndrome Differentiation and Treatment

The differentiation of hemorrhagic syndrome is to determine whether the case is the excess or deficiency type. The cases caused by hyperactivity of fire are referred to the excess type; while those caused by deficiency of yin with hyperactivity of fire or failure of deficient qi to con-

觉喉痒胸闷,一咯即出,血色鲜红,或夹泡沫,或痰血相兼,痰中带血;吐血者血随呕吐而出,常夹有食物残渣等胃内容物,血色多为咖啡色或紫暗色,大便多呈黑漆色;便血为粪中带血,其色或鲜红,或暗红,甚至黑如柏油样;尿血为小便中混有血液或夹有血丝;紫斑为肌肤出现青紫斑点,小如针尖,大者融合成片,压之不退色。

(3) 血、尿常规,大便潜血试验,血小板计数,出凝血时间,血管收缩时间,凝血酶原时间,毛细血管脆性试验及骨髓穿刺、纤维胃镜、上消化道钡餐造影、B超、胸部X线检查、支气管镜检或造影、胸腹部CT等检查,有助于进一步明确血证的病因。

(4) 除外生理性出血,经行衄血又名倒经、逆经,其发生与月经周期有密切关系,多于经行前期或经期出现。

【辨证论治】

血证的辨证主要是辨虚实,由火热亢盛所致者属于实证;由阴虚火旺及气虚不摄所致者,则属于虚证。而实证和虚证又常发生互相转化。如

trol blood are referred to the deficiency type. But excess and deficiency types often transform into each other. For instance, initially, adverse rising of qi by hyperactivity of fire leads to reckless movement of blood, but with the recurrence of bleeding, deficiency of blood occurs, resulting in accumulation of deficient fire inside the body; or impairment of qi by profuse bleeding causes deficiency of qi and yang, which fails to control the blood. In addition, with the accumulation of extravasated blood in the tissue spaces or stagnation of blood in the channels and viscera, blood stasis comes into being, which prevents the production of new blood and obstructs the circulation of qi and blood. As far as the treatment is concerned, it should primarily aim at dealing with blood, fire and qi. The treatment for blood includes controlling bleeding with astringents, by cooing blood and by eliminating blood stasis; the treatment for fire includes clearing away heat to purge fire for the case of excess-fire and nourishing yin to subdue fire for the case of deficient-fire; the treatment for qi includes clearing away heat from qifen and send the adverse qi downward for the excess type, and replenishing and warming qi for the deficiency type.

1. Epistaxis

(1) Pathogenic Heat Attacking the Lung

Chief Manifestations: Dry nose, nasal bleeding, dry mouth and throat, or feverish body, cough with scanty sputum, red tongue with thin coating, and rapid pulse.

Therapeutic Methods: To clear away lung heat and cool blood to stop bleeding.

Prescription: Modified Sang Ju Yin (Mori and Chrysanthemi Decoction), composed of Sangye (*Folium Mori*) 10 g, Juhua (*Flos Chrysanthemi*) 6 g, Bohe (*Herba Menthae*, to be decocted later) 6 g, Mudanpi (*Cortex Moutan Radicis*) 10 g, Zhizi (*Fructus Gardeniae*)

开始为火盛气逆,迫血妄行,但在反复出血之后,则会导致阴血亏损,虚火内生;或因出血过多,血去气伤,以致气虚阳衰,不能摄血。此外,出血之后,已离经脉而未排出体外的血液,留积体内,蓄结而为瘀血,瘀血又能妨碍新血的生长及气血的正常运行。血证的治疗应掌握治血、治火、治气三个原则。一曰治血,包括收敛止血、凉血止血和化瘀止血;二曰治火,实火当清热泻火,虚火当滋阴降火;三曰治气,实证当清气降气,虚证当补气温气。

1. 鼻衄

(1) 热邪犯肺证

主要证候 鼻燥衄血,口干咽燥,或兼有身热、咳嗽痰少等症,舌质红,苔薄,脉数。

治 法 清泄肺热,凉血止血。

方 药 桑菊饮加减:桑叶10 g,菊花6 g,薄荷(后下)6 g,牡丹皮10 g,栀子10 g,白茅根15 g,杏仁10 g,桔梗6 g,生甘草5 g。

10 g, Baimaogen (*Rhizoma Imperatae*) 15 g, Xingren
(*Semen Armeniacae Amarum*) 10 g, Jiegeng (*Radix
Platycodi*) 6 g and Shenggancao (*Radix Glycyrrhizae*)
5 g.

Modifications: For predominant lung heat with absence of superficial syndrome, remove Bohe and Jiegeng,
add Huangqin (*Radix Scutellariae*) 10 g and Zhizi
(*Fructus Gardeniae*) 10 g; for consumption of yin and
dry mouth and nose, add Xuanshen (*Radix Scrophulariae*) 12 g, Maimendong (*Radix Ophiopogonis*) 10 g and
Shengdihuang (*Radix Rehmanniae*) 12 g.

(2) Excess of Stomach Heat

Chief Manifestations: Bleeding in the nose or gum
with bright red blood, thirst with a desire for drink, dry
nose and mouth, foul breath, restlessness, constipation,
red tongue with yellow coating, rapid pulse.

Therapeutic Methods: To purge stomach fire and
cool blood to stop bleeding.

Prescription: Modified Yunü Jian (Jade Maid Decoction), composed of Shengshigao (*Gypsum Fibrosum*, to
be decocted first) 30 g, Shengdihuang (*Radix Rehmanniae*) 12 g, Maimendong (*Radix Ophiopogonis*)
10 g, Niuxi (*Radix Achyranthis Bidentatae*) 10 g, Mudanpi (*Cortex Moutan Radicis*) 10 g, Zhizi (*Fructus
Gardeniae*) 10 g, Oujie (*Nodus Nelumbinis Rhizomatis*) 10 g and Baimaogen (*Rhizoma Imperatae*) 15 g.

Modifications: For constipation, add Shengdahuang (*Radix et Rhizoma Rhei*) 6 g; for consumption
of yin, thirst, red tongue with little coating, add Tianhuafen (*Radix Trichosanthis*) 15 g, Shihu (*Herba Dendrobii*) 10 g and Yuzhu (*Rhizoma Polygonati Odorati*)
10 g.

(3) Flaming-up of Liver Fire

Chief Manifestations: Nasal bleeding, headache,

加　减　肺热盛而无表
证者,可去薄荷、桔梗,加黄芩
10 g,栀子10 g;阴伤较甚,口
鼻干燥显著者,加玄参12 g,麦
门冬10 g,生地黄12 g。

（2）胃热炽盛证

主要证候　鼻衄,或兼齿
衄,血色鲜红,口渴欲饮,鼻
干,口干臭秽,烦躁,便秘,舌
红,苔黄,脉数。

治　法　清胃泻火,凉血
止血。

方　药　玉女煎加减:
生石膏（先煎）30 g,生地黄
12 g,麦门冬10 g,牛膝10 g,牡
丹皮10 g,栀子10 g,藕节10 g,
白茅根15 g。

加　减　大便秘结者,加
生大黄6 g;阴伤较甚,口渴明
显,舌红苔少者,加天花粉
15 g,石斛10 g,玉竹10 g。

（3）肝火上炎证

主要证候　鼻衄,头痛,

dizziness, tinnitus, restlessness, irritability, red eyes, bitter mouth, red tongue with yellow coating, wiry and rapid pulse.

Therapeutic Methods: To purge liver fire and cool blood to stop bleeding.

Prescription: Modified Longdan Xiegan Tang (Gentianae Decoction for Purging Liver Fire), composed of Longdancao (*Radix Gentianae*) 5 g, Huangqin (*Radix Scutellariae*) 10 g, Shanzhi (*Fructus Gardeniae*) 10 g, Shengdihuang (*Radix Rehmanniae*) 12 g, Mudanpi (*Cortex Moutan Radicis*) 10 g, Baimaogen (*Rhizoma Imperatae*) 15 g, Xianhecao (*Herba Agrimoniae*) 12 g, Oujie (*Nodus Nelumbinis Rhizomatis*) 10 g, Cheqianzi (*Semenn Plantaginis*, wrapped) 10 g, Mutong (*Caulis Akebiae*) 3 g and Niuxi (*Radix Achyranthis Bidentatae*) 10 g.

Modification: For consumption of yin fluid, dry mouth and nose, red tongue with reduced saliva, thready and rapid pulse, remove Cheqianzi and Mutong, add Xuanshen (*Radix Scrophulariae*) 12 g, Nüzhenzi (*Fructus Ligustri Lucidi*) 10 g and Hanliancao (*Herba Ecliptae*) 10 g.

2. Gingival Hemorrhage

(1) Hyperactivity of Stomach Fire

Chief Manifestations: Bleeding from gum with bright red blood, inflammation of gum, headache, foul breath, red tongue with yellow coating, and bounding and rapid pulse.

Therapeutic Methods: To purge stomach fire and cool blood to stop bleeding.

Prescription: Modified Jiawei Qingwei San (Powder for Clearing away Stomach Heat with Additions) and Xiexin Tang (Decoction for Purging Heart Fire), composed of Huanglian (*Rhizoma Coptidis*) 3 g, Huangqin (*Radix*

目眩,耳鸣,烦躁易怒,两目红赤,口苦,舌红,苔黄,脉弦数。

治 法 清肝泻火,凉血止血。

方 药 龙胆泻肝汤加减:龙胆草5 g,黄芩10 g,栀子10 g,生地黄12 g,牡丹皮10 g,白茅根15 g,仙鹤草12 g,藕节10 g,车前子(包煎)10 g,木通3 g,牛膝10 g。

加 减 若阴液亏耗,口鼻干燥,舌红少津,脉细数者,可去车前子、木通,加玄参12 g,女贞子10 g,旱莲草10 g。

2. 齿衄

(1) 胃火炽盛证

主要证候 齿龈血色鲜红,齿龈红肿疼痛,头痛,口臭,舌红,苔黄,脉洪数。

治 法 清胃泻火,凉血止血。

方 药 加味清胃散合泻心汤加减:黄连3 g,黄芩10 g,生大黄(后下)5 g,生地黄12 g,牡丹皮10 g,藕节10 g,

Scutellariae) 10 g, Shengdahuang (*Radix et Rhizoma Rhei*, to be decocted later) 5 g, Shengdihuang (*Radix Rehmanniae*) 12 g, Mudanpi (*Cortex Moutan Radicis*) 10 g, Oujie (*Nodus Nelumbinis Rhizomatis*) 10 g and Daji (*Herba seu Radix Cirsii Japonici*) 10 g.

Modifications: For restlessness and thirst, add Shigao (*Gypsum Fibrosum*, to be decocted first) 30 g and Zhimu (*Rhizoma Anemarrhenae*) 10 g.

(2) Hyperactivity of Fire due to Deficiency of Yin

Chief Manifestations: Bleeding from gum with pink blood, gradual onset frequently induced by the attack of heat and overstrain, loose teeth, red tongue with little coating, thready and rapid pulse.

Therapeutic Methods: To nourish yin, subdue fire and cool blood to stop bleeding.

Prescription: Modified Liuwei Dihuang Wan (Pill of Six Drugs Containing Rehmannine) and Qiangen San (Rubiae Powder), composed of Shudihuang (*Radix Rehmanniae Preparata*) 12 g, Nüzhenzi (*Fructus Ligustri Lucidi*) 10 g, Hanliancao (*Herba Ecliptae*) 10 g, Niuxi (*Radix Achyranthis Bidentatae*) 10 g, Gouqizi (*Fructus Lycii*) 10 g, Baishaoyao (*Radix Paeoniae Alba*) 10 g, Mudanpi (*Cortex Moutan Radicis*) 10 g, Shengdihuang (*Radix Rehmanniae*) 12 g, Huangbai (*Cortex Phellodendri*) 10 g, Qiancao (*Radix Rubiae*) 10 g, Chaopuhuang (*Pollen Typhae*, stir-baked) 10 g and Oujie (*Nodus Nelumbinis Rhizomatis*) 10 g.

Modification: For predominant deficient fire manifested as low fever, feverish sensation over the palms and soles, add Digupi (*Cortex Lycii*) 10 g, Baiwei (*Radix Cynanchi Atrati*) 10 g and Zhimu (*Rhizoma Anemarrhenae*) 10 g.

大蓟10 g。

加 减 烦热口渴者,加生石膏(先煎)30 g,知母10 g。

（2）阴虚火旺证

主要证候 齿衄,血色淡红,起病较缓,常因受热及烦劳而诱发,齿摇不坚,舌质红,苔少,脉细数。

治 法 滋阴降火,凉血止血。

方 药 六味地黄丸合茜根散加减:熟地黄12 g,女贞子10 g,旱莲草10 g,牛膝10 g,枸杞子10 g,白芍药10 g,牡丹皮10 g,生地黄12 g,黄柏10 g,茜草10 g,炒蒲黄10 g,藕节10 g。

加 减 虚火较甚而见低热、手足心热者,加地骨皮10 g,白薇10 g,知母10 g。

3. Hemoptysis

(1) Dryness Heat Impairing the Lung

Chief Manifestations: Itching of the throat, cough with bloody sputum, dry mouth and nose, or feverish body, red tongue with reduced saliva, yellow and thin coating, rapid pulse.

Therapeutic Methods: To clear away heat, moisten the lung and calm the vessels to stop bleeding.

Prescription: Modified Sang Xing Tang (Mori and Armeniacae Amarum Decoction), composed of Sangye (*Folium Mori*) 10 g, Xingren (*Semen Armeniacae Amarum*) 10 g, Beimu (*Bulbus Fritillariae*) 6 g, Shashen (*Radix Adenophorae*) 10 g, Shengdihuang (*Radix Rehmanniae*) 12 g, Maimendong (*Radix Ophiopogonis*) 10 g, Zhizi (*Fructus Gardeniae*) 10 g, Baimaogen (*Rhizoma Imperatae*) 15 g and Oujie (*Nodus Nelumbinis Rhizomatis*) 10 g.

Modifications: For the case accompanied by fever, headache, cough, sore throat which are due to wind heat attacking the lung, add Jinyinhua (*Flos Lonicerae*) 15 g, Lianqiao (*Fructus Forsythiae*) 15 g and Niubangzi (*Fructus Arctii*) 6 g; for consumption of body fluid manifested as non-productive cough, or difficult expectoration of viscid sputum, red tongue with little coating and reduced saliva, add Xuanshen (*Radix Scrophulariae*) 10 g, Tianmendong (*Radix Asparagi*) 10 g and Tianhuanfen (*Radix Trichosanthis*) 12 g.

(2) Liver fire Attacking the Lung

Chief Manifestations: Paroxysmal cough with blood-tinged sputum or bright red blood, distending pain over the chest and hypochondrium, restlessness, irritability, bitter mouth, red tongue with yellow and thin coating, wiry and rapid pulse.

Therapeutic Methods: To purge liver fire, disperse

3. 咳血

(1) 燥热伤肺证

主要证候 喉痒咳嗽,痰中带血,口干鼻燥,或有身热,舌质红,少津,苔薄黄,脉数。

治 法 清热润肺,宁络止血。

方 药 桑杏汤加减:桑叶10 g,杏仁10 g,贝母6 g,沙参10 g,生地黄12 g,麦门冬10 g,栀子10 g,白茅根15 g,藕节10 g。

加 减 兼见发热、头痛、咳嗽、咽痛等风热犯肺之证,加金银花15 g,连翘15 g,牛蒡子6 g;津伤较甚,而见干咳无痰,或痰黏不易咯出,苔少舌红乏津者,可加玄参10 g,天门冬10 g,天花粉12 g。

(2) 肝火犯肺证

主要证候 咳嗽阵作,痰中带血或纯血鲜红,胸胁胀痛,烦躁易怒,口苦,舌质红,苔薄黄,脉弦数。

治 法 清肝泻肺,凉血

lung heat and cool blood to stop bleeding.

Prescription: Modified Xiebai San (Powder for Clearing away Lung Heat) and Dai Ge San (Powder of Indigo Naturalis and Concha Meretricis seu Cyclinae), composed of Sangbaipi (*Cortex Mori*) 10 g, Digupi (*Cortex Lycii*) 10 g, Mudanpi (*Cortex Moutan Radicis*) 10 g, Huangqin (*Radix Scutellariae*) 10 g, Haigeke (*Concha Meretricis seu Cyclinae*) 12 g, Qingdai (*Indigo Naturalis*, to be infused separately) 6 g, Oujie (*Nodus Nelumbinis Rhizomatis*) 10 g, Qiancao (*Radix Rubiae*) 10 g and Daji (*Herba seu Radix Cirsii Japonici*) 10 g.

Modification: For predominant liver fire, manifested as dizziness, red eyes, restlessness and irritability, add Zhizi (*Fructus Gardeniae*) 10 g and Longdancao (*Radix Gentianae*) 6 g.

(3) Lung Heat due to Yin Deficiency

Chief Manifestations: Cough with scanty blood-tinged sputum, or recurrent spitting of bright red blood, dry mouth and throat, flushed cheeks, hectic fever, night sweating, red tongue, thready and rapid pulse.

Therapeutic Methods: To nourish yin, moisten the lung, calm the vessels to stop bleeding.

Prescription: Modified Baihe Gujin Tang (Lilii Decoction for Strengthening Lung), composed of Baihe (*Buibus Lilii*) 10 g, Maimendong (*Radix Ophiopogonis*) 10 g, Xuanshen (*Radix Scrophulariae*) 10 g, Chuanbeimu (*Bulbus Fritillariae Cirrhosae*) 6 g, Shengdihuang (*Radix Rehmanniae*) 12 g, Baishaoyao (*Radix Paeoniae Alba*) 10 g and Oujie (*Nodus Nelumbinis Rhizomatis*) 10 g.

Modifications: For recurrent spitting of blood or spitting of profuse blood, add Ejiao (*Colla Corii Asini*, to be melted in the finished decoction) 10 g and Sanqifen (*Radix Noto ginseng*, powdered and to be taken sepa-

止血。

方　药　泻白散合黛蛤散加减：桑白皮10 g,地骨皮10 g,牡丹皮10 g,黄芩10 g,海蛤壳12 g,青黛（另冲）6 g,藕节10 g,茜草10 g,大蓟10 g。

加　减　肝火较甚,头晕目赤,心烦易怒者,加栀子10 g,龙胆草6 g。

（3）阴虚肺热证

主要证候　咳嗽痰少,痰中带血或反复咳血,血色鲜红,口干咽燥,颧红,潮热盗汗,舌质红,脉细数。

治　法　滋阴润肺,宁络止血。

方　药　百合固金汤加减：百合10 g,麦门冬10 g,玄参10 g,川贝母6 g,生地黄12 g,白芍药10 g,藕节10 g。

加　减　反复咳血及咳血量多者,加阿胶（烊化冲服）10 g,三七粉（另吞）3 g;潮热、颧红者,加青蒿10 g,鳖甲（先

rately) 3 g; for hectic fever and flushed cheeks, add Qinghao (*Herba Artemisiae Annuae*) 10 g, Biejia (*Carapax Trionycis*, to be decocted first) 15 g, Digupi (*Cortex Lycii*) 10 g and Baiwei (*Radix Cynanchi Atrati*) 6 g; for profuse night sweating, add Nuodaogen (*Rhizoma et Radix Oryzae Glutinosae*) 30 g and Muli (*Concha Ostreae*, to be decocted first) 25 g.

4. Hematemesis

(1) Excess of Stomach Heat

Chief Manifestations: Distention and fullness in the epigastrium and abdomen, even with pain in severe cases, spitting of bright red or dark purple blood often with food residue, foul breath, constipation, black stools, red tongue with yellow and greasy coating, smooth and rapid pulse.

Therapeutic Methods: To clear away stomach heat, purge fire and resolve blood stasis to stop bleeding.

Prescription: Modified Xiexin Tang (Decoction for Purging Heart Fire) and Shihui San (Powder of Ten Drugs Ashes), composed of Shengdahuang (*Radix et Rhizoma Rhei*, to be decocted later) 6 g, Huanglian (*Rhizoma Coptidis*) 3 g, Huangqin (*Radix Scutellariae*) 10 g, Zhizi (*Fructus Gardeniae*) 10 g, Qiancao (*Radix Rubiae*) 10 g, Cebaiye (*Cacumen Biotae*) 10 g, Mudanpi (*Cortex Moutan Radicis*) 10 g, Daji (*Herba seu Radix Cirsii Japonici*) 10 g and Xiaoji (*Herba Cirsii*) 10 g.

Modifications: For the adverse rising of stomach qi causing nausea and vomiting, add Daizheshi (*Haematitum*, to be decocted first) 15 g, Zhuru (*Caulis Bambusae in Taeniam*) 6 g and Xuanfuhua (*Flos Inulae*, wrapped) 6 g; for stomach yin damaged by heat, manifested as thirst, red and dry tongue, thready and rapid pulse, add Maimendong (*Radix Ophiopogonis*) 10 g,

煎)15 g,地骨皮10 g,白薇6 g;盗汗量多者,加糯稻根30 g,牡蛎(先煎)25 g。

4. 吐血

(1) 胃热壅盛证

主要证候 脘腹胀闷,甚则作痛,吐血色红或紫黯,常夹有食物残渣,口臭,便秘,大便色黑,舌质红,苔黄腻,脉滑数。

治 法 清胃泻火,化瘀止血。

方 药 泻心汤合十灰散加减:生大黄(后下)6 g,黄连3 g,黄芩10 g,栀子10 g,茜草10 g,侧柏叶10 g,牡丹皮10 g,大蓟10 g,小蓟10 g。

加 减 胃气上逆而见恶心呕吐者,可加代赭石(先煎)15 g,竹茹6 g,旋覆花(包煎)6 g;热伤胃阴而表现口渴、舌红而干、脉象细数者,加麦门冬10 g,石斛10 g,天花粉12 g。

Shihu (*Herba Dendrobii*) 10 g and Tianhuafen (*Radix Trichosanthis*) 12 g.

(2) Liver Fire Attacking the Stomach

Chief Manifestations: Spitting of bright red or dark purple blood, bitter mouth, pain over the hypochondria, restlessness, irritability, insomnia, dreamfulness, crimson tongue, wiry and rapid pulse.

Therapeutic Methods: To disperse liver fire, clear away stomach heat and cool blood to stop bleeding.

Prescription: Modified Longdan Xiegan Tang (Gentianae Decoction for Purging Liver Fire), composed of Longdancao (*Radix Gentianae*) 6 g, Huangqin (*Radix Scutellariae*) 10 g, Zhizi (*Fructus Gardeniae*) 10 g, Mudanpi (*Cortex Gardeniae*) 10 g, Shengdihuang (*Radix Rehmanniae*) 12 g, Oujie (*Nodus Nelumbinis Rhizomatis*) 10 g and Hanliancao (*Herba Ecliptae*) 10 g.

Modification: For severe pain over the hypochondria, add Yujin (*Radix Curcumae*) 10 g and Zhixiangfu (*Rhizoma Cyperi Preparata*) 10 g.

(3) Extravasation Caused by Deficiency of Qi

Chief Manifestations: Constant, intermittent spitting of dull pink blood, lassitude, palpitation, shortness of breath, pale complexion, pale tongue, thready and weak pulse.

Therapeutic Methods: To invigorate the spleen, nourish the heart, benefit qi and keep the blood flowing within the vessels.

Prescription: Modified Guipi Tang (Decoction for Invigorating Spleen and Nourishing Heart), composed of Huangqi (*Radix Astragali*) 12 g, Dangshen (*Radix Codonopsis*) 10 g, Baizhu (*Rhizoma Atractylodis Macrocephalae*) 10 g, Zhigancao (*Radix Glycyrrhizae*, roasted) 3 g, Danggui (*Radix Angelicae Sinensis*) 10 g,

（2）肝火犯胃证

主要证候　吐血色红或紫黯,口苦胁痛,心烦易怒,寐少梦多,舌质红绛,脉弦数。

治　法　泻肝清胃,凉血止血。

方　药　龙胆泻肝汤加减:龙胆草6 g,黄芩10 g,栀子10 g,牡丹皮10 g,生地黄12 g,藕节10 g,旱莲草10 g。

加　减　胁痛甚者,加郁金10 g,制香附10 g。

（3）气虚血溢证

主要证候　吐血缠绵不止,时轻时重,血色暗淡,神疲乏力,心悸气短,面色苍白,舌质淡,脉细弱。

治　法　健脾养心,益气摄血。

方　药　归脾汤加减:黄芪12 g,党参10 g,白术10 g,炙甘草3 g,当归10 g,白及6 g,乌贼骨15 g。

Baiji (*Rhizoma Bletillae*) 6 g and Wuzeigu (*Os Sepiellae seu Sepiae*) 15 g.

Modification: For deficiency of qi damaging yang and deficient cold in both the spleen and stomach, manifested as cold limbs, aversion to cold, loose stools, the treatment of warming the meridians should be adopted and Aiye (*Folium Artemisiae Argyi*) 10 g and Paojiang (*Rhizoma Zingiberis*, roasted in hot cinders) 3 g should be added.

5. Hemafecia

(1) Damp Heat in the Intestine

Chief Manifestations: Red blood in the stools, constipation or loose stools, or abdominal pain, bitter mouth, red tongue with yellow and greasy coating, soft-superficial and rapid pulse.

Therapeutic Methods: To clear away damp heat and cool blood to stop bleeding.

Prescription: Modified Diyu San (Sanguisorbae Powder) and Huaijiao Wan (Sophorae Pill), composed of Huanglian (*Rhizoma Coptidis*) 3 g, Huangqin (*Radix Scutellariae*) 10 g, Zhizi (*Fructus Gardeniae*) 10 g, Diyu (*Radix Sanguisorbae*) 10 g, Huaijiao (*Fructus Sophorae*) 10 g, Qiancao (*Radix Rubiae*) 10 g, Danggui (*Radix Angelicae Sinensis*) 10 g and Zhike (*Fructus Aurantii*) 6 g.

Modifications: For wind heat attacking the collaterals, manifested as profuse bleeding, add Jingjietan (*Herba Schizonepetae*, charred) 6 g; for accumulated damp heat and foul blood, add Cangzhu (*Rhizoma Atractylodis*) 10 g and Huangbai (*Cortex Phellodendri*) 10 g.

(2) Failure of Deficient Qi to Control Blood

Chief Manifestations: Red or dark purplish blood in the stools, poor appetite, lassitude, sallow complexion, palpitation, sleeplessness, pale tongue and thready pulse.

加　减　若气损及阳,脾胃虚寒,症见肢冷、畏寒、便溏者,治宜温经摄血,可加艾叶10 g,炮姜3 g。

5. 便血

(1) 肠道湿热证

主要证候　便血色红,大便不畅或稀溏,或有腹痛,口苦,舌质红,苔黄腻,脉濡数。

治　法　清化湿热,凉血止血。

方　药　地榆散合槐角丸加减:黄连3 g,黄芩10 g,栀子10 g,地榆10 g,槐角10 g,茜草10 g,当归10 g,枳壳6 g。

加　减　若风热灼络,血下如溅,加荆芥炭6 g;若湿热不清,血下污浊,加苍术10 g,黄柏10 g。

(2) 气虚不摄证

主要证候　便血色红或紫黯,食少,体倦,面色萎黄,心悸,少寐,舌质淡,脉细。

Therapeutic Methods: To benefit qi and keep the blood flowing within the vessels.

Prescription: Modified Guipi Tang (Decoction of Invigorating Spleen and Nourishing Heart), composed of Huangqi (*Radix Astragali*) 12 g, Dangshen (*Radix Codonopsis*) 10 g, Baizhu (*Rhizoma Atractylodis Macrocephalae*) 10 g, Zhigancao (*Radix Glycyrrhizae*, roasted) 3 g, Danggui (*Radix Angelicae Sinensis*) 10 g, Baiji (*Rhizoma Bletillae*) 6 g and Haipiaoxiao (*Os Sepiellae seu Sepiae*) 15 g.

Modification: For profuse bleeding, add Huaihua (*Flos Sophorae*) 10 g, Diyu (*Radix Sanguisorbae*) 10 g and Xianhecao (*Herba Agrimoniae*) 12 g.

(3) Deficient Cold in the Spleen and Stomach

Chief Manifestations: Dull purplish blood in the stools, or even dark blood in severe cases, dull abdominal pain, desire for hot drinks, lusterless complexion, lassitude, dislike of speaking, loose stools, pale tongue and thready pulse.

Therapeutic Methods: To invigorate the spleen, warm the middle energizer and nourish blood to stop bleeding.

Prescription: Modified Huangtu Tang (Terra Flava Usta Decoction), composed of Dangshen (*Radix Codonopsis*) 10 g, Baizhu (*Rhizoma Atractylodis Macrocephalae*) 10 g, Shufuzi (*Radix Aconiti Preparata*) 6 g, Zaoxintu (*Terra Flava Usta*) 10 g, Paojiang (*Rhizoma Zingiberis*, roasted in hot cinders) 3 g, Ejiao (*Colla Corii Asini*, to be melted in the finished decoction) 10 g, Shengdihuang (*Radix Rehmanniae*) 12 g, Baiji (*Rhizoma Bletillae*) 6 g and Haipiaoxiao (*Os Sepiellae seu Sepiae*) 15 g.

Modification: For predominant yang deficiency,

治　法　益气摄血。

方　药　归脾汤加减：黄芪12 g，党参10 g，白术10 g，炙甘草3 g，当归10 g，白及6 g，海螵蛸15 g。

加　减　便血量多者，加槐花10 g，地榆10 g，仙鹤草12 g。

（3）脾胃虚寒证

主要证候　便血紫黯，甚则黑色，腹部隐痛，喜热饮，面色不华，神倦懒言，便溏，舌质淡，脉细。

治　法　健脾温中，养血止血。

方　药　黄土汤加减：党参10 g，白术10 g，熟附子6 g，灶心土10 g，炮姜3 g，阿胶（烊化冲服）10 g，生地黄12 g，白及6 g，海螵蛸15 g。

加　减　阳虚较甚，畏寒

manifested as aversion to cold and cold limbs, add Lu-jiaoshuang (*Cornu Cervi Degelatinatum*) 10 g and Aiye (*Folium Artemisiae Argyi*) 6 g.

6. Hematuria

(1) Excessive Heat in the Lower Energizer

Chief Manifestations: A burning sensation in the urethra during urination, deep-colored urine, or bright red urine, restlessness, thirst, flushed face, aphtha, insomnia, red tongue, and rapid pulse.

Therapeutic Methods: To clear away heat, purge fire and cool blood to stop bleeding.

Prescription: Modified Xiaoji Yinzi (*Cirsii Decoction*), composed of Zhizi (*Fructus Gardeniae*) 10 g, Zhuye (*Herba Lophatheri*) 10 g, Mutong (*Caulis Akebiae*) 3 g, Huashi (*Talcum*, wrapped) 10 g, Shenggancao (*Radix Glycyrrhizae*) 3 g, Xiaoji (*Herba Cirsii*) 10 g, Shengdihuang (*Radix Rehmanniae*) 12 g, Puhuang (*Pollen Typhae*, wrapped) 10 g, Oujie (*Nodus Nelumbinis Rhizomatis*) 10 g, Danggui (*Radix Angelicae Sinensis*) 10 g and Hupofen (*Succinum*, powdered and to be infused separately) 0.5 g.

Modifications: For excessive heat, manifested as restlessness and thirst, add Huangqin (*Radix Scutellariae*) 10 g and Tianhuafen (*Radix Trichosanthis*) 12 g; for severe hematuria, add Huaihua (*Flos Sophorae*) 10 g and Baimaogen (*Rhizoma Imperatae*) 20 g; for urine with blood clots, add Taoren (*Semen Persicae*) 10 g, Honghua (*Flos Carthami*) 10 g and Niuxi (*Radix Achyranthis Bidentatae*) 10 g.

(2) Kidney Deficiency with Hyperactivity of Fire

Chief Manifestations: Scanty deep-colored urine with blood, dizziness, tinnitus, lassitude, flushed cheeks, hectic fever, soreness and weakness of the loins and

肢冷者,可加鹿角霜10 g,艾叶6 g。

6. 尿血

(1) 下焦热盛证

主要证候 小便黄赤灼热,尿血鲜红,心烦口渴,面赤口疮,夜寐不安,舌质红,脉数。

治 法 清热泻火,凉血止血。

方 药 小蓟饮子加减:栀子10 g,竹叶10 g,木通3 g,滑石(包煎)10 g,生甘草3 g,小蓟10 g,生地黄12 g,蒲黄(包煎)10 g,藕节10 g,当归10 g,琥珀粉(另冲)0.5 g。

加 减 热盛而心烦口渴者,加黄芩10 g,天花粉12 g;尿血较甚者,加槐花10 g,白茅根20 g;尿中夹有血块者,加桃仁10 g,红花10 g,牛膝10 g。

(2) 肾虚火旺证

主要证候 小便短赤带血,头晕耳鸣,神疲,颧红潮热,腰膝酸软,舌质红,脉

knees, red tongue, thready and rapid pulse.

Therapeutic Methods: To nourish yin, subdue fire and cool blood to stop bleeding.

Prescription: Modified Zhi Bai Dihuang Wan (Bolus of Anemarrhenae, Phellodendri and Rehmanniae), composed of Shengdihuang (*Radix Rehmanniae*) 12 g, Ejiao (*Colla Corii Asini*, to be melted in the finished decoction) 10 g, Hanliancao (*Herba Ecliptae*) 12 g, Shanyao (*Rhizoma Dioscoreae*) 12 g, Guiban (*Plastrum Testudinis*, to be decocted first) 15 g, Zhimu (*Rhizoma Anemarrhenae*) 10 g, Huangbai (*Cortex Phellodendri*) 10 g, Mudanpi (*Cortex Moutan Radicis*) 10 g, Xiaoji (*Herba Cirsii*) 12 g and Oujie (*Nodus Nelumbinis Rhizomatis*) 10 g.

Modification: For flushed cheeks and hectic fever, add Digupi (*Cortex Lycii*) 10 g and Baiwei (*Radix Cynanchi Atrati*) 12 g.

(3) Spleen Failing to Control Blood

Chief Manifestations: Prolonged hematuria, or even accompanied by bleeding from gum, hemokelidosis, poor appetite, fatigue, shortness of breath, weak voice, lusterless complexion, pale tongue, thready and weak pulse.

Therapeutic Methods: To invigorate the spleen and keep the blood flowing within the vessels.

Prescription: Modified Guipi Tang (Decoction for Invigorating Spleen and Nourishing Heart), composed of Huangqi (*Radix Astragali*) 12 g, Dangshen (*Radix Codonopsis*) 10 g, Baizhu (*Rhizoma Atratylodis Macrocephalae*) 10 g, Zhigancao (*Radix Glycyrrhizae*, roasted) 3 g, Danggui (*Radix Angelicae Sinensis*) 10 g, Fuling (*Poria*) 12 g, Yuanzhi (*Radix Polygalae*) 6 g, Guiyuanrou (*Arillus Longan*) 10 g and Suanzaoren (*Semen Ziziphi Spinosae*) 10 g.

细数。

治　法　滋阴降火,凉血止血。

方　药　知柏地黄丸加减:生地黄12 g,阿胶(烊化冲服)10 g,旱莲草12 g,山药12 g,龟版(先煎)15 g,知母10 g,黄柏10 g,牡丹皮10 g,小蓟12 g,藕节10 g。

加　减　颧红潮热者,加地骨皮10 g,白薇12 g。

(3) 脾不统血证

主要证候　久病尿血,甚或兼见齿衄、肌衄,食少,体倦乏力,气短声低,面色不华,舌质淡,脉细弱。

治　法　补脾摄血。

方　药　归脾汤加减:黄芪12 g,党参10 g,白术10 g,炙甘草3 g,当归10 g,茯苓12 g,远志6 g,桂圆肉10 g,酸枣仁10 g。

Modification: For collapse of middle energizer qi, manifested as bearing-down fullness of lower abdomen, add Shengma (*Rhizoma Cimicifugae*) 6 g and Chaihu (*Radix Bupleuri*) 6 g.

(4) Unconsolidation of Kidney Qi

Chief Manifestations: Prolonged hematuria with pale red blood in the urine, dizziness, tinnitus, lassitude, soreness of the lumbar spine, pale tongue, deep and weak pulse.

Therapeutic Methods: To replenish and restore kidney qi to stop bleeding.

Prescription: Modified Wubi Shanyao Wan (Powerful Dioscoreae Pill), composed of Dangshen (*Radix Codonopsis*) 10 g, Huangqi (*Radix Astragali*) 12 g, Baizhu (*Rhizoma Atractylodis Macrocephalae*) 10 g, Danggui (*Radix Angelicae Sinensis*) 10 g, Shudihuang (*Radix Rehmanniae Preparata*) 12 g, Shanyao (*Rhizoma Dioscoreae*) 12 g, Shanzhuyu (*Fructus Corni*) 10 g, Tusizi (*Semen Cuscutae*) 10 g, Duzhong (*Cortex Eucommiae*) 10 g, Bajitian (*Radix Morindae Officinalis*) 10 g, Lujiaoshuang (*Cornu Cervi Degelatinatum*) 10 g, Xianhecao (*Herba Agrimoniae*) 10 g, Puhuang (*Pollen Typhae* , wrapped) 10 g and Zizhucao (*Folium Callicarpae Formosanae*) 12 g.

Modification: For soreness of the lumbar spine with aversion to cold and timidness, add Lujiaopian (*Cornu Cervi* , sliced) 10 g and Gouji (*Rhizoma Cibotii*) 12 g.

7. Hemokelidosis

(1) Extravasation of Blood due to Blood Heat

Chief Manifestations: Bluish purple spots or patches of the skin, or accompanied by nose bleeding, bleeding from gum, hemafecia, hematuria, or fever, thirst, constipation, red tongue with yellow coating, wiry and

加　减　气虚下陷而见少腹坠胀者,可加升麻6 g,柴胡6 g。

(4) 肾气不固证

主要证候　久病尿血,血色淡红,头晕耳鸣,精神困惫,腰脊酸痛,舌质淡,脉沉弱。

治　法　补益肾气,固摄止血。

方　药　无比山药丸加减:党参10 g,黄芪12 g,白术10 g,当归10 g,熟地黄12 g,山药12 g,山茱萸10 g,菟丝子10 g,杜仲10 g,巴戟天10 g,鹿角霜10 g,仙鹤草10 g,蒲黄(包煎)10 g,紫珠草12 g。

加　减　腰脊酸痛,畏寒神怯者,加鹿角片10 g,狗脊12 g。

7. 紫斑

(1) 血热妄行证

主要证候　皮肤出现青紫斑点或斑块,或伴有鼻衄、齿衄、便血、尿血,或有发热,口渴,便秘,舌红,苔黄,脉

rapid pulse.

Therapeutic Methods: To clear away heat, remove toxic substance and cool blood to stop bleeding.

Prescription: Modified Shihui San (Powder of Ten Drugs Ashes), composed of Daji (*Herba seu Radix Cirsii Japonici*) 12 g, Xiaoji (*Herba Cirsii*) 12 g, Qiancaogen (*Radix Rubiae*) 10 g, Baimaogen (*Rhizoma Imperatae*) 20 g, Zonglütan (*Fibra Trachycarpi Vaginata*, charred) 10 g, Mudanpi (*Cortex Moutan Radicis*) 10 g, Zhizi (*Fructus Gardeniae*) 10 g and Shengdahuang (*Radix et Rhizoma Rhei*, to be decocted later) 6 g.

Modifications: For excessive heat, manifested as fever, extensive bleeding, add Shengshigao (*Gypsum Fibrosum*, to be decocted first) 30 g, Longdancao (*Radix Gentianae*) 3 g and Zicao (*Radix Arnebiae seu Lithospermi*) 12 g; for retention of heat in the stomach and intestines and stagnation of qi and blood, manifested as abdominal pain and hemafecia, add Baishaoyao (*Radix Paeoniae Alba*) 12 g, Shenggancao (*Radix Glycyrrhizae*) 3 g, Diyu (*Radix Sanguisorbae*) 10 g and Huaihua (*Flos Sophorae*) 10 g; for retention of heat in the meridians, accompanied by swollen and painful joint, add Qinjiao (*Radix Gentianae Macrophyllae*) 10 g, Mugua (*Fructus Chaenomelis*) 10 g and Sangzhi (*Ramulus Mori*) 15 g.

(2) Hyperactivity of Fire due to Deficiency of Yin

Chief Manifestations: Intermittent occurrence of bluish purple spots or patches of the skin, often accompanied by nose bleeding, bleeding from gum, or profuse menstruation, flushed cheeks, restlessness, thirst, feverish sensation of the palms and soles, or hectic fever, night sweating, red tongue with little coating, thready and rapid pulse.

弦数。

治　法　清热解毒,凉血止血。

方　药　十灰散加减:大蓟12 g,小蓟12 g,茜草根10 g,白茅根20 g,棕榈炭10 g,牡丹皮10 g,栀子10 g,生大黄(后下)6 g。

加　减　热毒炽盛,发热,出血广泛者,加生石膏(先煎)30 g,龙胆草3 g,紫草12 g;热壅胃肠,气血郁滞,症见腹痛、便血者,加白芍药12 g,生甘草3 g,地榆10 g,槐花10 g;邪热阻滞经络,兼见关节肿痛者,酌加秦艽10 g,木瓜10 g,桑枝15 g。

(2) 阴虚火旺证

主要证候　皮肤出现青紫斑点或斑块,时发时止,常伴鼻衄、齿衄,或月经过多,颧红,心烦,口渴,手足心热,或有潮热,盗汗,舌质红,苔少,脉细数。

Therapeutic Methods: To nourish yin, subdue fire and calm the vessels to stop bleeding.

Prescription: Modified Qiangen San (Rubiae Powder), composed of Qiancaogen (*Radix Rubiae*) 12 g, Huangqin (*Radix Scutellariae*) 10 g, Cebaiye (*Cacumen Biotae*) 10 g, Shengdihuang (*Radix Rehmanniae*) 12 g, Ejiao (*Colla Corii Asini*, to be melted in the finished decoction) 10 g, Shanzhuyu (*Fructus Corni*) 10 g and Guiban (*Plastrum Testudinis*, to be decocted first) 15 g.

Modifications: For predominant yin deficiency, add Xuanshen (*Radix Scrophulariae*) 10 g, Nüzhenzi (*Fructus Ligustri Lucidi*) 10 g and Hanliancao (*Herba Ecliptae*) 10 g; for hectic fever, add Digupi (*Cortex Lycii*) 10 g, Baiwei (*Radix Cynanchi Atrati*) 10 g and Qinjiao (*Radix Gentianae Macrophyliae*) 10 g.

(3) Failure of Deficient Qi to Control Blood

Chief Manifestations: Recurrent and persistent hemokelodosis, lassitude, dizziness, pale or sallow complexion, poor appetite, pale tongue, thready and weak pulse.

Therapeutic Methods: To replenish qi to stop bleeding.

Prescription: Modified Guipi Tang (Decoction for Invigorating Spleen and Nourishing Heart), composed of Huangqi (*Radix Astragali*) 12 g, Dangshen (*Radix Codonopsis*) 10 g, Baizhu (*Rhizoma Atractylodis Macrocephalae*) 10 g, Zhigancao (*Radix Glycyrrhizae*, roasted) 3 g, Danggui (*Radix Angelicae Sinensis*) 10 g, Shudihuang (*Radix Rehmanniae Preparata*) 12 g, Dazao (*Fructus Jujubae*) 5 pcs, Guiyuanrou (*Arillus Longan*) 10 g and Xianhecao (*Herba Agrimoniae*) 12 g.

Modifications: For soreness and weakness of the loins and knees due to insufficiency of kidney qi, add

治 法 滋阴降火,宁络止血。

方 药 茜根散加减:茜草根12 g,黄芩10 g,侧柏叶10 g,生地黄12 g,阿胶(烊化冲服)10 g,山茱萸10 g,龟版(先煎)15 g。

加 减 阴虚较甚者,可加玄参10 g,女贞子10 g,旱莲草10 g;潮热可加地骨皮10 g,白薇10 g,秦艽10 g。

(3) 气不摄血证

主要证候 反复发生肌衄,久病不愈,神疲乏力,头晕目眩,面色苍白或萎黄,食欲不振,舌质淡,脉细弱。

治 法 补气摄血。

方 药 归脾汤加减:黄芪12 g,党参10 g,白术10 g,炙甘草3 g,当归10 g,熟地黄12 g,大枣5 枚,桂圆肉10 g,仙鹤草12 g。

加 减 若兼肾气不足而见腰膝酸软者,可加山茱萸

Shanzhuyu (*Fructus Corni*) 10 g, Tusizi (*Herba Cuscutae*) 10 g and Xuduan (*Radix Dipsaci*) 10 g.

Other Treatments

1. Chinese Patent Drugs

(1) Longdan Xiegan Wan (Gentianae Pill for Purging Liver Fire): 6 g each time, twice daily; indicated for hematemesis and epistaxis due to hyperactivity of liver fire.

(2) Zhi Bai Dihuang Wan (Pill of Anemarrhenae, Phellodendri and Rehmanniae): 6 g each time, twice daily; indicated for bleeding resulting from yin deficiency and hyperactivity of fire.

(3) Renshen Guipi Wan (Ginseng Pill for Invigorating Spleen and Nourishing Heart): 6 g each time, twice daily; indicated for bleeding due to deficiency of the spleen.

(4) Yangyin Qingfei Wan (Bolus for Nourishing Yin and Clearing away Lung Heat): 1 - 2 boluses each time, twice daily; indicated for hemoptysis due to deficiency of lung yin and kidney yin, and hyperactivity of deficient fire leading to damage of lung collaterals.

(5) Weixuening Koufuye (Oral Liquids for Hemorrhage of Digestive Tract): 20 ml each time, twice daily; indicated for hemotemesis and hemafecia due to peptic ulcer.

(6) Reduqing (Tablet for Clearing away Toxic Heat): 4 - 6 tablets each time, twice or thrice daily; indicated for bleeding due to retention of heat and hyperactivity of fire in the triple energizer.

(7) Yunnan Baiyao (Yunnan White Medicinal Powder): 1 g each time, 3 times daily for oral use; indicated for various types of hemorrhagic syndrome.

2. Single-drug or Experiential Prescriptions

(1) Xianhecao (*Herba Agrimoniae*, fresh) 15 g,

10 g,菟丝子10 g,续断10 g。

【其他疗法】

1. 中成药

(1) 龙胆泻肝丸　每服6 g,每日 2 次。适用于肝火旺盛之吐血、衄血。

(2) 知柏地黄丸　每服6 g,每日 2 次。适用于阴虚火旺之出血。

(3) 人参归脾丸　每服6 g,每日 2 次。适用于脾虚不摄之出血。

(4) 养阴清肺丸　每服1~2 丸,每日 2 次。适用于肺肾阴虚,虚火内生,灼伤肺络之咯血。

(5) 胃血宁口服液　每次20 ml,每日 2 次。适用于消化性溃疡所致之吐血、便血。

(6) 热毒清　每服 4~6片,每日 2~3 次。适用于热毒内结、三焦火盛之出血。

(7) 云南白药　每服1 g,每日 3 次,口服。适用于各种出血。

2. 单验方

(1) 鲜仙鹤草15 g,小蓟

Xiaoji (*Herba Cirsii*) 15 g and Hanliancao (*Herba Eclip-tae*) 15 g. Mix and crush the herbs to get juice and take the juice once daily. It is indicated for epistaxis and gingi-val hemorrhage.

(2) Shengdihuang (*Radix Rehmanniae*) and Daji (*Herba seu Radix Cirsii Japonici*). Mix and crush the herbs to get juice, and take proper amount for individual cases. It is indicated for hemoptysis due to impairment of collaterals by lung heat.

(3) Shensanqi (*Radix Notoginseng*), Baiji (*Rhizo-ma Bletillae*) and Shengdahuang (*Radix et Rhizoma Rhei*). Mix and grind the herbs into fine powder in the proportion of 2∶2∶1, infuse the powder in warm boiled water for oral taking, 3 - 4.5 g each time, 3 - 4 times daily. It is indicated for hematemesis and hemafecia.

(4) Haipiaoxiao (*Os Sepiellae seu Sepiae*), Baiji (*Rhizoma Bletillae*) and Gancao (*Radix Glycyrrhizae*) in equal proportion. Mix and grind them into fine powder, and infuse the powder in warm boiled water for oral tak-ing, 3 g each time, 3 times daily. It is indicated for he-mafecia.

(5) Huaihua (*Flos Sophorae*) 50 g, Cebaiye (*Cacu-men Biotae*) 50 g, Jingjie (*Herba Schizonepetae*) 50 g and Chaozhike (*Fructus Aurantii*, stir-baked) 50 g. Mix and grind the herbs into powder for oral taking, 6 g each time, twice daily. It is indicated for bloody defeca-tion and discharge of bright red blood before defecation.

(6) Zhumagen (*Radix Boehmeriae*) 15 g, Shengdi-huang (*Radix Rehmanniae*) 10 g, Fuling (*Poria*) 10 g and Haipiaoxiao (*Os Sepiellae seu Sepiae*) 9 g. Decoct the herbs in water for oral use. It is indicated for protrac-ted hematuria.

(7) Baimaogen (*Rhizoma Imperatae*) 30 g. Decoct the herb in water for oral use, 1 dose daily. It is indicated

15 g,旱莲草15 g,三者共捣汁内服,每日 1 次。适用于血热妄行之口鼻衄血。

(2)生地黄汁、大蓟汁,混匀,适量内服。适用于肺热伤络之咳血。

(3)参三七、白及及生大黄,按 2∶2∶1 比例配成药末,每服 3～4.5 g,每日 3～4次,温开水调服。适用于吐血、便血。

(4)海螵蛸、白及、甘草各等量,研极细末,每次3 g,每日3 次,冲服。适用于便血。

(5)槐 花 50 g,侧 柏 叶50 g,荆芥50 g,炒枳壳50 g,做成内服散剂。每服6 g,每日 2次,温水送服。适用于肠风下血、便前出血。

(6)苎麻根15 g,生地黄10 g,茯苓10 g,海螵蛸9 g,煎汤服。适用于尿血不止。

(7)白茅根30 g,水煎服,每日 1 剂。适用于热证尿血。

for hematuria of the heat type.

(8) Qiancao (*Radix Rubiae*) 10 g, Baimaogen (*Rhizoma Imperatae*) 15 g and Huaihua (*Flos Sophorae*) 10 g. Decoct the herbs in water and take the decoction in two divided doses. It is indicated for hemokelidosis.

3. External Therapy

(1) Pound Dasuan (*Bulbus Allii*) into a paste and apply it to Yongquan point (KI 1). It is indicated for protracted epistaxis.

(2) Baicaoshuang (*Pulvis Fumi Cabonisatus*) and Xueyutan (*Crinis Carbonisatus*) of proper amount. Dip the cotton ball in the medicinal powder and tuck it into nostrils. It is indicated for epistaxis.

(3) Shengshigao (*Gypsum Fibrosum*) 30 g, Pengsha (*Borax*) 21 g, Bingpian (*Borneolum Syntheticum*) 1 g and Baijiangcan (*Bombyx Batryticatus*) 3 g. Mix and grind the drugs to fine powder and apply a bit of it to gum. It is indicated for bleeding from gum.

2.7.3 Anemia

General Description

Anemia is a kind of disease with the amount of hemoglobin in the peripheral circulation lower than the normal value. According to its pathogenesis, the disease can be divided into three types: defective blood formation, excessive destruction of red blood cell, and acute or chronic blood loss. Clinically, both acute and chronic blood loss are the common causes of anemia. Chronic hemorrhagic anemia is virtually iron-deficiency anemia. The major symptoms of anemia are sallow or pale complexion, pale finger nails, lips and palpebral conjunctiva, dizziness, tinnitus, palpitation and shortness of breath after exercises,

（8）茜草10 g,白茅根15 g,槐花10 g,水煎分2次服。适用于紫斑。

3. 外治法

（1）大蒜捣如泥,作饼,贴敷涌泉穴。适用于鼻衄不止。

（2）百草霜、血余炭适量,用棉花球蘸上药末塞入鼻内。适用于鼻衄。

（3）生石膏30 g,硼砂21 g,冰片1 g,白僵蚕3 g,共研极细末,取少许擦于齿龈。适用于齿衄。

第三节 贫血

【概述】

贫血中指外周血液中血红蛋白量低于正常值。按发病机理可分为造血不良、红细胞过度破坏及急慢性失血三类。不论急性或慢性出血都是临床上引起贫血的最常见原因。慢性失血性贫血实质上就是缺铁性贫血。贫血的主要症状为面色萎黄或苍白,指甲、口唇和睑结膜颜色苍白,头晕目花,耳鸣,活动后心

somnolence, lassitude, dry hair, hair loss, dry skin, or puffiness of the face, edema of the lower limbs, flat or fragile finger nails. In the serious case, hemorrhage and fever can be seen.

Anemia is referred to as "xue xu" (blood deficiency) in traditional Chinese medicine, and iron-deficiency anemia is similar to "wei huang" (sallow complexion) or "huang pang bing" (general edema with sallow skin). Aplastic anemia is characterized by general deficiency, so it is grouped into the category of "xu lao" (consumptive disease); and since it is often accompanied by hemorrhage, it is associated with "xue zheng" (hemorrhagic syndrome) to some extent.

There are a variety of causes of anemia, such as acute or chronic hemorrhage, intestinal parasitosis, disorders of the spleen and stomach, debility after illness or deficient constitution as well as the effect of some medicines or poisonous substances, which result in consumption of blood, or disorder of the spleen and kidneys leading to insufficient qi and blood, thus blood deficiency ensues.

Essentials for Diagnosis

(1) The patient has a history of suffering from hemorrhage, dysfunction of the gastrointestinal tract, denutrition, contact with or administration of the substances or medicines which are harmful to hematopoietic system, chronic infection, serious diseases of the heart, liver or kidneys, or malignant tumor.

(2) Physical examination: sallow complexion, pale lips and eyelids, pale flat or fragile finger nails, or mucocutaneous blood spots, jaundice, enlarged liver, spleen and lymph nodes can be seen.

(3) Laboratory examination may show decreased red blood cells and hemoglobin. If distinct decrease of leuko-

慌气短,困倦乏力,毛发干脱,皮肤干燥,或见面足浮肿,爪甲扁平或易脆裂。甚则可见出血、发热等症。

贫血,中医学统称"血虚",其中缺铁性贫血与"萎黄"、"黄胖病"相类似;再生障碍性贫血的全身虚弱情况较重,故多属于"虚劳"范围;同时因其常有出血的症状,故与"血证"也有一定的联系。

贫血的原因很多,如急、慢性出血,肠寄生虫病,脾胃不健,病后或素体虚弱,以及某些药物和毒物的影响等。由于以上因素,或使血液耗损,或影响脾肾功能,气血生化不足,而致血虚。

【诊断要点】

(1) 有失血,胃肠道功能障碍,营养缺乏,接触或使用过有害于造血组织的物质或药物,慢性感染,严重心、肝、肾疾病,及恶性肿瘤等病史。

(2) 体检见面色萎黄,口唇眼睑呈苍白色,爪甲色淡,形态扁平或脆裂。或有皮肤黏膜出血点,黄疸,肝、脾、淋巴结肿大等情况。

(3) 实验室检查可见外周血红细胞总数及血红蛋白量

cyte and thrombocytopenia is also found, it is indicated
that the disease may be aplastic anemia. When necessary,
bone marrow smear and other laboratory examinations are
recommended to ascertain the nature and causes of anemia.

Syndrome Differentiation and Treatment

Syndrome Differentiation should be made according
to the consumption of qi and blood, of yin and yang in the
viscera. Generally, if there is deficiency of qi and blood in
the heart and spleen, it is a mild case; if there is deficiency of liver yin and kidney yin or deficiency of spleen yang
and kidney yang, it is a severe case; and if there is deficiency of yin, yang, qi and blood, and the spleen, kidneys, heart and liver are diseased, it is a more severe
case. If the case with deficiency of healthy qi is attacked
by exogenous pathogenic factors, considerable attention
should be paid to the differentiation between the principal
deficiency and secondary excess, major and minor, insidious and acute. As far as the treatment is concerned, it
should primarily aim at nourishing blood, replenishing qi
and strengthening the spleen and kidneys. When nourishing blood is applied, replenishing qi to promote blood
production should also be considered; and more important, strengthening the spleen and kidneys, which are the
source of blood, should be applied at the same time. Nevertheless, the principles should vary with whether spleen
deficiency or kidney deficiency is prominent. If the case is
accompanied by deficiency of the heart and liver, both the
heart and the liver should be nourished at the same time.
If there is concurrence of principal deficiency and secondary excess, attention should be paid to the predominance
and urgency of both aspects. For the prolonged case of deficiency of blood with stagnation, it should be treated by

均减少。如白细胞及血小板
亦同时明显减少者,提示可能
为再生障碍性贫血。必要时
应作骨髓象或其他有关实验
室检查,以判断贫血的性质和
病因。

【辨证论治】

辨证应根据脏腑气血、阴
阳虚损的主次,区别其不同证
候。一般证属心脾气血亏虚
者,病情较轻,肝肾阴亏或脾
肾阳虚者,症情较重,更严重
者则阴阳气血俱虚,脾肾心肝
同病。若正虚感受外邪,还应
当注意本虚与标实之间的关
系,掌握病证的主次和缓急。
治疗应以养血益气,培补脾肾
为主要原则。既应补血,又要
重视益气以生血,同时更应培
补脾肾,以加强血液生化之
源,可根据脾虚或肾虚的主
次,分别处理。若心肝亦虚
者,当相应并补。本虚与标实
错见者,可根据其主次缓急,
酌情处理。如久病不复,血虚
挟瘀者,当于补气养血的同
时,适当加用活血化瘀的方
药,俾瘀祛新生,气血充旺。

replenishing qi and nourishing blood, with activating blood circulation to dissipate blood stasis as the supplementary treatment. In so doing, blood stasis is removed and new blood is produced, therefore, qi and blood is abundant.

1. Deficiency of Both Qi and Blood

Chief Manifestations: Sallow or pale complexion, lassitude, shortness of breath, poor appetite, palpitation, accompanied by insomnia, dizziness, or even fainting, pale or flat finger nails, pale and swollen tongue with thin coating, feeble and thready pulse.

Therapeutic Methods: To nourish blood and replenish qi.

Prescription: Modified Bazhen Tang (Decoction of Eight Precious Drugs) and Guipi Tang (Decoction for Invigorating Spleen and Nourishing Heart), composed of Dangshen (*Radix Codonopsis*) 15 g, Huangqi (*Radix Astragali*) 15 g, Baizhu (*Rhizoma Atractylodis Macrocephalae*) 10 g, Danggui (*Radix Angelicae Sinensis*) 10 g, Shudihuang (*adix Rehmanniae Preparatae*) 15 g, Chenpi (*Pericarpium Citri Reticulatae*) 10 g, Chaosuanzaoren (*Semen Ziziphi Spinosae*, stir-baked) 15 g, Guiyuanrou (*Cortex Cinnamomi*) 10 g, Zhigancao (*Radix Glycyrrhizae*, roasted) 6 g and Dazao (*Fructus Jujubae*) 10 pcs.

Modifications: For metrorrhagia or preceded cycle with profuse and reddish discharge in females, add Duanlonggu (*Os Draconis Usta*, to be decocted first) 20 g, Duanmuli (*Concha Ostreae Usta*, to be decocted first) 20 g and Xueyutan (*Crinis Carbonisatus*) 10 g; for severe palpitation, dreamfulness and timidness, add Yejiaoteng (*Caulis et Folium Polygoni Multiflori*) 15 g and Hehuanpi (*Cortex Albiziae*) 15 g; for night sweating and asthenic heat, add Digupi (*Cortex Lycii*) 15 g and

1. 气血两虚证

主要证候 面色萎黄或苍白,疲倦无力,气短,食少,心悸,兼有失眠,头昏晕,甚至有时欲倒,爪甲色淡或扁平如匙,舌质淡胖、苔薄,脉虚细。

治 法 养血补气。

方 药 八珍汤、归脾汤加减:党参15 g,黄芪15 g,白术10 g,当归10 g,熟地黄15 g,陈皮10 g,炒酸枣仁15 g,桂圆肉10 g,炙甘草6 g,大枣 10 枚。

加 减 妇女崩中漏下或月经超前,量多色淡者,加煅龙骨(先煎)20 g,煅牡蛎(先煎)20 g,血余炭10 g;心悸怔忡,多梦易惊者,加夜交藤15 g,合欢皮15 g;盗汗虚热者,可加地骨皮15 g,浮小麦 30 g。

Fuxiaomai (*Fructus Tritici Levis*) 30 g.

2. Deficiency of Liver Yin and Kidney Yin

Chief Manifestations: Pale complexion, flushed cheeks, dizziness, tinnitus, soreness and weakness of the loins and legs, often accompanied by low fever, dysphoria, feverish sensation over the palms and soles, night sweating, dry mouth, dry and fragile finger nails, dry skin with occasional petechia and ecchymosis, nose bleeding, gingival bleeding, menorrhagia, red tongue with thin coating, and thready, rapid and forceless pulse.

Therapeutic Methods: To tonify the liver and kidney, and nourish yin and blood.

Prescription: Modified Zuogui Wan (Bolus for Replening Kidney Yin) and Da Buyuan Jian (Potent Decoction for Replenishing Primordial Qi), composed of Shengdihuang (*Radix Rehmanniae*) 12 g, Shudihuang (*Radix Rehmanniae Preparata*) 12 g, Heshouwu (*Radix Polygoni Multiflori*) 10 g, Danggui (*Radix Angelicae Sinensis*) 10 g, Gouqizi (*Fructus Lycii*) 10 g, Nüzhenzi (*Fructus Ligustri Lucidi*) 10 g, Hanliancao (*Herba Ecliptae*) 12 g and Guiban (*Plastrum Testudinis*, to be decocted first) 15 g.

Modifications: For predominant asthenic heat, hectic fever, add Biejia (*Carapax Trionycis*, to be decocted first) 15 g, Digupi (*Cortex Lycii*) 12 g, Yinchaihu (*Radix Ste llariae*) 10 g and Qinghao (*Herba Artemisiae Annuae*) 10 g; for deficiency of qi, lassitude, add Taizishen (*Radix Pseudostellariae*) 12 g and Shanyao (*Rhizoma Dioscoreae*) 12 g; for hemorrhage or ecchymosis in the skin, add Daji (*Herba seu Radix Cirsii Japonici*) 10 g, Xiaoji (*Herba Cirsii*) 10 g, Xianhecao (*Herba Agrimoniae*) 12 g, Mudanpi (*Cortex Moutan Radicis*) 10 g, Chishaoyao (*Radix Paeoniae Rubra*) 10 g and Shuiniujiao (*Cornu Bubali*, to be decocted first) 30 g;

2. 肝肾阴虚证

主要证候 面白颧红,眩晕,耳鸣,腰酸腿软,常有低热,心烦,手足心热,盗汗,口干,指甲枯脆,皮肤干燥,或见皮肤瘀点、瘀斑、鼻衄、齿衄,妇女月经过多,舌质红、苔少,脉细数无力。

治　法 滋养肝肾,补益阴血。

方　药 左归丸、大补元煎加减:生地黄12 g,熟地黄12 g,何首乌10 g,当归10 g,枸杞子10 g,女贞子10 g,旱莲草12 g,龟版(先煎)15 g。

加　减 虚热明显,潮热,加鳖甲(先煎)15 g,地骨皮12 g,银柴胡10 g,青蒿10 g;气虚神疲,加太子参12 g,山药12 g;有出血或皮肤瘀斑者,加大蓟10 g,小蓟10 g,仙鹤草12 g,牡丹皮10 g,赤芍药10 g,水牛角(先煎)30 g;出血严重者,另用阿胶10 g 烊化冲服。

for serious hemorrhage, add Ejiao (*Colla Corii Asini*, to be melted and taken separately) 10 g.

3. Deficiency of Spleen Yang and Kidney Yang

Chief Manifestations: Pale complexion, pale lips and finger nails, emaciation or edema, dizziness, listlessness, shortness of breath, disinclination for speaking, soreness and weakness along the spinal column, aversion to cold, cold limbs, spontaneous sweating, poor appetite, loose stools, occasional nose bleeding and gingival bleeding, nocturnal emission and impotence in males, menoxenia in females, pale tongue, deep and thready pulse.

Therapeutic Methods: To warm and tonify the spleen and kidney, and benefit qi and nourish blood.

Prescription: Modified Yougui Wan (Bolus for Replenishing Kidney Yang) and Zhengyang Lilao Tang (Decoction for Salvaging Yang and Relieving Exhaustion), composed of Huangqi (*Radix Astragali*) 15 g, Baizhu (*Rhizoma Atractylodis Macrocephalae*) 10 g, Fuling (*Poria*) 15 g, Gancao (*Radix Glycyrrhizae*) 6 g, Shufuzi (*Radix Aconiti Preparata*) 10 g, Dafupi (*Pericarpium Arecae*) 10 g, Houpo (*Cortex Magnoliae Officinalis*) 6 g, Buguzhi (*Fructus Psoraleae*) 10 g, Tusizi (*Semen Cuscutae*) 15 g, Rougui (*Cortex Cinnamomi*) 6 g, Lujiaojiao (*Colla Cornus Cervi*, to be melted in the finished decoction) 10 g and Danggui (*Radix Angelicae Sinensis*) 10 g.

Modifications: For serious diarrhoea, add Chaoshanyao (*Rhizoma Dioscoreae*, stir-baked) 15 g and Chaobiandou (*Semen Dolichoris*, stir-baked) 10 g; for pronounced edema, add Zhuling (*Polyporus*) 10 g and Zexie (*Rhizoma Alismatis*) 10 g; for hemorrhage, add Paojiangtan (*Rhizoma Zingiberis Recens*, charred) 6 g, Xianhecao (*Herba Agrimoniae*) 15 g, Duanlonggu (*Os Draconis Usta*, to be decocted first) 30 g and Duanmuli

3. 脾肾阳虚证

主要证候　面色㿠白或苍白,口唇指甲淡白,消瘦或浮肿,头晕,精神委靡,少气懒言,腰脊酸楚,畏寒,肢冷,自汗,食少,便溏,偶见鼻衄、齿衄,男子遗精阳痿,女子月经不调,舌质淡,脉沉细。

治　法　温补脾肾,益气养血。

方　药　右归丸合拯阳理劳汤加减:黄芪15 g,白术10 g,茯苓15 g,甘草6 g,熟附子10 g,大腹皮10 g,厚朴6 g,补骨脂10 g,菟丝子15 g,肉桂6 g,鹿角胶(烊化冲服)10 g,当归10 g。

加　减　腹泻严重者,加炒山药15 g,炒扁豆10 g;水肿明显者,加猪苓10 g,泽泻10 g;若有出血,加炮姜炭6 g,仙鹤草15 g,煅龙骨(先煎)30 g,煅牡蛎(先煎)30 g。

(*Concha Ostreae Usta*, to be decocted first) 30 g.

Other Treatments

1. Chinese Patent Drugs

(1) Shouwu Pian (Polygoni Multiflori Tablet): 5 tablets each time, 3 times daily, taken with warm boiled water; indicated for weakness due to blood deficiency.

(2) Danggui Yangxue Gao (Angelicae Sinensis Extract for Nourishing Blood): 15 ml each time, 3 times daily; indicated for deficiency of both qi and blood.

(3) Liuwei Dihuang Wan (Pill of Six Drugs Containing Rehmannia): 6 g each time, twice daily; indicated for deficiency of liver yin and kidney yin.

2. Single-drug or Experiential Prescriptions

(1) Lüfan (*Melanteritum*) 6 g and Dazao (*Fructus Jujubae, kernel and peel removed*) 10 pcs. Grind Lüfan into powder and crush Dazao into a mash. Mix them thoroughly to make 40 pills. Take 1 pill each time, twice daily, 20 days as a course of treatment. It is indicated for iron-deficiency anemia.

(2) Xianhecao (*Herba Agrimoniae*) 30 g and Dazao (*Fructus Jujubae*) 10 pcs. Decoct the herbs in water and take the decoction in 2 doses. It is indicated for iron-deficiency anemia and aplastic anemia.

(3) Duanzaofan (*Melanterium Usta*) and Chaohuangdou (*Semen Sojae*, stir-baked) in the proportion of one to two. Grind them to fine powder and mix with jujube soup to make pills. Take 6 g each time, thrice daily. It is indicated for iron-deficiency anemia caused by ancylostomiasis.

(4) Hechefen (*Placenta Hominis*, powdered): 3 - 6 g each time, twice daily; indicated for anemia of all kinds.

(5) Niugusui (*Medulla Spinalis Bovis seu Bubali*) 24 g, Shanyao (*Rhizoma Dioscoreae*) 24 g, Taipanfen

【其他疗法】

1. 中成药

(1) 首乌片　每服 5 片，每日 3 次，温开水送服。适用于血虚体弱者。

(2) 当归养血膏　每服 15 ml，每日 3 次。适用于气虚血亏者。

(3) 六味地黄丸　每服 6 g，每日 2 次。适用于肝肾阴亏者。

2. 单验方

(1) 绿矾 6 g，研细；大枣 10 枚，去皮核，捣成枣泥。将绿矾放入枣泥中，捣匀，捻成 40 丸，每服 1 丸，每日 2 次，20 日为 1 个疗程。适用于缺铁性贫血。

(2) 仙鹤草 30 g，大枣 10 枚，水煎，分 2 次服。适用于缺铁性贫血和再生障碍性贫血。

(3) 煅皂矾 1 份，炒黄豆 2 份，研细末，枣汤泛为丸。每服 6 g，每日 3 次。适用于钩虫病引起的缺铁性贫血。

(4) 河车粉，每服 3～6 g，每日 2 次。适用于各种贫血。

(5) 牛骨髓 24 g，山药 24 g，胎盘粉 30 g，蜂蜜 24 g，共

(*Placenta Hominis*, powdered) 30 g and Honey (*Mel*) 24 g. Mix them together, put the mixture into a china jar and steam it in a pot. Take 2 spoonfuls each time, twice daily. It is indicated for aplastic anemia.

捣匀,入瓷罐中,放锅内蒸熟。每服 2 汤匙,每日 2 次。适用于再生障碍性贫血。

2.7.4　Thrombocytopenic Purpura

第四节　血小板减少性紫癜

General Description

【概述】

Thrombocytopenic purpura includes two types: primary and secondary. Primary thrombocytopenic purpura is a hemorrhagic disease caused by decrease of platelets for unknown cause and is related with immunity, while secondary thrombocytopenic purpura usually follows other diseases. Clinically, the disease is characterized by petechiae and ecchymosis in skin and mucosa or hemorrhage in viscera, absolute decrease of the number of platelets, the normal or increased number of megalocaryocytes in bone marrow accompanied by disturbance of maturity. This disease can be divided into acute type and chronic type according to the clinical manifestations and courses. Acute type is commonly found in children and the incidence in males is similar to that in females, while chronic type is often seen in young women and the ratio of incidence between males and females is 1 : 3 - 4. The severity of hemorrhage varies with the platelet count. In serious cases, there may be intracranial hemorrhage which may cause death.

According to the clinical manifestations, the disease is categorized as "xue zheng" (hemorrhagic syndrome), "fa ban" (purpura), "pu tao yi" (cyanosis), etc. Its cause lies in heat, toxic substance, blood stasis and deficiency. The major pathogenesis is that hyperactivity of heat and toxic substances or insufficiency of qi and yin

血小板减少性紫癜有原发性和继发性之分。原发性血小板减少性紫癜是原因不明的血小板减少,并与免疫因素有关的出血性疾病。继发性是由于其他疾病所致。本病的临床特征为皮肤和黏膜瘀点、瘀斑或内脏出血,血小板数绝对减少,骨髓巨核细胞数正常或增多并伴有成熟障碍。本病可分为急、慢性两类。急性型多见于儿童,男女发病率相近。慢性型以女性青年为多,男女发病率之比约 1:3～4。本病根据血小板计数的多少,其出血程度不一,重者可出现颅内出血,危及生命。

根据本病的临床表现,属于中医学"血证"、"发斑"、"葡萄疫"等范畴,其病因在于热、毒、瘀、虚。主要病机为热毒迫血,或气阴不足,血液不循常道,外溢血脉。

forces the blood to move recklessly, resulting in blood extravasating from vessels.

Essentials for Diagnosis

(1) In most cases, the patients have a previous history of viral infection 1 - 2 weeks prior to the onset of acute thrombocytopenic purpura. The onset of the disease is sudden, often manifested as fever and severe bleeding tendency. There may be hemorrhage in skin and mucosa, often accompanied by hemorrhage in gastrointestinal tract, urinary tract, respiratory tract, or even intracranial hemorrhage, which may cause death very often. But the disease is self-limited and is spontaneously cured within 4 - 6 weeks, at most half a year. In a few cases, the disease may progress to chronic type.

(2) The onset of chronic type is insidious. In most cases, there is bleeding tendency long before confirmed diagnosis. Generally, if platelet count is below $50 \times 10^9/L$, it is usually manifested as purpura, epistaxis, gingival bleeding, profuse menstruation, and accompanied by iron-deficiency anemia; if platelet count is below $30 \times 10^9/L$, hemorrhage in viscera can be found; if platelet count is below $10 \times 10^9/L$, intracranial hemorrhage may occur. Furthermore, it is persistent, with repeated attacks in the course of the disease.

(3) Laboratory examination shows platelet count decreased; red cell count and haemoglobin decreased in the case with loss of blood; leucocyte count normal, the bleeding time prolonged and coagulation time normal; the picture of bone marrow shows megalocaryocytes normal or increased with disturbance of maturity; in acute type megalocaryocytes are mostly granular while in chronic type, naked-nuclear; platelets few, antibody PAIgG, PAIgM, PAIgA, PAC$_3$ increased.

【诊断要点】

(1) 急性型在发病前1~2个星期常有病毒感染史。起病急骤,常伴有发热,出血倾向严重,不仅可见有皮肤、黏膜出血,同时可伴有胃肠道、泌尿道、呼吸道出血,甚至可出现颅内出血,而成为死亡的原因,但其有自限性,一般4~6个星期,最长半年内可自愈,少数可转变为慢性。

(2) 慢性型起病隐袭,多数在确诊前相当长的一段时间已有出血倾向。一般血小板计数在 $50 \times 10^9/L$ 以下,易见皮肤紫癜、鼻腔出血、牙龈出血,女性月经量多。常伴有缺铁性贫血,血小板计数在 $30 \times 10^9/L$ 以下,可伴见内脏出血,血小板计数在 $10 \times 10^9/L$ 以下可伴见颅内出血。病情可反复发作,缠绵不愈。

(3) 实验室检查可见血小板计数减少;有失血表现者,可见红细胞计数及血红蛋白减少;白细胞计数正常,出血时间延长,凝血时间正常;骨髓常规示巨核细胞数正常或增多,成熟障碍,急性者以颗粒型为主,慢性者以裸核为主,血小板少见或罕见。血小板相关抗体 PAIgG、PAIgM、PAIgA、PAC$_3$ 增高。

Syndrome Differentiation and Treatment

The differentiation of the disease is to clarify whether the case is the deficiency or the excess type. Acute type is usually referred to the excess type and the treatment should primarily aim at clearing away heat and cooling blood to stop bleeding; chronic type is usually referred to the deficiency type or the deficiency-excess type, so the treatment is nourishing yin and lowering fire, or benefiting qi and keeping the blood flowing within the vessels. For pronounced blood stasis, activating blood circulation to dissipate blood stasis should be the principal treatment.

1. Blood Attacked by Hyperactivity of Heat

Chief Manifestations: Abrupt onset with petechiae and purpuras in the skin, fever, thirst, often accompanied by gingival bleeding, epistaxis, even hematochezia, hematuria, red tongue with yellow coating and rapid pulse.

Therapeutic Methods: To cool blood to stop bleeding.

Prescription: Modified Xijiao Dihuang Tang (Cornu Rhinoceotis and Rehmanniae Decoction) and Qingying Tang (Decoction for Clearing away Heat in Yingfen), composed of Shuiniujiao (*Cornu Bubali*, to be decocted first) 30 g, Shengdihuang (*Radix Rehmanniae*) 15 g, Chishaoyao (*Radix Paeoniae Rubra*) 10 g, Mudanpi (*Cortex Moutan Radicis*) 10 g, Xuanshen (*Radix Scrophulariae*) 10 g, Zicao (*Radix Arnebiae seu Lithospermi*) 15 g, Shanglu (*Radix Phytolaccae*) 10 g, Yangtigen (*Radix Rumicis*) 10 g and Gancao (*Radix Glycyrrhizae*) 3 g.

Modifications: For pronounced hematuria, add Daji (*Herba seu Radix Cirsii Japonici*) 15 g, Xiaoji (*Herba*

【辨证论治】

本病临床辨证主要是辨虚实。急性者多属实证,治疗以清热凉血止血为主;慢性者多属虚证或虚实夹杂,治疗多用滋阴降火或益气摄血法。血瘀明显者,又当以活血化瘀为主。

1. 热盛迫血证

主要证候　起病急,来势快,皮肤出现紫斑、紫点,发热口渴,常伴牙龈、鼻腔出血,甚则便血、尿血,舌红,苔黄,脉数。

治　法　凉血止血。

方　药　犀角地黄汤合清营汤加减:水牛角30 g(先煎),生地黄15 g,赤芍药10 g,牡丹皮10 g,玄参10 g,紫草15 g,商陆10 g,羊蹄根10 g,甘草3 g。

加　减　尿血明显者,加大蓟15 g,小蓟15 g,仙鹤草

Cirsii）15 g and Xianhecao（*Herba Agrimoniae*）30 g;
for pronounced hemafecia, add Diyutan（*Radix Sanguisorbae*, charred）10 g and Huaihua（*Flos Sophorae*）
10 g; for constipation, add Shengdahuang（*Radix et Rhizoma Rhei*, to be decocted later）5 g.

2. Failure of Qi to Control Blood

Chief Manifestations: Slow onset of scattered purpuras which are aggravated by overwork, and appear and
fade intermittently, dizziness, lassitude, poor appetite,
sallow complexion, pale tongue with white coating,
thready and weak pulse.

Therapeutic Methods: To benefit qi, control blood
and stop bleeding.

Prescription: Modified Guipi Tang（Decoction for
Invigorating Spleen and Nourishing Heart）, composed of
Dangshen（*Radix Codonopsis*）15 g, Huangqi（*Radix
Astragali*）15 g, Baizhu（*Rhizoma Atractylodis Macrocephalae*）10 g, Zhigancao（*Radix Glycyrrhizae*, roasted) 10 g, Fuling（*Poria*）10 g, Xianhecao（*Herba Agrimoniae*）15 g, Qiancao（*Radix Rubiae*）10 g and Ji-
xueteng（*Caulis Spatholobi*）30 g.

Modifications: For insufficiency of kidney qi, add
Shanzhuyu（*Fructus Corni*）10 g, Nüzhenzi（*Fructus
Ligustri Lucidi*）10 g, Hanliancao（*Herba Ecliptae*）10 g
and Chuanxuduan（*Radix Dipsaci*）10 g; for cold hands
and feet, loose stools, white and smooth tongue coating
and deep pulse, add Paojiang（*Rhizoma Zingiberis*,
roasted in hot cinders）3 g and Baizhu（*Rhizoma Atractylodis Macrocephalae*）10 g.

3. Hyperactivity of Fire due to Deficiency of Yin

Chief Manifestations: Slow onset with longer
course, mild or serious ecchymosis at frequent intervals,
or accompanied by epistaxis, feverish sensation of the
palms, soles, and chest, dry mouth and throat, red

30 g;便血明显者,加地榆炭
10 g,槐花10 g;大便秘结者,
加生大黄(后下)5 g。

2. 气不摄血证

主要证候 起病缓慢,劳
累后加重,斑色暗淡,多呈散
在出现,时起时消,反复发作,
头昏乏力,食少纳减,面色萎
黄,舌淡,苔白,脉细弱。

治 法 益气摄血止血。

方 药 归脾汤加减:
党参15 g,黄芪15 g,白术10 g,
炙甘草10 g,茯苓10 g,仙鹤草
15 g,茜草10 g,鸡血藤30 g。

加 减 兼有肾气不足
者,加山茱萸10 g,女贞子
10 g,旱莲草10 g,川续断10 g;
手足不温,大便稀溏,苔白滑,
脉沉,加炮姜3 g,白术10 g。

3. 阴虚火旺证

主要证候 起病缓慢,病
程较长,皮肤紫斑时轻时重,
或伴鼻衄,五心烦热,口渴咽
干,舌光红无苔或花剥,脉

tongue without coating or geographic tongue, thready and rapid pulse.

Therapeutic Methods: To nourish yin and subdue fire to stop bleeding.

Prescription: Modified Qiangen San (Rubiae Powder), composed of Qiancaogen (*Radix Rubiae*) 15 g, Cebaiye (*Cacumen Biotae*) 10 g, Huangqin (*Radix Scutellariae*) 10 g, Shengdihuang (*Radix Rehmanniae*) 15 g, Ejiao (*Colla Corii Asini*, to be melted in the finished decoction) 10 g, Shenggancao (*Radix Glycyrrhizae*) 3 g, Nüzhenzi (*Fructus Ligustri Lucidi*) 10 g and Hanliancao (*Herba Ecliptae*) 10 g.

Modifications: For hectic fever, add Digupi (*Cortex Lycii*) 10 g and Yinchaihu (*Radix Stellariae*) 10 g; for night sweating, add Nuodaogen (*Rhizoma et Radix Oryzae Glutinosae*) 10 g and Bietaogan (*Fructus Pruni Immaturus*) 10 g; for severe dizziness, add Gouqizi (*Fructus Lycii*) 10 g and Heshouwu (*Radix Polygoni Multiflori*) 10 g.

4. Obstruction of Collaterals by Blood Stasis

Chief Manifestations: Prolonged and intractable purpura with dark purple ecchymosis, dim complexion, dark purple tongue, thready and unsmooth pulse.

Therapeutic Methods: To remove blood stasis and stop bleeding.

Prescription: Shixiao San Jiawei (Powder for Dissipating Blood Stasis with Additions), composed of Puhuang (*Pollen Typhae*, wrapped) 10 g, Wulingzhi (*Faeces Trogopterorum*) 10 g, Taoren (*Semen Persicae*) 10 g, Honghua (*Flos Carthami*) 3 g, Danggui (*Radix Angelicae Sinensis*) 10 g, Shudihuang (*Radix Rehmanniae Preparatae*) 10 g, Qiancao (*Radix Rubiae*) 10 g, Shanglu (*Radix Phytolaccae*) 10 g and Gancao (*Radix Glycyrrhizae*) 3 g.

细数。

治 法 滋阴降火止血。

方 药 茜根散加减: 茜草根15 g, 侧柏叶10 g, 黄芩10 g, 生地黄15 g, 阿胶(烊化冲服)10 g, 生甘草3 g, 女贞子10 g, 旱莲草10 g。

加 减 潮热明显, 加地骨皮10 g, 银柴胡10 g; 盗汗加糯稻根10 g, 瘪桃干10 g; 头晕甚者, 加枸杞子10 g, 何首乌10 g。

4. 瘀血阻络证

主要证候 病程日久, 迁延不愈, 紫斑色暗, 面色晦暗, 舌紫暗, 脉细涩。

治 法 化瘀止血。

方 药 失笑散加味: 蒲黄(包煎)10 g, 五灵脂10 g, 桃仁10 g, 红花3 g, 当归10 g, 熟地黄10 g, 茜草10 g, 商陆10 g, 甘草3 g。

Modifications: For blood stasis in the hypochondrium, add Zhi Biejia (*Carapax Trionycis*, roasted and to be decocted first) 15 g, Zhi Guiban (*Plastrum Testudinis*, roasted and to be decocted first) 15 g and Chaihu (*Radix Bupleuri*) 6 g; for constipation, add Juemingzi (*Semen Cassiae*) 10 g and Huomaren (*Fructus Cannabis*) 10 g; for lassitude, add Zhihuangqi (*Radix Astragali*, roasted) 12 g and Taizishen (*Radix Pseudostellariae*) 15 g.

Other Treatments

1. Chinese Patent Drugs

（1）Yunnan Baiyao (Yunnan White Medicinal Powder): 3 g each time, thrice daily, taken orally; indicated for pronounced hemorrhage.

（2）Dahuang Zhechong Wan (Pill of Rhei and Eupolyphaga seu Steleophaga): 3 g each time, thrice daily; indicated for obstruction of channel by blood stasis.

（3）Zhi Bai Dihuang Wan (Pill of Anemarrhenae, Phellodendri and Rehmanniae): 6 g each time, twice daily; indicated for hyperactivity of fire with deficiency of yin.

（4）Guipi Wan (Pill for Invigorating Spleen and Nourishing Heart): 6 g each time, twice daily; indicated for failure of qi to control blood.

2. Single-drug or Experiential Prescriptions

（1）Huashengyi (*Testa Arachidis Hypogaeae*) 30 g and Dazao (*Fructus Jujubae*) 10 pcs. Decoct the herbs in water for oral administration, 1 dose daily, 5 - 7 days as a course of treatment. It is indicated for mild thrombocytopenic purpura.

（2）Malantou (*Herba Kalimeridis Indicae*) 15 g. Clean and mash the herb to collect juice, take the juice with warm boiled water, 1 dose daily, 7 days as a course of treatment. It is indicated for thrombocytopenic purpura with predominant heat.

加 减 胁下结块,加炙鳖甲(先煎)15 g,炙龟版(先煎)15 g,柴胡6 g;大便秘结者,加决明子10 g,火麻仁10 g;乏力明显者,加炙黄芪12 g,太子参15 g。

【其他疗法】

1. 中成药

（1）云南白药 每服3 g,每日 3 次,口服。适用于本病出血明显者。

（2）大黄䗪虫丸 每服3 g,每日 3 次。适用于本病瘀血阻络证。

（3）知柏地黄丸 每服6 g,每日 2 次。适用于本病阴虚火旺证。

（4）归脾丸 每服6 g,每日 2 次。适用于本病气不摄血证。

2. 单验方

（1）花生衣30 g,大枣 10枚。水煎服,每日 1 剂,5～7日为 1 个疗程。适用于血小板减少性紫癜轻症。

（2）马兰头15 g,洗净,捣烂绞汁,以温水冲服。每日 1剂,7 日为 1 个疗程。适用于本病证候偏热者。

(3) Luxiancao (*Herba Pyrolae*) 100 g, Huanyangcao (*Radix Rhodiolae Yunnanensis*) 100 g and Danshen (*Radix Salviae Miltiorrhizae*) 50 g. Decoct the herbs in water for oral administration, 1 dose daily, 10 days as a course of treatment. It is indicated for the prolonged case of thrombocytopenic purpura.

(4) Quyu Huaban Tang (Decoction for Removing Blood Stasis and Petechia), composed of Danggui (*Radix Angelicae Sinensis*) 10 g, Chishaoyao (*Radix Paeoniae Rubra*) 15 g, Chuanxiong (*Rhizoma Chuanxiong*) 12 g, Jixueteng (*Caulis Spatholobi*) 30 g, Yimucao (*Herba Leonuri*) 12 g, Puhuang (*Pollen Typhae*, wrapped) 10 g, Wulingzhi (*Faeces Trogopterorum*) 10 g, Taoren (*Semen Persicae*) 10 g, Honghua (*Flos Carthami*) 10 g, Xiangfu (*Rhizoma Cyperi*) 10 g and Zhihuangqi (*Radix Astragali*, roasted) 20 g. Decoct all the herbs in water for oral administration, 1 dose daily, and take the decoction in 2 doses. It is indicated for thrombocytopenic purpura with blood stasis.

(5) Dai Ge San (Powder of Indigo Naturalis and Concha Meretricis seu Cyclinae): composed of Gefen (*Pulvis Concha Meretricis*, unprepared) 30 g and Qingdai (*Indigo Naturalis*) 30 g. Mix them thoroughly, take 3 - 5 g each time, twice daily. It is indicated for thrombocytopenic purpura due to hyperactive liver fire impairing lung yin, complicated by cough with hemoptysis.

(6) Baixian Xiaodian Tang (Decoction of Dictamni and Agrimoniae for Relieving Purpura): composed of Baixianpi (*Cortex Dictamni*) 50 g, Xuejianchou (*Herba Chenopodii Hybridi*) 30 g, Qiancao (*Radix Rubiae*) 25 g, Xianhecao (*Herba Agrimoniae*) 15 g, Mudanpi (*Cortex Moutan Radicis*) 20 g, Diyutan (*Radix Sanguisorbae*, charred) 20 g, Shengdihuangtan (*Radix Rehmanniae*, charred) 20 g, Jinyinhua (*Flos Lonicerae*)

(3) 鹿衔草100 g,还阳草100 g,丹参50 g,水煎服,每日1剂,10 日为 1 个疗程。适用于本病日久不愈者。

(4) 祛瘀化斑汤　当归10 g,赤芍药15 g,川芎12 g,鸡血藤30 g,益母草12 g,蒲黄(包煎)10 g,五灵脂10 g,桃仁10 g,红花10 g,香附10 g,炙黄芪20 g。水煎服,每日 1 剂,分2 次服。适用于本病血瘀证。

(5) 黛蛤散　蛤粉(生)30 g,青黛30 g,和匀。每服3～5 g,每日 2 次。适用于本病木火刑金犯肺,伴咳嗽咯血者。

(6) 白仙消癜汤　白鲜皮50 g,血见愁30 g,茜草25 g,仙鹤草15 g,牡丹皮20 g,地榆炭20 g,生地黄炭20 g,金银花20 g,丹参30 g,参三七20 g,羚羊角粉1 g(另冲),紫草20 g。水煎服,每日 1 剂,分 2 次服。适用于本病血热型。

20 g, Danshen (*Radix Salviae Miltiorrhizae*) 30 g, Shensanqi (*Radix Notoginseng*) 20 g, Lingyangjiaofen (*Cornu Saigae Tataricae*, powdered and to be infused separately) 1 g and Zicao (*Radix Arnebiae seu Lithospermi*) 20 g. Decoct the herbs in water and take the decoction in 2 doses. It is indicated for thrombocytopenic purpura with blood heat.

(7) Zidian Tang (Decoction for Relieving Purpura): composed of Shengdihuang (*Radix Rehmanniae*) 15 g, Baimaogen (*Rhizoma Imperatae*) 60 g, Mudanpi (*Cortex Moutan Radicis*) 9 g, Baishaoyao (*Radix Paeoniae Alba*) 9 g, Xianhecao (*Herba Agrimoniae*) 15 g, Heishanzhi (*Fructus Gardeniae*, stir-baked) 9 g, Xiaoji (*Herba Cirsii*) 30 g, Oujie (*Nodus Nelumbinis Rhizomatis*) 15 g, Jinyinhua (*Flos Lonicerae*) 15 g, Heye (*Folium Nelumbinis*) 9 g and Shensanqifen (*Radix Notoginseng*, powdered and to be infused separately) 3 g. Decoct the herbs in water and take the decoction in 2 doses. It is indicated for thrombocytopenic purpura with endogenous heat caused by yin deficiency.

(8) Ziyin Yiqi Liangxue Tang (Decoction for Nourishing Yin, Replenishing Qi and Cooling Blood), composed of Shengdihuang (*Radix Rehmanniae*) 30 g, Sangbaipi (*Cortex Mori*) 30 g, Baimaogen (*Rhizoma Imperatae*) 30 g, Niuxixi (*Radix Rumicis Patientiae*) 15 g and Dangshen (*Radix Codonopsis*) 10 g. Decoct the herbs in water and take the decoction in 2 doses. It is indicated for thrombocytopenic purpura with insufficiency of both qi and yin.

2.7.5 Leukopenia

General Description

Leukopenia is a kind of disease with the number of

（7）紫癜汤　生地黄 15 g，白茅根 60 g，牡丹皮 9 g，白芍药 9 g，仙鹤草 15 g，黑山栀 9 g，小蓟 30 g，藕节 15 g，金银花 15 g，荷叶 9 g，参三七粉（另冲）3 g。水煎服，每日 1 剂，分 2 次服。适用于本病阴虚内热之证。

（8）滋阴益气凉血汤　生地黄 30 g，桑白皮 30 g，白茅根 30 g，牛西西 15 g，党参 10 g。水煎服，每日 1 剂，分 2 次服。适用于本病气阴不足者。

第五节　白细胞减少症

【概述】

外周血液中白细胞总数

the white blood cells in the peripheral circulation lower than 4.0×10^9/L. In most cases, the disease is related to the decrease of granulocytes because the granulocyte is the major component of the white blood cell in the peripheral circulation. Granulocytopenia is defined as the absolute number of granulocytes is reduced below 1.8×10^9/L. And if white cell count is lower than 2.0×10^9/L, and the number of neutrophils is lower than 0.5×10^9/L or even is reduced to zero and there are pronounced corresponding symptoms, agranulocytopenia appears.

The disease is caused by physical, chemical, medical or biologic factors, while some diseases, congenital constitution as well as some unknown reasons may contribute to the decrease of the production of white blood cells, acceleration of their destruction or even abnormality of distribution. It may be divided into five types, namely, decrease of granulocyte multiplication, disturbance of granulocyte maturity, shortening of granulocyte survival time, abnormality of granulocyte distribution and compound type.

According to its clinical manifestations, this disease is grouped into the categories of "xu lao" (consumptive disease) and "xu sun" (deficiency impairment), which is mostly caused by insufficiency of qi and blood, consumption of essence and blood, or deficiency of healthy qi leading to weakness of resistance.

Essentials for Diagnosis

(1) There may be a family history or a contact history of physical and chemical injurant or drugs that may induce this disease.

(2) It usually has a gradual onset, with mild and nonspecific symptoms, such as lassitude, dizziness, palpitation, poor appetite, insomnia or no obvious constitutional

低于 4.0×10^9/L,称为白细胞减少症。因为粒细胞是外周血中白细胞的主要组成部分,故白细胞减少在大多数情况下是由粒细胞减少所致。粒细胞绝对值低于 1.8×10^9/L 时,即称粒细胞减少症。若白细胞计数低于 2.0×10^9/L,中性粒细胞低于 0.5×10^9/L 甚或消失,临床症状严重者,则称粒细胞缺乏症。

本症是由于物理、化学、药物、生物因素,某些疾病、先天体质性因素,以及一些不明原因使白细胞生成减少、破坏加速或分布异常。本病可分为五型,即粒细胞增生减低型、粒细胞成熟障碍型、粒细胞存活时间缩短型、粒细胞分布异常型及复合型。

根据本病的主要临床表现,属中医学"虚劳"、"虚损"等范畴。多为气血不足或精血亏损,正气内虚而卫外不固。

【诊断要点】

(1) 有本病的家族史,或有理化有害物质接触史,或使用过可能诱发本病的药物。

(2) 本病一般起病缓慢,症状较轻,可有周身乏力、倦怠、头晕、心慌、食欲不振、失

symptoms. Acute agranulocytopenia has an abrupt onset, manifested as rigor, high fever, sore throat, headache, painful joints, extreme lassitude, etc.

(3) The patient may be sick with such signs as congestion and edema of pharyngeal mucosa, swollen tonsil and submaxillary lymph nodes. And necrotic ulcer of the mucosa of the mouth, throat, anus and rectum can also be seen in acute agranulocytopenia.

(4) Blood routine test: Leukocyte count decreases distinctly. Bone marrow smear reveals hyperplasia of the hematopoietic cells, especially the proliferation and differentiation of granulocytes.

(5) This disease should be distinguished from acute leukaemia, aplastic anaemia, myeloproliferative syndrome and malignant histiocytosis.

Syndrome Differentiation and Treatment

Laukopenia is usually referred to deficiency syndrome, or deficiency accompanied by excess syndrome. Clinically, it is divided into five types, namely, deficiency of spleen qi and stomach qi, deficiency of both the heart and spleen, deficiency of spleen yang and kidney yang, deficiency of liver yin and kidney yin and deficiency of healthy qi and excess of pathogenic factors. As for the treatment, it should primarily aim at replenishing qi and blood as well as benefiting the liver and kidneys.

1. Deficiency of Spleen Qi and Stomach Qi

Chief Manifestations: Sleepiness, lassitude, shortness of breath, dislike for speaking, weakness of four limbs, loss of appetite, abdominal distension and fullness,

眠等非特异性症状,亦可无明显不适感。急性粒细胞缺乏症则起病急骤,有寒战、高热、咽痛、头痛、关节疼痛、极度疲乏等症状。

(3) 体征可有咽部黏膜充血、水肿,扁桃体及颌下淋巴结肿大。急性粒细胞缺乏症尚可见到口腔、咽部及肛门、直肠等处黏膜坏死性溃疡。

(4) 血常规检查,白细胞计数明显减少。骨髓象检查可了解造血细胞的增生情况,尤其是粒细胞系统的增殖与分化。

(5) 本病应注意与急性白血病、再生障碍性贫血、骨髓增生异常综合征、恶性组织细胞增生症等疾病相鉴别。

【辨证论治】

本病辨证多属虚证,或虚中夹实。临床主要分为脾胃气虚、心脾两虚、脾肾阳虚、肝肾阴虚、正虚邪盛五证。治疗以补气血、益肝肾为原则。

1. 脾胃气虚证

主要证候 困乏倦怠,少气懒言,四肢无力,食少纳呆,脘腹胀满,大便溏薄,舌质淡

loose stools, pink and swollen tongue with teeth marks on its margin, thin and white or thick and white coating, and weak pulse.

Therapeutic Methods: To invigorate the spleen, nourish the stomach and replenish middle energizer qi.

Prescription: Modified Jiawei Sijunzi Tang (Four Mild-Drug Decoction with Additions), composed of Dangshen (*Radix Codonopsis*) 10 g, Huangqi (*Radix Astragali*) 30 g, Baizhu (*Rhizoma Atractylodis Macrocephalae*) 12 g, Fuling (*Poria*) 12 g, Baibiandou (*Semen Lablae Album*) 12 g and Zhigancao (*Radix Glycyrrhizae*, roasted) 6 g.

Modifications: For abdominal distension and fullness, which is aggravated after eating, add Muxiang (*Radix Aucklandiae*) 10 g and Chenpi (*Pericarpium Citri Reticulatae*) 6 g; for dry mouth, remove Baizhu and add Shanyao (*Rhizoma Dioscoreae*) 12 g; for red tongue, add Taizishen (*Rhizoma Pedicularidis Davidii*) 10 g or Xiyangshen (*Radix Panacis Quinquefolii*) 10 g.

2. Deficiency of Both the Heart and Spleen

Chief Manifestations: Sallow complexion, lassitude, poor appetite, loose stools, palpitation, shortness of breath, insomnia, amnesia, pale swollen tongue with thin and white coating, thready and weak pulse.

Therapeutic Methods: To replenish qi, nourish blood, invigorate the spleen and nourish the heart.

Prescription: Modified Guipi Tang (Decoction for Invigorating Spleen and Nourishing Heart), composed of Dangshen (*Radix Codonopsis*) 10 g, Huangqi (*Radix Astragali*) 30 g, Danggui (*Radix Angelicae Sinensis*) 15 g, Baizhu (*Rhizoma Atractylodis Macrocephalae*) 12 g, Fushen (*Sclerotium Poriae Circum Radicem Pini*) 15 g, Guiyuanrou (*Arillus Longan*) 15 g, Suanzaoren (*Semen Ziziphi Spinosae*) 12 g, Yuanzhi (*Radix*

红,舌体胖大有齿痕,苔薄白或白厚,脉弱。

治　法　健脾养胃,补益中气。

方　药　加味四君子汤加减:党参10 g,黄芪30 g,白术12 g,茯苓12 g,白扁豆12 g,炙甘草6 g。

加　减　脘腹胀满,食后尤甚者,加木香10 g,陈皮6 g;口干者,去白术,加山药12 g;舌质偏红者,加太子参10 g,或西洋参10 g。

2. 心脾两虚证

主要证候　面色萎黄,神倦乏力,不思饮食,纳少便溏,心悸气短,失眠健忘,舌质淡,舌体胖大,苔薄白,脉细弱。

治　法　益气补血,健脾养心。

方　药　归脾汤加减:党参10 g,黄芪30 g,当归15 g,白术12 g,茯神15 g,桂圆肉15 g,酸枣仁12 g,远志12 g,木香10 g,炙甘草5 g,生姜3 片。

Polygalae) 12 g, Muxiang (*Radix Aucklandiae*) 10 g, Zhigancao (*Radix Glycyrrhizae*, roasted) 5 g and Shengjiang (Rhizoma Zingiberis Recens) 3 pcs.

Modifications: For loss of appetite, add Shanzha (*Fructus Crataegi*) 10 g; for loose stools, add Chaoyiyiren (*Semen Coicis*, stir-baked) 15 g and Fuling (*Poria*) 15 g; for insomnia and dreamfulness, add Baiziren (*Semen Biotae*) 12 g and Danshen (*Radix Salviae Miltiorrhizae*) 15 g; for palpitation and amnesia, add Shichangpu (*Rhizoma Acori Tatarinowii*) 8 g; for red tip of the tongue and dry mouth, remove Shengjiang and Dangshen and add Taizishen (*Radix Pseudostellariae*) 20 g.

3. Deficiency of Spleen Yang and Kidney Yang

Chief Manifestations: Pale complexion, listlessness, aversion to cold, cold limbs, pain and coldness over the back and loins, copious clear urine or frequent urination at night, dyspeptic diarrhea, impotence, nocturnal emission, praecox ejaculation, pale swollen tongue with teeth marks on its margin, white coating and deep, even-soft pulse.

Therapeutic Methods: To replenish qi, invigorate the spleen, warm the kidney and strengthen yang.

Prescription: Modified Baoyuan Tang (Decoction for Preserving Primordial Qi) and Yougui Wan (Bolus for Replenishing Kidney Yang), composed of Hongshen (*Radix Ginseng Rubra*, to be decocted separately) 10 g, Huangqi (*Radix Astragali*) 25 g, Rougui (*Cortex Cinnamomi*) 6 g, Zhifuzi (*Radix Aconiti Preparata*) 6 g, Duzhong (*Cortex Eucommiae*) 12 g, Tusizi (*Semen Cuscutae*) 15 g, Shudihuang (*Radix Rehmanniae Preparata*) 15 g, Shanyao (*Rhizoma Dioscoreae*) 12 g, Shanzhuyu (*Fructus Corni*) 12 g, Gouqizi (*Fructus Lycii*) 10 g, Danggui (*Radix Angelicae Sinensis*) 12 g,

加　减　食少纳呆者,加山楂10 g;大便溏薄者,加炒薏苡仁15 g,茯苓15 g;失眠多梦,夜寐不安者,加柏子仁12 g,丹参15 g;心悸健忘者,加石菖蒲8 g;舌尖红,口干者,去生姜、党参,加太子参20 g。

3. 脾肾阳虚证

主要证候　面色㿠白,精神委靡,畏寒肢冷,腰背冷痛,小便清长或夜尿频多,下利清谷,阳痿,遗精早泄,舌淡体胖有齿痕,苔白,脉沉缓。

治　法　益气健脾,温肾壮阳。

方　药　保元汤合右归丸加减:红参(另煎)10 g,黄芪25 g,肉桂6 g,制附子6 g,杜仲12 g,菟丝子15 g,熟地黄15 g,山药12 g,山茱萸12 g,枸杞子10 g,当归12 g,鹿角胶(烊化冲服)10 g。

Lujiaojiao（*Colla Cornus Cervi*, to be melted in the finished decoction）10 g.

Modifications: For poor appetite and loose stools, add Sharen（*Fructus Amomi*, to be decocted later）6 g, Fuling（*Poria*）15 g and Baizhu（*Rhizoma Atractylodis Macrocephalae*）10 g; for impotence and nocturnal emission, add Yinyanghuo（*Herba Epimedii*）12 g and Buguzhi（*Fructus Psoraleae*）12 g; for pain and coldness over the back and loins, and cold hands and feet, add Sangjisheng（*Herba Taxilli*）12 g.

4. Deficiency of Liver Yin and Kidney Yin

Chief Manifestations: Dizziness, tinnitus, dry eyes, flushed cheeks, dry mouth and throat, soreness and weakness in the loins and knees, feverish sensation of the palms, soles, and chest, night sweating, nocturnal emission in males, scanty menstruation in females, red margin and tip of the tongue with little coating, thready and rapid pulse.

Therapeutic Methods: To replenish essence, nourish blood, and tonify the kidney and liver.

Prescription: Modified Erzhi Wan（Erzhi Pill）and Zuogui Wan（Bolus for Replenishing Kidney Yin）, composed of Shudihuang（*Radix Rehmanniae Preparata*）20 g, Nüzhenzi（*Fructus Ligustri Lucidi*）15 g, Hanliancao（*Herba Ecliptae*）15 g, Gouqizi（*Fructus Lycii*）12 g, Tusizi（*Semen Cuscutae*）12 g, Guibanjiao（*Colla Plastri Testudinis*, to be melted in the finished decoction）15 g, Lujiaojiao（*Colla Cornus Cervi*, to be melted in the finished decoction）10 g and Shanzhuyu（*Fructus Corni*）12 g.

Modifications: For dizziness and tinnitus, add Baijili（*Fructus Tribuli*）15 g and Juhua（*Flos Chrysanthemi*）10 g; for soreness and weakness in the loins and knees, add Heshouwu（*Radix Polygoni Multiflori*）12 g

加　减　食欲不振,纳少便溏者,加砂仁(后下)6 g,茯苓15 g,白术10 g;阳痿遗精者,加淫羊藿12 g,补骨脂12 g;腰背冷痛,四末不温者,桑寄生12 g。

4. 肝肾阴虚证

主要证候　头晕耳鸣,双目干涩,两颧发红,咽干口渴,腰膝酸软,五心烦热,夜寐盗汗,男子遗精,女子经少,舌边尖红,苔少,脉细数。

治　法　填精益肾,养血补肝。

方　药　二至丸合左归丸加减:熟地黄20 g,女贞子15 g,旱莲草15 g,枸杞子12 g,菟丝子12 g,龟版胶(烊化冲服)15 g,鹿角胶(烊化冲服)10 g,山茱萸12 g。

加　减　头晕耳鸣较著者,加白蒺藜15 g,菊花10 g;腰膝酸软无力者,加何首乌12 g,牛膝12 g;咽干口渴者,

and Niuxi (*Radix Achyranthis Bidentatae*) 12 g; for dry
mouth and throat, remove Lujiaojiao and Shudihuang, add
Shengdihuang (*Radix Rehemanniae*) 10 g, Nanshashen
(*Radix Adenophorae*) 10 g and Maimendong (*Radix
Ophiopogonis*) 10 g; for feverish sensation of the palms,
soles and chest, night sweating, add Zhimu (*Rhizoma
Anemarrhenae*) 10 g and Mudanpi (*Cortex Moutan
Radicis*) 10 g.

5. Deficiency of Healthy Qi and Excess of Pathogenic Factors

Chief Manifestations: Persistent sthenic fever,
flushed face, red eyes, swollen and painful throat, extreme thirst, irritability, even mania and delirium, dry
stools, scanty dark urine, crimson tongue with yellow
coating, bounding and rapid pulse.

Therapeutic Methods: To clear away heat and toxic
substances, and support healthy qi to eliminate pathogenic
factors.

Prescription: Modified Baihu Jia Renshen Tang
(White Tiger Decoction with Ginseng) and Wuwei Xiaodu
Yin (Antiphlogistic Decoction of Five Ingredients), composed of Pugongying (*Herba Taraxaci*) 20 g, Shengshigao (*Gypsum Fibrosum*) 30 g, Hongshen (*Radix Ginseng Rubra*, to be decocted separatedly) 10 g, Jinyinhua
(*Flos Lonicerae*) 15 g, Yejuhua (*Flos Chrysanthemi
Indici*) 15 g, Zhimu (*Rhizoma Anemarrhenae*) 10 g,
Huangqin (*Radix Scutellariae*) 15 g, Zihuadiding (*Herba Violae*) 12 g and Shenggancao (*Radix Glycyrrhizae*)
6 g.

Modifications: For severe sore throat, add Shandougen (*Radix Sophorae Tonkinensis*) 5 g and Banlangen (*Radix Isatidis*) 10 g; for high fever with coma, add
Shuiniujiao (*Cornu bubali*, to be decocted first) 30 g,
Shengdihuang (*Radix Rehemanniae*) 20 g and Mudanpi

去鹿角胶、熟地黄,加生地黄
10 g,南沙参10 g,麦门冬10 g;
五心烦热,夜寐盗汗者,加知
母10 g,牡丹皮10 g。

5. 正虚邪盛证

主要证候 壮热不退,面
红目赤,咽喉肿痛,口渴多饮,
心中懊恼,甚则躁狂谵妄,大
便干结,小便短赤,舌红绛,苔
黄,脉洪数。

治 法 清热解毒,扶正
祛邪。

方 药 白虎加人参汤
合五味消毒饮加减:蒲公英
20 g,生石膏30 g,红参(另煎)
10 g,金银花15 g,野菊花15 g,
知母10 g,黄芩15 g,紫花地丁
12 g,生甘草6 g。

加 减 咽喉肿痛甚者,
加山豆根5 g,板蓝根10 g;高
热神昏者,加水牛角(先煎)
30 g,生地黄20 g,牡丹皮15 g;
烦渴多饮者,加天花粉15 g,天

(*Cortex Moutan Radicis*) 15 g; for extreme thirst, add Tianhuafen (*Radix Trichosanthis*) 15 g and Tianmendong (*Radix Asparagi*) 15 g; for constipation, abdominal fullness and rigidity, add Shengdahuang (*Radix et Rhizoma Rhei*, to be decocted later) 6 g and Zhishi (*Fructus Aurantii Immaturus*) 10 g.

Other Treatments

1. Chinese Patent Drugs

(1) Shengxue Zibu Pian (Tonic Tablet for Hemopoiesis): 5 tablets each time, 3 times daily; indicated for various types of leukopenia.

(2) Ejiao Buxue Gao (Extract of Colla Corii Asini for Replenishing Blood): 20 g each time, twice daily; indicated for various types of leukopenia.

(3) Jixueteng Gao (Spatholobi Extract): 6-10 g each time, twice daily; indicated for various types of leukopenia.

(4) Shen Qi Gao (Ginseng and Astragali Extract): 9 g each time, twice daily; indicated for leukopenia caused by failure of deficient qi to generate blood.

(5) Jianxue Chongji (Blood-Tonifying Granule): 1 sachet each time, 3 times daily; indicated for leukopenia caused by radiotherapy, chemotherapy, organic solvent or unknown causes.

(6) Qi Zao Chongji (Astragali and Jujubae Granule): 15 - 30 g each time, 3 times daily; indicated for leukopenia caused by deficiency of qi and blood.

(7) Guipi Wan (Pill for Invigorating Spleen and Nourishing Heart): 6 g each time, twice daily; indicated for leukopenia caused by deficiency of both the heart and spleen.

(8) Buzhong Yiqi Wan (Pill for Strengthening Middle Energizer and Benefiting Qi): 6 g each time, twice daily; indicated for leukopenia caused by deficiency of the spleen

门冬15 g；大便秘结，脘腹坚满者，加生大黄（后下）6 g，枳实10 g。

【其他疗法】

1. 中成药

（1）生血滋补片　每服5片，每日3次。适用于各种白细胞减少症。

（2）阿胶补血膏　每服20 g，每日2次。适用于各种白细胞减少症。

（3）鸡血藤膏　每服6～10 g，每日2次。适用于各种白细胞减少症。

（4）参芪膏　每服9 g，每日2次。适用于气虚不能生血之白细胞减少症。

（5）健血冲剂　每服1袋，每日3次。适用于放疗、化疗后，有机溶剂及不明原因所致的白细胞减少症。

（6）芪枣冲剂　每服15～30 g，每日3次。适用于气血两虚之白细胞减少症。

（7）归脾丸　每服6 g，每日2次。适用于心脾两虚之白细胞减少症。

（8）补中益气丸　每服6 g，每日2次。适用于脾胃虚弱，中气不足之白细胞减

and stomach and insufficiency of middle energizer qi.

(9) Bushen Qiangshen Pian (Tablet for Invigorating Kidney and Strengthening Health): 5 tablets each time, 3 times daily; indicated for leukopenia caused by insufficiency of kidney qi and consumption of kidney essence.

(10) Zhiling Jiaonang (Zhiling Capsule): 2 - 4 capsules each time, twice daily; indicated for leukopenia caused by deficiency of the spleen and kidney, and insufficiency of healthy qi.

2. Single-drug or Experiential Prescriptions

(1) Shengbai Tang (Decoction for Leukopenia): Lianzi (*Semen Nelumbinis*) 10 g, Suanzaoren (*Semen Aiaiphi Spinosae*) 12 g, Baizhu (*Rhizoma Atractylodis Macrocephalae*) 30 g, Shanyao (*Rhizoma Dioscoreae*) 30 g, Shudihuang (*Radix Rehmanniae Preparata*) 30 g, Baishaoyao (*Radix Paeoniae Alba*) 10 g and Gancao (*Radix Glycyrrhizae*) 6 g. Decoct the herbs in water for oral administration, 1 dose daily and 6 days being a course of treatment. It is indicated for leukopenia caused by deficiency of qi and blood and deficiency of both the heart and spleen.

(2) Shengxue Ling (Decoction for Hemopoiesis): Dahuang (*Radix et Rhizoma Rhei*, to be decocted later) 6 - 9 g, Zhechong (*Eupolyphaga seu Steleophaga*) 4. 5 - 6 g, Xiangfu (*Rhizoma Cyperi*) 10 g, Baizhu (*Rhizoma Atractylodis Macrocephalae*) 15 g, Gancao (*Radix Glycyrrhizae*) 15 g, Fuling (*Poria*) 15 g, Huangqi (*Radix Astragali*) 20 g and Shengdihuang (*Radix Rehmanniae*) 30 g. Decoct the herbs in water for oral administration, 1 dose daily. It is indicated for leukopenia caused by anticancer drugs.

(3) Jijia Shengbai Tang (Decoction of Spatholobi and Squama Manitis for Leukopenia): composed of Jixueteng (*Caulis Spatholobi*) 30 g, Paochuanshanjia (*Squama Manitis*, to be decocted first) 10 g, Nüzhenzi (*Fructus*

少症。

（9）补肾强身片　每服 5 片,每日 3 次。适用于肾气不足、肾精亏损之白细胞减少症。

（10）至灵胶囊　每服 2～4 粒,每日 2 次。适用于脾肾两虚、正气不足的白细胞减少症。

2. 单验方

（1）升白汤　莲子 10 g,酸枣仁 12 g,白术 30 g,山药 30 g,熟地黄 30 g,白芍药 10 g,甘草 6 g,水煎服,每日 1 剂,6 日为 1 个疗程。适用于气血双亏、心脾两虚的白细胞减少症。

（2）生血灵　大黄（后下）6～9 g,䗪虫 4.5～6 g,香附 10 g,白术 15 g,甘草 15 g,茯苓 15 g,黄芪 20 g,生地黄 30 g。水煎服,每日 1 剂。适用于抗癌药物所致的白细胞减少症。

（3）鸡甲升白汤　鸡血藤 30 g,炮穿山甲（先煎）10 g,女贞子 15 g,黄芪 15 g,补骨脂 15 g,淫羊藿 15 g,茯苓 10 g,白

Ligustri Lucidi）15 g, Huangqi（*Radix Astragali*）15 g, Buguzhi（*Fructus Psoraleae*）15 g, Yinyanghuo（*Herba Epimedii*）15 g, Fuling（*Poria*）10 g and Baizhu（*Rhizoma Atractylodis Macrocephalae*）20 g. Decoct the herbs in water for oral administration, 1 dose daily and 3 weeks being a course of treatment. It is indicated for Leukopenia caused by deficiency of spleen qi and kidney qi.

（4）Guben Yangxue Tang（Decoction for Strengthening Body Resistence and Nourishing Blood）: composed of Huangqi（*Radix Astragali*）15 - 30 g, Yinyanghuo（*Herba Epimedii*）12 g, Buguzhi（*Fructus Psoraleae*）15 g, Danggui（*Radix Angelicae Sinensis*）15 g, Jixueteng（*Caulis Spatholobi*）30 g, Danshen（*Radix Salviae Miltiorrhizae*）15 g, Huzhang（*Rhizoma Polygoni Cuspidati*）15 g and Dazao（*Fructus Jujubae*）4 pcs. Decoct the herbs in water for oral administration, 1 dose daily. It is indicated for leukopenia caused by deficiency of both the spleen and kidney.

（5）Chidou Shengxue Fang（Phaseoli Decoction for Hemopoiesis）: composed of Chixiaodou（*Semen Phaseoli*）30 g, Heidadou（*Semen Sojae*）30 g, Biandou（*Semen Dolichoris*）10 g, Buguzhi（*Fructus Psoraleae*）10 g, Yinyanghuo（*Herba Epimedii*）10 g, Danshen（*Radix Salviae Miltiorrhizae*）10 g, Kushen（*Radix Sophorae Flavescentis*）6 g and Chaihu（*Radix Bupleuri*）6 g. Decoct the herbs in water for oral administration, 1 dose daily. It is indicated for leukopenia caused by radiotherapy or chemotherapy.

2.7.6　Hidrosis Syndrome

General Description

Hidrosis syndrome refers to the disorder of secretion of sweat caused by imbalance of yin and yang, and weak-

术20 g。水煎服,每日 1 剂,3 个星期为 1 个疗程。适用于脾肾气虚之白细胞减少症。

（4）固本养血汤　黄芪 15～30 g,淫羊藿12 g,补骨脂 15 g,当归15 g,鸡血藤30 g,丹参15 g,虎杖15 g,大枣 4 枚。水煎服,每日 1 剂。适用于脾肾不足之白细胞减少症。

（5）赤豆生血方　赤小豆 30 g,黑大豆30 g,扁豆10 g,补骨脂10 g,淫羊藿 10 g,丹参 10 g,苦参6 g,柴胡6 g。水煎服,每日 1 剂。适用于放疗、化疗等所致白细胞减少症。

第六节　汗证

【概述】

汗证是指由于阴阳失调,腠理不固,而致汗液外泄失常

ness of body surface. Frequent sweating in the daytime, not affected by environmental factors and aggravated on slight exertion, is known as spontaneous sweating; sweating that occurs during sleep but stops upon wakening is called night sweating or sleep sweating.

The etiology of hidrosis syndrome is related to debility due to prolonged illness and excessive pathogenic heat. In terms of and pathogenesis, hidrosis syndrome is caused by insufficiency of lung qi, disharmony of ying-qi and wei-qi, insufficiency of heart blood, deficient yin and hyperactive fire, and accumulation of pathogenic heat.

Hidrosis syndrome, in western medicine, may be seen in hyperthyroidism, vegetative nerve functional disturbance, rheumatic fever and tuberculosis.

Essentials for Diagnosis

(1) Sweating over the head, neck, chest, or four limbs, or all over the body that is not affected by environmental conditions. Frequent sweating in the daytime aggravated on slight exertion is spontaneous sweating; continuous sweating that occurs during sleep and ceases on wakening is night sweating.

(2) Spontaneous sweating and night sweating may be seen in some other diseases, but they are among the symptoms and signs of those diseases. Sweating, in this case, is not the main manifestation. So it is necessary to make a clear distinction between hidrosis syndrome and other diseases in which spontaneous sweating and night sweating are present.

(3) Examinations such as blood sedimentation, T_3, T_4, basal metabolism rate, chest X-ray, sputum smear, and ASO test should be taken to rule out the possibilities of hyperthyroidism, pulmonary tuberculosis, rheumatic fever, etc.

的病证。其中,不因外界环境因素的影响,而白昼时时汗出,动辄益甚者,称为自汗;寐中汗出,醒来自止者,称为盗汗,亦称为寝汗。

汗证的病因与久病体虚、邪热偏盛有关,病机主要有肺气不足、营卫不和、心血不足、阴虚火旺、邪热郁蒸等。

汗证可见于西医学中的甲状腺功能亢进症、植物神经功能紊乱、风湿热、结核病等。

【诊断要点】

(1) 不受外界环境影响,在头面、颈胸,或四肢、全身出汗者。昼日汗出溱溱,动则益甚为自汗;睡眠中汗出津津,醒后汗止为盗汗。

(2) 其他疾病引起的自汗、盗汗除外。作为其他疾病过程中出现的自汗、盗汗,因疾病的不同,各具有该疾病的症状及体征,且出汗大多不居于突出地位。

(3) 查血沉、T_3、T_4、基础代谢率、胸部 X 线摄片、痰涂片、抗"O"等,以排除甲状腺功能亢进症、肺结核、风湿热等。

Syndrome Differentiation and Treatment

It is essential to classify spontaneous sweating and night sweating into yin, yang, deficiency and excess types. Generally, deficiency types are more common than excess ones. Cases of spontaneous sweating are usually attributive to qi deficiency or yang deficiency while those of night sweating attributive to yin deficiency generating internal heat. If sweating is due to hyperactivity of liver fire or accumulation of damp heat, it is of the excess type.

The treatment for the deficiency type should aim at replenishing qi, nourishing yin, consolidating the body surface and checking sweating; for the excess type, clearing away heat in the liver and dissipating dampness to regulate ying qi should be adopted. As for the case with coexistence of deficiency and excess, it must be first determined whether deficiency or excess is predominant and consideration should be given to both in the treatment.

1. Weakness of the Lung and Weiqi

Chief Manifestations: Sweating which is exacerbated by slight exertion, aversion to wind, susceptibility to common colds, lassitude, lusterless complexion, thready and weak pulse, and thin and white tongue coating.

Therapeutic Methods: To replenish qi and consolidate body surface.

Prescription: Modified Yupingfeng San (Jade Screen Powder), composed of Shenghuangqi (*Radix Astragali*) 12 g, Fangfeng (*Radix Saposhnikoviae*) 6 g, Baizhu (*Rhizoma Atractylodis Macrocephalae*) 10 g, Dangshen (*Radix Codonopsis*) 12 g, Dazao (*Fructus Jujubae*) 5 pcs and Gancao (*Radix Glycyrrhizae*) 5 g.

Modifications: For profuse sweating, add Fuxiaomai (*Fructus Tritici Levis*) 15 g, Nuodaogen (*Rhizoma et Radix Oryzae Glutinosae*) 20 g and Duanmuli (*Concha Ostreae Usta*) 15 g; for predominant qi deficiency,

【辨证论治】

自汗、盗汗的辨证首先应区别阴阳虚实。一般来说,自汗盗汗均属 虚多实少之证。其中自汗多属气虚、阳虚;盗汗多属阴虚内热。而因肝火、湿热等邪热郁蒸而汗出者则属实证。治疗原则,虚证当益气养阴,固表敛汗;实证宜清肝泻热,化湿和营。如有虚实兼夹,还应分辨主次,适当兼顾治疗。

1. 肺卫不固证

主要证候 汗出恶风,稍劳汗出尤甚,易于感冒,体倦乏力,面色少华,脉细弱,苔薄白。

治 法 益气固表。

方 药 玉屏风散加减:生黄芪12 g,防风6 g,白术10 g,党参12 g,大枣5 枚,甘草5 g。

加 减 汗出多者,可加浮小麦15 g,糯稻根20 g,煅牡蛎15 g。气虚甚者,党参加至20 g,黄芪加至24 g。

increase Dangshen (*Radix Codonopsis*) to 20 g and Huangqi (*Radix Astragali*) to 24 g.

2. Disharmony between Ying Qi and Wei Qi

Chief Manifestations: Sweating with aversion to wind, general aching, intermittent chills and fever, or half-body or localized sweating, thin and white tongue coating, and even-soft pulse.

Therapeutic Methods: To regulate ying-qi and wei-qi.

Prescription: Modified Guizhi Tang (Cinnamomi Decoction), composed of Guizhi (*Ramulus Cinnamomi*) 6 g, Baishaoyao (*Radix Paeoniae Alba*) 12 g, Fuling (*Poria*) 12 g, Shengjiang (*Rhizoma Zingiberis Recens*) 5 pcs and Gancao (*Radix Glycyrrhizae*) 3 g.

Modifications: For profuse sweating, add Duanlonggu (*Os Draconis Usta*) 15 g and Duanmuli (*Concha Ostreae Usta*) 15 g to stop sweating; for sweating complicated with qi deficiency, add Huangqi (*Radix Astragali*) 12 g; for sweating complicated with yang deficiency, add Shufuzi (*Radix Aconiti Preparata*) 6 g; for half-body or localized sweating, add Dazao (*Fructus Jujubae*) 5 pcs and Fuxiaomai (*Fructus Tritici Levis*) 12 g.

3. Insufficiency of Heart Blood

Chief Manifestations: Spontaneous sweating or night sweating, palpitation, insomnia, lassitude, short breath, lusterless complexion, pale tongue, and thready pulse.

Therapeutic Methods: To tonify blood and nourish the heart.

Prescription: Modified Guipi Tang (Decoction for Invigorating Spleen and Nourishing Heart), composed of Huangqi (*Radix Astragali*) 12 g, Dangshen (*Radix Codonopsis*) 10 g, Baizhu (*Rhizoma Atractylodis Macrocephalae*) 10 g, Zhigancao (*Radix Glycyrrhizae*,

2. 营卫不和证

主要证候　汗出恶风,周身酸楚,时寒时热,或表现半身、某局部出汗,苔薄白,脉缓。

治　法　调和营卫。

方　药　桂枝汤加减:桂枝 6 g,白芍药 12 g,茯苓 12 g,生姜 5 片,甘草 3 g。

加　减　汗出多者,酌加煅龙骨 15 g,煅牡蛎 15 g,固涩敛汗。兼气虚者,加黄芪 12 g。兼阳虚者,加熟附子 6 g。如半身或局部出汗者,可加大枣 5 枚,浮小麦 12 g。

3. 心血不足证

主要证候　自汗或盗汗,心悸少寐,神疲气短,面色不华,舌质淡,脉细。

治　法　补血养心。

方　药　归脾汤加减:黄芪 12 g,党参 10 g,白术 10 g,炙甘草 3 g,当归 10 g,熟地黄 12 g,大枣 5 枚,桂圆肉 10 g。

roasted) 3 g, Danggui (*Radix Angelicae Sinensis*) 10 g, Shudihuang (*Radix Rehmanniae Preparata*) 12 g, Dazao (*Fructus Jujubae*) 5 pcs and Guiyuanrou (*Arillus Longan*) 10 g.

　　Modifications: For profuse sweating, add Duanmuli (*Concha Ostreae Usta*, to be decocted first) 20 g, Wuweizi (*Fructus Schisandrae*) 6 g and Fuxiaomai (*Fructus Tritici Levis*) 12 g; for severe blood deficiency, add Zhiheshouwu (*Radix Polygoni Multiflori Preparata*) 10 g and Gouqizi (*Fructus Lycii*) 10 g.

4. Deficiency of Yin and Hyperactivity of Fire

　　Chief Manifestations: Night sweating, or spontaneous sweating, feverish sensation in the palms, soles and chest, or accompanied by afternoon fever, flushed cheeks, thirst, red tongue with little coating, and thready, rapid pulse.

　　Therapeutic Methods: To nourish yin and subdue fire.

　　Prescription: Modified Danggui Liuhuang Tang (Angelicae Sinensis Decoction with Six Ingredients), composed of Danggui (*Radix Angelicae Sinensis*) 10 g, Shengdihuang (*Radix Rehmanniae*) 12 g, Shudihuang (*Radix Rehmanniae Preparata*) 12 g, Huangqin (*Radix Scutellariae*) 10 g, Huanglian (*Rhizoma Coptidis*) 3 g, Huangbo (*Cortex Phellodendri*) 10 g, Baishaoyao (*Radix Paeoniae Alba*) 10 g, Taizishen (*Radix Pseudostellariae*) 10 g, Wuweizi (*Fructus Schisandrae*) 6 g and Wumei (*Fructus Mume*) 6 g.

　　Modifications: For profuse sweating, add Muli (*Concha Ostreae*)30 g, Fuxiaomai (*Fructus Tritici Levis*) 15 g and Nuodaogen (*Rhizoma et Radix Oryzae Glutinosae*) 20 g to stop sweating; for severe afternoon fever, add Qinjiao (*Radix Gentiannae Macrophyllae*) 10 g, Yinchaihu (*Radix Stellariae*) 10 g and Baiwei

　　加　减　汗出多者,加煅牡蛎20 g,五味子6 g,浮小麦12 g;血虚甚者,加制何首乌10 g,枸杞子10 g。

4. 阴虚火旺证

　　主要证候　夜寐盗汗,或有自汗,五心烦热,或兼午后潮热,两颧色红,口渴,舌红少苔,脉细数。

　　治　法　滋阴降火。

　　方　药　当归六黄汤加减:当归10 g,生地黄12 g,熟地黄12 g,黄芩10 g,黄连3 g,黄柏10 g,白芍药10 g,太子参10 g,五味子6 g,乌梅6 g。

　　加　减　汗出多者,加牡蛎30 g、浮小麦15 g、糯稻根20 g以固涩敛汗;潮热甚者,加秦艽10 g、银柴胡10 g、白薇10 g以清退虚热。

(*Radix Cynanchi Atrati*) 10 g to clear away asthenic heat.

5. Accumulation of Pathogenic Heat

Chief Manifestations: Continuous sweating with yellow-stained sweat, flushed face with a hot sensation, restlessness, bitter mouth, yellow urine, thin and yellow tongue coating, wiry and rapid pulse.

Therapeutic Methods: To clear away heat in the liver and dissipate dampness to regulate ying qi.

Prescription: Modified Longdan Xiegan Tang (Gentianae Decoction for Purging Liver Fire), composed of Huangqin (*Radix Scutellariae*) 10 g, Zhizi (*Fructus Gardeniae*) 10 g, Mutong (*Caulis Akebiae*) 3 g, Zexie (*Rhizoma Alismatis*) 12 g, Cheqianzi (*Semen Plantaginis*, wrapped) 10 g, Shengdihuang (*Radix Rehmanniae*) 12 g and Nuodaogen (*Rhizoma et Radix Oryzae Glutinosae*) 20 g.

Modifications: For severe interior heat and scanty urine, add Yinchen (*Herba Artemisiae Scopariae*) 10 g; for less predominant damp heat retention, flushed face and less pronounced thirst, add Huangbai (*Cortex Phellodendri*) 10 g, Cangzhu (*Rhizpma Atractylodis*) 10 g, Yiyiren (*Semen Coicis*) 12 g and Niuxi (*Radix Achyranthis Bidentatae*) 10 g.

Other Treatments

1. Chinese Patent Drugs

(1) Yupingfeng San (Jade Screen Powder): 6 g each time, twice daily; applicable to spontaneous sweating due to qi deficiency.

(2) Longdan Xiegan Wan (Gentianae Pill for Purging Liver Fire): 6 g each time, twice daily; applicable to spontaneous sweating and night sweating due to retained damp heat in the liver and gallbladder.

2. Single-drug or Experiential Prescriptions

(1) Maimendong (*Radix Ophiopogonis*) 12 g,

5. 邪热郁蒸证

主要证候 蒸蒸汗出,汗液易使衣服黄染,面赤烘热,烦躁,口苦,小便色黄,舌苔薄黄,脉象弦数。

治 法 清肝泄热,化湿和营。

方 药 龙胆泻肝汤加减:黄芩10 g,栀子10 g,木通3 g,泽泻12 g,车前子(包煎)10 g,生地黄12 g,糯稻根20 g。

加 减 里热较甚,小便短赤,加茵陈10 g;湿热内蕴而热势不盛,面赤烘热、口苦等症不显著者,可加黄柏10 g,苍术10 g,薏苡仁12 g,牛膝10 g。

【其他疗法】

1. 中成药

(1) 玉屏风散 每服6 g,每日 2 次。适用于气虚自汗。

(2) 龙胆泻肝丸 每服6 g,每日 2 次。适用于肝胆湿热所致之自汗、盗汗。

2. 单验方

(1) 麦门冬、乌梅、五味子

Wumei（*Fructus Mume*）12 g, Wuweizi（*Fructus Schisandrae*）12 g and Dazao（*Fructus Jujubae*）10 pcs. Decoct the above herbs in water and take the decoction in 2 divided doses. It is applicable to night sweating due to yin deficiency.

(2) Equal amounts of Chaihu（*Radix Bupleuri*）and Huhuanglian（*Rhizoma Picrorhizae*）. Grind the above herbs into powder and infuse the powder for oral taking. It is applicable to night sweating due to yin deficiency.

(3) Xianhecao（*Herba Agrimoniae*）30 g and Dazao（*Fructus Jujubae*）15 g. Decoct the herbs in water and take the decoction. It is applicable to night sweating.

(4) Huangqi（*Radix Astragali*）15 g, Fuxiaomai（*Fructus Tritici Levis*）15 g and Dazao（*Fructus Jujubae*）5 pcs. Decoct the herbs in water and take the decoction, 1 dose a day. It is applicable to spontaneous sweating due to qi deficiency.

(5) Mahuanggen（*Radix Ephedrae*）10 g, Muli（*Concha Ostreae*）20 g and Fuxiaomai（*Fructus Tritici Levis*）20 g. Decoct the herbs in water and take the decoction, 1 dose a day. It is applicable to spontaneous sweating.

(6) Wumei（*Fructus Mume*）10 pcs, Fuxiaomai（*Fructus Tritici Levis*）15 g, Sangye（*Folium Mori*）10 g and Dazao（*Fructus Jujubae*）5 pcs. Decoct the herbs in water for oral use. It is applicable to night sweating due to yin deficiency.

(7) Bietaogan（*Fructus Pruni Immaturus*）10 pcs, Fuxiaomai（*Fructus Tritici Levis*）15 g and Dazao（*Fructus Jujubae*）5 pcs. Decoct the herbs in water for oral use, 1 dose a day. It is applicable to night sweating.

3. External Therapy

(1) Grind Wubeizi（*Galla Chinensis*）into powder and add a little water to make paste. Then apply the paste

各12 g,大枣 10 枚,水煎服,每日 1 剂,分 2 次服。适用于阴虚盗汗。

(2) 柴胡、胡黄连各等分,研末冲服。适用于阴虚盗汗。

(3) 仙鹤草 30 g,大枣 15 g,煎服。适用于盗汗。

(4) 黄芪 15 g,浮小麦 15 g,大枣 5 枚,水煎服,每日 1 剂。适用于气虚自汗。

(5) 麻黄根 10 g,牡蛎 20 g,浮小麦 20 g,水煎服,每日 1 剂。适用于自汗。

(6) 乌梅 10 枚,浮小麦 15 g,桑叶 10 g,大枣 5 枚,水煎服。适用于阴虚盗汗。

(7) 瘪桃干 10 枚,浮小麦 15 g,大枣 5 枚,水煎服,每日 1 剂。适用于盗汗。

3. 外治法

(1) 五倍子研粉,加水少许搅成糊状,睡前置于脐部。

to the umbilical region at bed-time and fix it with gauze. It is applicable to night sweating.

(2) Equal amounts of Wubeizi (*Galla Chinensis*) and Baifan (*Alumen*). Grind the above herbs into fine powder, mix up the powder with warm water to make paste. Apply the paste to the umbilical region and fix it with gauze. Change the dressing every other day. It is applicable to night sweating.

(3) Mahuanggen (*Radix Ephedrae*) 50 g, Duanmuli (*Concha Ostreae Usta*) 50 g, Chishizhi (*Halloysitum Rubrum*) 25 g and Longgu (*Os Draconis*) 25 g. Grind the above herbs into fine powder, wrap the powder with a piece of thin, tough silk for dabbing the hidrotic part.

(4) Duanmuli (*Concha Ostreae Usta*) 50 g, Huashi (*Talcum*) 90 g, Mahuanggen (*Radix Ephedrae*) 150 g, Gongdingxiang (*Gemma Caryophylli*) 30 g and Songxiang (*Colophonium*) 60 g. Grind the above herbs into fine powder, wrap 15 g of the powder with a piece of thin, tough silk and dab the hidrotic part until sweating stops.

(5) Baifan (*Alumen*) 20 g and Gegen (*Radix Puerariae*) 20 g. Decoct the herbs in water and wash the hands and feet with the decoction several times a day. It is applicable to polyhidrosis of hands and feet.

2.7.7 Edema

General Description

Edema, marked by swelling of the head, face, eyelids, limbs, abdomen and back, and even the whole body, is a morbid condition caused by invasion of pathogenic factors, improper diet, or overstrain which result in failure of the lungs to regulate the water passage, failure of the spleen to transport and transform body fluids, fail-

并用纱布固定。适用于盗汗。

（2）五倍子、白矾等分为末,以温水调湿填脐中,外用纱布固定,隔日取之。适用于盗汗。

（3）麻黄根、煅牡蛎各50 g,赤石脂、龙骨各25 g,共研细末,以绢包扑汗用。

（4）煅牡蛎50 g,滑石90 g,麻黄根150 g,公丁香30 g,净松香60 g,共研细末,以绢包15 g,扑汗处,汗止为度。

（5）白矾20 g,葛根20 g,煎水洗手足,每日数次。适用于手足汗多。

第七节　水肿

【概述】

水肿是指因感受外邪、饮食失调或劳倦过度,使肺失通调,脾失转输,肾失开合,膀胱气化不利,导致体内水液潴留,泛滥肌肤,表现以头面、眼睑、四肢、腹背,甚至全身浮肿

ure of the kidneys to regulate water metabolism, and failure of the urinary bladder to control urination, thus giving rise to abnormal fluid retention in the body and further involving the muscles and skin.

Invasion of pathogenic wind, retention of noxious dampness, retention of water and dampness, improper diet, prolonged illness, stress and excessive sexual activities are considered as the main causes of edema. It usually occurs when the function of qi activity is impaired. In terms of viscera, the transportation and transformation of body fluids are related to the lungs, spleen and kidneys, but more closely to the kidneys. Besides, if there exists blood stasis and the functioning of the triple energizers is impaired, edema will be obstinate and unresponsive to treatment.

Edema may be seen in acute and chronic glomerulonephritis, nephrotic syndrome, congestive heart failure, endocrine disturbance and dystrophy in western medicine.

Essentials for Diagnosis

(1) Edema usually begins from eyelids or lower limbs, and then spreads to four limbs and the entire body. In mild cases, there may be light swelling around the eyelids or in the tibia while in severe cases, generalized swelling, abdominal fullness and enlargement, asthmatic breathing with inability to lie supine may be present. In even more severe cases, retention of urine, nausea, vomiting, foul breath, nasal bleeding, atrophy of the gum or even headache, convulsion, coma and delirium may occur.

(2) The patient may have a history of tonsillitis, palpitation, septicemia or purpura, or invalidism.

(3) Urine routine examination, 24-hour quantitative

为特征的一类病证。

水肿的病因主要有风邪外袭、湿毒浸淫、水湿浸渍、饮食不当、久病劳欲等。水肿的发生,主要是全身气化功能障碍的表现。就脏腑而言,人体水液的运化,主要与肺、脾、肾有关,但与肾的关系更为密切。此外,瘀血阻滞、三焦水道不利,往往可使水肿顽固难愈。

水肿与西医学中的急慢性肾小球肾炎、肾病综合征、充血性心力衰竭、内分泌失调,以及营养障碍等疾病所出现的水肿较为相近。

【诊断要点】

(1) 水肿先从眼睑或下肢开始,继及四肢和全身。轻者仅眼睑或足胫浮肿,重者全身皆肿,甚则腹大胀满,气喘不能平卧。更严重者可见尿闭、恶心呕吐、口有秽味、鼻衄牙宣,甚则头痛、抽搐、神昏、谵语等危象。

(2) 可有乳蛾、心悸、疮毒、紫癜以及久病体虚病史。

(3) 尿常规、24 小时尿蛋

determination of urinary protein, blood routine examination, determination of blood sedimentation rate, plasma albumin, creatinine, urea nitrogen in blood and humoral immunity, as well as electrocardiography, cardiac functional test and B-type ultrasonic examination for the kidneys are the necessary means in the diagnosis of edema.

Syndrome Differentiation and Treatment

To make the diagnosis of edema, it is essential to clarify whether the complaint is edema of the yang type or edema of the yin type. Usually the yang-type edema is characterized by a short duration, a rapid development, more pronounced edema on the head and face with the skin shiny and thin. However, the yin-type edema is marked by a longer duration, a gradual development, more pronounced pitted edema of lower limbs, sallow and grayish skin. The treatment for the yang-type should aim at eliminating pathogenic factors, with such methods as diaphoresis and diuresis. When necessary, purgation should be used. For the yin-type, it is advisable to support healthy qi to eliminate pathogenic factors, for instance, to promote diuresis by invigorating the spleen and warming the kidneys. If edema is persistent, promoting diuresis by activating blood circulation and dissipating blood stasis is recommended as the accessory treatment.

1. Invasion by Wind and Overflow of Water

Chief Manifestations: Acute onset, edema starting from the eyelids, followed by four limbs and the whole body, aversion to cold, fever, soreness of the limbs and joints, dysuria, etc. In cases with predominant wind heat, there may also be swelling and pain in the throat, red tongue, superficial, smooth and rapid pulse. In cases with predominant wind cold, aversion to cold, cough, dyspnea, thin white tongue coating, and superficial, smooth or superficial, tense pulse may be present.

白定量、血常规、血沉、血浆白蛋白、血尿素氮、肌酐、体液免疫以及心电图、心功能测定、肾 B 超等检查,以助明确诊断。

【辨证论治】

水肿的辨证主要应辨别阳水、阴水。阳水病程较短,病势较急,浮肿主要在头面部,皮肤光亮而薄,呈凹陷性水肿,按之易复;阴水病程较长,病势缓,浮肿部位主要在下肢,皮肤萎黄、灰滞,亦呈凹陷性水肿,但按之难复。阳水治疗以祛邪为主,常用治法为发汗、利小便,必要时可酌用攻逐法。阴水一般需扶正祛邪并进,多以健脾温肾利水为主;若水肿日久不退,宜配用活血化瘀利水法。

1. 风水泛滥证

主要证候 眼睑浮肿,继则四肢及全身皆肿,来势迅速,多有恶寒、发热、肢节酸楚、小便不利等症。偏于风热者,伴咽喉红肿疼痛,舌质红,脉浮滑数。偏于风寒,兼恶寒,咳喘,舌苔薄白,脉浮滑或浮紧。

Therapeutic Methods: To eliminate wind, disperse lung qi, circulate water to relieve edema.

Prescription: Modified Yuebi Jia Zhu Tang (Yuebi Decoction with Atractylodis Macrocephalae), composed of Mahuang (*Herba Ephedrae*) 6 g, Shigao (*Gypsum Fibrosum*, to be decocted first) 30 g, Xingren (*Semen Armeniacae Amarum*) 10 g, Baizhu (*Rhizoma Atractylodis Macrocephalae*) 10 g, Fuling (*Poria*) 12 g and Zexie (*Rhizoma Alismatis*) 12 g.

Modifications: For predominance of wind heat, add Lianqiao (*Fructus Forsythiae*) 15 g, Jiegeng (*Radix Platycodi*) 6 g, Banlangen (*Radix Isatidis*) 15 g and Xianmaogen (*Rhizoma Imperatae*, fresh) 12 g; for predominance of wind cold, remove Shigao and add Zisuye (*Folium Perillae*) 10 g, Guizhi (*Ramulus Cinnamomi*) 6 g and Fangfeng (*Radix Saposhnikoviae*) 6 g; for severe cough and dyspnea, add Qianhu (*Radix Peucedani*) 10 g and Ziyuan (*Radix Asteris*) 10 g; for sweating with aversion to wind and deficiency of wei qi, add Fangji (*Radix Stephaniae Tetrandrae*) 10 g and Huangqi (*Radix Astragali*) 15 g.

2. Retention of Noxious Dampness

Chief Manifestations: Edema of the eyelids followed by generalized edema, dysuria, pyogenic infection, or even ulceration of skin, fever with aversion to wind, red tongue with thin yellow coating, and superficial, rapid or smooth, rapid pulse.

Therapeutic Methods: To disperse lung qi, remove toxic substance, and promote diuresis to relieve edema.

Prescription: Modified Mahuang Lianyao Chixiaodou Tang (Decoction of Ephedrae, Forsythiae and Phaseoli) and Wuwei Xiaodu Yin (Antiphlogistic Decoction of Five Ingredients), composed of Mahuang (*Herba Ephedrae*) 6 g, Xingren (*Semen Armeniacae Amarum*) 10 g,

治　法　疏风宣肺,行水消肿。

方　药　越婢加术汤加减:麻黄6 g,石膏(先煎)30 g,杏仁10 g,白术10 g,茯苓12 g,泽泻12 g。

加　减　若属风热偏盛,可加连翘15 g,桔梗6 g,板蓝根15 g,鲜茅根12 g;若风寒偏盛,去石膏,加紫苏叶10 g,桂枝6 g,防风6 g;若咳喘较甚,可加前胡10 g,紫菀10 g;若见汗出恶风,卫阳已虚,加防己10 g,黄芪15 g。

2. 湿毒浸淫证

主要证候　眼睑浮肿,延及全身,小便不利,身发疮痍,甚则溃烂,恶风发热,舌质红,苔薄黄,脉浮数或滑数。

治　法　宣肺解毒,利湿消肿。

方　药　麻黄连轺赤小豆汤合五味消毒饮加减:麻黄6 g,杏仁10 g,桑白皮10 g,赤小豆12 g,金银花15 g,连翘15 g,野菊花15 g,蒲公英15 g,

Sangbaipi (*Cortex Mori*) 10 g, Chixiaodou (*Semen Phaseoli*) 12 g, Jinyinhua (*Flos Lonicerae*) 15 g, Lian-qiao (*Fructus Forsythiae*) 15 g, Yejuhua (*Flos Chrysanthemi Indici*) 15 g, Pugongying (*Herba Taraxaci*) 15 g, Zihuadiding (*Herba Violae*) 15 g and Zibeitiankui (*Herba Senecionis Nudicaulis*) 15 g.

Modifications: For predominant dampness with skin ulceration, add Kushen (*Radix Sophorae Flavescentis*) 15 g and Tufuling (*Rhizoma Smilacis Glabrae*) 15 g; for predominant wind with itching, add Baixianpi (*Cortex Dictamni*) 12 g and Difuzi (*Fructus Kochiae*) 12 g; for blood heat with red and swollen skin, add Mudanpi (*Cortex Moutan Radicis*) 10 g and Chishaoyao (*Radix Paeoniae Rubra*) 10 g; for constipation, add Sheng-dahuang (*Radix et Rhizoma Rhei*, to be decocted later) 6 g and Mangxiao (*Natrii Sulfas*, to be infused separately) 6 g.

3. Retention of Water and Dampness

Chief Manifestations: Pitted edema of the whole body, scanty urine, heaviness of the body, feeling of oppression in the chest, poor appetite, nausea, greasy white tongue coating, and deep, even-soft pulse.

Therapeutic Methods: To invigorate the spleen, eliminate dampness, activate yang and promote diuresis.

Prescription: Modified Wupi Yin (Five Peels Decoction) and Weiling Tang (Poria Decoction for Regulating Stomach), composed of Cangzhu (*Rhizoma Atractylodis*) 10 g, Houpo (*Cortex Magnoliae Officinalis*) 10 g, Chenpi (*Pericarpium Citri Reticulatae*) 6 g, Guizhi (*Ramulus Cinnamomi*) 6 g, Fuling (*Poria*) 12 g, Zexie (*Rhizoma Alismatis*) 12 g, Shengjiangpi (*Cortex Zingiberis Rhizomatis*) 3 g and Dafupi (*Pericarpium Arecae*) 12 g.

Modification: For severe edema with asthma, add

紫花地丁15 g,紫背天葵15 g。

加 减 若湿盛而皮肤糜烂者,加苦参15 g,土茯苓15 g;若风盛而瘙痒者,加白鲜皮12 g,地肤子12 g;若血热而红肿,加牡丹皮10 g,赤芍药10 g;若大便不通,加生大黄(后下)6 g,芒硝(另冲)6 g。

3. 水湿浸渍证

主要证候 全身水肿,按之没指,小便短少,身体困重,胸闷,纳呆,泛恶,苔白腻,脉沉缓。

治 法 健脾化湿,通阳利水。

方 药 五皮饮合胃苓汤加减:苍术10 g,厚朴10 g,陈皮6 g,桂枝6 g,茯苓12 g,泽泻12 g,生姜皮3 g,大腹皮12 g。

加 减 若肿甚而喘,可

Mahuang (*Herba Ephedrae*) 5 g, Xingren (*Semen Armeniacae Amarum*) 10 g and Tinglizi (*Semen Lepidii seu Descurainiae*) 10 g.

4. Excess of Damp Heat

Chief Manifestations: General edema with the skin shiny and taut, fullness in the chest and abdomen, restless fever, thirst, scanty deep yellow urine, or dry stools, red tongue with yellow greasy coating, and deep, rapid or soft-superficial, rapid pulse.

Therapeutic Methods: To clear away heat, promote diuresis and regulate qi circulation.

Prescription: Modified Shuzao Yinzi (Decoction for Diuresis), composed of Mutong (*Caulis Akebiae*) 6 g, Zexie (*Rhizoma Alismatis*) 12 g, Fulingpi (*Cortex Sclerotii Poriae*) 12 g, Chixiaodou (*Semen Phaseoli*) 12 g, Huangbo (*Cortex Phellodendri*) 10 g, Zhuling (*Polyporus*) 12 g, Shanglu (*Radix Phytolaccae*) 6 g, Binglang (*Semen Arecae*) 10 g, Cangzhu (*Rhizoma Atractylodis*) 10 g and Shengyiyiren (*Semen Coicis*) 12 g.

Modifications: For abdominal flatulence and constipation, add Shengdahuang (*Radix et Rhizoma Rhei*, to be decocted later) 6 g and Tinglizi (*Semen Lepidii seu Descurainiae*) 10 g; for retention of damp heat in the urinary bladder damaging the blood vessels, manifested as painful urination and hematuria, add Daji (*Herba seu Radix Cirsii Japonici*) 12 g, Xiaoji (*Herba Cirsii*) 12 g and Baimaogen (*Rhizoma Imperatae*) 20 g; for severe edema accompanied by chest oppression, asthmatic breathing, inability to lie supine, and wiry, forceful pulse, add Tinglizi (*Semen Lepidii seu Descurainiae*) 10 g, Xingren (*Semen Armeniacae Amarum*) 10 g and Fangji (*Radix Stephaniae Tetrandrae*) 10 g; for long-standing retention of damp heat transforming into dryness which further damages yin, manifested as dry mouth and throat

加麻黄5 g,杏仁10 g,葶苈子10 g。

4. 湿热壅盛证

主要证候 遍体浮肿,皮肤绷急光亮,胸脘痞闷,烦热口渴,小便短赤,或大便干结,舌红,苔黄腻,脉沉数或濡数。

治　法 清热利湿,疏利气机。

方　药 疏凿饮子加减:木通6 g,泽泻12 g,茯苓皮12 g,赤小豆12 g,黄柏10 g,猪苓12 g,商陆6 g,槟榔10 g,苍术10 g,生薏苡仁12 g。

加　减 若腹部胀满,大便不通者,加生大黄(后下)6 g,葶苈子10 g;若湿热之邪下注膀胱,伤及血络,症见尿痛、尿血者,加大蓟12 g,小蓟12 g,白茅根20 g;若肿势严重,兼胸闷气喘,不能平卧,脉弦有力者,加葶苈子10 g,杏仁10 g,防己10 g;若湿热久羁,化燥伤阴,症见口燥咽干,大便干结,可加猪苓10 g,滑石(包煎)12 g,麦门冬10 g,阿胶(烊化冲服)10 g。

and dry stools, add Zhuling (*Polyporus*) 10 g, Huashi
(*Talcum*, wrapped) 12 g, Maimendong (*Radix Ophiopogonis*) 10 g and Ejiao (*Colla Corii Asini*, to be melted
and infused separately) 10 g.

5. Deficiency of Spleen Yang

Chief Manifestations: General pitted edema which
is more pronounced below the loins, abdominal flatulence,
impaired appetite, loose stools, lusterless complexion,
lassitude, cold limbs, small amount of urine, pale tongue
with greasy white coating or smooth white coating, and
deep, even-soft or deep, weak pulse.

Therapeutic Methods: To warm and invigorate
spleen yang so as to promote diuresis.

Prescription: Modified Shipi Yin (Decoction for Invigorating Spleen), composed of Zhifuzi (*Radix Aconiti
Lateralis Preparata*) 6 g, Ganjiang (*Rhizoma Zingiberis*) 3 g, Caoguo (*Fructus Tsaoko*) 6 g, Baizhu (*Rhizoma Atractylodis Macrocephalae*) 10 g, Fuling (*Poria*)
12 g, Jiaomu (*Semen Zanthoxyli*) 6 g, Houpo (*Cortex
Magnoliae Officinalis*) 6 g, Muxiang (*Radix Aucklandiae*) 10 g and Dafupi (*Pericarpium Arecae*) 12 g.

Modifications: For short breath and weak voice,
add Dangshen (*Radix Codonopsis*) 12 g and Huangqi (*Radix Astragali*) 15 g; for small amount of urine, add Guizhi
(*Ramulus Cinnamomi*) 6 g and Zexie (*Rhizoma Alismatis*) 12 g.

6. Deficiency of Kidney Yang

Chief Manifestations: General pitted edema which
is more pronounced below the loins, palpitation, short
breath, soreness and heaviness in the loins, decreased
quantity of urine, cold limbs, aversion to cold, lassitude,
pale or grayish dim complexion, pale and swollen tongue
with white coating, deep and thready or deep, slow and
forceless pulse.

5. 脾阳虚衰证

主要证候 身肿,腰以下
为甚,按之凹陷不易恢复,脘
腹胀闷,纳减便溏,面色不华,
神倦肢冷,小便短少,舌质淡,
苔白腻或白滑,脉沉缓或
沉弱。

治 法 温运脾阳,以利
水湿。

方 药 实脾饮加减:
制附子6 g,干姜3 g,草果6 g,
白术10 g,茯苓12 g,椒目6 g,
厚朴6 g,木香10 g,大腹皮
12 g。

加 减 若气短声弱,可
加党参12 g,黄芪15 g;若小便
短少,可加桂枝6 g,泽泻12 g。

6. 肾阳衰微证

主要证候 面浮身肿,腰
以下尤甚,按之凹陷不起,心
悸,气促,腰部酸重,尿量减
少,四肢厥冷,怯寒神疲,面色
㿠白或灰滞,舌质淡胖,苔白,
脉沉细或沉迟无力。

Therapeutic Methods: To warm the kidney, assist yang, activate qi to promote diuresis.

Prescription: Modified Jisheng Shenqi Wan (Pill for Replenishing Kidney Qi from Prescriptions for Saving Life) and Zhenwu Tang (Zhenwu Decoction), composed of Zhifuzi (*Radix Aconiti Lateralis Preparata*) 6 g, Rougui (*Cortex Cinnamomi*) 3 g, Bajitian (*Radix Morindae Officinalis*) 10 g, Yinyanghuo (*Herba Epimedii*) 10 g, Baizhu (*Rhizoma Atractylodis Macrocephalae*) 10 g, Fuling (*Poria*) 12 g, Zexie (*Rhizoma Alismatis*) 12 g, Cheqianzi (*Semen Plantaginis*, wrapped) 12 g, Niuxi (*Radix Achyranthis Bidentatae*) 10 g and Shanyao (*Rhizoma Dioscoreae*) 12 g.

Modifications: If there is palpitation, cyanotic lips, feeble pulse, or slow-irregular and intermittent pulse, increase Zhifuzi to 12 g and add Guizhi (*Ramulus Cinnamomi*) 6 g, Zhigancao (*Radix Glycyrrhizae*, roasted) 3 g and Danshen (*Radix Salviae Miltiorrhizae*) 12 g. If there is asthmatic breathing, sweating, and superficial, feeble and rapid pulse, add Hongshen (*Radix Ginseng Rubra*, to be decocted separately) 10 g, Gejiefen (*Pulvis Gecko*, powdered and to be infused separately) 1 g, Wuweizi (*Fructus Schisandrae*) 6 g, Shanzhuyu (*Fructus Corni*) 10 g, Muli (*Concha Ostreae*, to be decocted first) 15 g and Longgu (*Os Draconis*, to be decocted first) 15 g. If deficiency of kidney yang is persistent, it impairs yin, giving rise to deficiency of kidney yin. In this case, there appear such manifestations as recurrence of edema, lassitude, soreness in the loins, nocturnal emmission, dry mouth and throat, feverish sensation in the palms, soles and chest, red tongue and thready, rapid pulse. The treatment then should aim at nourishing kidney yin and promoting diuresis concurrently. The alternative prescription is: Shanyao (*Rhizoma Dioscoreae*) 12 g,

治　法　温肾助阳,化气行水。

方　药　《济生》肾气丸合真武汤加减:制附子6 g,肉桂3 g,巴戟天10 g,淫羊藿10 g,白术10 g,茯苓12 g,泽泻12 g,车前子(包煎)12 g,牛膝10 g,山药12 g。

加　减　若心悸、唇绀、脉虚或结代,重用制附子12 g,再加桂枝6 g,炙甘草3 g,丹参12 g;若见喘促、汗出、脉虚浮而数,加红参(另煎)10 g,蛤蚧粉(另冲)1 g,五味子6 g,山茱萸10 g,牡蛎(先煎)15 g,龙骨(先煎)15 g。若因肾阳久衰,阳损及阴,可导致肾阴亏虚,症见水肿反复发作,精神疲惫,腰酸遗精,口燥咽干,五心烦热,舌红,脉细数等,治宜滋补肾阴为主,兼利水湿,可改用山药12 g,山茱萸10 g,枸杞子12 g,牡丹皮10 g,泽泻12 g,茯苓12 g。

Shanzhuyu (*Fructus Corni*) 10 g, Gouqizi (*Fructus Lycii*) 12 g, Mudanpi (*Cortex Moutan Radicis*) 10 g, Zexie (*Rhizoma Alismatis*) 12 g and Fuling (*Poria*) 12 g.

Other Treatments

1. Chinese Patent Drugs

(1) Jingui Shenqi Wan (Pill for Replenishing Kidney Qi from Golden Cabinet): 6 g each time, twice daily, per os; applicable to edema due to deficiency of kidney yang.

(2) Renshen Jianpi Wan (Ginseng Pill for Invigorating Spleen): 6 g each time, twice daily, per os; applicable to edema due to deficiency of the spleen and stomach.

(3) Shen Ling Baizhu Wan (Pill of Ginseng, Poria and Atractylodis Macrocephalae): 6 g each time, twice daily, per os; applicable to edema due to deficiency of qi and blood, stagnation of qi and retention of dampness which result from deficiency of the spleen with failure to generate blood.

(4) Liuwei Dihuang Wan (Pill of Six Drugs Containing Rehmanniae): 6 g each time, twice daily, per os; applicable to edema due to deficiency of kidney yin.

(5) Kongxian Dan (Pill for Controlling Phlegm Fluid): Take the pills at a draught on empty stomach every morning with the dosage gradually increased from 1.5 g to 4.5 g and decreased when the pills take effect. In case of stomachache and diarrhea, suspend the pills immediately. It is applicable to the case with strong constitution suffering from pronounced edema and scanty urine.

(6) Dahuang Zhechong Wan (Pill of Rhei and Eupolyphaga seu Steleophaga): 3 g each time, thrice daily, per os; applicable to edema with blood stasis.

2. Single-drug or Experiential Prescriptions

(1) Grind the stir-baked Hulupiao (*Pericarpium Lagenariae Sicerariae*) 30 g into fine powder, mix the powder with rice gruel and take it every day. It is applica-

【其他疗法】

1. 中成药

(1)《金匮》肾气丸　每服6 g,每日 2 次,口服。适用于肾阳不足之水肿。

(2) 人参健脾丸　每服6 g,每日 2 次,口服。适用于脾胃虚弱之水肿。

(3) 参苓白术丸　每服6 g,每日 2 次,口服。适用于脾虚化源不足,气血亏虚,气滞湿停之水肿。

(4) 六味地黄丸　每服6 g,每日 2 次,口服。适用于肾阴亏虚之水肿。

(5) 控涎丹　每日用量1.5～4.5 g,晨起空腹顿服。剂量从小到大,见效后即减量。腹痛、腹泻明显者立即停药。适用于水肿明显,小便量少,而身体壮实者。

(6) 大黄䗪虫丸　每服3 g,每日 3 次,口服。适用于水肿而有瘀血者。

2. 单验方

(1) 葫芦瓢30 g,微炒后研为末,每日和入粥中服用。适用于水肿不消,小便量

ble to persistent edema with scanty urine.

(2) Decoct Yumixu (*Stylus Zeae Maydis*) 50 g with 600 ml of water for 20 – 30 minutes or to 300 – 400 ml of the decoction. Filter the decoction for oral taking, 1 dose a day. It is applicable to edema with scanty urine.

(3) Stew a carp (about 500 g) in water with ginger (30 g), spring onion (60 g) and Shenghuangqi (Radix Astragali) 50 g. Take the soup and also the carp without putting in any salt. It is applicable to edema with difficulty in urination, shortness of breath and lassitude.

(4) Decoct Yimucao (*Herba Leonuri*, *dried*) 125 g in 800 ml of water to collect 300 ml of the decoction. Take the decoction in 4 divided doses, once every 3 hours. It is applicable to kidney disease with edema and difficulty in urination.

(5) Cook a Donggua (*Fructus Benincasae*) (2,000 g) and Chixiaodou (*Semen Phaseoli*) 120 g thoroughly and take them in 2 divided doses every day. It is applicable to edema with difficulty in urination.

3. External Therapy

(1) Decoct Zisuye (*Folium Perillae*) 500 g in water and wash the body with the decoction, once or twice a week. It is applicable to edema on the head and face.

(2) Crush 2 – 3 river snails with 15 g of salt into a mash and apply the mash to the navel and the area two fingers in width below the navel, once daily. It is applicable to edema with ascites or retention of urine.

少者。

（2）玉米须 50 g，加水 600 ml，用温水煎煮 20～30 分钟，或煎至 300～400 ml，经过滤后口服，每日 1 剂。适用于小便量少者。

（3）生黄芪50 g，鲤鱼 1 条（500 g左右），生姜30 g，葱60 g，炖汤不放盐，喝汤吃鱼。适用于水肿，小便不利，气短乏力者。

（4）益母草125 g，晒干，加水800 ml，煎至 300 ml，去渣分 4 次服，隔 3 小时服 1 次。适用于肾病水肿，小便不利。

（5）冬瓜 1 只（重约 2 000 g），赤小豆120 g，将冬瓜和赤小豆共煮烂，每日分 2 次服完。适用于水肿，小便不利。

3. 外治法

（1）紫苏叶500 g，煎汤全身淋洗，每星期 1～2 次。适用于水肿以头面为甚者。

（2）田螺肉 2～3 只，细盐 15 g，捣烂敷脐和脐下两指处，日换 1 次。适用于水肿伴有腹水或尿闭者。

2.8 Other Diseases

2.8.1 Simple Obesity

General Description

Obesity is an increase of body weight 20% higher than the normal standard. It is caused by over-intake of heat energy which is beyond the requirement of the human body and stored as excessive fat in the body. Usually it falls into two categories: simple obesity and secondary obesity. Simple obesity has no obvious endocrine-metabolic disturbance but comes into being from childhood. Clinically it is manifested as overweight and fatigue accompanied by abdominal flatulence, heavy limbs, fullness over the chest, short breath, palpitation and hyperhidrosis. Though it may be seen at any age, obesity is mostly seen in middle aged and older groups. With the improvement of the living standards, more and more people suffer from obesity and its related diseases such as hyperlipemia, coronary atherosclerotic heart disease, hypertension, diabetes, fatty liver, cholelithiasis, apoplexy, etc., which has already aroused universal concern. Secondary obesity may have the symptoms of primary diseases like hypothalamic syndrome and Cushing's syndrome. Some related nervous, mental and endocrine examinations should be made to determine the diagnosis.

Obesity results from endogenous and exogenous

第八章 其他病证

第一节 单纯性肥胖

【概述】

肥胖是由于进食热量多于人体消耗量而以脂肪形式储存于体内,使体重超过标准体重20%以上,通常分为单纯性和继发性两大类。单纯性肥胖一般指无明显内分泌代谢病因,自幼年起即有肥胖者。临床表现以体态肥胖,疲倦乏力为主,并且多见腹胀肢沉,胸闷气促,心悸多汗等症。本病虽可见于任何年龄组,但尤以中年以后多见。随着人们生活水平的提高,肥胖症与之相关的病证,如高脂血症、冠状动脉粥样硬化性心脏病、高血压病、糖尿病、脂肪肝、胆石症、中风等日渐增多,故已引起普遍关注。继发性肥胖可有原发病的症状,如下丘脑综合征、库欣综合征等,应作神经、精神、内分泌等方面的有关检查明确诊断。

本病的病因和发病机理

factors. The former refers to various intrinsic factors (heredity, neuropychosis, metabolism, endocrine) which affect the regulation of the fat metabolism, and the latter includes hyperphagia and hypoactivity.

According to its clinical manifestations, obesity pertains to the categories of "fei pang" (overweight) or "tan yin" (fat man). Its etiology is related to congenital disposition, over-intake of greasy food, prolonged lying or sitting, deficiency of healthy qi due to protracted illness, and emotional upset. It mainly involves the spleen and muscles, but is closely related to the deficiency of kidney qi. Generally, its pathogenesis is principal deficiency and secondary excess. Principal deficiency is marked by qi deficiency, mostly deficiency of spleen qi and kidney qi, which may be accompanied with deficiency of heart qi and spleen qi and failure of the liver and gallbladder to control dispersion; secondary excess is mainly the retention of turbid phlegm and fat accompanied with dampness, blood stasis and qi stagnation.

Essentials for Diagnosis

(1) Overweight: Standard weight (kg) = [height (cm) − 100] × 0.9. If the actual body weight exceeds the standard weight by 20% and muscularity and water retention are excluded, this can be diagnosed as obesity.

(2) Fat accumulation: Fat accumulation can be estimated by the thickness of skin fold. The average thickness of subscapular skin fold of a normal person aged 25 is 14.2 mm. The average thickness of skin fold of the deltoid region of a 25-year-old male is 10.4 mm, and that of a 25-year-old female is 17.5 mm.

(3) It may be accompanied with the following symp-

可归纳为内因和外因两方面。内因为内在的各种因素(遗传、神经精神、物质代谢、内分泌)对脂肪代谢等调节失常所致。外因则以饮食过多而活动过少为主。

根据本病的临床表现,当属于中医学"肥胖"、"痰饮"等范畴。其病因与先天禀赋、过食肥甘、久卧久坐、久病正虚、情志所伤有关。病位主要在脾与肌肉,但与肾气虚衰关系密切。病机总属本虚标实,本虚以气虚为主,多见脾肾气虚,可兼见心脾气虚及肝胆疏泄失调;其标实以痰浊膏脂为主,兼有水湿、瘀血、气滞等。

【诊断要点】

(1) 超出标准体重   标准体重(kg) = 〔身高(cm) − 100〕× 0.9,若实际体重超过标准体重 20%,排除肌肉发达或水分潴留因素,即可诊断肥胖。

(2) 脂肪堆积程度   可用皮褶度估计。25 岁正常人肩胛下皮褶厚度平均为 14.2 mm;三角肌部位皮褶厚度,25 岁男性平均为 10.4 mm,女性平均为 17.5 mm。

(3) 可伴有神疲乏力,嗜

toms: listlessness, lassitude, drowsiness, palpitation, hyperorexia, hypologia, short breath, dyspnea, big belly and abdominal distension, or amenorrhea, impotence, aversion to heat, profuse sweating, pain of the back and loins, and arthragia.

Syndrome Differentiation and Treatment

The syndrome differentiation for this disease is mainly to determine which is predominant: principal deficiency or secondary excess. Accumulation of heat in the spleen and stomach, internal retention of phlegm and stagnation of qi and blood are characteristic of secondary excess, while dysfunction of the spleen in transportation and transformation, deficiency of spleen yang and kidney yang are typical of principal deficiency. The treatment is based on the principle of supporting healthy qi and eliminating pathogenic factors. The following methods can be adopted accordingly: recuperating and invigorating the spleen and kidney, dispersing the stagnated liver qi and gallbladder qi, dissipating dampness and eliminating phlegm, promoting diuresis to remove blood stasis, promoting digestion and purging fu-organs.

1. Accumulation of Heat in the Spleen and Stomach

Chief Manifestations: Polyphagia, polyorexia, fat physique, abdominal fullness and distention, rosy cheeks, dry mouth with bitter taste, restlessness, dizziness, burning pain and upset in the stomach relieved after eating, red tongue with yellow and greasy coating, wiry and smooth pulse.

Therapeutic Methods: To purge stomach fire and promote digestion as the auxiliary treatment.

Prescription: Modified Xiao Chengqi Tang (Decoction for Mild Purgation) and Baohe Wan (Lenitive Pill), composed of Shengdahuang (*Radix et Rhizoma Rhei*, to

睡心悸,食欲亢进,少气懒言,气短气喘,腹大胀满,或闭经,阳痿,怕热多汗,腰背痛,关节痛等症状。

【辨证论治】

本病辨证主要辨其标本虚实的主次。脾胃积热、痰浊内盛和气滞血瘀证以标实为主,脾虚不运、脾肾阳虚证以本虚为主。治疗以扶正驱邪为原则,根据标本虚实,分别采取调补脾肾、疏肝利胆、化湿祛痰、利水化瘀、消导通腑等法。

1. 脾胃积热证

主要证候　多食,消谷善饥,形体肥胖,脘腹胀满,面色红润,口干口苦,心烦头昏,胃脘灼痛嘈杂,得食则缓,舌质红,苔黄腻,脉弦滑。

治　法　清胃泻火,佐以消导。

方　药　小承气汤合保和丸加减:生大黄(后下)10 g,枳实10 g,泽泻15 g,焦山

be decocted later) 10 g, Zhishi (*Fructus Aurantii Immaturus*) 10 g, Zexie (*Rhizoma Alismatis*) 15 g, Jiaoshanzha (*Fructus Crataegi*, charred) 10 g, Jiaoliuqu (*Massa Medicata Fermentata*, charred) 12 g, Fuling (*Poria*) 15 g, Zhibanxia (*Rhizoma Pinelliae Preparata*) 10 g and Jineijin (*Corium Stomachicum Galli*) 10 g.

Modifications: For excessive stomach heat, add Huanglian (*Rhizoma Coptidis*) 5 g and Zhizi (*Radix Gardeniae*) 10 g; for bitter taste in the mouth and distending pain over the hypochondrium, add Yinchen (*Herba Artemisiae Scopariae*) 15 g and Caojueming (*Semen Cassiae*) 15 g.

2. Dysfunction of the Spleen in Transportation

Chief Manifestations: Fat physique, listlessness, lassitude, bodily heaviness, chest distress and abdominal distention, slight edema of limbs which is alleviated in the morning and aggravated in the evening and after over-work, normal or impaired appetite, indulgence in eating and drinking, dysuria, loose stools or constipation, swollen pale tongue with teeth marks on its margin, thin and white or white and greasy coating, soft-superficial and thready pulse.

Therapeutic Methods: To invigorate the spleen, benefit qi, promote diuresis and eliminate dampness.

Prescription: Modified Shen Ling Baizhu San (Powder of Ginseng, Poria and Atractylodis Macrocephalae) and Fangji Huangqi Tang (Decoction of Stephaniae Tetrandrae and Astragali), composed of Huangqi (*Radix Astragali*) 15 g, Dangshen (*Radix Codonopsis*) 12 g, Cangzhu (*Rhizoma Atractylodis*) 10 g, Baizhu (*Rhizoma Atractylodis Macrocephalae*) 10 g, Fangji (*Radix Stephaniae Tetrandrae*) 10 g, Fuling (*Poria*) 15 g, Cheqianzi (*Semen Plantaginis*, wrapped) 15 g, Zexie

楂10 g,焦六曲12 g,茯苓15 g,制半夏10 g,鸡内金10 g。

加 减 胃热盛者,加黄连5 g,栀子10 g;口苦,胁肋胀痛者,加茵陈15 g,草决明15 g。

2. 脾虚不运证

主要证候 肥胖臃肿,神疲乏力,身体困重,胸闷脘胀,四肢轻度浮肿,晨轻暮重,劳累后明显,饮食如常或偏少,既往多有暴饮暴食史,小便不利,便溏或便秘,舌淡胖边有齿印,苔薄白或白腻,脉濡细。

治 法 健脾益气,渗利水湿。

方 药 参苓白术散合防己黄芪汤加减:黄芪15 g,党参12 g,苍术10 g,白术10 g,防己 10 g,茯苓15 g,车前子(包煎)15 g,泽泻15 g,桂枝10 g,甘草6 g。

(*Rhizoma Alismatis*) 15 g, Guizhi (*Ramulus Cinnamomi*) 10 g and Gancao (*Radix Glycyrrhizae*) 6 g.

Modifications: For swollen limbs, add Dafupi (*Pericarpium Arecae*) 10 g and Sangbaipi (*Cortex Mori Radicis*) 10 g; for abdominal distention and loose stools, add Chenpi (*Pericarpium Citri Reticulatae*) 10 g and Laifuzi (*Semen Raphani*) 10 g; for short breath, aversion to cold and cold limbs, add Rougui (*Cortex Cinnamomi*, to be decocted later) 3 g; for lack of appetite, add Foshou (*Fructus Citri Sarcodactylis*) 6 g, Jiaoshanzha (*Fructus Crataegi*, charred) 10 g and Shenqu (*Massa Medicata Fermentata*) 12 g.

3. Internal Retention of Phlegm

Chief Manifestations: Fat physique, bodily heaviness, lassitude of limbs, thoracic fullness, phlegm accumulation, dizziness, vomiting and lack of appetite, dry mouth with no desire for drinking, preference for greasy food and liquor, listlessness and somnolence, white and greasy or white and smooth tongue coating, smooth pulse.

Therapeutic Methods: To dry dampness, resolve phlegm, regulate qi and eliminate mass.

Prescription: Modified Erchen Tang (Erchen Decoction) and Zexie Tang (Alismatis Decoction), composed of Chenpi (*Pericarpium Citri Reticulatae*) 10 g, Fuling (*Poria*) 15 g, Zhibanxia (*Rhizoma Pinelliae Preparata*) 10 g, Shichangpu (*Rhizoma Acori Talarinowii*) 10 g, Zhiyuanzhi (*Radix Polygalae*, roasted) 6 g, Zexie (*Rhizoma Alismatis*) 15 g, Dongguapi (*Exocarpium Benincasae*) 10 g and Gualoupi (*Pericarpium Trichosanthis*) 15 g.

Modification: For restlessness, sleeplessness, lack of appetite, constipation, red tongue with yellow coating, smooth and rapid pulse, add Zhuru (*Caulis Bambusae in Taeniam*) 6 g, Huangqin (*Radix Scutellariae*) 10 g and

加　减　肢肿甚者,加大腹皮10 g,桑白皮10 g;腹胀便溏者,加陈皮 10 g,莱菔子10 g;气短乏力,畏寒肢冷者,加肉桂(后下)3 g;纳谷不香者,加佛手6 g,焦山楂10 g,神曲12 g。

3. 痰浊内盛证

主要证候　形盛体胖,身体重着,肢体困倦,胸膈痞满,痰涎壅盛,头晕目眩,呕不欲食,口干而不欲饮,嗜食肥甘醇酒,神疲嗜卧,苔白腻或白滑,脉滑。

治　法　燥湿化痰,理气消痞。

方　药　二陈汤合泽泻汤加减:陈皮10 g,茯苓15 g,制半夏10 g,石菖蒲10 g,炙远志6 g,泽泻15 g,冬瓜皮10 g,瓜蒌皮15 g。

加　减　心烦不寐,纳少、便秘,舌红,苔黄,脉滑数者,加竹茹6 g,黄芩10 g,制大黄6 g。

Zhidahuang (*Radix et Rhizoma Rhei Preparata*) 6 g.

4. Deficiency of Spleen Yang and Kidney Yang

Chief Manifestations: Fat physique, facial edema, listlessness and somnolence, short breath, abdominal distention, loose stools, spontaneous perspiration, dyspnea which becomes worse on exertion, aversion to cold, cold limbs, edema of lower limbs, oliguria during the day and nocturia, pale swollen tongue with thin and white coating, deep and thready pulse.

Therapeutic Methods: To warm and tonify the spleen and kidney, induce diuresis and relieve fluid retention.

Prescription: Modified Zhenwu Tang (Zhenwu Decoction) and Ling Gui Zhu Gan Tang (Decoction of Poria, Cinnamomi, Atractylodis Macrocephlae and Glycyrrhizae), composed of Huangqi (*Radix Astragali*) 15 g, Dangshen (*Radix Codonopsis*) 10 g, Fuling (*Poria*) 10 g, Baizhu (*Rhizoma Atractylodis Macrocephalae*) 10 g, Baishaoyao (*Radix Paeoniae Alba*) 12 g, Ganjiang (*Rhizoma Zingiberis*) 6 g, Zhifuzi (*Radix Aconiti Lateralis Preparata*) 10 g, Guizhi (*Ramulus Cinnamomi*) 6 g and Cheqianzi (*Semen Plantaginis*, wrapped) 10 g.

Modifications: For serious spontaneous perspiration, add Duanlonggu (*Os Draconis Usta*) 20 g and Duanmuli (*Concha Ostreae Usta*) 20 g; for oliguria and edema of limbs, add Zexie (*Rhizoma Alismatis*) 12 g, Zhuling (*Polyporus*) 10 g and Dafupi (*Pericarpium Arecae*) 10 g; for abdominal distention and loose stools, add Houpo (*Cortex Magnoliae Officinalis*) 6 g, Chenpi (*Pericarpium Citri Reticulatae*) 6 g, Cangzhu (*Rhizoma Atractylodis*) 10 g and Laifuzi (*Semen Raphani*) 10 g; for aversion to cold and cold limbs, add Buguzhi (*Fructus Psoraleae*) 10 g, Xianmao (*Rhizoma Curculiginis*)

4. 脾肾阳虚证

　　主要证候　形体肥胖,颜面虚浮,神疲嗜卧,气短乏力,腹胀便溏,自汗气喘,动则更甚,畏寒肢冷,下肢浮肿,尿昼少夜频,舌淡胖,苔薄白,脉沉细。

　　治　法　温补脾肾,利水化饮。

　　方　药　真武汤合苓桂术甘汤加减:黄芪15 g,党参10 g,茯苓10 g,白术10 g,白芍药12 g,干姜6 g,制附子10 g,桂枝6 g,车前子(包煎)10 g。

　　加　减　自汗量多者,加煅龙骨20 g,煅牡蛎20 g;尿少肢肿者,加泽泻12 g,猪苓10 g,大腹皮10 g;腹胀便溏者,加厚朴6 g,陈皮6 g,苍术10 g,莱菔子10 g;畏寒肢冷者,加补骨脂10 g,仙茅10 g,淫羊藿10 g,益智仁10 g。

10 g, Yinyanghuo (*Herba Epimedii*) 10 g and Yizhiren (*Fructus Alpiniae Oxyphyllae*) 10 g.

5. Qi Stagnation and Blood Stasis

Chief Manifestations: Full-grown physique, purplish red face or dull red face, chest distress and hypochondric distention, restlessness, irritability, sleeplessness or restless sleep, constipation, purplish red tongue with petechia or ecchymosis, or with engorged sublingual veins, deep and wiry pulse or unsmooth pulse.

Therapeutic Methods: To activate blood circulation and dissipate blood stasis.

Prescription: Modified Xuefu Zhuyu Tang (Decoction for Removing Blood Stasis in Chest) and Tao Hong Siwu Tang (Four-Ingredient Decoction with Persicae and Carthami), composed of Danggui (*Radix Angelicae Sinensis*) 10 g, Shengdihuang (*Radix Rehmanniae*) 10 g, Taoren (*Semen Persicae*) 10 g, Honghua (*Flos Carthami*) 10 g, Chuanxiong (*Rhizoma Chuanxiong*) 10 g, Chishaoyao (*Radix Paeoniae Rubra*) 10 g, Chaihu (*Radix Bupleuri*) 6 g, Zhike (*Fructus Aurantii*) 10 g, Jiegeng (*Radix Platycodi*) 6 g, Shenggancao (*Radix Glycyrrhizae*) 6 g and Chuanniuxi (*Radix Cyathulae*) 10 g.

Modifications: For stagnated heat in the body, manifested as nestlessness, irritability, dryness and bitter taste in the mouth, and constipation, add Yinchen (*Herba Artemisiae*) 10 g, Zhizi (*Radix Gardeniae*) 10 g, Zhidahuang (*Radix et Rhizoma Rhei Preparata*) 6 g and Huangqin (*Radix Scutellariae*) 10 g; for stagnation of qi, chest distress, shortness of breath, abdominal fullness and distention, add Yujin (*Radix Curcumae*) 10 g, Houpo (*Cortex Magnoliae Officinalis*) 6 g, Chenpi (*Pericarpium Citri Reticulatae*) 6 g and Laifuzi (*Semen Raphani*) 10 g.

5. 气滞血瘀证

主要证候 体形丰满,面色紫红或暗红,胸闷胁胀,心烦易怒,夜不能寐或夜寐不安,大便秘结,舌暗红或有瘀点、瘀斑,或舌下瘀筋,脉沉弦或涩。

治 法 活血祛瘀,行气散结。

方 药 血府逐瘀汤合桃红四物汤加减:当归10 g,生地黄10 g,桃仁10 g,红花10 g,川芎10 g,赤芍药10 g,柴胡6 g,枳壳10 g,桔梗6 g,生甘草6 g,川牛膝10 g。

加 减 瘀热内结,表现心烦易怒,口干口苦,大便秘结者,加茵陈10 g,栀子10 g,制大黄6 g,黄芩10 g;气机郁滞,胸闷气粗,脘腹胀满者,加郁金10 g,厚朴6 g,陈皮6 g,莱菔子10 g。

Other Treatments

1. Chinese Patent Drugs

（1）Jianfei Wan (Weight-Reducing Bolus): 1 bolus each time, twice or thrice daily; indicated for obesity with retention of phlegm-dampness in the body.

（2）Qingshen Jianfei Pian (Weight-Reducing Tablet): 5 tablets each time, 3 times a day; indicated for obesity with retention of dampness and stagnation of blood due to deficiency of qi.

（3）Kangling Heji (Healthful and Effective Mixture): 100 ml each time, twicea day; indicated for obesity with retention of dampness and stagnation of blood due to deficiency of qi.

（4）Sanhua Jianfei Cha (Three-Flower Tea for Reducing Weight): 1 sachet each time, 3 times a day; indicated for obesity with retention of dampness and stagnation of blood due to stagnation of qi.

（5）Baijin Wan (Baijin Pill): 6 g each time, 3 times a day; indicated for obesity with retention of phlegm-dampness in the body.

（6）Fangfeng Tongsheng Wan (Saposhnikoviae Pill for Dispersing Superficies): 6 g each time, 3 times a day; indicated for obesity with retention of dampness due to stomach heat.

2. Single-drug or Experiential Prescriptions

（1）Heye Tang (Nelumbinis Decoction): composed of Heye (*Folium Nelumbinis*) 10 g, Cangzhu (*Rhizoma Atractylodis*) 10 g, Baizhu (*Rhizoma Atractylodis Macrocephalae*) 10 g, Huangbai (*Cortex Phellodendri*) 10 g, Niuxi (*Radix Achyranthis Bidentatae*) 10 g, Yiyiren (*Semen Coicis*) 15 g, Huangqi (*Radix Astragali*) 15 g, Guizhi (*Ramulus Cinnamomi*) 10 g, Mugua (*Fructus Chaenomelis*) 10 g, Fuling (*Poria*) 10 g, Zexie (*Rhizoma Alismatis*) 12 g, Shanzha (*Fructus*

【其他疗法】

1. 中成药

（1）减肥丸　每服1丸，每日2～3次。适用于痰湿内阻之肥胖症。

（2）轻身减肥片　每服5片，每日3次。适用于气虚湿阻血瘀之肥胖症。

（3）康灵合剂　每服100 ml，每日2次。适用于气虚湿阻血瘀之肥胖症。

（4）三花减肥茶　每服1包，每日3次。适用于气滞湿阻血瘀之肥胖症。

（5）白金丸　每服6 g，每日3次。适用于痰湿内阻之肥胖症。

（6）防风通圣丸　每服6 g，每日3次。适用于胃热湿阻之肥胖症。

2. 单验方

（1）荷叶汤　荷叶10 g，苍术10 g，白术10 g，黄柏10 g，牛膝10 g，薏苡仁15 g，黄芪15 g，桂枝10 g，木瓜10 g，茯苓10 g，泽泻12 g，山楂10 g，车前草10 g，虎杖15 g，夏枯草10 g，甘草5 g。每日1剂，水煎服。适用于胃热气滞湿阻之肥胖症。

Crataegi) 10 g, Cheqiancao (*Herba Plantaginis*) 10 g, Huzhang (*Rhizoma Polygoni Cuspidati*) 15 g, Xiakucao (*Spica Prunellae*) 10 g and Gancao (*Radix Glycyrrhizae*) 5 g. Decoct the above drugs in water for oral administration, one dose a day. It is indicated for obesity with stagnation of qi and retention of dampness due to stomach heat.

(2) Xiaofei Yin (Weight-Reducing Decoction): composed of Heye (*Folium Nelumbinis*) 15 g, Zexie (*Rhizoma Alismatis*) 15 g and Shanzha (*Fructus Crataegi*) 15 g. Decoct the drugs in water and take the decoction as the substitute for tea, one dose a day. It is indicated for simple obesity.

(3) Jianfei Qingshenle (Decoction for Reducing Weight): composed of Loulu (*Radix Rhapontici*) 10 g, Juemingzi (*Semen Cassiae*) 15 g, Heye (*Folium Nelumbinis*) 10 g, Zexie (*Rhizoma Alismatis*) 12 g, Fangji (*Radix Stephaniae Tetrandrae*) 10 g, Shengdihuang (*Radix Rehmanniae*) 12 g, Dangshen (*Radix Codonopsis*) 10 g, Shuiniujiao (*Cornu Bubali*, to be decocted first) 20 g, Huangqi (*Radix Astragali*) 15 g and Wugong (*Scolopendra*) 3 g. Decoct the above drugs in water for oral administration, one dose a day. It is indicated for simple obesity.

(4) Caojueming (*Semen Cassiae*). Grind the herb into fine powder after it is stir-baked and take 3 - 5 g each time, twice or thrice a day. It is indicated for obesity complicated with hyperlipidemia.

(5) Qinggong Jianfei Xianyao Cha (Qing-Dynasty Palace Wonder Drink for Reducing Weight), composed of Heye (*Folium Nelumbinis*) 10 g, Zisuye (*Folium Perillae*) 10 g, Shanzha (*Fructus Crataegi*) 10 g and appropriate amount of oolong tea. Steep the herbs in water and drink the tea once a day. It is indicated for obesity

(2) 消肥饮 荷叶15 g,泽泻15 g,山楂15 g,代茶饮,每日 1 剂。适用于单纯性肥胖。

(3) 减肥轻身乐 漏芦10 g,决明子15 g,荷叶10 g,泽泻12 g,防己10 g,生地黄12 g,党参10 g,水牛角20 g(先煎),黄芪15 g,蜈蚣3 g,水煎服,每日1剂。适用于单纯性肥胖。

(4) 草决明,炒熟研末,每服3～5 g,每日2～3次。适用于肥胖合并高脂血症。

(5) 清宫减肥仙药茶 荷叶10 g,紫苏叶10 g,山楂10 g,加乌龙茶适量,泡水代茶。每日 1 次。适用于肥胖症合并高脂血症。

complicated with hyperlipidemia.

3. External Therapy

（1）Muzeicao（*Herba Equiseti Hiemalis*）30 g, Kuandonghua（*Flos Farfarae*）20 g, Cheqiancao（*Herba Plantaginis*）30 g, Shichangpu（*Rhizoma Acori Tatarinowii*）20 g, Juhua（*Flos Chrysanthemi*）15 g and Shengdahuang（*Radix et Rhizoma Rhei*）30 g. Decoct the above herbs in 2,000 ml of water for 20 minutes. Remove the dregs and pour the decoction into a bathtub. Keep adding warm water while fuming and bathing the body, 30 minutes a time, twice or thrice a week, ten times being a course of treatment. It is indicated for obesity.

（2）Heye（*Folium Nelumbinis*）15 g, Fangji（*Radix Stephaniae Tetrandrae*）10 g, Baiziren（*Semen Biotae*）15 g and Zexie（*Rhizoma Alismatis*）10 g. Decoct the herbs in 3,000 ml of water for 15 minutes. Remove the dregs, mix the decoction with 3,000 ml of hot water and bathe the whole body, 30 minutes at a time, twice or thrice a week, ten times being a course of treatment. It is indicated for those with fat physique, dizziness, restlessness, oliguria and edema.

2.8.2　Hyperlipoproteinemia

General Description

Hyperlipemia refers to the elevated concentration of lipids in the plasma. When the plasma lipoprotein concentration exceeds the normal maximum, it is called hyperlipoproteinemia. As plasma lipid is liposoluble, it must be combined with protein to form a water-soluble compound that can circulate in the body. Therefore hyperlipemia is usually manifested as hyperlipoproteinemia and the follow-

3. 外治法

（1）木贼草30 g,款冬花20 g,车前草30 g,石菖蒲20 g,菊花15 g,生大黄30 g。上药加水2 000 ml,煎沸20分钟,去渣取汁,加入浴盆中趁热先熏后洗,洗浴时不断加热水。每次30分钟,每星期2～3次,连续10次为1个疗程。适用于肥胖者。

（2）荷叶15 g,防己10 g,柏子仁15 g,泽泻10 g。上药加水3 000 ml,煮沸15分钟,去渣取汁,兑热水3 000 ml,洗浴全身。每次30分钟,每星期2～3次,连续10次为1个疗程。适用于体形肥胖、头晕心烦、尿少浮肿者。

第二节　高脂蛋白血症

【概述】

血浆脂质浓度超过正常高限时称高脂血症。血浆脂蛋白浓度超过正常高限时称高脂蛋白血症。由于血浆脂质为脂溶性,必须与蛋白质结合为水溶性复合物而运行全身,故高脂血症常表现为高脂

ing physical signs are commonly seen: xanthoma of eye-lid, xanthoma of tendon, subcutaneous nodular xanthoma and arteriosclerosis, or overweight and fundus lipidosis. This disease is the pathologic base of coronary atherosclerotic heart disease, hypertension, diabetes, fatty liver, cholelithiasis, apoplexia, etc. and becomes the main risk factor that endangers the health of mankind.

The causes of this disease fall into two main categories: primary and secondary. Primary hyperlipemia arises from congenital metabolic defect of lipid and lipoprotein (or hereditary defect) and from certain environmental factors (including diet, nutrition and drugs) through some unknown mechanism. Secondary hyperlipemia arises from certain diseases such as diabetes, liver diseases, kidney diseases, thyroid diseases and the effect of some factors such as wine drinking, obesity, diet, life style, etc.

This disease is included in the categories of "tan zheng" (phlegm syndrome), "shi zhuo" (damp retention), "xuan yun" (vertigo), "fei pang" (obesity) and others in TCM. Its causes are related to congenital disposition, improper diet, seven emotional disorders, debility after prolonged illness, and overstrain. The main pathogenesis is deficiency of the liver, spleen and kidney, internal stagnation of phlegm-dampness, blockage of the vessels and disharmony between yin and yang, qi and blood.

Essentials for Diagnosis

(1) At present, there are not yet international or national unified criteria for hyperlipoproteinemia. Generally, the total cholesterol (TC) > 6.465 mmol/L is considered

蛋白血症。其临床主要证候为眼睑黄色瘤、肌腱黄色瘤、皮下结节状黄色瘤及动脉硬化的体征，或有肥胖、眼底脂质沉着。本病是冠状动脉粥样硬化性心脏病、高血压病、糖尿病、脂肪肝、胆石症、中风等病症的病理基础，成为危害人类健康的主要因素。

本病的病因可分为原发性和继发性两大类。原发性者由于脂质和脂蛋白代谢先天性缺陷（或遗传性缺陷），以及某些环境因素（包括饮食、营养和药物等）通过未知的机理而引起的。继发性者主要继发于某种疾病，如糖尿病、肝脏疾病、肾脏疾病、甲状腺疾病以及饮酒、肥胖、饮食以及生活方式等因素的影响。

根据本病的临床表现，当属于中医学"痰证"、"湿浊"、"眩晕"、"肥胖"等范畴。其病因与禀赋不足、饮食不节、七情所伤、久病体弱、劳逸失当有关。主要病机为肝脾肾虚，痰湿内阻，脉络瘀滞，阴阳气血失调。

【诊断要点】

（1）高脂蛋白血症的标准，目前国际和国内尚无统一标准，一般将总胆固醇

as hypercholesterolemia, and triglycerides (TG)＞2.258 mmol/L as hypertriglyceridemia.

(2) In lipoprotein electrophoresis, the increased β-lipoprotein (LDL) and pre-β-lipoprotein (VLDC) has the function of promoting the atherosclerosis.

(3) In addition to the analysis of blood lipids, the following are also helpful to the diagnosis of this disease: case history, family history, clinical manifestations (such as xanthoma, arcus senilis, etc.), and some other laboratory tests such as electrocardinographic examination, blood sugar determination, thyroid, liver and kidney function tests, etc.

Syndrome Differentiation and Treatment

Clinically, it is necessary to differentiate the deficiency type from the excess type. Internal retention of phlegm-dampness, blockage by phlegm and blood stasis, and liver qi stagnation are mostly of the excess type, while deficiency of spleen yang and kidney yang and deficiency of liver yin and kidney yin are of the deficiency type. The treatment is based on the principle of invigorating the spleen, revolving phlegm and dispelling dampness. In accordance with different cases, the treatments of clearing away heat, dispersing the stagnant liver qi, normalizing gallbladder function, nourishing the kidney and liver, and activating blood circulation can also be used.

1. Internal Retention of Phlegm Dampness

Chief Manifestations: Fat physique, dizziness, distention and heavy sensation of the head, blurred vision, abdominal distress and distention, nausea, profuse sputum, blockage of the throat by sputum, numbness of limbs, heavy sensation of the body, eyelid edema, loose

（TC）＞6.465 mmol/L 定为高胆固醇血症，三酰甘油（TG）＞2.258 mmol/L 定为高三酰甘油血症。

（2）血脂蛋白电泳中，β-脂蛋白（LDL）和前β脂蛋白（VLDC），其含量增高有促使动脉粥样硬化的作用。

（3）除血脂分析外，病史、家族史、临床表现（如黄色瘤、老年环等）以及其他实验室检查，如心电图，血糖，甲状腺及肝、肾功能，对本病的诊断也有一定的帮助。

【辨证论治】

本病临床应辨其虚实的主次，痰湿内盛、痰瘀交阻证和肝郁气滞证多实，脾肾阳虚和肝肾阴虚证属虚。治疗以健脾化痰除湿为基本大法，据情结合清热、疏肝、利胆、补肾、养肝、活血等法。

1. 痰湿内盛证

主要证候　形体肥胖，头晕胀重，视物昏花，脘腹闷胀，恶心欲吐，痰多，喉间痰凝，肢体麻木，身沉体倦，目睑浮胀，便溏不爽，舌质淡红，苔白腻，

stools, light red tongue with white and greasy coating, smooth or soft-superficial pulse.

Therapeutic Methods: To dissipate dampness, eliminate phlegm, lift lucid yang and lower turbid yin.

Prescription: Modified Erchen Tang (Erchen Decoction) and Banxia Baizhu Tianma Tang (Decoction of Pinelliae, Atratylodis Macrocephalae and Gastrodiae), composed of Fabanxia (*Rhizoma Pinelliae Preparata*) 10 g, Cangzhu (*Rhizoma Atractylodis*) 10 g, Baizhu (*Phizoma Atractylodis Macrocephalae*) 10 g, Tianma (*Rhizoma Gastrodiae*) 10 g, Chenpi (*Pericarpium Citri Reticulatae*) 10 g, Houpo (*Cortex Magnoliae Officinalis*) 6 g, Fuling (*Poria*) 10 g, Zexie (*Rhizoma Alismatis*) 10 g, Cheqianzi (*Semen Plantaginis*, wrapped) 12 g, Heye (*Folium Nelumbinis*) 10 g, Chaihu (*Radix Bupleuri*) 6 g and Shengma (*Rhizoma Cimicifugae*) 6 g.

Modifications: For dizziness and vomiting, add Daizheshi (*Hematitum seu Ochra*, to be decocted first) 20 g, Xuanfuhua (*Flos Inulae*, wrapped) 10 g and Zhuru (*Caulis Bambusae in Taeniam*) 10 g; for chest distress, sensation of suffocation and thoracic fullness, add Xiebai (*Bulbus Allii Macrostemi*) 6 g, Gualoupi (*Pericarpium Trichosanthis*) 10 g, Shichangpu (*Rhizoma Acori Tatarinowii*) 6 g and Zhike (*Fructus Aurantii*) 10 g.

2. Blockage by Phlegm and Blood Stasis

Chief Manifestations: Dizziness, distention and heavy sensation of the head or headache, tiredness with preference for sleep, chest distress, cold back, sensation of suffocation, precordial dull pain or stabbing pain which becomes severe in rainy days and muggy days or during the night, fat physique, heavy and numb limbs, dark purple tongue with ecchymosis and greasy coating, un-

脉滑或濡。

治　法　化湿祛痰,升清降浊。

方　药　二陈汤合半夏白术天麻汤加减:法半夏10 g,苍术10 g,白术10 g,天麻10 g,陈皮10 g,厚朴6 g,茯苓10 g,泽泻10 g,车前子(包煎)12 g,荷叶10 g,柴胡6 g,升麻6 g。

加　减　头晕欲仆,呕恶泛吐者,加代赭石(先煎)20 g,旋覆花(包煎)10 g,竹茹10 g;胸闷、气窒、痞满者,加薤白6 g,瓜蒌皮10 g,石菖蒲6 g,枳壳10 g。

2. 痰瘀交阻证

主要证候　头晕胀重或疼痛,疲困喜卧,胸闷背冷,有窒息感,心前区闷痛或刺痛,尤以阴雨天和闷热天或夜间明显,形体肥胖,肢体麻木沉重,舌紫暗有瘀斑,苔腻,脉涩或弦滑。

smooth or wiry and smooth pulse.

Therapeutic Methods: To dissipate phlegm, relieve stagnation, and promote blood circulation to dredge meridians.

Prescription: Modified Gualou Xiebai Banxia Tang (Decoction of Trichosanthis, Allii Macrostemi and Pinelliae) and Tao Hong Siwu Tang (Four-Ingredient Decoction with Persicae and Carthami), composed of Gualoupi (*Pericarpium Trichosanthis*) 10 g, Xiebaitou (*Bulbus Allii Macrostemi*) 6 g, Fabanxia (*Rhizoma Pinelliae Preparata*) 10 g, Taoren (*Semen Persicae*) 10 g, Honghua (*Flos Carthami*) 10 g, Shensanqi (*Radix Notoginseng*) 10 g, Chuanxiong (*Rhizoma Chuanxiong*) 10 g, Chishaoyao (*Radix Paeoniae Rubra*) 10 g, Gegen (*Radix Puerariae*) 10 g and Gansong (*Rhizoma et Radix Nardostachydis*) 10 g.

Modifications: For thick greasy and slippery tongue coating, add Huoxiang (*Herba Agastaches*) 10 g, Peilan (*Herba Eupatorii*) 10 g, Houpo (*Cortex Magnoliae Officinalis*) 10 g and Cangzhu (*Rhizoma Atractylodis*) 10 g; for cold sensation in the chest and back, add Chishizhi (*Halloysitum Rubrum*) 10 g, Guizhi (*Ramulus Cinnamomi*) 10 g, Xixin (*Herba Asari*) 3 g and Ganjiang (*Rhizoma Zingiberis*) 5 g; for chest distress and short breath, add Taizishen (*Radix Pseudostellariae*) 10 g, Shichangpu (*Rhizoma Acori Tatarinowii*) 6 g and Zhike (*Fructus Aurantii*) 10 g; for stabbing pain in the chest radiating to the shoulders and the back, and cyanotic hands, feet and lips, add Danshen (*Radix Salviae Miltiorrhizae*) 12 g, Puhuang (*Pollen Typhae*, wrapped) 10 g and Wulingzhi (*Faeces Trogopterorum*) 10 g.

3. Stagnation of Liver Qi

Chief Manifestations: Dizziness and blurred vision, irritability, hypochondriac distension with eruct-

治　法　化痰宣痹，活血通脉。

方　药　瓜蒌薤白半夏汤合桃红四物汤加减：瓜蒌皮10 g，薤白头6 g，法半夏10 g，桃仁10 g，红花10 g，参三七10 g，川芎10 g，赤芍药10 g，葛根10 g，甘松10 g。

加　减　舌苔厚腻而水滑者，加藿香10 g，佩兰10 g，厚朴10 g，苍术10 g；胸背部有冷感者，加赤石脂10 g，桂枝10 g，细辛3 g，干姜5 g；心胸憋闷，气短者，加太子参10 g，石菖蒲6 g，枳壳10 g；胸部刺痛放射至肩背部，手足和口唇青紫者，加丹参12 g，蒲黄（包煎）10 g，五灵脂10 g。

3. 肝郁气滞证

主要证候　头晕目眩，性急易怒，胁胀嗳气，胃中嘈杂

ation, gastric upset, loose stools with bowel sound, abundant wind from bowels, thin white or thin yellow tongue coating, thready and wiry pulse.

Therapeutic Methods: To Soothe liver qi, invigorate the spleen and regulate stomach qi.

Prescription: Modified Chaihu Shugan San (Bupleuri Powder for Soothing Liver Qi), composed of Chaihu (*Radix Bupleuri*) 10 g, Baizhu (*Rhizoma Atractylodis Macrocephalae*) 10 g, Baishaoyao (*Radix Paeoniae Alba*) 10 g, Zhike (*Fructus Aurantii*) 10 g, Gancao (*Radix Glycyrrhizae*) 5 g, Chenpi (*Pericerpium Citri Reticulatae*) 6 g, Fabanxia (*Rhizoma Pinelliae Preparata*) 10 g, Fuling (*Poria*) 10 g, Zexie (*Rhizoma Alismatis*) 10 g, Zisugeng (*Caulis Perillae*) 10 g, Zisuye (*Folium Perillae*) 6 g, Huanglian (*Rhizoma Coptidis*) 3 g, Wuzhuyu (*Fructus Evodiae*) 2 g, Guya (*Fructus Oryzae Germinatus*) 10 g, Maiya (*Fructus Hordei Germinatus*) 10 g and Bohe (*Herba Menthae*) 6 g.

Modifications: For increase of body weight, add Huzhang (*Rhizoma Polygoni Cuspidati*) 15 g, Yujin (*Radix Curcumae*) 10 g, Shengshanzha (*Fructus Crataegi*) 10 g, Heye (*Folium Nelumbinis*) 10 g and Yiyiren (*Semen Coicis*) 15 g; for pronounced hypochondriac distending pain, add Qingpi (*Pericarpium Citri Reticulatae Viride*) 6 g, Lulutong (*Fructus Liguidambaris*) 10 g, Chuanlianzi (*Fructus Meliae Toosendan*) 10 g and Yanhusuo (*Rhizoma Corydalis*) 10 g; for sore throat, difficulty in expectorating sticky sputum, cough in the morning and occasional vomiting, add Lü'emei (*Flos Mume*) 5 g, Muhudie (*Semen Oroxyli*) 5 g, Shegan (*Rhizoma Belamcandae*) 10 g and Gualoupi (*Pericarpium Trichosanthis*) 10 g; for dizziness, feverish face, red eyes with distending pain, bitter mouth, polyphagia, polyorexia, fat physique and elevation of blood pressure,

或肠鸣便溏,矢气频多,舌苔薄白或薄黄,脉细弦。

治 法 疏肝理气,健脾和胃。

方 药 柴胡疏肝散加减:柴胡10 g,白术10 g,白芍药10 g,枳壳10 g,甘草5 g,陈皮6 g,法半夏10 g,茯苓10 g,泽泻10 g,紫苏梗10 g,紫苏叶6 g,黄连3 g,吴茱萸2 g,谷芽10 g,麦芽10 g,薄荷6 g。

加 减 体重显增,形体渐胖者,加虎杖15 g,郁金10 g,生山楂10 g,荷叶10 g,薏苡仁15 g;胁肋胀痛显著者,加青皮6 g,路路通10 g,川楝子10 g,延胡索10 g;咽痛,痰黏咯吐不畅,晨间咳嗽,时作呕恶者,加绿萼梅5 g,木蝴蝶5 g,射干10 g,瓜蒌皮10 g;头晕面烘,目赤胀痛,口苦,多食善饥,形体肥胖,血压明显增高者,加石膏(先煎)30 g,玄参10 g,决明子15 g,制大黄10 g,瓜蒌皮10 g。

add Shigao (*Gypsum Fibrosum*, to be decocted first)
30 g, Xuanshen (*Radix Scrophulariae*) 10 g, Juemingzi
(*Semen Cassiae*) 15 g, Zhidahuang (*Radix et Rhizoma
Rhei Preparata*) 10 g and Gualoupi (*Pericarpium Trichosanthis*) 10 g.

4. Deficiency of Spleen Yang and Kidney Yang

Chief Manifestations: Dizziness, tinnitus, deafness, facial edema, swelling limbs, listlessness, cold body
and limbs, cold and sore waist and knees, loss of appetite, loose stools, fatigue, impotence, prospermia, hyposexuality, pale swollen tongue with thin and white coating, deep and thready pulse.

Therapeutic Methods: To warm and tonify the
spleen and kidney, eliminate dampness and resolve
phlegm.

Prescription: Modified Fuzi Lizhong Tang (Aconiti
Lateralis Decoction for Regulating Middle Energizer) and
Yougui Yin (Decoction for Replenishing Kidney Yang),
composed of Zhifuzi (*Radix Aconiti Lateralis Prepara-
ta*) 10 g, Ganjiang (*Rhizoma Zingiberis*) 6 g, Fuling
(*Poria*) 10 g, Baizhu (*Rhizoma Atractylodis Macro-
cephalae*) 10 g, Dangshen (*Radix Codonopsis*) 10 g,
Shanzhuyu (*Fructus Corni*) 10 g, Lujiaopian (*Cornu
Cervi*, sliced) 10 g, Bajitian (*Radix Morindae Officina-
lis*) 10 g, Shanyao (*Rhizoma Dioscoreae*) 12 g, Gouqizi
(*Fructus Lycii*) 10 g, Yinyanghuo (*Herba Epimedii*)
10 g and Zexie (*Rhizoma Alismatis*) 15 g, Zhigancao
(*Radix Glycyrrhizae*, roasted) 6 g.

Modifications: For dizziness, head distension, gid-
diness, occasional vomiting and comparatively high blood
pressure, add Cishi (*Magnetitum*, to be decocted first)
30 g, Gouteng (*Ramulus Uncariae cum Uncis*, to be
decocted later) 15 g, Tianma (*Rhizoma Gastrodiae*)
10 g and Fabanxia (*Rhizoma Pinelliae Preparata*) 10 g;

4. 脾肾阳虚证

主要证候　头晕昏沉,耳鸣耳聋或面浮肢肿,精神委靡,形寒肢冷,腰膝酸冷,纳减便溏,体倦乏力,阳痿早泄,性欲减退,舌质淡胖,苔薄白,脉沉细。

治　法　温补脾肾,祛湿化浊。

方　药　附子理中汤合右归饮加减:制附子10 g,干姜6 g,茯苓10 g,白术10 g,党参10 g,山茱萸10 g,鹿角片10 g,巴戟天10 g,山药12 g,枸杞子10 g,淫羊藿10 g,泽泻15 g,炙甘草6 g。

加　减　头晕作胀,目眩,时有呕恶,血压较高者,加磁石(先煎)30 g,钩藤(后下)15 g,天麻10 g,法半夏10 g;形寒背冷,咳喘动则尤甚者,加苍术10 g,白芥子10 g,紫苏

for cold body and back, cough with dyspnea which is worse on exertion, add Cangzhu (*Rhizoma Atractylodis*) 10 g, Baijiezi (*Semen Sinapis Albae*) 10 g, Zisuzi (*Fructus Perillae*) 10 g, Xixin (*Herba Asari*) 3 g and Tusizi (*Semen Cuscutae*) 10 g; for impaired appetite, loose stools and diarrhea before dawn, add Buguzhi (*Fructus Psoraleae*) 10 g, Roudoukou (*Semen Myristicae*) 10 g, Weihezi (*Fructus Chebulae*, roasted in hot cinders) 10 g and Yizhiren (*Fructus Alpiniae Oxyphyllae*) 10 g; for clear and long urination and profuse urine at night, add Yizhiren (*Fructus Alpiniae Oxyphyllae*) 10 g, Jinyingzi (*Fructus Rosae Laevigatae*) 10 g and Sangpiaoxiao (*Oötheca Mantidis*) 10 g.

5. Deficiency of Liver Yin and Kidney Yin

Chief Manifestations: Dizziness, heavy head and light feet, dry eyes, blurred vision, tinnitus, hypoacusis, dreamful sleep, dry mouth and throat, feverish sensation of the palms, soles and chest, sore and weak knees and loins, tremulous and numb limbs, emaciation, debility, red tongue with little coating or with fissures, thready, rapid and weak pulse.

Therapeutic Methods: To nourish yin, suppress yang and promote blood circulation.

Prescription: Modified Qi Ju Dihuang Wan (Rehmanniae Bolus with Lycii and Chrysanthemi), composed of Juhua (*Flos Chrysanthemi*) 10 g, Gouqizi (*Fructus Lycii*) 10 g, Shanzhuyu (*Fructus Corni*) 10 g, Shengdihuang (*Radix Rehmanniae*) 10 g, Fuling (*Poria*) 10 g, Mudanpi (*Cortex Moutan Radicis*) 10 g, Sangshenzi (*Fructus Mori*) 10 g, Heizhima (*Semen Sesami Nigrum*) 10 g, Zhiheshouwu (*Radix Polygoni Multiflori Preparata*) 10 g, Huangjing (*Rhizoma Polygonati*) 10 g, Sangjisheng (*Herba Taxilli*) 10 g, Shengshanzha (*Fructus Crataegi*) 10 g, Huainiuxi (*Radix Achyran-*

子10 g,细辛3 g,菟丝子10 g;纳减便溏,五更泻者,加补骨脂10 g,肉豆蔻10 g,煨诃子10 g,益智仁10 g;小便清长,夜尿量多者,加益智仁10 g,金樱子10 g,桑螵蛸10 g。

5. 肝肾阴虚证

主要证候　头晕,晕甚欲仆,头重足轻,两目干涩,视物昏花,耳鸣重听,少寐多梦,口干咽燥,五心烦热,腰膝酸软,手颤肢麻,形瘦体弱。舌红少苔,或有裂纹,脉细数而弱。

治　法　滋阴潜阳,活血通脉。

方　药　杞菊地黄丸加减:菊花10 g,枸杞子10 g,山茱萸10 g,生地黄10 g,茯苓10 g,牡丹皮10 g,桑椹子10 g,黑芝麻10 g,制何首乌10 g,黄精10 g,桑寄生10 g,生山楂10 g,怀牛膝10 g,磁石(先煎)30 g。

this Bidentatae) 10 g and Cishi (*Magnetitum*, to be de-cocted first) 30 g.

Modifications: For dizziness accompanied with tremor and numbness of limbs, elevation of blood pres-sure, add Luobumaye (*Folium Apocyni Veneti*) 10 g, Huaihua (*Flos Sophorae*) 10 g, Xixiancao (*Herba Sieg-esbeckiae*) 15 g, Shengmuli (*Caro Ostreae*, to be decoc-ted first) 30 g and Guiban (*Plastrum Testudinis*, to be decocted first) 15 g; for dry stools and infrequent evacua-tion, add Xuanshen (*Radix Scrophulariae*) 10 g, Rou-congrong (*Herba Cistanchis*) 10 g and Danggui (*Radix Angelicae Sinensis*) 10 g; for dark purple tongue with ec-chymosis, high viscosity of blood, accompanied by coro-nary heart disease and angina pectoris, add Taoren (*Se-men Persicae*) 10 g, Danshen (*Radix Salviae Miltior-rhizae*) 10 g, Shensanqifen (*Radix Notoginseng*, to be powdered and infused separately) 3 g and Chuanxiong (*Rhizoma Chuanxiong*) 10 g; for hectic fever, flushed cheeks and burning sensation of the skin, add Biejia (*Carapax Trionycis*, to be decocted first) 15 g, Qinghao (*Herba Artemisiae Annuae*) 12 g, and Baiwei (*Radix Cynanchi Atrati*) 10 g.

Other Treatments

1. Chinese Patent Drugs

(1) Shouwu Pian (Polygoni Multiflori Tablet): 0.25 g each time, 3 times a day; indicated for hyperchol-esterolemia with deficiency of liver yin and kidney yin.

(2) Jiaogulan Zongdai Jiaonang (Gynostemma Glyco-sides Capsule): 40 mg each time, 3 times a day; indicated for hypercholesterolemia and hypertriglyceridemia.

(3) Shanzha Chongji (Crataegi Granules): 1 sachet each time, 3 times a day; indicated for hypercholesterol-emia and high LDL.

(4) Tongmai Jiangzhi Pian (Tablet for Activating

加　减　头晕伴手颤肢麻,血压升高显著者,加罗布麻叶10 g、槐花10 g、豨莶草15 g、生牡蛎(先煎)30 g、龟版(先煎)15 g;大便干结,数日一行者,加玄参10 g、肉苁蓉10 g、当归10 g;舌紫暗有瘀斑,血黏度高,伴冠心病、心绞痛者,加桃仁10 g、丹参10 g、参三七粉(另冲)3 g、川芎10 g;潮热颧红,肌肤灼热者,加鳖甲(先煎)15 g、青蒿12 g、白薇10 g。

【其他疗法】

1. 中成药

(1) 首乌片　每服0.25 g,每日3次。适用于肝肾阴虚、胆固醇增高者。

(2) 绞股蓝总甙胶囊　每服40 mg,每日3次。适用于总胆固醇、三酰甘油增高者。

(3) 山楂冲剂　每服1袋,每日3次。适用于胆固醇和低密度脂蛋白增高者。

(4) 通脉降脂片　每服4

Blood and Lowering Blood Lipid): 4 tablets each time, 3 times a day; indicated for hypertriglyceridemia and hyper-β-lipoproteinemia.

(5) Zexie Jiangzhi Pian (Alismatis Tablet for Lowering Blood Lipid): 4 tablets each time, 3 times a day; indicated for various types of hyperlipemia.

(6) Baijin Wan (Baijin Pill): 6 g each time, twice a day; indicated for various types of hyperlipemia.

2. Single-drug or Experiential Prescriptions

(1) Shanzha (*Fructus Crataegi*) 15 g and Maiya (*Fructus Hordei Germinatus*) 15 g. Decoct the herbs in water and take the decoction once or twice a day. It is indicated for hypercholesterolemia.

(2) Shanzha Jiangzhi Pian (Crataegi Tablet for Lowering Blood Lipid): composed of Shanzha (*Fructus Crataegi*) 30 g, Gegen (*Radix Puerariae*) 15 g and Mingfan (*Alumen*) 1.2 g. Prepare the drugs into tablets as one-day dose, and take the tablets in three times, four weeks being a course of treatment. It is indicated for hypercholesterolemia.

(3) Jiangzhi Tang (Decoction for Lowering Blood Lipid): composed of Heshouwu (*Radix Polygoni Multiflori*) 15 g, Gouqizi (*Fructus Lycii*) 10 g and Caojueming (*Semen Cassiae*) 30 g. Decoct the drugs in water and take the decoction in two divided doses, two months being a course of treatment. It is indicated for hypercholesterolemia.

(4) Shouwu Jiangzhi Tang (Polygoni Multiflori Decoction for Lowering Blood Lipid): composed of Shengheshouwu (*Radix Polygoni Multiflori*) 15 g, Juhua (*Flos Chrysanthemi*) 10 g, Shudihuang (*Radix Rehmanniae Preparata*) 15 g, Maimendong (*Radix Ophiopogonis*) 15 g, Yejiaoteng (*Caulis et Folium Polygoni*

片,每日 3 次。适用于三酰甘油、β 脂蛋白增高者。

(5) 泽泻降脂片　每服 4 片,每日 3 次。适用于高脂血症各证型。

(6) 白金丸　每服 6 g,每日 2 次。适用于高脂血症各证型。

2. 单验方

(1) 山楂 15 g,麦芽 15 g,水煎服,每日 1～2 次。适用于胆固醇增高者。

(2) 山楂降脂片　山楂 30 g,葛根 15 g,明矾 1.2 g,为 1 日量,制成片剂,分 3 次服,疗程为 4～6 个星期。适用于胆固醇增高者。

(3) 降脂汤　何首乌 15 g,枸杞子 10 g,草决明 30 g,水煎分 2 次服,疗程 2 个月。适用于胆固醇增高者。

(4) 首乌降脂汤　生何首乌 15 g,菊花 10 g,熟地黄 15 g,麦门冬 15 g,夜交藤 15 g,鸡冠花 10 g,北沙参 15 g,玄参 15 g,合欢皮 15 g,白芍药 10 g。水煎服,每日 1 剂。适用于胆固

Multiflori) 15 g, Jiguanhua (*Inflorescentia Celosiae Cristatae*) 10 g, Beishashen (*Radix Glehniae*) 15 g, Xuanshen (*Radix Scrophulariae*) 15 g, Hehuanpi (*Cortex Albiziae*) 15 g and Baishaoyao (*Radix Paeoniae Alba*) 10 g. Decoct the drugs in water for oral administration, one dose a day. It is indicated for hypercholesterolemia.

(5) Yinchen Zexie Yin (Decoction of Artemisiae Scopariae and Alismatis): composed of Yinchen (*Herba Artemisiae Scopariae*) 15 g, Zexie (*Rhizoma Alismatis*) 15 g and Gegen (*Radix Puerariae*) 15 g. Decoct the drugs in water for oral administration. It is indicated for hypertriglyceridemia and hyper-β-lipoproteinemia.

3. External Therapy

(1) Baijiezi (*Semen Sinapis Albae*) 30 g, Danxing (*Arisaema cum Bile*) 15 g, Baifan (*Alumen*) 15 g, Chuanxiong (*Rhizoma Chuanxiong*) 10 g, Yujin (*Radix Curcumae*) 10 g and proper amount of ginger juice. Grind the first five drugs into fine powder, mix the powder with ginger juice to make a paste. Then put the paste on the patient's navel and cover it with gauze and fix it with adhesive tape. Change the dressing once a day, 15 days as a course of tresatment. Usually the medicine takes effect in about 5 - 7 days and if it is applied for one or two months in succession the recurrence of the disease can be avoided. It is indicated for the case of hyperlipemia with accumulation of turbid phlegm in the body.

(2) Wuzhuyu (*Fructus Evodiae*, prepared with bile) 100 g, Longdancao (*Radix Gentianae*) 50 g, Tuliuhuang (*Sulfer*) 20 g, Zhusha (*Cinnabaris*) 15 g and Mingfan (*Alumen*) 30 g. Grind the drugs into powder, sift the powder and mix it with proper amount of Xiaojigen (*Radix Cirsii*) juice to make a paste. Apply it to the acupoints of Shenque (CV 8) and Yongquan (KI1) on both

（5）茵陈泽泻饮　茵陈15 g,泽泻15 g,葛根15 g,水煎服。适用于三酰甘油、β脂蛋白增高者。

3. 外治法

（1）白芥子30 g,胆星15 g,白矾15 g,川芎10 g,郁金10 g,姜汁适量。将前5味研末,用生姜汁调和如膏状,把膏药贴在患者的脐孔上,外用纱布覆盖,胶布固定,每日换药1次,15日为1个疗程。通常5～7日可奏效,连用1～2个月可防止复发。适用于高脂血症痰浊内蕴者。

（2）吴茱萸(胆汁拌制)100 g,龙胆草50 g,土硫黄20 g,朱砂15 g,明矾30 g,小蓟根汁适量。将前5味药研碎为末,过筛,加入小蓟根汁调和成糊,敷于神阙及双侧涌泉穴,每穴用10～15 g,上盖纱

sides, 10 - 15 g for each acupoint. Then cover it with gauze and fix it with adhesive tape. Change the dressing once every other day, one month as a course of treatment. It is indicated for hyperlipemia.

(3) Heye (*Folium Nelumbinis*) 15 g, Fangji (*Radix Stephaniae Tetrandrae*) 10 g, Baiziren (*Semen Platycladi*) 15 g and Zexie (*Rhizoma Alismatis*) 10 g. Boil the above drugs in 3,000 ml of water for 15 minutes, then remove the dregs and add 3,000 ml of warm water to the decoction and use it to bathe the body for 30 minutes. Take the medicated bath twice or thrice a week and ten times in succession make up a course of treatment. It is indicated for the case of hyperlipemia with fat physique, dizziness, dysphoria, oliguria, and edema.

(4) Danshen Shouwu Xiji (Medicated Liquid of Salviae Miltiorrhizae and Polygoni Multiflori): composed of Danshen (*Radix Salviae Miltiorrhizae*) 30 g, Heshouwu (*Radix Polygoni Multiflori*) 30 g, Shanzha (*Fructus Crataegi*) 30 g and Muxiang (*Radix Aucklaneliae seu Saussureae seu Vladimiriae*) 10 g. Soak the drugs in 3,000 ml of water for one hour and boil for 15 minutes. Remove the dregs, pour the hot decoction into a basin and bathe the body for 30 minutes. Take the medicated bath 3 times a week and 10 times in succession make up a course of treatment. One dose can be used twice. It is indicated for hyperlipemia with blurred vision, tinnitus, soreness of waist, weakness of legs, palpitation and numbness of the limbs.

(5) Xiakucao (*Spica Prunellae*) 30 g, Gouteng (*Ramulus Uncariae cum Uncis*) 20 g, Sangye (*Folium Mori*) 15 g and Juhua (*Flos Chrysanthemi*) 20 g. Decoct the above drugs and use the decoction to immerse the feet for 10 - 15 minutes, twice a day, 10 - 15 days being a course of treatment. It is indicated for hyperlipemia.

布,胶布固定,2 日换 1 次,1 个月为 1 个疗程。适用于高脂血症者。

(3) 荷叶15 g,防己10 g,柏子仁15 g,泽泻10 g。上药加水 3 000 ml,煮沸 15 分钟,去渣取汁,兑热水 3 000 ml,洗浴全身。每次 30 分钟,每周 2～3次,连续 10 次为 1 个疗程。适用于高脂血症体形肥胖,头晕心烦,尿少浮肿者。

(4) 丹参首乌洗剂　丹参 30 g,何首乌30 g,山楂30 g,木香10 g。上药加水 3 000 ml,浸泡 1 小时,煮沸 15 分钟,去渣取汁,将药倒入盆内,趁热浸浴。每次薰洗 30 分钟,每星期 3 次,10 次为 1 个疗程,每剂可用 2 次。适用于高脂血症,眩目耳鸣,腰酸腿软,心悸肢麻者。

(5) 夏枯草30 g,钩藤 20 g,桑叶15 g,菊花20 g。上药共煎水洗脚,每日 1～2 次,每次 10～15 分钟,10～15 日为 1 个疗程。适用于高脂血症者。

2.8.3　Diabetes Mellitus

General Description

Diabetes mellitus is a common endocrine metabolic disease. It is characterized by abnormal increase of blood sugar concentration, glycosuria and decrease of glucose tolerance. Clinically, there is no symptom at the early stage, and polyphagia, polydipsia, polyuria, thirst, susceptibility to hunger, tiredness, and emaciation may appear later. Serious cases may have ketoacidosis and hyperosmotic nonketonic coma. There are also some common complications and concomitant diseases, such as acute infection, tuberculosis, atherosclerosis, renal and retinal angionosis, neuropathy, etc. The disease can be found at any age, but it is more common in the middle-aged and old people. The morbidity increases with the age, with higher morbidity found in the people aged 45 and older and the highest in the people aged 60. The morbidity of diabetes in western countries is as high as 2% to 5%. In China it is 1.5% to 2.3% and the total number of patients suffering from diabetes is estimated to be about 20 million. Since it causes damages to many organs of the human body, bringing about higher mortality rate and disability rate, and seriously affecting the people's health and life quality, diabetes has been listed as the third serious disease following cardiovascular disease and tumor in many countries in the world.

The disease is closely related to the advance of age, obesity, reduction of physical labor and the habit of taking food of high caloric, high fat and high protein. Its basic physiopathologic changes are caused by the absolute or

第三节　糖尿病

【概述】

糖尿病是一种常见的内分泌代谢性疾病。其基本特征是血糖浓度异常升高,糖尿,葡萄糖耐量减低。本病早期临床多无症状,到了症状期才出现多饮、多食、多尿、口渴、易饥饿、疲乏、消瘦等症状。严重者发生酮症酸中毒、高渗昏迷等。常见的并发症及伴随症有急性感染、肺结核、动脉粥样硬化、肾和视网膜等大小血管病变以及神经病变等。本病可发生于任何年龄,多见于中老年人。患病率随年龄而增长,至45岁后明显上升,至60岁达到高峰。西方发达国家糖尿病的发病率高达2%～5%,中国为1.5%～2.3%,估计患病总人数约达2千万。由于糖尿病可造成对人体多脏器的损害,其死亡率、致残率较高,严重影响了人民的身体健康及生活质量,故在世界上许多国家已将其列为继心血管疾病和肿瘤之后的第三大疾病。

本病的发生与年龄的增高、肥胖、体力劳动的减少及高热量、高脂肪、高蛋白的饮食习惯等关系较为密切。其

relative insufficiency of insulin secretion, leading to metabolic disturbance of carbohydrate, protein, fat, water and electrolyte, and even the acid-base imbalance in severe cases.

According to its clinical manifestations, diabetes is categorized in TCM as "xiao ke" or "xiao dan", both of which mean diabetes. It is attributed to yin-deficiency diathesis, improper diet, emotional disorders, overstrain and excessive sexual activities. The main pathogenesis lies in consumption of yin fluid leading to endogenous dryness-heat in the body, with yin deficiency as the principal aspect and dryness-heat as the secondary aspect, and often with the presence of blood stasis and phlegm retention. If prolonged yin deficiency impairs yang, this will result in deficiency of both yin and yang as well as deficiency of both qi and yin.

Essentials for Diagnosis

(1) The onset of the disease is slow and the patients are mostly of middle and old age or have the family history of the disease.

(2) Polydipsia, polyphagia, polyuria, emaciation, and weakness. There may also be pruritus vuluae or pruritus cutanea, numbness of limbs, sensory disturbance of extremities, blurred vision, lumbago, hyposexuality, irregular menstruation, impotence, sterility, etc.

(3) Laboratory examination reveals fasting blood-glucose>7.0 mmol/L, or blood-glucose two hours after meal>11.1 mmol/L, decrease of sugar tolerance, fasting urine sugar positive over three times in succession.

(4) Insulin determination, insulin release test, serum c-peptide determination, glycosylized hemoglobin determination, ketonuria test, and urinometry are helpful to

基本生理病理改变是由于胰岛素分泌绝对或相对不足引起的代谢紊乱,包括糖、蛋白质、脂肪、水及电解质等,严重时常导致酸碱平衡失常。

根据本病的临床表现,当属于中医学"消渴"、"消瘅"范畴。其病因与素体阴虚、饮食不节、情志失调、劳欲过度有关。主要病机为阴津亏损,燥热内生,且以阴虚为本,燥热为标,常可见瘀血痰浊;日久阴损及阳,可见气阴两虚和阴阳两虚。

【诊断要点】

(1) 起病缓慢,以中老年人居多,或有家族史。

(2) 多饮,多食,多尿,消瘦无力。还可出现外阴或皮肤瘙痒、四肢麻木、肢端感觉障碍、视物模糊、腰痛、性欲减退、月经不调、阳痿不育等。

(3) 实验室检查空腹血糖>7.0 mmol/L,或餐后 2 小时血糖>11.1 mmol/L,糖耐量减低,空腹尿糖定性检查连续 3 次以上出现阳性。

(4) 胰岛素测定、胰岛素释放试验、血清 C-肽测定、糖基化血红蛋白测定、尿酮体、

the diagnosis of the disease.

Syndrome Differentiation and Treatment

The syndrome differentiation of the disease should aim at the predominance of yin deficiency or dryness-heat. Generally at the onset, yin deficiency predominates. As the disease progresses, there appears the coexistence of yin deficiency and dryness-heat, and yin deficiency predominates again at the late stage. Clinically, the disease is classified as the following syndromes: fluid consumption due to lung heat, excessive fire in the stomach, deficiency of kidney yin, deficiency of both qi and yin, and deficiency of both yin and yang. The treatment is based on the principle of eliminating heat by nourishing yin, moistening dryness and promoting fluid production. According to the condition of the principal and secondary aspects, deficiency and excess, as well as the location of pathological changes of the disease, the following methods are respectively adopted: clearing heat and purging fire, resolving phlegm to activate meridians, promoting blood circulation to remove blood stasis, removing dampness, nourishing the kidney to replenish yin, invigorating the spleen to tonify qi, replenishing both yin and yang, etc.

1. Fluid Consumption due to Lung Heat

Chief Manifestations: Polydipsia, thirst right after drinking, dry tongue and mouth, polyuria, insufficient saliva, red tongue with yellow thin coating, bounding and rapid pulse.

Therapeutic Methods: To clear away heat to moisten the lung, promote saliva production to quench thirst.

Prescription: Modified Xiaoke Fang (Diabetes Prescription) and Erdong Tang (Ophiopogonis and Asparagi Decoction), composed of Shengdihuang (*Radix Rehmanniae*) 10 g, Maimendong (*Radix Ophiopogonis*)

尿比重的检测有助于本病的诊断。

【辨证论治】

本病辨证主要是辨其阴虚与燥热的主次,一般病变初起以阴虚为主,进一步发展则阴虚与燥热互见,后期以阴虚为主。临床主要分为肺热津伤、胃火炽盛、肾阴亏损、气阴两虚和阴阳两虚证。治疗以养阴清热、润燥生津为基本原则,根据标本虚实主次、病变部位,分别采用清热泻火、化痰通络、活血化瘀、祛湿降浊、滋肾养阴、健脾益气、阴阳并补等法。

1. 肺热津伤证

主要证候 烦渴多饮,随饮随渴,口舌干燥,尿频量多,舌红少津,苔薄黄,脉洪数。

治 法 清热润肺,生津止渴。

方 药 消渴方合二冬汤加减:生地黄10 g,麦门冬10 g,北沙参10 g,天门冬10 g,知母10 g,天花粉20 g,黄连

10 g, Beishashen (*Radix Glehniae*) 10 g, Tianmendong
(*Radix Asparagi*) 10 g, Zhimu (*Rhizoma Anemarrhe-nae*) 10 g, Tianhuafen (*Radix Trichosanthis*) 20 g,
Huanglian (*Rhizoma Coptidis*) 5 g, Huangqin (*Radix Scutellariae*) 10 g and Gegen (*Radix Puerariae*) 10 g.

Modifications: For cases with extreme thirst, add Shi-hu (*Herba Dendrobii*) 10 g; for dry feces, add Jue-mingzi (*Semen Cassiae*) 15 g; for polydipsia with a desire for drinking, yellow dry tongue coating, and bounding large pulse, add Taizishen (*Radix Pseudostellariae*) 10 g and Shi-gao (*Gypsum Fibrosum*, to be decocted first) 30 g.

2. Excessive Fire in the Stomach

Chief Manifestations: Polyphagia with susceptibility to hunger, emaciation, dry mouth, thirst, constipation, red tongue with dry yellow coating, and smooth, solid and forceful pulse.

Therapeutic Methods: To clear away stomach heat, moisten dryness, nourish yin and produce fluid.

Prescription: Yunü Jian Jiawei (Jade Maid Decoction with Additions), composed of Shengshigao (*Gypsum Fibrosum*, to be decocted first) 30 g, Zhimu (*Rhizoma Anemarrhenae*) 10 g, Shengdihuang (*Radix Rehmanniae*) 10 g, Maimendong (*Radix Ophiopogonis*) 10 g, Zhizi (*Radix Gardeniae*) 10 g, Niuxi (*Radix Achyranthis Bidentatae*) 10 g and Xuanshen (*Radix Scrophulariae*) 10 g.

Modifications: For constipation, add Mangxiao (*Natrii Sulfas seu Mirabititum*, infused) 10 g and Zhi-dahuang (*Radix et Rhizoma Rhei Preparata*) 10 g; for swollen and painful gum with flaring up of stomach fire, add Huanglian (*Rhizoma Coptidis*) 5 g.

3. Deficiency of Kidney Yin

Chief Manifestations: Polyuria, cloudy urine, dry mouth and lips, emaciation, sore and weak knees and

5 g,黄芩10 g,葛根10 g。

加　减　口干甚者,加石斛10 g;大便干燥者,加决明子15 g;若烦渴引饮,苔黄燥,脉洪大者,加太子参10 g,石膏(先煎)30 g。

2. 胃火炽盛证

主要证候　多食易饥,形体消瘦,口干口渴,大便秘结,舌红,苔黄干燥,脉滑实有力。

治　法　清胃润燥,养阴增液。

方　药　玉女煎加味:生石膏(先煎)30 g,知母10 g,生地黄10 g,麦门冬10 g,栀子10 g,牛膝10 g,玄参10 g。

加　减　大便秘结者,加芒硝(冲)10 g,制大黄10 g;胃火上炎,牙龈肿痛者,加黄连5 g。

3. 肾阴亏损证

主要证候　尿频量多,混浊如脂膏,口干唇燥,形体瘦

loins, red tongue with little coating, deep, thready and rapid pulse.

Therapeutic Methods: To nourish yin and strengthen the kidney.

Prescription: Modified Liuwei Dihuang Tang (Decoction of Six Drugs Containing Rehmanniae), composed of Shengdihuang (*Radix Rehmanniae*) 10 g, Shanyurou (*Fructus Corni*) 10 g, Gouqizi (*Fructus Lycii*) 10 g, Shanyao (*Rhizoma Dioscoreae*) 10 g, Fuling (*Poria*) 10 g, Zexie (*Rhizoma Alismatis*) 10 g and Mudanpi (*Cortex Moutan Radicis*) 10 g.

Modifications: For cases with restless sleep, seminal emission, red tongue, thready and rapid pulse, add Huangbai (*Cortex Phellodendri*) 10 g, Zhimu (*Rhizoma Anemarrhenae*) 10 g, Longgu (*Os Draconis*, to be decocted first) 30 g, Muli (*Concha Ostreae*, to be decocted first) 30 g and Guiban (*Plastrum Testudinis*, to be decocted first) 15 g; for large amount of turbid urine, add Yizhiren (*Fructus Alpiniae Oxyphyllae*) 10 g, Fupenzi (*Fructus Rubi*) 10 g and Wuweizi (*Fructus Schisandrae*) 10 g; for drowsiness, short breath, pale red tongue, add Dangshen (*Radix Codonopsis*) 10 g and Huangqi (*Radix Astragali*) 10 g.

4. Deficiency of Both Qi and Yin

Chief Manifestations: No obvious polydipsia, polyuria or polyphagia but dry mouth and throat, lassitude, palpitation, short breath, spontaneous sweating, night sweating, feverish sensation of the chest, palms and soles, insomnia, dreamfulness, scanty dark yellow urine, constipation, red tongue with reduced saliva, swollen tongue or with teeth marks, thin coating or geographic tongue, wiry and thready pulse or smooth and rapid pulse.

Therapeutic Methods: To replenish qi and nourish yin.

弱,腰膝酸软,舌质红少苔,脉沉细数。

　　治　法　滋阴固肾。

　　方　药　六味地黄汤加减:生地黄10 g,山茱萸10 g,枸杞子10 g,山药10 g,茯苓10 g,泽泻10 g,牡丹皮10 g。

　　加　减　烦躁失眠,遗精,舌红,脉细数者,加黄柏10 g,知母10 g,龙骨(先煎)30 g,牡蛎(先煎)30 g,龟版(先煎)15 g;尿量多而混浊者,加益智仁10 g,覆盆子10 g,五味子10 g;困倦,气短,舌淡红者,加党参10 g,黄芪10 g。

4. 气阴两虚证

　　主要证候　无明显的多饮、多尿、多食症状,仅有口干咽干,倦怠乏力,心悸气短,自汗盗汗,五心烦热,失眠多梦,小便短赤,大便秘结,舌红少津,舌体胖或有齿印,苔薄或花剥,脉弦细或滑数。

　　治　法　益气养阴。

Prescription: Modified Shengmai San (Powder for Reinforcing Qi and Nourishing Yin) and Zengye Tang (Decoction for Increasing Fluid), composed of Taizishen (*Radix Pseudostellariae*) 10 g, Shengdihuang (*Radix Rehmanniae*) 10 g, Xuanshen (*Radix Scrophulariae*) 10 g, Maimendong (*Radix Ophiopogonis*) 10 g, Wuweizi (*Fructus Schisandrae*) 10 g, Gegen (*Radix Puerariae*) 10 g, Tianhuafen (*Radix Trichosanthis*) 15 g, Baishaoyao (*Radix Paeoniae Alba*) 10 g and Huangjing (*Rhizoma Polygonati*) 10 g.

Modifications: For yin deficiency with obvious polyphagia, polydipsia and polyuria, add Shigao (*Gypsum Fibrosum*, to be decocted first) 30 g, Zhimu (*Rhizoma Anemarrhenae*) 10 g and Shudihuang (*Radix Rehmanniae Preparata*) 12 g; for short breath and lassitude, remove Taizishen, add Huangqi (*Radix Astragali*) 15 g and Dangshen (*Radix Codonopsis*) 10 g.

5. Deficiency of Both Yin and Yang

Chief Manifestations: Frequent urination with cloudy urine (*as frequent as once after each drink*), dark face, sore and weak loins and knees, cold body, aversion to cold, impotence, pale tongue with white coating, deep thready and forceless pulse.

Therapeutic Methods: To warm yang and nourish the kidney to induce astringency.

Prescription: Modified Shenqi Wan (Bolus for Invigorating Kidney Qi), composed of Zhifuzi (*Radix Aconiti Lateralis Preparata*) 10 g, Rougui (*Cortex Cinnamomi*, to be decocted later) 3 g, Shudihuang (*Radix Rehmanniae Preparata*) 10 g, Mudanpi (*Cortex Moutan Radicis*) 10 g, Zexie (*Rhizoma Alismatis*) 10 g, Fuling (*Poria*) 10 g, Jinyingzi (*Fructus Rosae Laevigatae*) 10 g, Fupenzi (*Fructus Rubi*) 10 g, Xuanshen (*Radix Scrophulariae*) 10 g, Zhihuangjing (*Rhizoma*

方　药　生脉散合增液汤加减：太子参10 g，生地黄10 g，玄参10 g，麦门冬10 g，五味子10 g，葛根10 g，天花粉15 g，白芍药10 g，黄精10 g。

加　减　以阴虚为主，且三多症状较明显者，加石膏（先煎）30 g，知母10 g，熟地黄12 g；气短乏力明显者，去太子参，加黄芪15 g，党参10 g。

5. 阴阳两虚证

主要证候　小便频数，混浊如膏，甚至饮一溲一，面色黧黑，腰膝酸软，形寒畏冷，阳痿，舌质淡，苔白，脉沉细无力。

治　法　温阳滋肾固涩。

方　药　肾气丸加减：制附子10 g，肉桂（后下）3 g，熟地黄10 g，牡丹皮10 g，泽泻10 g，茯苓10 g，金樱子10 g，覆盆子10 g，玄参10 g，制黄精10 g，淫羊藿10 g。

Polygonati Preparata) 10 g and Yinyanghuo (*Herba Epimedii*) 10 g.

Modifications: For severe soreness and weakness of the loins, add Duzhong (*Cortex Eucommiae*) 10 g, Niuxi (*Radix Achyranthis Bidentatae*) 10 g and Xuduan (*Radix Dipsaci*) 10 g; for aversion to cold, add Lujiaopian (*Cornu Cervi, sliced*) 10 g and Ziheche (*Placenta Hominis*) 10 g; for sickly, dimmish black and lusterless complexion, add Heshouwu (*Radix Polygoni Multiflori*) 10 g, Gouqizi (*Fructus Lycii*) 10 g and Gusuibu (*Rhizoma Drynariae*) 10 g; for loose stools, add Buguzhi (*Fructus Psoraleae*) 10 g and Yizhiren (*Fructus Alpiniae Oxyphyllae*) 10 g.

6. Deficiency of Both Qi and Blood

Chief Manifestations: Prolonged course of illness, lassitude, drowsiness, weakness, short breath, hypologia, pale lips and nails, lusterless hair, emaciation, dry mouth, thirst, cloudy and sweet urine, emaciation with good appetite or anorexia with abdominal distension, inclination for sitting and dislike for moving, palpitation, insomnia, white and dry tongue coating with reduced saliva, thready and weak pulse.

Therapeutic Methods: To tonify blood, replenish qi, moisten dryness and promote fluid production.

Prescription: Modified Guipi Tang (Decoction for Invigorating Spleen and Nourishing Heart) and Shengyu Tang (Specific Decoction for Recovery), composed of Huangqi (*Radix Astragali*) 15 g, Dangshen (*Radix Codonopsis*) 10 g, Baizhu (*Rhizoma Atractylodis Macrocephalae*) 10 g, Shanyao (*Rhizoma Dioscoreae*) 10 g, Fuling (*Poria*) 10 g, Shudihuang (*Radix Rehmanniae Preparata*) 12 g, Shengdihuang (*Radix Rehmanniae*) 10 g, Danggui (*Radix Angelicae Sinensis*) 10 g, Baishaoyao (*Radix Paeoniae Alba*) 10 g, Gegen (*Radix*

加　减　腰酸软甚者,加杜仲10 g,牛膝10 g,续断10 g;畏寒怕冷者,加鹿角片10 g,紫河车10 g;面容憔悴,黧黑无华者,加何首乌10 g,枸杞子10 g,骨碎补10 g;大便溏泄者,加补骨脂10 g,益智仁10 g。

6. 气血两虚证

主要证候　病程日久,神疲困倦,疲乏无力,少气懒言,唇甲淡白,毛发不荣,形体消瘦,口干口渴,尿混浊味甜,能食而消瘦,或食少而腹胀,喜坐少动,心悸少寐,苔白而干燥少津,脉细弱。

治　法　补血益气,润燥生津。

方　药　归脾汤合圣愈汤加减:黄芪15 g,党参10 g,白术10 g,山药10 g,茯苓10 g,熟地黄12 g,生地黄10 g,当归10 g,白芍药10 g,葛根10 g,天花粉20 g。

Puerariae) 10 g and Tianhuafen (*Radix Trichosanthis*) 20 g.

Modifications: For severe blood deficiency, add Ejiao (*Colla Corii Asini*, to be melted and infused) 10 g and Zihechefen (*Placenta Hominis*, powdered and to be infused) 10 g and increase the dosage of Dangshen and Huangqi to 30 g each to replenish qi and promote blood generation; for impaired appetite and loose stools, remove Danggui and add Chaoyiyiren (*Semen Coicis*, stir-baked) 15 g, Weimuxiang (*Radix Aucklaneliae*, roasted in fresh cinders) 10 g and Zexie (*Rhizoma Alismatis*) 15 g.

7. Phlegm Stagnation and Blood Stasis

Chief Manifestations: Fat physique, heavy head and body, localized stabbing pain on certain part of the body, dark purple lips and extremities, or numbness of limbs, sensation of stickiness and greasiness in the mouth, loss of appetite, dark purple tongue with ecchymosis, thick and greasy coating, smooth or unsmooth pulse.

Therapeutic Methods: To resolve phlegm, activate blood, remove blood stasis and dredge meridians.

Prescription: Modified Wendan Tang (Decoction for Clearing away Gallbladder Heat) and Tao Hong Siwu Tang (Four-Ingredient Decoction with Persicae and Carthami), composed of Huanglian (*Rhizoma Coptidis*) 5 g, Zhuru (*Caulis Bambusae in Taeniam*) 10 g, Danxing (*Arisaema cum Bile*) 10 g, Zhishi (*Fructus Aurantii Immaturus*) 10 g, Taoren (*Semen Persicae*) 10 g, Honghua (*Flos Carthami*) 10 g, Danggui (*Radix Angelicae Sinensis*) 10 g, Chuanxiong (*Rhizoma Chuanxiong*) 10 g, Guijianyu (*Ramulus Euonymi Alati*) 15 g, Shuizhi (*Hirudo*) 3 g, Zelan (*Herba Lycopi*) 10 g and Zhibaijiangcan (*Bombyx Batryticatus*, roasted) 10 g.

加　减　血虚甚者,加阿胶(烊化冲服)10 g,紫河车粉(冲服)10 g,并重用党参30 g,黄芪30 g,以补气生血;食少便溏者,去当归,加炒薏苡仁15 g,煨木香10 g,泽泻15 g。

7. 痰瘀阻滞证

主要证候　形体肥胖,头身沉重,身体某部固定刺痛,口唇或肢端紫暗,或肢体麻木,口中黏腻,饮食乏味,舌苔厚腻,舌质紫暗有瘀斑,脉滑或涩。

治　法　化痰活血,逐瘀通络。

方　药　温胆汤合桃红四物汤加减:黄连5 g,竹茹10 g,胆星10 g,枳实10 g,桃仁10 g,红花10 g,当归10 g,川芎10 g,鬼箭羽15 g,水蛭3 g,泽兰10 g,炙白僵蚕10 g。

Modifications: For blood stasis in the brain, add Yujin (*Radix Curcumae*) 10 g and Shichangpu (*Rhizoma Acori Graminei*) 10 g; for blood stasis in the heart, add Gualou (*Fructus Trichosanthis*) 10 g and Gegen (*Radix Puerariae*) 10 g; for blood stasis in the back and shoulders, add Pianjianghuang (*Rhizoma Curcumae Longae*, *sliced*) 10 g and Guizhi (*Ramulus Cinnamomi*) 10 g; for blood stasis in the lower limbs, add Niuxi (*Radix Achyranthis Bidentatae*) 10 g and Hai'ercha (*Catechu*) 10 g; for qi deficiency, add Huangqi (*Radix Astragali*) 10 g and Taizishen (*Radix Pseudostellariae*) 10 g; for qi stagnation, add Chenpi (*Pericarpium Citri Reticulatae*) 10 g, Zhike (*Fructus Aurantii*) 10 g and Muxiang (*Radix Aucklaneliae*) 10 g; for qi depression, add Xiangfu (*Rhizoma Cyperi*) 10 g and Chaihu (*Radix Bupleuri*) 6 g.

Other Treatments

1. Chinese Patent Drugs

(1) Xiaoke Wan (Diabetes Pill): 5 - 10 pills each time, 3 times per day; indicated for diabetes with deficiency of both qi and yin, especially effective for incipient diabetes and diabates of mild, moderate and stable types.

(2) Jiangtangshu (Pill for Reducing Blood Sugar): 4 - 6 pills each time, 3 times per day; indicated for diabetes with deficiency of both qi and yin accompanied with blood stasis.

(3) Yuquan Wan (Jade Spring Pill): 6 g (60 pills) each time, 4 times per day, taken with warm boiled water, one month being a course of treatment; indicated for diabetes with deficient yin and reduced saliva.

(4) Shen Qi Jiangtang Pian (Ginseng and Astragali Tablet for Reducing Blood Sugar): 3 tablets each time, 3 times per day, taken with warm boiled water, one month being a course of treatment; indicated for diabetes with

加 减 瘀阻在脑者,加郁金10 g,石菖蒲10 g;瘀阻在心者,加瓜蒌10 g,葛根10 g;瘀阻在肩背者,加片姜黄10 g,桂枝10 g;瘀在下肢者,加牛膝10 g,孩儿茶10 g;兼有气虚者,加黄芪10 g,太子参10 g;兼气滞者,加陈皮10 g,枳壳10 g,木香10 g;兼气郁者,加香附10 g,柴胡6 g。

【其他疗法】

1. 中成药

(1) 消渴丸 每服5～10粒,每日3次。适用于糖尿病证属气阴两虚者。对初发病,轻、中型及稳定型疗效较好。

(2) 降糖舒 每服4～6粒,每日3次。适用于糖尿病证属气阴两虚,夹有瘀血者。

(3) 玉泉丸 每服6 g(60粒),每日4次,温开水送服。1个月为1个疗程。适用于糖尿病证属阴亏津少者。

(4) 参芪降糖片 每服3片,每日3次,温开水送服。连服1个月为1个疗程。适用于糖尿病证属气阴不足,脾肾

deficiency of qi and yin, deficiency of both spleen and kidney, and contraindicated for excessive heat syndrome.

(5) Kelening Jiaonang (Kelening Capsule): 4 capsules each time, 3 times per day, three months being a course of treatment; indicated for diabetes with deficiency of both qi and yin.

(6) Liuwei Dihuang Wan (Pill of Six Drugs Containing Rehmanniae) 6 - 9 g each time, twice per day; indicated for diabetes with yin deficiency of liver yin and kidney yin and used with caution for spleen deficiency with anorexia and loose stools.

(7) Jingui Shenqi Wan (Pill for Invigorating Kidney Qi from Golden Cabinet): 9 g each time, twice or thrice daily, taken with warm boiled water or dilute salty water; indicated for diabetes with kidney-yang deficiency.

(8) Tangniaole Jiaonang (Diabetes Capsule): 3 - 4 capsules (0.3 g per capsule) each time, 3 times per day; indicated for diabetes with deficiency of both qi and yin.

2. Single-drug or Experiential Prescriptions

(1) Huanglian Jiangtang Yin (Coptidis Decoction for Reducing Sugar): composed of Huanglian (*Rhizoma Coptidis*) 3 g, Tianhuafen (*Radix Trichosanthis*) 15 g, Shengdihuang (*Radix Rehmanniae*) 12 g, Ouzhi (*Rhizoma Nelumbinis*, liquidized) 90 ml and 120 ml of cow milk. First, decoct Huanglian, Tianhuafen and Shengdihuang, then remove the dregs from the decoction. Boil the cow milk, pour it together with Ouzhi to the decoction and take the decoction in divided doses. It is indicated for diabetes with deficiency of both qi and yin and endogenous heat.

(2) Ningtang Yin (Decoction for Controlling Blood Sugar): composed of Jiaogulan (*Rhizoma seu Herba Gynostemmatis Pentaphylli*) 15 g, Tianhuafen (*Radix*

两虚者。凡有热实证者，禁用。

（5）渴乐宁胶囊　每服4粒,每日3次,3个月为1个疗程。适用于糖尿病证属气阴两虚者。

（6）六味地黄丸　每服6～9g,每日2次。适用于糖尿病证属肝肾阴虚者。脾虚食少便溏者慎用。

（7）《金匮》肾气丸　每服9g,每日2～3次,温开水或淡盐水送服。适用于糖尿病证属肾阳不足者。

（8）糖尿乐胶囊　每服3～4粒,每粒0.3g,每日3次。适用于糖尿病证属气阴两虚者。

2. 单验方

（1）黄连降糖饮　黄连3g,天花粉15g,生地黄12g,藕汁90ml,牛乳120ml。先煎黄连、天花粉、生地黄,煎后去渣,将牛乳煮沸,与藕汁一并冲入,频服。适用于糖尿病证属气阴两虚内热者。

（2）宁糖饮　绞股蓝15g,天花粉15g,葛根15g,焦山楂15g,玄参15g,紫丹参

Trichosanthis) 15 g, Gegen (*Radix Puerariae*) 15 g, Jiaoshanzha (*Fructus Crataegi, charred*) 15 g, Xuanshen (*Radix Scrophulariae*) 15 g, Zidanshen (*Radix Salviae Miltiorrhizae*) 20 g, Huangqi (*Radix Astragali*) 30 g, Baimaogen (*Rhizoma Imperatae*) 30 g and Cangzhu (*Rhizoma Atractylodis*) 10 g. Decoct the drugs in water for oral administration, 1 dose per day, 30 days being a course of treatment. It is indicated for diabetes with deficiency of both qi and yin accompanied with blood stasis.

(3) Bugu Huayu Tang (Decoction for Tonifying Bone and Removing Blood Stasis): composed of Heizhima (*Semen Sesami Nigrum*) 10 g, Sangye (*Folium Mori*) 10 g, Shengdihuang (*Radix Rehmanniae*) 10 g, Renshen (*Radix Ginseng*) 10 g, Shuizhi (*Hirudo*) 10 g and Lizhihe (*Semen Litchi*) 10 g. Decoct the drugs in water for oral administration, one dose per day, one month being a course of treatment. It is indicated for diabetes cases of old age.

(4) Digu Taojiao Yin (Decoction of Lycii Radicis and Resina Persicae): composed of Digupi (*Cortex Lycii Radicis*) 30 g and Taoshujiao (*Resina Persicae*) 15 g. Decoct the drugs in water for oral administration, once per day. It is indicated for the diabetes with excessive heat and blood stasis.

(5) Wenshen Huayu Tang (Decoction for Warming Kidney and Removing Blood Stasis): composed of Lujiaoshuang (*Cornu Cervi Degelatinatum*) 30 - 50 g, Shengdihuang (*Radix Rehmanniae*) 20 g, Shudihuang (*Radix Rehmanniae Preparata*) 20 g, Gouqizi (*Fructus Lycii*) 15 g, Biejia (*Carapax Trionycis, to be decocted first*) 15 g, Shenghuangqi (*Radix Astragali*) 30 g, Cangzhu (*Rhizoma Atractylodis*) 10 g, Danshen (*Radix Salviae Miltiorrhizae*) 30 g, Chuanxiong (*Rhi-*

20 g,黄芪30 g,白茅根30 g,苍术10 g。水煎服。每日 1 剂,30 日为 1 个疗程。适用于糖尿病证属气阴两虚挟有瘀血者。

(3) 补骨化瘀汤 黑芝麻10 g,桑叶10 g,生地黄10 g,人参10 g,水蛭10 g,荔枝核10 g。水煎服。每日 1 剂,1 个月为 1 个疗程。适用于老年糖尿病者。

(4) 地骨桃胶饮 地骨皮30 g,桃树胶15 g。水煎服,每日 1 次。适用于糖尿病证属热盛血瘀者。

(5) 温肾化瘀汤 鹿角霜30～50 g,生地黄20 g,熟地黄20 g,枸杞子15 g,鳖甲(先煎)15 g,生黄芪30 g,苍术10 g,丹参30 g,川芎10 g,桃仁10 g。水煎服。每日 1 剂,分2～3次服,1 个月为 1 个疗程。适用于中老年糖尿病者。

zoma *Chuanxiong*) 10 g and Taoren (*Semen Persicae*) 10 g. Decoct the drugs in water, one dose per day, and take the decoction in 2 – 3 divided doses, one month being a course of treatment. It is indicated for diabetes cases of middle and old age.

(6) Yuhu Wan (Jade Pot Pill): composed of Renshen (*Radix Ginseng*) and Gualou (*Fructus Trichosanthis*). Take equal quantity of each of the above drugs and grind them into fine powder, then make the powder into pills as big as phoenix tree seeds. Take 30 pills each time with warm boiled water. It is indicated for diabetes with polydipsia.

(7) Yitang Tang (Decoction for Restraining Blood Sugar): composed of Shengshigao (*Gypsum Fibrosum*, to be decocted first) 30 g, Shanyao (*Rhizoma Dioscoreae*) 30 g, Maimendong (*Radix Ophiopogonis*) 20 g, Tianhuafen (*Radix Trichosanthis*) 20 g, Shudihuang (*Radix Rehmanniae Preparata*) 20 g, Shihu (*Herba Dendrobii*) 15 g, Bixie (*Rhizoma Dioscoreae Hypoglaucae*) 15 g, Fupenzi (*Fructus Rubi*) 15 g, Tusizi (*Semen Cuscutae*) 15 g, Sangpiaoxiao (*Oötheca Mantidis*) 15 g, Yizhiren (*Fructus Alpiniae Oxyphyllae*) 10 g and Wubeizi (*Galla Chinensis*) 6 g. Decoct the above drugs in water for oral administration, one dose daily. It is indicated for diabetes with yin deficiency and dry heat.

(8) Modified Qiwei Baizhu San (Seven-Ingredient Powder Containing Atractylodis Macrocephalae): composed of Dangshen (*Radix Codonopsis*) 10 g, Gegen (*Radix Puerariae*) 10 g, Shanyao (*Rhizoma Dioscoreae*) 10 g, Baizhu (*Rhizoma Atractylodis Macrocephalae*) 10 g, Wumei (*Fructus Mume*) 5 – 10 g, Fuling (*Poria*) 12 g, Huoxiang (*Herba Agastaches*) 10 g, Yiyiren (*Semen Coicis*) 15 g, Guya (*Fructus Oryzae Germinatus*) 10 g, Maiya (*Fructus Hordei Germinatus*)

(6) 玉壶丸 人参、瓜蒌根各等分。上药共研细末,为丸,如梧桐子大,每服 30 丸,温水送服。适用于糖尿病饮水无度者。

(7) 抑糖汤 生石膏(先煎) 30 g, 山药 30 g, 麦门冬 20 g, 天花粉 20 g, 熟地黄 20 g, 石斛 15 g, 萆薢 15 g, 覆盆子 15 g, 菟丝子 15 g, 桑螵蛸 15 g, 益智仁 10 g, 五倍子 6 g。水煎服,每日 1 剂。适用于糖尿病证属阴虚燥热者。

(8) 加减七味白术散 党参 10 g, 葛根 10 g, 山药 10 g, 白术 10 g, 乌梅 5 ～ 10 g, 茯苓 12 g, 藿香 10 g, 薏苡仁 15 g, 谷芽 10 g, 麦芽 10 g, 炙甘草 3 g。水煎服,每日 1 剂。适用于糖尿病脾虚者。

10 g and Zhigancao (*Radix Glycyrrhizae*, roasted) 3 g. Decoct the above drugs in water for oral administration, one dose daily. It is indicated for diabetes with spleen deficiency.

3. External Therapy

（1）Huangjing (*Rhizoma Polygonati*) 30 g and Digupi (*Cortex Lycii Radicis*) 30 g. Add 3,000 ml of water to the drugs, leave the drugs soaked for 30 minutes and boil them for 30 minutes. Remove the dregs, pour the medicinal liquid into the bath basin and add 3,000 ml of warm water to it. Then use the liquid to bathe the body for 30 minutes each time, one dose and one bath per day, 15 days being a course of treatment. It is indicated for diabetes with deficient yin and excessive endogenous heat.

（2）Huanglian (*Rhizoma Coptidis*) 50 g. Add 2,500 ml of water to it, boil it for 30 minutes, remove the dregs and add 3,000 ml of warm water to the medicinal liquid. Then use it to bathe the body for 30 minutes each time, once or twice every day, 15 days being a course of treatment. It is indicated for diabetes with excessive stomach heat.

（3）Shigao (*Gypsum Fibrosum*) 5 g, Zhimu (*Rhizoma Anemarrhenae*) 2 g, Shengdihuang (*Radix Rehmanniae*) 0.6 g, Dangshen (*Radix Codonopsis*) 0.6 g, Gancao (*Radix Glycyrrhizae*) 1 g, Xuanshen (*Radix Scrophulariae*) 1 g, Tianhuafen (*Radix Trichosanthis*) 0.2 g, Huanglian (*Rhizoma Coptidis*) 0.3 g, small amount of Jingmi (*Semen Oryzae Sativae*) and Melbine Hydrochloride 40 mg. Extract all the above drugs except Melbine Hydrochloride, make them into powder and keep the powder at a cool place. To apply the medicine, use a wet towel to wipe clean the navel, get 250 mg of the medicinal powder and mix it thoroughly with melbine hydrochloride; then apply it to the navel, cover it with absorb-

3. 外治法

（1）黄精 30 g,地骨皮 30 g,加水 3 000 ml,浸泡 30 分钟后,煮沸 30 分钟,去渣,取药液,倒入浴盆中,兑入 3 000 ml 温水,浸浴全身,每次 30 分钟,每日 1 剂,浸洗 1 次,15 日为 1 个疗程。适用于糖尿病证属阴虚内热者。

（2）黄连 50 g,加水 2 500 ml,煎煮 30 分钟,去渣,取药液,倒入浴盆中,兑入温水 3 000 ml,浸泡洗浴全身,每次 30 分钟,每日 1～2 次,15 日为 1 个疗程。适用于糖尿病胃热较盛者。

（3）石膏 5 g,知母 2 g,生地黄 0.6 g,党参 0.6 g,甘草 1 g,玄参 1 g,天花粉 0.2 g,黄连 0.3 g,粳米少许,盐酸二甲双胍 40 mg。上方除盐酸二甲双胍外经提炼制成粉剂,放阴凉处。用时用湿毛巾将脐擦净,取药粉 250 mg,加盐酸二甲双胍混匀,敷入药粉,盖以药棉,外用胶布固定,每 5～7 日换药 1 次,6 次为 1 个疗程。适用于糖尿病证属气阴两虚内热偏盛者。

ent cotton and fix it with adhesive tape. Change the medicine every 5 - 7 days, 6 times being a course of treatment. It is indicated for diabetes with deficiency of both qi and yin and excessive endogenous heat.

2.8.4 Hyperthyroidism

General Description

Hyperthyroidism is a disease caused by excessive quantities of hormone secreted by thyroid acinar cells due to an auto-immune disorder and other factors. The chief clinical manifestations are polyphagia, emaciation, aversion to heat, profuse sweating, palpitation, irritability, ocular proptosis, thyroid enlargement, etc. In view of its causes, the disease can be classified into many types. The most common one is diffuse goiter with hyperthyroidism, thyroid enlargement and exophthalmus, which makes up 88% of the disease. And following it there is nodular goiter with hyperthyroidism. The disease occurs more often in females and the ratio of incidence between males and females is about 1 : 4 - 6. It may be found in any age group, but more often in those aged 20 - 40.

Hyperthyroidism is an autoimmune disease, related to mental upset or a history of mental trauma. Its pathogenesis is still not completely known. Generally it is believed that hyperthyroidism is caused by the existence of thyroid stimulus antibody (TSAb).

According to the clinical manifestations of the disease, it is categorized in TCM as "ying qi" (goiter), "zhong xiao" (polyphagia), "gan yu" (hepatic stagnation), "gan huo" (hepatic fire) and "xin ji" (palpitation).

第四节 甲状腺功能亢进症

【概述】

甲状腺功能亢进症是由于自身免疫反应等因素致使甲状腺腺泡细胞分泌过多的相应激素而引起的疾病。主要临床表现为多食、消瘦、畏热、多汗、心悸、激动、眼球突出、甲状腺肿大等。按病因不同可分为许多类型,最常见的占本病 88% 的为弥漫性甲状腺肿大伴功能亢进,有甲状腺肿及突眼。其次为结节性甲状腺肿伴功能亢进。本病多见于女性,男女之比约为1:4~6,各年龄组均可发病,以20~40 岁为多见。

本病的发生与精神刺激或创伤病史有关,是一种自身免疫性疾病。其发病机理至今尚未完全明了。一般认为由于患者体内存在有甲状腺刺激抗体(TSAb)所致。

根据本病的临床表现,当属于中医学"瘿气"、"中消"、"肝郁"、"肝火"、"心悸"范畴。其病因为情志不遂、饮食水土

Its etiological factors are emotional upset, improper diet and unsuitable living conditions, yin-deficiency constitution, etc. At the onset, it is attributed to qi stagnation, liver fire, stagnant phlegm and blood stasis, pertaining to excess type. The prolonged case is often marked by yin deficiency or deficiency of both qi and yin and often involves the liver, heart, spleen and kidney, pertaining to deficiency type.

Essentials for Diagnosis

(1) The main clinical manifestations are aversion to heat, polyhidrosis, irritability, increased appetite, emaciation, diarrhea, tachycardia, ocular proptosis and thyroid enlargement. Tremor and murmur can be found on the gland.

(2) Laboratory examination reveals increase of total T_3 and T_4. Thyrotropin-Releasing Hormone (TRH) stimulation test shows no increase of thyroid-stimulating hormone (TSH). The iodine intake rate of thyroid increases with an early peak. Immunologic examination can find abnormity of anti-thyroid globulin antibody, anti-microsome antibody and immune globulin.

(3) Radioactive nuclein CT scanning can exclude thyroid adenoma and other causes of thyroid enlargement.

Syndrome Differentiation and Treatment

It is important to differentiate between the deficiency type and excess type of the disease. The case at the onset is often of the excess type mostly due to qi stagnation, liver fire, stagnant phlegm and blood stasis. The prolonged case belongs to the deficiency type, often characterized by yin deficiency or deficiency of both qi and yin. Clinically, the disease is categorized into the following syndromes: qi and phlegm stagnation, liver fire attacking the stomach,

失宜、素体阴虚等。初起多实，因气郁肝火，痰凝血瘀所致；久病属虚，多见阴虚或气阴两虚，常涉及肝、心、脾、肾等脏。

【诊断要点】

（1）临床主要表现为怕热多汗，易激动，饮食量大，消瘦，腹泻，心动过速，眼征及甲状腺肿大，在甲状腺部位查到震颤及血管杂音。

（2）实验室检查可见血清总 T_3、T_4 升高，促甲状腺激素释放激素（TRH）兴奋试验、促甲状腺激素（TSH）不升高，甲状腺摄碘率升高且高峰提前。免疫学检查可发现抗甲状腺球蛋白抗体、抗微粒体抗体和免疫球蛋白异常。

（3）放射性核素 CT 扫描可排除甲状腺腺瘤及其他甲状腺肿大。

【辨证论治】

本病辨证主要是辨虚实，初起多实，多因气郁肝火、痰凝血瘀所致；久病属虚，多见阴虚或气阴两虚。临床主要分为气郁痰阻、肝火犯胃、气阴两虚、心肝阴虚证和甲状腺危象证。治疗以理气化痰、清热泻火、软坚散结为基本原

deficiency of both qi and yin, deficiency of heart yin and liver yin, and thyroid crisis. The treatment is based on the principles of regulating qi to resolve phlegm, clearing away heat and purging fire, and softening hardness and dissipating mass. For the prolonged case with blood stasis, the principle of promoting blood circulation to remove blood stasis should be added. While for hyperactive liver fire affecting yin, tonifying yin should be taken as the main principle. In case of deficiency of spleen qi and stomach qi, tonifying qi and invigorating the spleen should be adopted.

1. Qi and Phlegm Stagnation

Chief Manifestations: Thyroid enlargement which feels soft and painless, distending sensation in the neck, sensation of obstruction in the throat, irritability, chest distress, hypochondriac pain, trembling fingers, patient's condition influenced by emotions, pale red tongue with thin and white coating, wiry and smooth pulse.

Therapeutic Methods: To regulate qi, alleviate mental depression, resolve phlegm and remove the goiter.

Prescription: Modified Chaihu Shugan Yin (Bupleuri Decoction for Soothing Liver Qi), Composed of Chaihu (*Radix Bupleuri*) 6 g, Qingpi (*Pericarpium Citri Reticulatae Viride*) 10 g, Chenpi (*Pericarpium Citri Reticulatae*) 10 g, Baishaoyao (*Radix Paeoniae Alba*) 10 g, Xiangfu (*Rhizoma Cyperi*) 10 g, Yujin (*Radix Curcumae*) 10 g, Shengmuli (*Concha Ostreae*, to be decocted first) 30 g, Chuanxiong (*Rhizoma Chuanxiong*) 10 g, Zhebeimu (*Bulbus Fritillariae*) 10 g and Fabanxia (*Rhizoma Pinelliae Preparata*) 10 g, Chaobaijiezi (*Semen Sinapis*, stir-baked) 10 g.

Modifications: For discomfort in the throat and neck, add Jiegeng (*Radix Platycodi*) 10 g, Zhidanxing

则。病久有血瘀征象者应佐以活血化瘀；肝火亢盛伤阴者，又当滋阴降火为主；若出现脾胃气虚者，则应益气健脾。

1. 气郁痰阻证

主要证候 甲状腺肿大，质软不痛，颈部觉胀，喉间有如物堵塞感，急躁易怒，胸闷胁痛，手指微颤，病情波动与情绪有关，舌质淡红，舌苔薄白，脉弦滑。

治 法 理气舒郁，化痰消瘿。

方 药 柴胡疏肝饮加减：柴胡6 g，青皮10 g，陈皮10 g，白芍药10 g，香附10 g，郁金10 g，生牡蛎(先煎)30 g，川芎10 g，浙贝母10 g，法半夏10 g，炒白芥子10 g。

加 减 咽、颈不适者，加桔梗10 g，制胆星10 g，牛蒡

(*Arisaema cum Bile*) 10 g, Niubangzi (*Fructus Arctii*) 10 g and Shegan (*Rhizoma Belamcandae*) 10 g; for restlessness and insomnia, remove Chaihu and Qingpi, add Mudanpi (*Cortex Moutan Radicis*) 10 g and Zhizi (*Fructus Gardeniae*) 10 g; for dry mouth, red eyes, constipation and reddish urine, remove Chaihu, Qingpi and Fabanxia, add Longdancao (*Radix Gentianae*) 6 g, Xiakucao (*Spica Prunellae*) 10 g, Zexie (*Rhizoma Alismatis*) 15 g and Zhidahuang (*Radix et Rhizoma Rhei Preparata*) 6 g; for polyorexia, remove Chaihu, add Huanglian (*Rhizoma Coptidis*) 5 g, Shengshigao (*Gypsum Fibrosum*, to be decocted first) 20 g and Beishashen (*Radix Glehniae*) 10 g; for poor appetite and loose stools, add Baizhu (*Rhizoma Atractylodis Macrocephalae*) 10 g, Fuling (*Poria*) 15 g and Shanyao (*Rhizoma Dioscoreae*) 12 g.

2. Liver Fire Attacking the Stomach

Chief Manifestations: Moderate thyroid enlargement which feels soft and smooth, severe thirst, polydipsia, profuse sweating, ocular proptosis, trembling fingers, facial hotness, polyorexia, emaciation, constipation, red tongue with yellow coating, wiry and rapid pulse.

Therapeutic Methods: To purge liver fire and stomach fire, promote fluid production to quench thirst.

Prescription: Modified Zhizi Qinggan Tang (Gardeniae Decoction for Clearing Liver Fire), composed of Zhizi (*Radix Gardeniae*) 10 g, Mudanpi (*Cortex Moutan Radicis*) 10 g, Longdancao (*Radix Gentianae*) 6 g, Shengshigao (*Gypsum Fibrosum*, to be decocted first) 30 g, Zhimu (*Rhizoma Anemarrhenae*) 10 g, Maimendong (*Radix Ophiopogonis*) 10 g, Xuanshen (*Radix Scrophulariae*) 10 g, Chaihu (*Radix Bupleuri*) 6 g, Chishaoyao (*Radix Paeoniae Rubra*) 10 g, Danggui

子10 g,射干10 g;心烦少寐者,去柴胡、青皮,加牡丹皮10 g,栀子10 g;口干目赤,便结溲赤者,去柴胡、青皮、法半夏,加龙胆草6 g,夏枯草10 g,泽泻15 g,制大黄6 g;消谷善饥者,去柴胡,加黄连5 g,生石膏(先煎)20 g,北沙参10 g;纳差,便溏者,加白术10 g,茯苓15 g,山药12 g。

2. 肝火犯胃证

主要证候 甲状腺中等度肿大,质软光滑,烦渴多饮,多汗,眼突指颤,面部烘热,多食善饥,消瘦,便秘,舌质红,苔黄,脉弦数。

治 法 清泻肝胃,生津止渴。

方 药 栀子清肝汤加减:栀子10 g,牡丹皮10 g,龙胆草6 g,生石膏(先煎)30 g,知母10 g,麦门冬10 g,玄参10 g,柴胡6 g,赤芍药10 g,当归10 g,川芎10 g,钩藤20 g,白蒺藜10 g,生牡蛎(先煎)30 g。

(*Radix Angelicae Sinensis*) 10 g, Chuanxiong (*Rhizoma Chuanxiong*) 10 g, Gouteng (*Ramulus Uncariae cum Uncis*) 20 g, Baijili (*Fructus Tribuli*) 10 g, and Shengmuli (*Concha Ostreae*, to be decocted first) 30 g.

Modifications: For constipation, add Yuliren (*Semen Pruni*) 10 g and Huomaren (*Semen Cannabis*) 10 g; for distending sensation in the eyes and obvious exophthalmus, add Chongweizi (*Fructus Leonuri*) 10 g, Juemingzi (*Semen Cassiae*) 15 g, Xiakucao (*Spica Prunellae*) 10 g, Juhua (*Flos Chrysanthemi*) 10 g, Zhebeimu (*Bulbus Fritillariae*) 10 g and Danshen (*Radix Salviae Miltiorrhizae*) 12 g; for trembling fingers, add Shijueming (*Concha Haliotidis*, to be decocted first) 20 g; for thyroid enlargement with nodules, add Xiakucao (*Spica Prunellae*) 10 g, Shancigu (*Pseudobulbus Cremastrae seu Pleiones*) 10 g, Biejia (*Carapax Trionycis*, to be decocted first) 15 g and Danshen (*Radix Salviae Miltiorrhizae*) 10 g.

3. Deficiency of Both Qi and Yin

Chief Manifestations: Palpitation, short breath, restlessness, sleeplessness, lassitude, impaired appetite, loose stools, spontaneous sweating, emaciation, mild thyroid enlargement, red tongue with little coating, deep and thready pulse or thready rapid and forceless pulse.

Therapeutic Methods: To replenish qi, nourish yin, and remove the goiter.

Prescription: Shengmai San Jiawei (Powder for Reinforcing Qi and Nourishing Yin with Additions), composed of Taizishen (*Radix Pseudostellariae*) 10 g, Maimendong (*Radix Ophiopogonis*) 10 g, Wuweizi (*Fructus Schisandrae*) 10 g, Shengguiban (*Plastrum Testudinis*, to be decocted first) 15 g, Tianmendong (*Radix Asparagi*) 10 g, Huangjing (*Rhizoma Polygonati*) 10 g, Baiziren (*Semen Platycladi*) 10 g, Baizhu

加　减　便秘者,加郁李仁10 g,火麻仁10 g;双眼作胀,眼球突出明显者,加茺蔚子10 g,决明子15 g,夏枯草10 g,菊花10 g,浙贝母10 g,丹参12 g;手指颤抖者,加石决明(先煎)20 g;甲状腺肿大有结节者,加夏枯草10 g,山慈姑10 g,鳖甲(先煎)15 g,丹参10 g。

3. 气阴两虚证

主要证候　心悸气短,心烦不寐,神疲乏力,纳少便溏,自汗消瘦,甲状腺轻度肿大,舌质红,少苔,脉沉细或细数无力。

治　法　益气养阴,消瘿散结。

方　药　生脉散加味:太子参10 g,麦门冬10 g,五味子10 g,生龟版(先煎)15 g,天门冬10 g,黄精10 g,柏子仁10 g,白术10 g,山药12 g,茯神10 g,远志6 g。

(*Rhizoma Atractylodis Macrocephalae*) 10 g, Shanyao
(*Rhizoma Dioscoreae*) 12 g, Fushen (*Sclerotium Poriae circum Radicem Pini*) 10 g and Yuanzhi (*Radix Polygalae*) 6 g.

Modifications: For spontaneous perspiration, add
Duanlonggu (*Os Draconis Usta*, to be decocted first)
30 g, Duanmuli (*Concha Ostreae Usta*, to be decocted
first) 30 g and Fuxiaomai (*Fructus Tritici Levis*) 10 g;
for marked thyroid enlargement with nodules, add Honghua (*Flos Carthami*) 10 g, Taoren (*Semen Persicae*)
10 g and Danshen (*Radix Salviae Miltiorrhizae*) 12 g;
for abdominal distension and impaired appetite, add Sharen
(*Fructus Amomi*, to be decocted later) 3 g, Baikouren
(*Fructus Amoni Rotundus*, to be decocted later) 3 g,
Guya (*Fructus Oryzae Germinatus*) 10 g and Maiya
(*Fructus Hordei Germinatus*) 10 g.

4. Deficiency of Heart Yin and Liver Yin

Chief Manifestations: Thyroid enlargement which
feels soft, palpitation, restlessness, sleeplessness, profuse sweating, trembling fingers, dizziness, red tongue
with thin coating, thready and rapid pulse.

Therapeutic Methods: To nourish yin and blood,
tranquilize the mind and nourish the liver.

Prescription: Modified Buxin Dan (Powder for Tonifying Heart) and Yiguan Jian (Ever-effective Decoction
for Nourishing Liver and Kidney), composed of Shengdihuang (*Radix Rehmanniae*) 10 g, Xuanshen (*Radix
Scrophulariae*) 10 g, Maimendong (*Radix Ophiopogonis*) 10 g, Tianmendong (*Radix Asparagi*) 10 g, Taizishen (*Radix Pseudostellariae*) 10 g, Fuling (*Poria*)
10 g, Wuweizi (*Fructus Schisandrae*) 10 g, Danggui
(*Radix Angelicae Sinensis*) 10 g, Danshen (*Radix
Salviae Miltiorrhizae*) 10 g, Suanzaoren (*Semen Ziziphi Spinosae*) 10 g, Baiziren (*Semen Platycladi*) 10 g,

加　减　自汗者,加煅龙
骨(先煎)30 g,煅牡蛎(先煎)
30 g,浮小麦10 g;甲状腺肿大
明显,有结节者,加红花10 g,
桃仁10 g,丹参12 g;腹胀食少
者,加砂仁(后下)3 g,白蔻仁
(后下)3 g,谷芽10 g,麦芽
10 g。

4. 心肝阴虚证

主要证候　甲状腺肿大,
质软,心悸不安,心烦不寐,多
汗,指颤,头晕目眩,舌质红,
苔薄,脉细数。

治　法　滋养阴血,宁心
柔肝。

方　药　补心丹合一贯
煎加减:生地黄10 g,玄参
10 g,麦门冬10 g,天门冬10 g,
太子参10 g,茯苓10 g,五味子
10 g,当归10 g,丹参10 g,酸枣
仁10 g,柏子仁10 g,远志6 g,
枸杞子10 g,川楝子10 g。

Yuanzhi (*Radix Polygalae*) 6 g, Gouqizi (*Fructus Lycii*) 10 g and Chuanlianzi (*Fructus Meliae Toosendan*) 10 g.

Modifications: For trembling fingers, add Gouteng (*Ramulus Uncariae cum Uncis*) 20 g, Baijili (*Fructus Tribuli*) 10 g and Baishaoyao (*Radix Paeoniae Alba*) 10 g; for tinnitus, soreness and weakness of the loins and knees, add Guiban (*Plastrum Testudinis*, to be decocted first) 15 g, Sangjisheng (*Herba Taxilli*) 10 g, Niuxi (*Radix Achyranthis Bidentatae*) 10 g, Cishi (*Magnetitum*, to be decocted first) 20 g and Tusizi (*Semen Cuscutae*) 10 g; for profuse sweating, add Muli (*Concha Ostreae*, to be decocted first) 30 g, Fuxiaomai (*Fructus Tritici Levis*) 10 g and Lianzixin (*Plumula Nelumbinis*) 10 g.

In the case of thyroid crisis, manifested as thyroid enlargement, exophthalmus, high fever, or even hyperpyrexia, increase of blood pressure, tachycardia as fast as 160 - 200 beats per minute, accompanied with restlessness, profuse sweating, nausea, vomiting, jaundice, abdominal pain, diarrhea, even coma and delirium, crimson tongue, thready and rapid pulse, the case should be treated by clearing away the heat at yingfen and xuefen and clearing away heart fire for resuscitation. The prescription adopted is modified Xijiao Dihuang Tang (Cornu Rhinocerotis and Rehmanniae Decoction), which is composed of Xijiaofen (*Cornu Rhinocerotis*, powdered and to be infused separately) 1 g or Shuiniujiaopian (*Cornu Bubali*, sliced and to be decocted first) Shengdihuang (*Radix Rehmanniae*) 10 g, Mudanpi (*Cortex Moutan Radicis*) 10 g, Chishaoyao (*Radix Paeoniae Rubra*) 10 g, Xuanshen (*Radix Scrophulariae*) 10 g, Huanglian (*Rhizoma Coptidis*) 5 g, Yujin (*Radix Curcumae*) 10 g, Shigao (*Gypsum Fibrosum*, to be decocted first) 30 g and

加　减　手指颤抖者,加钩藤20 g,白蒺藜10 g,白芍药10 g;耳鸣,腰膝酸软者,加龟版(先煎)15 g,桑寄生10 g,牛膝10 g,磁石(先煎)20 g,菟丝子10 g;心烦多汗者,加牡蛎(先煎)30 g,浮小麦10 g,莲子心10 g。

若出现甲状腺危象,症见甲状腺肿大,眼突,常发高热,有时可有过高热,血压增高,心率快,每分钟可达160～200次左右。伴有烦躁不安,大汗淋漓,恶心呕吐,黄疸,腹痛腹泻,甚至神昏谵语,舌红绛,脉细数。治以清营凉血,清心开窍。方用犀角地黄汤加减。药用犀角粉(另冲)1 g或水牛角片(先煎)30 g,生地黄10 g,牡丹皮10 g,赤芍药10 g,玄参10 g,黄连5 g,郁金10 g,石膏(先煎)30 g,竹叶10 g。热盛神昏谵语者,鼻饲安宫牛黄丸(加温开水化后)1粒,或牛黄清心丸(加温开水化后)1粒。

Zhuye (*Folium Phyllostachydis Henonis*) 10 g. For coma and delirium due to excessive heat, use nasal feeding of one bolus of Angong Niuhuang Wan (Calculus Bovis Bolus for Resuscitation, resolved in warm water), or one bolus of Niuhuang Qingxin Wan (Calculus Bovis Bolus for Clearing away Heart Fire, resolved in warm water).

Other Treatments

1. Chinese Patent Drugs

(1) Jiakang Pian (Hyperthyroidism Tablet): 0.25 g/tablet, 4 - 5 tablets each time, 3 - 4 times per day, 15 days as a course of treatment; indicated for hyperthyroidism, either incipient or recurrent cases.

(2) Kunming Shanhaitang Pian (Tripterygium Hypoglaucum Tablet): 0.25 g/tablet, 1 - 3 tablets each time, 3 times per day; indicated for all types of hyperthyroidism.

(3) Liuwei Dihuang Wan (Bolus of Six Drugs Containing Rehmanniae): 1 bolus each time, twice a day; indicated for hyperthyroidism with deficiency of liver yin and kidney yin.

(4) Tianwang Buxin Dan (Tianwang Bolus for Tonifying Heart): 1 bolus each time, twice a day; indicated for hyperthyroidism with deficiency of heart yin and liver yin.

(5) Xiaoying Wan (Goiter-Removing Bolus): 1 bolus each time, 3 times a day; indicated for hyperthyroidism with stagnation of qi and phlegm.

(6) Yikang Wan (Bolus for Inhibiting Hyperthyroidism): 1 bolus each time, twice a day; indicated for hyperthyroidism with deficiency of heart yin and liver yin and endogenous deficient wind.

【其他疗法】

1. 中成药

（1）甲亢片　0.25 g/片，每服4～5片，每日3～4次，15日为1个疗程，可连服3～4个疗程。适用于甲状腺功能亢进症，对初发、复发患者均有效。

（2）昆明山海棠片0.25 g/片，每服1～3片，每日3次。适用于甲状腺功能亢进症各证型。

（3）六味地黄丸　每服1丸，每日2次。适用于甲状腺功能亢进症肝肾阴虚者。

（4）天王补心丹　每服1丸，每日2次。适用于甲状腺功能亢进症心肝阴虚者。

（5）消瘿丸　每服1丸，每日3次。适用于甲状腺功能亢进症气滞痰凝者。

（6）抑亢丸　每服1丸，每日2次。适用于甲状腺功能亢进症心肝阴虚，虚风内动者。

2. Single-drug or Experiential Prescriptions

（1） Huangqi （*Radix Astragali*） 20 g, Xuanshen （*Radix Scrophulariae*） 20 g and Shancigu （*Pseudobulbus Cremastrae seu Pleionies*） 20 g. Decoct the drugs in water for oral administration, 1 dose per day and take the decoction in 2 divided doses. It is indicated for hyperthyroidism with deficiency of both qi and yin.

（2） Pingjia Tang （Decoction for Relieving Hyperthyroidism）: composed of Huangqi （*Radix Astragali*） 15 g, Dangshen （*Radix Codonopsis*） 10 g, Maimendong （*Radix Ophiopogonis*） 10 g, Baishaoyao （*Radix Paeoniae Alba*） 10 g, Xiakucao （*Spica Prunellae*） 10 g, Shengdihuang （*Radix Rehmanniae*） 10 g, Danshen （*Radix Salviae Miltiorrhizae*） 10 g, Muli （*Concha Ostreae*, to be decocted first） 20 g, Suzi （*Fructus Perillae*） 10 g, Wuweizi （*Fructus Schisandrae*） 10 g, Xiangfu （*Rhizoma Cyperi*） 10 g and Baijiezi （*Semen Sinapis Albae*） 10 g. Decoct the drugs in water for oral administration, one dose per day and take the decoction in 2 divided doses. It is indicated for hyperthyroidism with deficiency of both qi and yin and stagnation of phlegm and qi.

（3） Xiaozhong Jialiu Wan （Detumescence Bolus for Goiter）: composed of Xiakucao （*Spica Prunellae*） 30 g, Danggui （*Radix Angelicae Sinensis*） 30 g, Zhenzhumu （*Concha Margaritifera Usta*） 30 g, Shengmuli （*Concha Ostreae*） 30 g, Kunbu （*Thallus Laminariae et Eckloniae*） 15 g and Danshen （*Radix Salviae Miltiorrhizae*） 15 g. Grind the above drugs together into fine powder, and make boluses （9 g each） with honey. Take 1 bolus, twice a day. This is indicated for goiter with phlegm stagnation and blood stasis.

（4） Take a piece of pig thyroid or goat thyroid, dry and grind it into powder. Take 0.1 - 0.2 g of the powder in two doses per day. It is indicated for hyperthyroidism

2. 单验方

（1）黄芪20 g,玄参20 g,山慈姑20 g。水煎服,每日1剂,分2次服。适用于甲状腺功能亢进症气阴两虚者。

（2）平甲汤　黄芪15 g,党参10 g,麦门冬10 g,白芍药10 g,夏枯草10 g,生地黄10 g,丹参10 g,牡蛎(先煎)20 g,苏子10 g,五味子10 g,香附10 g,白芥子10 g,水煎服,每日1剂,分2次服。适用于甲状腺功能亢进症气阴两虚,痰气瘀阻者。

（3）消肿甲瘤丸　夏枯草30 g,当归30 g,珍珠母30 g,生牡蛎30 g,昆布15 g,丹参15 g。共研细末,加蜜制丸,每丸重9 g,每服1丸,每日2次。适用于痰瘀阻滞,甲状腺肿大者。

（4）猪靥或羊靥1具,研粉,每日服0.1～0.2 g,分2次服。适用于甲状腺功能亢进

of various types.

(5) Liuye Gao (Salicis Babylonicae Extract): Cut Liuye (*Folium Salicis Balylonicae*) 500 g into small pieces, add 1,500 ml of water to it and decoct it twice, then remove the dregs, cook the decoction on a slow fire into extract. Add proper amount of honey to the extract and mix them thoroughly for use. Take 5 g, 3 times per day. It is indicated for hyperthyroidism of various types.

3. External Therapy

(1) Wubeizi (*Galla Chinensis*) 30 - 50 g. Put it into a marmite, stir-bake it until it becomes yellow, then grind it into powder after it becomes cool. Before going to bed in the evening, mix the powder with rice vinegar to make a paste and apply it to the affected part, then wash it off the next morning, seven times being a course of treatment. It is indicated for hyperthyroidism with stagnation of qi and phlegm and protracted stagnation generating fire.

(2) Chuanwu (*Radix Aconiti*) 60 g, Caowu (*Radix Aconiti Kusnezoffii*) 50 g, Ruxiangmian (*Olibanum*, powdered) 60 g, Moyaomian (*Myrrha*, powdered) 60 g, Jixingzi (*Semen Impatientis*) 160 g, Shensanqi (*Radix Notoginseng*) 30 g, Mahuang (*Herba Ephedrae*) 30 g, Rouguimian (*Cortex Cinnamomi*, to be powdered and decocted later) 30 g, Quanxie (*Scorpio*) 30 g, Baizhi (*Radix Angelicae Dahuricae*) 60 g, Chuanxiong (*Rhizoma Chuanxiong*) 30 g, Shengmaqianzi (*Semen Strychni*) 30 g, Dingxiangmian (*Gemma Caryophylli*, powdered) 30 g and Zicao (*Radix Arnebiae seu Lithospermi*) 30 g. Put these drugs into 3,600 ml of sesame oil and fry them until they turn scorched. Filter and heat the sesame oil to 240℃ and then withdraw the fire. Add 1,200 grams of heated Zhangdan (*Minium*) to it and mix them thoroughly. After it is coagulated, soak it in cold water

（5）柳叶膏　柳叶500 g，切碎，加水1 500 ml，煎2次，去渣，文火收膏，加适量蜂蜜调匀即成。每服5 g，每日3次。适用于甲状腺功能亢进症各证型。

3. 外治法

（1）五倍子30～50 g，放入砂锅内炒黄，冷却后研成末，晚上睡觉时用米醋调成膏状敷于患处，次日晨洗掉，7次为1个疗程。适用于本病气郁痰聚或郁久化火者。

（2）川乌60 g，草乌50 g，乳香面60 g，没药面60 g，急性子160 g，参三七30 g，麻黄30 g，肉桂面（后下）30 g，全蝎30 g，白芷60 g，川芎30 g，生马钱子30 g，丁香面30 g，紫草30 g。将上药置于3 600 ml芝麻油中煎至药枯，滤净，加热至240度撤火，兑入加热之章丹1 200 g，搅匀，凝结后放入冷水中浸15～20日，每日换水1次。用时加温摊纸或布上，大者5～6 g，小者2～3 g，作成膏药，外贴，5～7日换药1次。适用于本病甲状腺肿大明显者。

for 15 - 20 days and change the water once a day. Warm and spread it on a piece of paper or cloth to make an ointment, 5 - 6 g for a large one or 2 - 3 g for a small one. Apply it to the affected part and change it once every 5 - 7 days. It is indicated for hyperthyroidism with noticeable thyroid enlargement.

2.8.5 Acquired Immune Deficiency Syndrome（AIDS）

General Description

AIDS is a special disease of acquired immune deficiency. It is caused by the infection of human immunodeficiency virus （HIV）, therefore it is called Acquired Immune Deficiency Syndrome. The major clinical manifestations are fever, night sweating, emaciation, lassitude, cough, diarrhea, rash, generalized lymphadenectasis, etc. The disease is a new type of infectious disease which has caught the greatest attention in the world today. As its mortality rate is extremely high and the two-year survival rate is less than 30%, it is known as the "super cancer" and the "new pestilence in the 20th century". The disease is transmitted by way of sexual intercourse, injection, mother-to-infant, etc. Its incubation period is several months to half a year, and even as long as seven years. When the virus attacks the immune system of the human body, it completely destroys the immune function and makes the human body lose its resistance against various kinds of viruses, bacteria, protozoa and fungi, therefore aids patients easily die of various kinds of infections.

第五节　艾滋病

【概述】

艾滋病是一种特殊的后天免疫缺陷性疾病,是由于感染人类免疫缺陷病毒(HIV)所致。由于本病是后天获得性免疫系统被损害或缺陷而引起,故又称为"获得性免疫缺陷综合征"。临床主要表现为发热、盗汗、消瘦、乏力、咳嗽、腹泻、皮疹、全身淋巴结肿大等。本病是当代最引人注目的一种新型传染病,病死率极高,其两年存活率在 30% 以下,被当今世界称为"超级癌症"及"20 世纪新瘟疫"。本病主要通过性交、注射及母婴等途径传染。其潜伏期为数月至半年,最长可达 7 年之久。病毒可攻击人体的免疫系统,使机体的免疫功能遭到彻底破坏,失去对各病毒、细菌、原虫及真菌等的抵抗力和防卫能力,极易发生各种感染而致命。

In accordance with its clinical manifestations, this disease at the initial and intermediate stages, belongs to the categories of "wen bing" (seasonal febrile disease) and "yi bing" (epidemic disease) in TCM. The disease at later stage is similar to "acute tuberculosis". It is caused by unclean copulation, perverse behavior or contact with epidemic pathogenic factor. When healthy qi is insufficient, the epidemic pathogenic factor would seize a chance to attack the human body and therefore AIDS occurs. As the pathogenic factor is extremely serious, it may directly attack yingfen and xuefen upon the onset of the disease. The incubation period of the disease is long and the disease is terribly serious and lingering. After the seasonal febrile syndrome presents, lung qi and lung yin are often damaged and then the spleen, heart, liver, and kidney are involved with appearance of defeciency syndrome.

Essentials for Diagnosis

(1) A history of homosexuality or multipartner heterosexuality; the spouse's or sexual partners' antibody against HIV positive; a history of taking drugs through intravenous injection; having used blood product of factor Ⅷ or blood without anti-HIV test; a history of contact with AIDS patients or with HIV-infected persons; or a history of syphilis, gonorrhoea, nongonococcal urethritis, etc.

(2) Clinical manifestations of the upper respiratory tract infection such as fever, lassitude, sore throat, and general malaise; headache, rash, meningocephalitis, or acute polyneuritis in some cases; lymphadenectasis in the neck, armpit and occiput, and splenomegaly.

(3) In laboratory examination, the total count of peripheral leukocytes and lymphocytes is decreased after the

根据本病患者的临床表现,早中期可属于中医学的"温病"、"疫病"范畴,晚期则与虚劳中的"急痨"相似。主要由交合不洁或乖逆,触染淫秽疫毒而致。当机体正气不足时,毒邪则可乘虚而入,发为艾滋病。由于疫毒深重,病发即直入营血。本病潜伏期长,病势凶顽而缠绵,继温热证之后,往往先伤肺之气阴,然后深入脾、心、肝、肾诸脏腑渐见虚损诸象。

【诊断要点】

(1) 有同性恋或异性恋者有多个性伴侣史,或配偶或性伴侣抗 HIV 抗体阳性;有静脉吸毒史;用过Ⅷ因子等血液制品或未经抗 HIV 检测的血液;或有与艾滋病患者或 HIV 感染者有密切接触史;或有过梅毒、淋病、非淋菌性尿道炎等性病史。

(2) 临床表现有发热、乏力、咽痛、全身不适等上呼吸道感染症状;个别有头痛、皮疹、脑膜脑炎或急性多发性神经炎;颈、腋及枕部淋巴结肿大,脾肿大。

(3) 实验室检查外周血白细胞及淋巴细胞总数起病后

onset, and later the total count of lymphocytes increases with the appearance of heteromorphous lymphocytes. The ratio of $CD_4/CD_3 > 1$.

（4）Anti-HIV positive.

Syndrome Differentiation and Treatment

As AIDS patients' immune function is seriously defective and the clinical manifestation is deficiency of healthy qi, strengthening healthy qi should be taken as the main principle in the treatment. This disease is also apt to be complicated by many kinds of fatal opportunistic infection so that there often appear acute symptoms of secondary aspect of the disease. At this time urgent measures should be taken to treat the symptoms of secondary aspect. At the early stage of Aids, healthy qi is usually deficient with pathogenic factors hanging on in the body, therefore the treatment should be strengthening healthy qi and eliminating the pathogenic factor at the same time. During the intermediate stage, phlegm and stasis are often accompanied with toxic heat. The methods of clearing away heat and toxic substance, resolving phlegm, removing stasis, and dissipating mass should be used and supplemented by strengthening healthy qi. During the late stage, as the disease has been protracted, healthy qi is seriously deficient and there are often complications of superficial nodules and tumors, therefore strengthening healthy qi should be used as the major method and supplemented with some medicines for eliminating pathogenic factors.

1. Warm Pathogenic Factor Attacking the Lung and Damaging Yin

Chief Manifestations: Sore throat, fever, cough without sputum, or blood-stained sputum, short breath, chest pain, rash, pruritus, emaciation, fatigue, night sweating, red dry tongue, thin and yellow coating and thready pulse.

下降,以后淋巴细胞总数上升可见异型淋巴细胞。CD_4/CD_3 比值>1。

（4）抗 HIV 阳性。

【辨证论治】

艾滋病患者的免疫功能严重缺陷。临床表现为正气亏虚,故治疗当以扶正培本为主。仅本病又易并发多种致命的机会性感染而呈现标急之象,这时便应予急则治标。一般艾滋病患者早期多为正虚而感邪,应扶正祛邪兼施;中期多挟热毒痰瘀,宜用清热解毒、化痰行瘀、软坚散结诸法,并适当配以扶正;后期因病延日久,正气大虚,且多并发痰核、肿瘤,故应以扶正为主,再适当配用祛邪之品。

1. 温邪犯肺伤阴证

主要证候 咽痛发热,咳呛无痰或痰中带血,气促胸痛,皮疹瘙痒,形瘦神疲,寐中汗出,舌红少津,苔薄黄,脉细。

Therapeutic Methods: To nourish yin, clear away heat, moisten the lung to promote fluid production.

Prescription: Modified Maimendong Yin (Ophiopogonis Decoction) and Baihe Gujin Tang (Lilii Decoction for Strengthening Lung), composed of Taizishen (*Radix Pseudostellariae*) 12 g, Xuanshen (*Radix Scrophulariae*) 10 g, Shengdihuang (*Radix Rehmanniae*) 12 g, Shudihuang (*Radix Rehmanniae Praeparata*) 12 g, Baihe (*Bulbus Lilii*) 10 g, Zhimu (*Rhizoma Anemarrhenae*) 10 g, Maimendong (*Radix Ophiopogonis*) 10 g, Fushen (*Sclerotium Poriae circum Radicem Pini*) 10 g, Baishaoyao (*Radix Paeoniae Alba*) 12 g, Danggui (*Radix Angelicae Sinensis*) 10 g, Zhebeimu (*Bulbus Fritillariae Thunbergii*) 10 g, Gualou (*Fructus Trichosanthis*) 10 g, Jiegeng (*Radix Platycodi*) 6 g and Shenggancao (*Radix Glycyrrhizae*) 5 g.

Modifications: For persistent cough, add Madouling (*Fructus Aristolochiae*) 12 g and Dai Ge San (Powder of Indigo Naturalis and Concha Meretricis Cyclinae, wrapped) 10 g; for intense chest pain, add Zelan (*Herba Lycopi*) 10 g and Shixiao San (Powder for Dissipating Blood Stasis, wrapped) 10 g; for prolonged bloody sputum, add Qiancao (*Radix Rubiae*) 10 g and Baimaogen (*Rhizoma Imperatae*) 20 g.

2. Middle Energizer Deficiency with Heat Retention in the Stomach and Intestines

Chief Manifestations: Lingering fever, emaciation, short breath, lassitude of limbs, abdominal pain, diarrhea, yellow and thin stools sometimes with pus and blood, tensemus, nausea, vomiting, white and greasy tongue coating, and soft-superficial, thready pulse.

Therapeutic Methods: To replenish qi, invigorate the spleen, clean the intestines and dissipate dampness.

Prescription: Modified Buzhong Yiqi Tang (Decoc-

治 法 养阴清热,润肺生津。

方 药 麦门冬饮合百合固金汤加减:太子参12 g,玄参10 g,生地黄12 g,熟地黄12 g,百合10 g,知母10 g,麦门冬10 g,茯神10 g,白芍药12 g,当归10 g,浙贝母10 g,瓜蒌10 g,桔梗6 g,生甘草5 g。

加 减 咳呛不止者,加马兜铃12 g,黛蛤散(包煎)10 g;胸疼剧烈者,加泽兰10 g,失笑散(包煎)10 g;痰红不止者,加茜草10 g,白茅根20 g。

2. 中虚热蕴胃肠证

主要证候 身热缠绵,形羸少气,四肢疲惫,腹痛便泄,泻下黄稀或便下脓血,里急后重,恶心呕吐,苔白腻,脉濡细。

治 法 益气健脾,清肠化湿。

方 药 补中益气汤合

tion for Strengthening Middle Energizer and Benefiting Qi) and Baitouweng Tang (Pulsatillae Decoction), composed of Shenghuangqi (*Radix Astragali*) 12 g, Dangshen (*Radix Codonopsis*) 10 g, Shengma (*Rhizoma Cimicifugae*) 6 g, Chaihu (*Radix Bupleuri*) 10 g, Baitouweng (*Radix Pulsatillae*) 10 g, Qinpi (*Cortex Fraxini*) 10 g, Huanglian (*Rhizoma Coptidis*) 5 g, Huangqin (*Radix Scutellariae*) 10 g, Huangbai (*Cortex Phellodendri*) 10 g, Guan-zhong (*Rhizoma Dryopteris Crassirhizomae*) 10 g, Molihua (*Flos Jasmini Sambac*) 6 g and Baishaoyao (*Radix Paeoniae Alba*) 12 g.

Modifications: For vomiting and loss of appetite, add Zhibanxia (*Rhizoma Pinelliae Preparata*) 10 g, Zisugeng (*Caulis Perillae*) 6 g and Shengjiang (*Rhizoma Zingiberis Recens*) 3 g; for abdominal pain, add Muxiang (*Radix Aucklaneliae*) 10 g and Chaofangfeng (*Radix Saposhnikoviae*, stir-baked) 6 g; for persistent diarrhea, add Hongteng (*Caulis Sargentodoxae*) 15 g and Xianhecao (*Herba Agrimoniae*) 15 g.

3. Excessive Heat and Phlegm Causing Coma

Chief Manifestations: Fever, headache, nausea, vomiting, coma or restlessness and delirium, stiff neck, convulsion, or dementia, or epileptoid seizure, yellow and greasy tongue coating, thready and rapid pulse or smooth and rapid pulse.

Therapeutical Methods: To clear away heart fire for resuscitation, cool the liver and stop wind.

Prescription: Modified Xi Huang Xuanqiao Tang (Decoction of Cornu Rhinocerotis and Calculus Bovis for Resuscitation), composed of Shuiniujiao (*Cornu Bubali*, to be decocted first) 30 g, Gouteng (*Ramulus Uncariae cum Uncis*) 12 g, Lianqiao (*Fructus Forsythiae*) 15 g, Lingyangjiaofen (*Cornu Saigae Tataricae*, to be powdered and infused separately) 0.5 g, Chuanbeimu (*Bul-

白头翁汤加减：生黄芪12 g，党参10 g，升麻6 g，柴胡10 g，白头翁10 g，秦皮10 g，黄连5 g，黄芩10 g，黄柏10 g，贯众10 g，茉莉花6 g，白芍药12 g。

加　减　呕吐不食者，加制半夏10 g，紫苏梗6 g，生姜3 g；腹痛不止者，加木香10 g，炒防风6 g；泻下不止者，加红藤15 g，仙鹤草15 g。

3. 热盛痰蒙窍闭证

主要证候　发热头痛，恶心呕吐，神识昏昧或烦躁谵语，项强惊厥，四肢抽搐或神情痴呆，或癫痫样发作，苔黄腻，脉细数或滑数。

治　法　清心开窍，凉肝熄风。

方　药　犀黄宣窍汤加减：水牛角（先煎）30 g，钩藤12 g，连翘15 g，羚羊角粉（另冲）0.5 g，川贝母10 g，石菖蒲6 g。

bus Fritillariae Cirrhosae) 10 g and Shichangpu (*Rhi-zoma Acori Tatarinowii*) 6 g.

Modification: For damage of peripheral nerves, pain of limbs and difficulty in motion, add Huzhang (*Rhi-zoma Polygoni Cuspidati*) 15 g, Cansha (*Feculae Bom-bycis*, wrapped) 12 g, Quanxie (*Scorpio*) 3 g and Bai-jiangcan (*Bombyx Batryticatus*) 10 g.

4. Deficiency of Spleen Yang and Kidney Yang

Chief Manifestations: Fever or lingering low fever, emaciation, lassitude, palpitation, short breath, dizziness, soreness and pain of loins and knees, impaired appetite, nausea, frequent hiccup, frequent diarrhea or morning diarrhea, continuous abdominal pain, cold body and limbs, spontaneous sweating, night sweating, luster-less hair and complexion, pale nails, rash, pruritus, or thrush, deep thready pulse or thready rapid pulse, pale swollen tongue or with petechia, thin and white coating or with white patches.

Therapeutic Methods: To invigorate the spleen, lift lucid yang, warm the kidney and astringe the intestines.

Prescription: Modified Da Taohua Tang (Taohua Decoction for Warming Middle Energiaer and Relieving Diarrhea) and Qijun Tang (Qijun Decoction), composed of Renshen (*Radix Ginseng*, to be decocted separately) 10 g, Huangqi (*Radix Astragali*) 15 g, Baizhu (*Rhizoma Atractylodis Macrocephalae*) 10 g, Ganjiang (*Rhizoma Zingiberis*) 3 g, Shufuzi (*Radix Aconiti Preparata*) 6 g, Rougui (*Cortex Cinnamomi*) 3 g, Danggui (*Radix Angelicae Sinensis*) 10 g, Baishaoyao (*Radix Paeoniae Alba*) 12 g, Roudoukou (*Semen Myristicae*) 10 g, Chishizhi (*Halloysitum Rubrum*) 10 g, Duan-longgu (*Os Draconis Usta*) 30 g, Duanmuli (*Concha Ostreae Usta*) 30 g, Fuling (*Poria*) 10 g and Zhigancao

加 减 周围神经损害，出现肢体疼痛、行动困难者，加虎杖15 g，蚕沙（包煎）12 g，全蝎3 g，白僵蚕10 g。

4. 脾肾阳气虚弱证

主要证候 发热或低热缠绵，形削神倦，心悸气促，头目眩晕，腰膝酸痛，纳呆泛恶或呃逆连声，泻下无度或五更泄泻，腹痛绵绵，肢冷形寒，自汗盗汗，毛悴色夭，爪甲苍白，皮疹瘙痒，或见鹅口疮，脉沉细无力或细数，舌淡胖或有紫斑，苔薄白或舌上有白色斑块覆盖。

治 法 健脾升清，温肾涩肠。

方 药 大桃花汤合启峻汤加减：人参（另煎）10 g，黄芪15 g，白术10 g，干姜3 g，熟附子6 g，肉桂3 g，当归10 g，白芍药12 g，肉豆蔻10 g，赤石脂10 g，煅龙骨30 g，煅牡蛎30 g，茯苓12 g，炙甘草5 g。

(*Radix Glycyrrhizae*, roasted) 5 g.

Modifications: For lingering fever, remove Rougui, add Guizhi (*Ramulus Cinnamomi*) 10 g; for persistent vomiting, add Zhibanxia (*Rhizoma Pinelliae Preparata*) 10 g and Shengjiang (*Rhizoma Zingiberis Recens*) 3 g; for persistent hiccup, add Gongdingxiang (*Gemma Caryophylli*) 5 g and Shidi (*Calyx Kaki*) 5 g; for persistent diarrhea, add Weihezi (*Fructus Chebulae*, roasted in fresh cinders) 6 g and Shiliupi (*Pericarpium Granati*) 10 g.

Other Treatments

1. Chinese Patent Drugs

(1) Huangqijing Koufuye (Oral Liquid of Astragali Essence): 10 ml each time, twice a day; indicated for deficiency qi and blood with external deficiency, spontaneous perspiration and weakness of limbs.

(2) Jingui Shenqi Wan (Pill for Invigorating Kidney Qi from *Golden Cabinet*): 6 g each time, twice a day; indicated for deficiency of kidney yang with dizziness, tinnitus, sore and weak knees and loins.

(3) Shengmai Yin (Oral Liquid for Reinforcing Qi and Nourishing Yin): 10 ml each time, 3 times a day; indicated for deficiency of qi and yin.

(4) Liuwei Dihuang Wan (Pill of Six Drugs Containing Rehmanniae): 6 g each time, twice a day; indicated for deficiency of kidney yin with dizziness, tinnitus, sore and weak knees and loins, bone-heat syndrome and fever, night sweating and nocturnal emission.

2. Single Drug or Experiential Prescriptions

(1) Juhua (*Flos Chrysanthemi*) 30 g. Decoct it in water and take the decoction in 2 doses. It is indicated for AIDS at prodromal stage and the related syndromes with fever.

加　减　身热缠绵者,去肉桂,加桂枝10 g;呕吐不止者,加制半夏10 g,生姜3 g;呃逆不止者,加公丁香5 g,柿蒂5 g;泄泻不止者,加煨诃子6 g,石榴皮10 g。

【其他疗法】
1. 中成药
(1) 黄芪精口服液　每次10 ml,每日2次,口服。适用于气虚血少,表虚自汗,四肢乏力者。

(2)《金匮》肾气丸　每次6 g,每日2次。适用于肾阳不足,头晕目眩,腰膝酸软者。

(3) 生脉饮　每次10 ml,每日3次,口服。适用于气阴不足之证。

(4) 六味地黄丸　每次6 g,每日2次,口服。适用于肾阴亏虚,头晕耳鸣,腰膝酸软,骨蒸潮热,盗汗遗精者。

2. 单验方
(1) 菊花30 g,水煎分2次服。适用于艾滋病前驱期及相关综合征期见发热者。

（2）Yiyiren（*Semen Coicis*）30 g. Decoct it in water and take the decoction in 2 doses. It is indicated for the related syndromes of AIDS with diarrhea.

（3）Tufuling（*Rhizoma Smilacis Glabrae*）30 g. Decoct it in water and take the decoction in 2 doses. It is indicated for AIDS with skin damage.

（2）薏苡仁30 g，水煎分 2 次服。适用于艾滋病相关综合征见腹泻者。

（3）土茯苓30 g，水煎分 2 次服。适用于艾滋病伴见皮肤损害者。

Postscript

The compilation of *A Newly Compiled Practical English-Chinese Library of TCM* was started in 2000 and published in 2002. In order to demonstrate the academic theory and clinical practice of TCM and to meet the requirements of compilation, the compilers and translators have made great efforts to revise and polish the Chinese manuscript and English translation so as to make it systematic, accurate, scientific, standard and easy to understand. Shanghai University of TCM is in charge of the translation. Many scholars and universities have participated in the compilation and translation of the Library, i.e. Professor Shao Xundao from Xi'an Medical University (former Dean of English Department and Training Center of the Health Ministry), Professor Ou Ming from Guangzhou University of TCM (celebrated translator and chief professor), Henan College of TCM, Guangzhou University of TCM, Nanjing University of TCM, Shaanxi College of TCM, Liaoning College of TCM and Shandong University of TCM.

The compilation of this Library is also supported by the State Administrativqe Bureau and experts from other universities and colleges of TCM. The experts on the Compilation Committee and Approval Committee have directed the compilation and translation. Professor She

后 记

《(英汉对照)新编实用中医文库》(以下简称《文库》)从2000年中文稿的动笔,到2002年全书的付梓,完成了世纪的跨越。为了使本套《文库》尽可能展示传统中医学术理论和临床实践的精华,达到全面、系统、准确、科学、规范、通俗的编写要求,全体编译人员耗费了大量的心血,付出了艰辛的劳动。特别是上海中医药大学承担了英语翻译的主持工作,得到了著名医学英语翻译家、原西安医科大学英语系主任和卫生部外语培训中心主任邵循道教授,著名中医英语翻译家、广州中医药大学欧明首席教授的热心指导,河南中医学院、广州中医药大学、南京中医药大学、陕西中医学院、辽宁中医学院、山东中医药大学等中医院校英语专家的全力参与,确保了本套《文库》具有较高的英译水平。

在《文库》的编撰过程中,我们始终得到国家主管部门领导和各中医院校专家们的关心和帮助。编纂委员会的国内外学者及审定委员会的

Jing, Head of the State Administrative Bureau and Vice-Minister of the Health Ministry, has showed much concern for the Library. Professor Zhu Bangxian, head of the Publishing House of Shanghai University of TCM, Zhou Dunhua, former head of the Publishing House of Shanghai University of TCM, and Pan Zhaoxi, former editor-in-chief of the Publishing House of Shanghai University of TCM, have given full support to the compilation and translation of the Library.

With the coming of the new century, we have presented this Library to the readers all over the world, sincerely hoping to receive suggestions and criticism from the readers so as to make it perfect in the following revision.

Zuo Yanfu
Pingju Village, Nanjing
Spring 2002

专家对编写工作提出了指导性的意见和建议。尤其是卫生部副部长、国家中医药管理局局长佘靖教授对本书的编写给予了极大的关注,多次垂询编撰过程,并及时进行指导。上海中医药大学出版社社长兼总编辑朱邦贤教授,以及原社长周敦华先生、原总编辑潘朝曦先生及全体编辑对本书的编辑出版工作给予了全面的支持,使《文库》得以顺利面世。在此,一并致以诚挚的谢意。

在新世纪之初,我们将这套《文库》奉献给国内外中医界及广大中医爱好者,恳切希望有识之士对《文库》存在的不足之处给予批评、指教,以便在修订时更臻完善。

左言富
于金陵萍聚村
2002 年初春

A Newly Compiled Practical English-Chinese Library of Traditional Chinese Medicine

（英汉对照）新编实用中医文库

Basic Theory of Traditional Chinese Medicine	中医基础理论
Diagnostics of Traditional Chinese Medicine	中医诊断学
Science of Chinese Materia Medica	中药学
Science of Prescriptions	方剂学
Internal Medicine of Traditional Chinese Medicine	中医内科学
Surgery of Traditional Chinese Medicine	中医外科学
Gynecology of Traditional Chinese Medicine	中医妇科学
Pediatrics of Traditional Chinese Medicine	中医儿科学
Traumatology and Orthopedics of Traditional Chinese Medicine	中医骨伤科学
Ophthalmology of Traditional Chinese Medicine	中医眼科学
Otorhinolaryngology of Traditional Chinese Medicine	中医耳鼻喉科学
Chinese Acupuncture and Moxibustion	中国针灸
Chinese Tuina (Massage)	中国推拿
Life Cultivation and Rehabilitation of Traditional Chinese Medicine	中医养生康复学